# HEARING
# AND
# DEAFNESS

# CONTRIBUTORS

B. M. Anderman, Ed. D., Chief, Audiology and Speech Pathology, Department of Medicine and Surgery, Veterans Administration.

R. Carhart, Ph.D., Professor of Audiology, Professor of Otolaryngology and Maxillofacial Surgery; Director of the Auditory Research Laboratory, Northwestern University.

H. Davis, M.D., Research Associate, Central Institute for the Deaf, Professor Emeritus of Physiology and Research, Professor of Otolaryngology, School of Medicine, Washington University.

E. P. Fowler, Jr., M.D., was Professor of Otolaryngology, College of Physicians and Surgeons, Columbia University; Director of the Ear, Nose and Throat Service, Presbyterian Hospital, New York.

R. Goldstein, Ph.D., Professor of Communicative Disorders, College of Letters and Science, and the Department of Rehabilitative Medicine, School of Medicine, University of Wisconsin.

I. J. Hirsh, Ph.D., Director of Research, Central Institute for the Deaf; Professor of Psychology, Washington University.

H. S. Lane, Ph.D., Principal, Central Institute for the Deaf; Professor of Education, Washington University.

A. F. Niemoeller, Sc.D., Research Associate, Central Institute for the Deaf; Associate Professor of Electrical Engineering, Washington University.

M. D. Pauls (Hardy), Ph.D., Associate Professor of Laryngology and Otology; Associate Professor of Environmental Medicine, Division of Audiology and Speech, The Johns Hopkins Medical Institutions.

D. A. Ramsdell, Ph.D., was Chief, Clinical Psychology Section, Veterans Administration, Boston.

S. R. Silverman, Ph.D., Director, Central Institute for the Deaf; Professor of Audiology, Washington University.

McCay Vernon, Ph.D., Professor of Psychology, Western Maryland College

T. E. Walsh, M.R.C.S., L.R.C.P., Professor Emeritus of Otolaryngology, School of Medicine, Washington University.

B. R. Williams, LL.D., Chief, Communication Disorders Branch, Division of Disability Services, Rehabilitation Services Administration, Social and Rehabilitation Services, Department of Health, Education, and Welfare.

# HEARING
# AND
# DEAFNESS

## THIRD EDITION

### Hallowell Davis, M.D.
### S. Richard Silverman, Ph.D.
#### CENTRAL INSTITUTE FOR THE DEAF

**HOLT, RINEHART AND WINSTON**
New York   Chicago   San Francisco   Atlanta
Dallas   Montreal   Toronto   London   Sydney

# PREFACE

What really is deafness? Is it a number on a decibel scale that describes the severity of hearing impairment? Is it a disease like mumps or measles or meningitis? Is it an ankylosed stapes? Is it a piece of tissue in the auditory system that would be judged to be abnormal if viewed under a microscope? Is it an affliction to be conquered by the ingenious scientist? Is it the burden of a child whose parent hopes persistently and fervently that the scientist will be successful, and soon? Is it a special mode of communication? Is it something that is encountered occasionally in the man or woman whose fingers fly and whose utterances are arrhythmic and strident? Is it a cause to which diligent, skillful and patient teachers have committed themselves for generations? Is it the agony of isolation from a piece of the real world? Is it the joy of accomplishment that mocks the handicap? Is it the bright mind and the potentially capable hands for which the economy has no use because they are uncultivated? Is it a crystallization of attitudes of a distinctive group whose deafness, modes of communication, and other associated attributes (such as previous education) that they have in common cause them to band together to achieve social and economic self-realization? Of course, it is all of these and more, depending on who asks the question and why.

In seeking the answer to the question, each one of us has his own motives, his own purposes, and his own responsibilities. The public official is concerned with the magnitude and severity of the problem, ways of organizing to solve it, legislative needs, and costs; the physician and the investigator study causes and pathology of deafness, its "psychology" and its management; the educator considers the physical plant, personnel requirements, and methods of instruction and communication; the rehabilitator is sensitive to training and job opportunities; and the deaf person himself and those close to him seek the opportunity for him to be all he can and wants to be. As in the legend of the three blind men, it is difficult to perceive and comprehend the whole elephant.

The third edition of *Hearing and Deafness* is intended to be a comprehensive textbook for those who wish to explore the needs and possible remedies for deafness, for students of audiology who are preparing to be audiologists or for work in closely related fields. For others it may be useful as a reference book or as a summary of the present status and state-of-the-art of audiology. It emphasizes principles. It does not go into fine details of anatomy, of surgical technique, of the administration of particular tests of hearing, or of methods of instruction or counseling of the deaf. It provides a guide to the literature in the form of lists of suggested readings at the end of each chapter. These lists consist chiefly of other books and summary or survey articles in addition to a few specific citations of original sources. Brief characterizations of these other books or articles should assist the student in his search for further information.

We have tried not to burden the book with unnecessary mathematical or electronic detail or with unnecessary medical terminology, although more of it has been introduced in this revision. The student must certainly learn the meanings of the more common professional and technical terms. To help him identify and understand the technical terms more readily, the editors have made free use of italics and quotation marks to tag such words when they first appear and when their meaning can easily be understood from the context. A glossary presents systematically some definitions that are scattered in the text, particularly those that are relatively new or recently standardized.

*Hearing and Deafness* originated as a "guide for laymen"—laymen who were personally interested in impairments of hearing. Dr. Hallowell Davis edited the first edition, but most of the chapters were prepared by specialists in various fields, from surgery, psychology, electronics, speechreading to education of the deaf and others. The various authors read and criticized one another's chapters, and Dr. Davis wrote several chapters and gave some unity to the whole. The first edition served its purpose well, but it unexpectedly served another purpose equally well, namely that of a textbook for students in the new academic and professional fields of audiology. The second edition was revised to improve and update the book as a text, with less emphasis on the needs of an individual who is trying to understand his own handicap or to use a hearing aid and with more emphasis on the basic sciences. Military audiology was replaced by industrial audiology, and so on. In the third edition this development has continued, with considerable expansion of the treatment of acoustics, psychoacoustics, neurophysiology, genetics, audiometry, the handicaps of hearing, and the education of deaf children, and a new emphasis on social problems and government involvement with education and the handicapped. Some of the less relevant material has been condensed or eliminated to allow for the expansions.

In the present revision of the chapters on conservation of hearing, audiometry, special auditory tests, and standards and medicolegal rules, we have included rather extensive direct quotations from certain authoritative statements or reviews that have been published so far only in technical journals or pamphlets. The presentation, which is more detailed and technical than that of the more familiar material, was chosen for the benefit of those who are professionally engaged in some branch of audiology. We hope that these more technical chapters will be interesting to casual readers also, but the difference in treatment represents more than the personal caprice of their authors. It reflects the difference in the availability elsewhere of information on these particular topics.

It is inevitable and even desirable that there be some overlap in a book dealing with so broad a field as audiology, especially when chapters are written by different authors. Such overlap emphasizes both the points that are repeated and the interrelations among the topics. Examples will be found in the chapters on speechreading and auditory training, on hearing handicap in the adult and in the child, and in the several chapters (2, 7, 9, 16) in which use is made of the recent National Health Survey.

In the table of contents the chapters have been grouped as before into six sections. From the titles of the sections it is obvious that the general sequence of the book is from physics, psychophysics, biology, medicine, and surgery to modern studies of impaired hearing and hearing aids and thence to special education and rehabilitation of adults with impaired hearing. The emphasis then shifts to the problems of the education of deaf and hard-of-hearing children and finally to employment and vocational guidance of adults. In general, the sequence is from inanimate nature to the individual human to complex social problems.

The sequence is probably as familiar as it is arbitrary. It has a disadvantage in that it places some of the more difficult technical chapters first. Readers with educational and social interests may skip boldly to their own territory at once. After all, something has to come first, and the present arrangement has the advantage of explaining basic terms and ideas, such as the decibel and hearing loss, before they are used in other contexts.

In spite of the shift from physical to biological to social, there is one theme that runs evenly throughout the book. It could not be concentrated in any one place, and nearly every chapter must be read to learn all we have to say about it. That theme is *psychology*. Hearing, our main topic, is certainly a province of psychology. Communication may use physical tools and have social aspects, but it is basically a psychological process. Tests of hearing are also squarely in the province of the psychologist. The reaction of the individual to deafness and the basic problems of self-adjustment, of education, and of vocational guidance are clearly psychological. At first glance, it may seem that psychology has been slighted and that only one chapter deals with a single and rather special aspect of psychology. On the contrary, the entire book is permeated with it. In fact, the psychological aspects of the various sections give our book its unity.

## SURVEY BY CHAPTERS

The following survey of the third edition by chapters is intended to give the reader a brief topical summary of the substance of each chapter and thus supplement the table of contents as a guide to selective reading. For those who are historically minded it may be interesting to compare this survey with the corresponding surveys in the first and the second editions. The transformation of the book from a guide for layman to a textbook for professionals will be very evident. At the same time the great changes in some chapters, in contrast with the very minor changes in others, reflect the usual uneven rate of progress in any technical or professional field. In some areas there are breakthroughs and periods of rapid advance. Elsewhere, particularly if advance was rapid in a previous decade, the picture is much the same as it was ten or even 22 years ago, but we assure our readers that even the most static of our chapters have been reviewed carefully.

### Audiology

Audiology is now well established as an area of scientific interest and also of service to the public. A professional organization, the American Speech and Hearing Association, sets examinations and issues certificates of qualification. Audiology ranges from audiology as a paramedical specialty closely related to otology, to an independent profession related to handicaps, resulting from impaired hearing, in learning or utilizing language skills. At the present time the audiologist performs his services in a variety of organizational frameworks.

### Acoustics and Psychoacoustics

This chapter has been almost entirely rewritten and expanded to provide an adequate foundation for a modern medical audiologist. The first part reviews the fundamentals of acoustics with particular emphasis on the analysis and measurement of sound. It gives a necessary foundation for intelligent use of the sound-level meter and also the various types of electric audiometer.

The second part of the chapter is a survey of psychoacoustics. It deals with the abilities of the human listener as a detector and analyzer of sounds. Particular attention is given to the sensitivity of hearing and also to the data and concepts of psychoacoustics that do or might form the basis of audiometric tests of hearing.

### Anatomy and Physiology of the Auditory System

Our knowledge of the gross anatomy of the ear has not changed much in 22 years and the drawings prepared for the first edition of *Hearing and Deafness* still rank with the best. The microscopic anatomy of the sense organ and how the sense organ acts as a mechanical analyzer of sound and a transducer of sound energy to nerve impulses are discussed in some detail. In particular Dr. Davis describes the "auditory sensory unit" and its "tuning curve." These concepts are the basis of his later interpretations of sensory-neural hearing loss.

Dr. Davis has also added a discussion of the organization of the central auditory system, its development, and some principles of central nervous activity in general. Dr. Davis writes with authority in this chapter as he has investigated the biophysics and neurophysiology of the auditory nervous system for nearly 40 years.

### Abnormal Hearing and Deafness

This chapter, originally written by Drs. Davis and Fowler for the second edition, has been expanded considerably by Dr. Davis with the advice and assistance of many able medical colleagues. Both conductive and sensory-neural hearing loss are analyzed in terms of biophysics and physiology. The sections on otosclerosis and noise-exposure are brought up to date. Two new sections discuss genetics and congenital defects such as those from maternal rubella. A theory is presented that attributes difficulty in learning language ("dyslogomathia") to early sensory deprivation. The section on functional deafness is revised, but Dr. Davis's original account of psychogenic deafness is retained.

### The Medical Treatment of Hearing Loss and the Conservation of Hearing

Partly as a memorial to the late Dr. E. P. Fowler, Jr., this chapter has been retained as revised in 1960, with only minor updatings. It includes an important section on Conservation of Hearing in Noise, with extensive direct quotations from the guide by that title issued by the Committee on Conservation of Hearing of the American Academy of Ophthalmology and Otolaryngology.

### Surgical Treatment of Hearing Loss

Dr. Walsh describes the role of surgery in dealing with malformations and also infections of the ear, and the effects of these operations on hearing. He gives particular attention to the surgical procedures aimed at improving hearing, such as myringoplasty, tympanoplasty, fenestration, stapes mobilization and stapedectomy.

He discusses not only the theoretical improvement that is possible but the chances of attaining a particular result, based on follow-up studies of his own cases.

## Audiometry: Pure Tone and Simple Speech Tests

The standard tuning fork tests, effectively used by otologists but often neglected by audiologists, are described more fully than in previous editions. Pure-tone audiometry is discussed with particular reference to the new international (ISO) reference zero levels. The draft proposal for a new USA Standard for Audiometers, which almost certainly will be adopted before this chapter appears in print, provided the outline for and the definitions in this chapter. (In anticipation of the adoption of the new USA Standard, which includes the ISO zero reference levels, this edition of *Hearing and Deafness* uses exclusively the ISO reference levels.)

Speech audiometry, with its word tests and articulation scores, is described and evaluated. In 1947 and 1960 we had great hopes for speech audiometry, but now our assessment is more sober. Speech audiometry seems to be firmly established and it makes a real contribution to audiological practice, but the difficulties in the way of standardization and precise measurements are formidable. Nearly all of the word and sentence lists in current use are given in the Appendix with brief statements of the character and particular usefulness of each. Their use in general is directed toward the phonemic study of language and to articulation testing of speech-communication systems quite as much as to clinical audiometry.

## Other Auditory Tests

Here we consider various additional audiometric tests that are in current use, including loudness balance, the SISI test, and fast tone decay. They are all useful aids to otological or neurological diagnosis, to the detection of feigning (malingering), or to the educational assessment of children. Our emphasis is on principles: for details of technique we rely on other books to which references are given.

New additions in the third edition are a description of the new "evoked-response audiometry," and also a discussion of the nature of tests appropriate to otoneurological problems. We explain why evoked-response audiometry will probably replace electrodermal and classical electroencephalic audiometry as a test of the auditory system in young or uncooperative children.

## Hearing Handicap, Standards for Hearing, and Medicolegal Rules

The present revision of this chapter reviews systematically the use of audiometry to assess the fitness or the handicap of an individual with respect to his hearing. The general criterion of handicap, endorsed by several important medically oriented groups including the American Medical Association, is "one's personal efficiency in everyday living, particularly in the hearing of speech." Numerical values for this criterion are given in extensive verbatim quotations from the "Guide for the Classification and Evaluation of Hearing Handicap" published by the American Academy of Ophthalmology and Otolaryngology. These values are then compared with information on the prevalence of hearing handicap, taken from reports on the recent (1960–1963) National Health Survey. For standards of hearing and screening levels the current U.S. Army regulation (AR 40-501) serves as an illustration.

Various medicolegal rules for calculating the compensation appropriate for various degrees of hearing impairment are summarized and an extensive list of pertinent references is given.

Dr. Davis introduces his concept of "actuarial hearing thresholds," meaning the expected median threshold for a given age and sex. He discusses the delicate problems of "normal hearing" and of multiple causation of a hearing impairment.

All of these rules and discussions are presented in terms of the new ISO reference zero levels for pure-tone audiometry.

### Hearing Aids

The design objectives for hearing aids remain the same in 1969 as they were in 1947, but light weight, small size, and inconspicuousness have now been much more fully realized, thanks to the transistor, the mercury battery, and the printed circuit. In modern miniature instruments only an expert can make an internal repair. We have therefore eliminated from this chapter all details of circuitry.

Dr. Niemoeller, who replaces Mr. Gordon Taylor as coauthor of this chapter, is Associate Professor of Electrical Engineering and also Research Associate at Central Institute for the Deaf. He writes from firsthand experience concerning the principles of operation of a hearing aid, the advantages and disadvantages of group aids for schoolchildren, ear-level hearing aids, and the compromises necessary in selecting the "best" instrument for an individual.

### Counseling about Hearing Aids

Dr. Davis and Dr. Silverman have revised and reduced this chapter by eliminating such items as the list of "accepted" hearing aids and the Troubleshooting Chart. Together they consider the many practical questions that arise as to who should wear a hearing aid, on which ear, and whether it should be body-worn or an ear-level instrument, and so on. They incorporate the principles developed in the previous chapter into a set of directions and suggestions addressed to the prospective user. This material also constitutes advice to an audiologist on how to compare instruments with one another while using a minimum of equipment.

### Speechreading

Dr. Pauls has made a number of modifications in revising this chapter, but the principles remain as they were in 1947. The process is called speechreading, not lipreading, because so much information is obtained from gestures, facial expression, and attention to the entire situation. Speechreading and a hearing aid supplement one another beautifully if the deaf person has any residual hearing. Dr. Pauls closes with a series of very practical suggestions for all who are hard of hearing.

### Auditory Training

An entirely new chapter under the old title has been written by Dr. Ira J. Hirsh, Director of Research at Central Institute for the Deaf and Professor of Psychology at Washington University. Dr. Hirsh discusses, as a psychologist, various aspects of hearing and auditory perception, pattern recognition, and the perception of speech. He considers the problems of rehabilitating the adult who has lost part of his hearing and of auditory training in the use of a hearing aid. He also considers the auditory education of the deaf child, with its additional difficulties, and the controversy whether the approach to it should be unisensory or multisensory.

### Development and Conservation of Speech

The title of the chapter has been expanded to reflect its discussion of the original development of speech in childhood and the differences between the methods of teaching speech to deaf as opposed to hard-of-hearing children. Dr. Carhart also considers the problems relating to speech that arise for the hard-of-hearing adult.

The remaining chapters of the book deal with problems rather than with techniques. The problems differ according to the age at which the impairment occurs and its severity. The second and third editions reflect the shift of problems from a wartime to a peacetime basis.

### From Aristotle to Bell—and Beyond (1969)

Dr. Silverman surveys the gradual development of our present social attitude toward the deaf and particularly the deaf-mutes. The deaf are no longer regarded as imbeciles. Deaf children are handicapped children in need of special education. Dr. Silverman recounts the parts played by the pioneers in the education of the deaf. He also notes the important increasing involvement of the federal government of the United States of America in this and related problems. Here he writes from the vantage point of one who has advised and also participated in implementing some of these developments.

### Deaf Children

For the second edition Dr. Silverman, with the collaboration of Dr. Lane, entirely rewrote the original chapter, using much material from his chapter in the *Handbook of Speech Pathology* (Lee Travis, ed.) Once again we are indebted to Dr. Travis and to the publishers, Appleton Century-Crofts, Inc., for their courtesy in allowing reuse of the substance and often entire sections of Dr. Silverman's chapter in the revised edition of their Handbook.

The chapter reviews several historic controversies between different schools of thought and should provide a starting point for any future discussions of the methods of education of deaf children, whether by the oral, manual, or combined method.

### Hard-of-Hearing Children

Dr. Silverman, with the collaboration of Dr. Davis, has revised this chapter extensively. Five classes of children are defined according to their hearing levels for speech. For each class a different regimen, with or without special education, hearing aids, or auditory training, is required. The next topic is the *identification of the young hearing-impaired child*. Auditory screening of neonates is evaluated, and the concept is developed of a *high-risk register* of children to be examined often and carefully. Educational needs and procedures are summarized, and the need for psychological, educational, and vocational guidance is stressed.

### The Psychology of the Hard-of-Hearing and the Deafened Adult

Dr. Ramsdell wrote this chapter in 1946 on the basis of his experiences as psychologist at the Army Rehabilitation Center at Deshon General Hospital. He took his cue from the oft-repeated statement by deafened soldiers that "the world has gone dead," and he proceeded with a thoughtful and original psychological analysis. Nothing has appeared since 1947 to amplify or to controvert his observations and interpretations. The present chapter, unchanged from the second edition, is a memorial to Dr. Ramsdell, who died in 1965.

### The Veterans Administration's Audiology Program

Dr. Anderman can write authoritatively about this program, for he is Chief of Audiology and Speech Correction in the Veterans Administration. He tells of the objectives, the size, and the general plan of the program, with its Veterans Administration Audiology Clinics distributed over the country, reinforced by numerous university and hospital clinics that cooperate on a contract basis. He notes the special interest of the Veterans Administration in "nonorganic deafness" and in the most efficient large-scale procurement and individual distribution of hearing aids.

The only changes in this edition have been to bring various names and numbers up to date. A list of the Veterans Administration Audiology and Speech Pathology Clinics of a regional nature is given in the Appendix.

### Vocational Guidance for the Deaf

The first author of this chapter, Mr. Boyce R. Williams, is deaf and, as Consultant, Deaf and the Hard of Hearing, in the Office of Vocational Rehabilitation, Department of Health, Education and Welfare, he holds an important government position concerned with vocational guidance for the deaf. He therefore writes with special enthusiasm, authority, and understanding of the subject. His coauthor is Dr. McCay Vernon, a research psychologist located at Western Maryland College. Their new chapter combines the subject matter of three separate chapters in the first edition on social and economic problems of the aurally handicapped.

Mr. Williams and Dr. Vernon survey the facilities available for the assistance of the deaf. They also examine the handicap of deafness and show how it makes the deaf person a unique client for the vocational counselor. The problems of psychological evaluation and intelligence testing of the deaf are examined at some length. They also note that present social and economic trends toward greater urbanization and relatively greater demand for "white-collar workers" threaten serious additional difficulties for the deaf and for their counselors in the future.

The source of data used in our graphs and tables is usually noted in the accompanying legend or in an occasional footnote.

We have already noted that we have tried to confine our Suggested Readings at the end of each chapter to secondary sources of a general or survey character. Also we have named in the text only a few of the distinguished workers in the cause of the deaf and the hard of hearing, chiefly workers of previous generations. Nevertheless, as many chapters of the third edition were expanded to include more and more new technical detail, we have mentioned the names of more and more investigators and have included their writings in our reading lists. Many of these investigators are still active. Here the purpose is not to single out a few for special honor but to enable the student to identify the appropriate citation in the list of suggested readings or to serve as a guide for those who wish to go directly to the scientific literature. Actually the serious student of audiology must learn who are or recently have been important contributors to the development of the science and profession of audiology, including many whose names do not appear in our citations or text.

In this revision some of the original authors are no longer represented. Two of them, Dr. Edmund P. Fowler, Jr. and Donald A. Ramsdell, have died, but much of what they wrote is retained. Other authors are newcomers, notably Dr. Ira J. Hirsh, formerly Director of Research at Central Institute for the Deaf and presently Dean of Faculty of Arts and Sciences at Washington University (St. Louis), and Arthur F. Niemoeller, also a member of the Research Staff at Central Institute for the Deaf. Dr. S. Richard Silverman, Director of Central Institute for the Deaf and co-editor of the second edition, has continued as co-editor. He has edited or rewritten the second half of the book dealing with hearing aids, speech, language, education, and social problems. Dr. Davis has written the expansions of the first half of the book. Dr. Davis is Director Emeritus of Research at Central Institute for the Deaf. The third edition, even more than the second, is a product of and strongly reflects the point of view of the staff of Central Institute for the Deaf. We thank our colleagues in other institutions for their contributions, both old and new, and we hope that our point of view is not too one-sided; it has the advantage of being unified.

Hallowell Davis
S. Richard Silverman

*St. Louis, Missouri*
*November 1969*

# FOREWORD TO THE
# FIRST EDITION

Granted that the first handicap of deafness lies in communication, it has often seemed to me that a close second might be the attitude of hearing people toward it and that the former would be considerably lessened if we could do something to improve the latter.

Man's need for communication with his fellow man is possibly his greatest need and the fulfillment of his other needs and desires is largely dependent upon, or at the last greatly facilitated by, his ability to satisfy this basic one. The development of language, both spoken and written, as a means of communication is one of mankind's greatest achievements. Yet, because from birth we hearing people effortlessly, almost unconsciously, have *absorbed* this magnificent tool simply because we are lucky enough to hear, we take it very much for granted and tend to belittle, to shun, or to look somewhat askance at anyone who has had to fashion, bit by bit, word by word, sound by sound, a workable, even though imperfect, language tool for himself.

By turns I have been amused, annoyed, angry, and frustrated by this attitude and its various manifestations. However, I have tried to remind myself that people are like this because they don't know any better. Some thought and perhaps a little effort often *are* required to understand the speech and to follow the language of a deaf or severely hard-of-hearing person. It often *does* entail more attention than we usually give to our casual conversations to enable the deaf or hard-of-hearing person, who must depend mainly upon our lip movements, to understand what we are saying. I find very few people who are willing to give this attention or make this effort. Perhaps most people's impatience, even their rudeness, is partly due to this too swiftly paced, this tabloid, he-who-runs-may-read age and partly to a natural laziness of mind. However, I believe a great deal of it is due to almost complete lack of understanding of the problems faced by those with a hearing loss and to the narrowness and fear and insecurity bred of ignorance.

There is no other subject that vitally affects the lives of so many people on which there is so little positive information and so much fuzzy and widespread misinformation and misunderstanding. I doubt if over five per cent of our population has ever read anything authentic on the deaf or the hard of hearing. And yet the impression that the deaf have no vocal chords and so cannot speak is widespread. It might surprise you to know how many people ask if the deaf learn to read Braille.

A great many of the misconceptions concerning the deaf undoubtedly can be traced to that inaccurate and unfortunate term "deaf and dumb." The implications it has given rise to in the minds of generations of hearing children and the attitudes it has engendered, not to mention the devastation it has caused in the hearts of parents, are incalculable. Fortified with those words alone, many people are almost determined in their belief that the totally deaf cannot possibly speak.

Education for the deaf, speech reading, and speech are not new. Speech has been taught in this country for close to a century. And yet, accurate, not to mention easy-to-read, articles or books for the layman, this fellow whom we must reach, whose attitudes we must change, are so few as to be almost non-existent. I often have said that educators of the deaf talk to other educators of the deaf, write for other educators of the deaf in magazines for educators of the deaf and nothing reaches the layman—the layman who one day may be the totally unprepared mother or father of a little deaf baby, the layman who himself may become deaf or hard of hearing.

So my spirits leapt when I read the title of this book, *Hearing and Deafness: A Guide for Laymen.* Here at last is information, correct, easy to read, covering nearly every phase of the problem in a manner suited to that numerically large and needy group of people—laymen.

*Hearing and Deafness* should do much to change an attitude and, in consequence, be the means of greatly lessening the handicap of deafness.

I feel very honored and happy to be able to have even such a small finger in this notable work.

Louise Tracy

*The John Tracy Clinic*
*Los Angeles, California*
*August 1947*

# INTRODUCTION TO THE
# FIRST EDITION

If there is another book which fulfills the aims and purposes of this one, I have not seen it. In my opinion the resolution of the editor

. . . to answer the thousand and one questions that are continually being asked by all sorts of people about the nature of hearing and the problem of deafness, . . .

has been most effectually carried out.

When one desires to read something concerning his own problem, he turns naturally to pertinent articles that are easy to get and simple to understand. A large number of such writings on the treatment of deafness has recently appeared in some of our popular magazines. These commentaries, written ostensibly in an informative vein but produced plainly for "reader appeal," were composed by professional lay writers who have constantly before them two cardinal questions in journalism: (1) Is it new or unusual? and (2) Does it have human or dramatic appeal?

These articles, semi-scientific in character but produced in journalistic style and given extensive circulation, seem to have aroused in an untold number of persons an interest in their deafness that long had remained dormant, and that never would have been so completely stimulated, had it not been for the journalist and his manner of writing.

Similarly, new interests in the problems of deafness, new operations to restore hearing, new electrical apparatus to give more perfect sound reception to improperly functioning ears, new methods of ensuring the preservation of speech, and a new understanding of the mental attributes of the hard of hearing have made almost mandatory the publication of an up-to-date, authoritative, and comprehensible reference work that covers the field of *audiology* both as a textbook and as a guide.

*Hearing and Deafness: A Guide for Laymen* is just such a text. Not without a dash of the "new and unusual" and not without its human appeal, this "guide" contains factual and instructive discussions of various phases of audiology. In the early pages we are informed that the sequence of chapters is "from inanimate nature to the individual human to complex social problems" and that in spite of this shift "there is one theme that runs evenly throughout the book." That theme, we are told, is *psychology*. Unquestionably, this topic reaches its climax when we are enlightened concerning the importance of "auditory backgrounds" which are responsible for that "comfortable sense-of-being-a-part-of-a-living-active-world," and also when we recognize the significance of the *three psychological levels of hearing*. Furthermore, suspicion, so characteristic a feature of the hard of hearing, is admirably discussed and is a matter that should be thoroughly understood by all deafened persons who retain it.

Every otologist, every teacher of the deaf, every social worker, every chapter of the American Hearing Society, and every other person "concerned with auditory rehabilitation or with the conservation of hearing" should welcome the publication of this book, for in what other compact form can one find reliable answers to such questions as (1) "Why did I lose my hearing?" (2) "Is my deafness bad enough to require the use of a hearing aid?" (3) "Should I buy a bone or air conduction instrument?" and (4) "In which ear should I wear the 'aid'?"

Or if the problem involves a congenitally deaf child, we have replies to such queries as (1) "Why doesn't my child talk?" (2) "Will he be able to talk?" and (3) "What about his education?"

Among the other "thousand and one questions that are continually being asked" and that have received such impressive answers are (1) "Why do I hear a buzzer when I cannot hear a doorbell or telephone?" (2) "Will the fenestration operation cure my deafness?" (3) "Does industry discriminate against the hard of hearing?" (4) "Why do people stop talking when I come into the room?" and (5) "Why does the intense stillness so depress me?"

Further perusing the pages of this work, we become interested in the variations of normal hearing, and in finding out just what Miss Brown, Mr. Jones, and Mrs. Smith can expect from the use of a hearing aid. And while the mechanically minded inquirers are running their fingers up and down the "Cause, Test and Remedy" columns of the "Troubleshooting Chart," and as the speech-reading class is memorizing the twelve suggestions for "ease of communication," the daring among us are venturing to trespass upon that special preserve where the more erudite disquisitions are lurking.

Surely this work, so extensive in scope, so practical in application and so expert in composition will serve a real need. Conceived, as it is, in the spirit of altruism and occupying, as it does, a niche not held by any other work, it deserves highest commendation and should be in the hands of all the thousands upon thousands of those who ask the questions and want to get the correct answers.

C. Stewart Nash
*President*
*American Hearing Society*
*Rochester, New York*
*September 5, 1947*

# CONTENTS

## PART THREE    AUDITORY TESTS AND HEARING AIDS

## PART SIX   SOCIAL AND ECONOMIC PROBLEMS

## APPENDIX

# PART ONE
# AUDIOLOGY

# CHAPTER 1

# AUDIOLOGY

## HALLOWELL DAVIS, M.D.

You who read this book may be deaf yourself, or perhaps your hearing is not as keen as it used to be; or you may have a parent or a friend whose hearing is failing. Possibly your child is deaf and needs special teaching so that he may understand and be understood. Imperfect hearing is so common that sooner or later it comes close to everyone. Perhaps you are beginning your training to become a professional audiologist. But, whether you want to help yourself or want to help others, or are merely curious, you want to know what can go wrong with hearing and what can be done about it.

Five hundred years ago you might have consulted for guidance the writings of St. Albertus Magnus, teacher of Thomas Aquinas and the dominant figure in Latin learning and natural science of the thirteenth century, who wrote: "Lion's brain, if eaten, causes madness; but remedies deafness, if inserted in the ear with some strong oil." [1] And another widely respected

authority, St. Hildegard of Bingen (about 1125), held that "deafness may be remedied by cutting off a lion's right ear and holding it over the patient's ear just long enough to say, 'Hear, *adimacus,* by the living God and the keen virtue of a lion's hearing,' " and that "the heart of a weasel, dried and placed with wax in the ear, benefits headache or deafness." [2]

This book not only attempts to guide a student in problems relating to hearing and deafness. It also gives a survey of a general field of knowledge and of social endeavor centering around hearing. "Audiology," meaning the science of hearing, seems to be a useful name for this field, even though linguistic purists may object to adding a Greek suffix to a Latin root. The word is probably inevitable. We shall use it in a very broad sense. For some purposes it may be helpful to speak more specifically of "medical audiology" when medical aspects of impaired hearing are our primary concern. The government use of the term (as in the title "Consultant in Audiology")

[1] Lynn Thorndike, *A History of Magic and Experimental Science* (New York: Columbia University Press, 1923), II, 561.

[2] *Ibid.*, pp. 145–146.

is in a definitely medical context. It is particularly useful here, however, because it indicates an interest in the *function* of the ear, and not only in *diseases* of the ear. The diseases of the ear, the recognized province of *otology,* may be a threat to life, and hearing then becomes secondary. *Audiology* considers the ear as an *aid* to life.

Since 1946 audiology has become a profession as well as an area of knowledge. Numerous "clinical audiologists" are engaged in testing hearing in hospitals, in special clinics and other institutions, and in private offices. Many of these men and women are members of the American Speech and Hearing Association. This association has established a Committee on Clinical Certification which sets examinations in hearing and issues certificates of qualification both in speech and in hearing.

Clinical audiologists test hearing and may make recommendations concerning the use and choice of hearing aids. They do not, however, sell hearing aids. According to the code of ethics of the American Speech and Hearing Association, it is considered unethical for a member to engage directly in the sale of hearing aids or even to test hearing in a center that would benefit directly from the sale of a particular hearing aid. The business of distribution and sale of hearing aids is handled by hearing aid dealers.

The development of audiology and specifically of clinical audiology has led to many and serious discussions of the relation of audiology to otology. How far do the rights and responsibilities of the clinical audiologist, with his special training and experience, go—particularly in the directions of making a diagnosis, in recommending the use of a hearing aid, and in planning a course of education or rehabilitation? In the medical area he is clearly dependent on and subordinate to the physician, but other areas are his own. Where is the boundary?

Probably the best statement of a point of view that seems to be more and more widely accepted was drafted in 1955 by a committee, under the cochairmanship of Dr. Gordon Hoople and Dr. Raymond Carhart, concerned with this problem. The report of this committee has never been published in full, but permission has been granted to reproduce from it the following:

## A Statement of Orientation

We have learned a great deal during the past quarter century about (1) how to measure sound; (2) how to assess hearing; (3) how to study the physiology, biophysics, and psychophysics of the auditory system; (4) how to deal with hearing impairments by surgical or medical means; and (5) how to educate and to rehabilitate persons with impaired hearing. Representatives from many disciplines are now concerned with the facts of hearing and the problems of hearing loss. Their various activities have come to carry the label "audiology."

Audiology is the science of hearing. In other words, audiology is undergirded by the competences and methods of many fields. Among the contributing fields are (1) physics, which studies acoustic events as one manifestation of matter and motion; (2) medicine, which is concerned with the human organism in sickness and health; (3) psychology, which deals with responses of the organism to stimuli; (4) education, which seeks to modify and guide the behavior of the organism; and (5) sociology, which attacks the problems of fitting the individual into his culture. Audiology, then, is not a particular academic discipline of professional activity. It is the mobilizing of professional skills to cope with the phenomena of hearing. Thus, when an individual concentrates his training, his competence, and his experience on problems of auditory communication, he is working in the field of audiology. His interest may be to investigate auditory phenomena, his chosen task may be to train others to work in the field, or his goal may be to serve clinically those persons who suffer impaired hearing.

Current emphasis among those who use the term "audiology" is heavily clinical. Consequently, important problems of inter-professional relationships have arisen. Among these is the question of how to achieve optimal inter-action between otologists and clinical audiologists, as we shall in this report designate specialists in managing non-medical aspects of auditory impairment.

The two committees agreed that otology and clinical audiology have distinctive yet related tasks. These tasks may be described as follows:

1. Otology has basic responsibility for the biological function of hearing. *It alone rightfully undertakes the work of diagnosing diseases of the ear, of specifying the causation of hearing impairment, and of treating pathologies of the auditory mechanism.*

2. Clinical audiology deals with hearing as a foundation to the learning and the utilizing of language skills. *The emphasis is upon understanding the social functions of hearing and upon increasing the ability of handicapped individuals to cope with the communicational demands of everyday life.*

3. The two fields share responsibility for jointly planning the proper sequence in management of the individual patient. Information on the patient should be exchanged freely. Moreover, decisions regarding otological management of the patient should always precede decisions on audiological management, since maximal social efficiency can be achieved only after biological function has been restored as fully as possible.

Audiology in relation to otology is concerned with diagnostic tests of hearing and the evaluation of the results of medical or surgical efforts to improve hearing. Actually the otologist himself may perform many simple diagnostic tests. He becomes an audiologist the moment he picks up a tuning fork. The more complicated tests, however, and particularly those that require electronic equipment and sound-proof booths, the otologist usually delegates to a professional specialist. This audiologist is usually not himself a physician, but he is one of an increasing number of "paramedical specialists" who have special training and competence in particular complex

chemical or physical diagnostic procedures. He shares with the otologist a biological orientation toward hearing, and it is important for him to understand the anatomy and physiology of the ear and the nature of the various diseases and disorders of the ear in order to adapt his tests intelligently to the needs of a particular patient and to help the otologist evaluate the results of the tests. The final responsibilities of diagnosis and of treatment, however, still rest with the physician.

Another orientation of the audiologist, however, is toward assessing the hearing handicap of his client and assisting him to overcome the handicap by means other than medicine or surgery—once the medical management of the case has been established. He gives advice concerning hearing aids and evaluates their effectiveness and, from special knowledge of the possibilities of special education or rehabilitative training, he participates in decisions concerning education and the improved utilization of language skills. Just as the otologist may perform simple audiological diagnostic tests so the educator, the clinical psychologist, the speech pathologist, and even the hearing-aid dealer may perform simple audiological tests to evaluate a hearing handicap. The audiologist, however, is equipped and trained to perform more accurate and extensive tests. If he knows the fundamental principles of hearing aids, of special education of the deaf, and of the rehabilitation of the deaf and hard of hearing, he can also perform the very important service of evaluating his patient's handicap and guiding the appropriate audiological management.

The relations of otology and other specialties with audiology are clear enough in principle although they have been obscured by the variety of organizations under which audiological services have been made available. There is nevertheless a fundamental unity in audiology because its tests are all psychological tests. They are based squarely on the branch of psychology known as psychophysics and more particularly on psychoacoustics. Thus a firm foundation in psychoacoustics, including familiarity with the principles of acoustics and with the electronic equipment appropriate to psychoacoustics, is essential for all audiologists, whatever their orientation may be.

## CONTRIBUTIONS OF AUDIOLOGY

The contributions of audiology are not trivial. Recent developments in medicine, in electronics, in our social point of view, and in education have greatly increased its importance. Surgery can now improve hearing in otosclerosis and other middle-ear conditions, but the conditions must be correctly diagnosed and evaluated. Auditory tests now assist the neurologist as well as the otologist. Hearing aids are efficient electroacoustic instruments, and with increasing miniaturization are becoming more and more acceptable to potential users; but candidates for hearing aids still need advice. Deaf children apparently suffer from a specific handicap, not from a general mental inferiority, and even profoundly deaf children can be taught to speak and to read speech. This is most effectively done if special instruction is begun early, and the audiologist plays a very important part in the early identification and assessment of deaf babies and preschool children. Of course older children and adults also benefit from improved opportunities for rehabilitation. Identification and assessment are both easier than with babies, but the assessment must be correct. Actually the identification of children with hearing handicaps requires a cooperative effort of physicians, audiologists, educators, and an informed public.

## THE ADMINISTRATIVE PATTERNS OF AUDIOLOGY

Within the last 25 years there have been significant events and changes of attitude toward the handicaps of hearing. It is now recognized that with special education the deaf can and do become or remain fully responsible members of society. The federal government of the United States is becoming increasingly involved in problems of medical care, education and rehabilitation, including those of the hearing-handicapped. Particularly relevant is the establishment of the National Advisory Committee on the Education of the Deaf, the National Technical Institute for the Deaf, and a Bureau of Education for the Handicapped.

The establishment of these new federal agencies has added to the diversity in the administrative framework through which audiological services are offered. Audiological activities have quite often been conducted as part of the program of a university department of speech, of education, or of psychology. Again these activities have frequently been organized as a subdivision of a department of otolaryngology. Under these circumstances, audiology has been included within the services of departments of rehabilitation, of public health, or within programs for crippled children, within the services of a hospital, or within the private practice of the otolaryngologist. Finally, clinical audiology has been made an independent enterprise in a few instances.

In view of the many ways in which audiological services are being made available, it is probably unwise to specify any particular organizational or administrative pattern as the only proper one. The contemporary situation is furnishing a trial of the effectiveness of the various patterns. We may expect the most desirable organizational practices to evolve only if we avoid premature opinions and encourage sympathetic insight among all those who have a part in the development and administration of programs in audiology.

# PART TWO
# HEARING AND HEARING LOSS

# CHAPTER 2

## ACOUSTICS
## AND
## PSYCHOACOUSTICS

### HALLOWELL DAVIS, M.D.

"Sound is what we hear." So says the man just in from the street.

"No," says a physicist, "sound is a form of energy. It is an organized movement of molecules; it is a series of waves of pressure in the air or water or whatever medium is transmitting the sound."

"Yes," says a psychologist, "but you should add that sound is a sensation, something that exists only within ourselves. The sensation is aroused when sound waves tickle our ears and send nerve impulses running to the brain along the auditory nerve. We all know what sound is like in experience. It is real but intangible. We can't weigh it on a pair of scales, measure it with a meter, or even take it out and look at it."

And while the physicist glares at the psychologist, the man from the street raises the old question: If a bomb explodes in the midst of the Sahara Desert or at the South Pole with no man or other living creature there to hear, will there be any sound?

"Of course there will," says the physicist.

"Impossible," says the psychologist. "Didn't I tell you. . . ." And so it goes.

### WHAT IS SOUND

The sort of argument recorded above was once taken quite seriously, until it was realized that words and their meanings are not created in Heaven but are consciously or unconsciously made by man for his own use. And often very clumsy, foggy, and ambiguous he makes them! The word "sound" is used, and we shall so use it, to mean *both* the physicist's pressure waves and moving molecules and the psychologist's subjective sensation in the mind of the listener. And now that we realize that the word has a double meaning, there need actually be no confusion. Which meaning is intended is usually quite clear. The physicist's sound can be measured by apparatus, and it can do work; it can push small objects back and forth or generate heat. The other kind of sound is all in our minds and may be high-pitched or low-pitched, loud or faint, pleasant or unpleasant. These at-

9

tributes cannot be measured by thermometers or voltmeters, but they can be appreciated by a listener; and a listener can tell us a lot about his sensations and about the relations among them: which of two sounds is louder, which is higher in pitch, and so on.

Between the physical sound of pressure waves and our insubstantial but intensely real sensations lie our ears, our nerves, and our brains. The physiologist, who thinks of sound in the physical sense, studies how the sound waves are gathered by the external ear, conducted by the middle ear, and concentrated and analyzed in the inner ear, as well as how they set up nerve impulses in the auditory nerve. He follows the nerve impulses up to the gray matter of the brain and can tell us something of how their pattern in time (and in distribution among the thousands of nerve fibers in the auditory pathways) corresponds to the original pattern of the physicist's sound waves. But no one can say how the patterns of nerve impulses generate our subjective sensations.

The psychologist who wants to relate sensations to objects and events in the physical world gets little help from the physiologist. He must go back to the beginning and compare the loudness, the pitch, or the unpleasantness of the sensations as reported by his subjects with the intensity, the frequency, the wave form, the temporal pattern, or other measurable attribute of the physical sound. This sort of study is known as *psychophysics,* and much of what we shall have to say about sound and hearing will be statements of just these relationships between the objective and the subjective aspects of sound. The relationships are not properties of physical sound but the relation between physical sound and the properties of human beings, particularly of their ears and their brains.

The physicist's sound is a form of energy. It can be "created" only by transformation from another form of energy, and it in turn can do work and be transformed into still other forms. Specifically, it is an organized movement to and fro of the molecules of a gas, or liquid, or solid. Small solid objects, such as particles of dust in the air, move bodily with the air molecules and help us to visualize the organized movement of the molecules.

Solid objects may "vibrate," one part moving back and forth in relation to other parts. The to-and-fro motion of the vibrating part is much the same as the motion of the air molecules in sound waves except that the molecules of the bell, the tuning fork, or the violin string are stuck together and must move as a mass. The branch of physics that deals with this vibratory form of energy, whether in air, in water, or in solid objects, is known as *acoustics.*

### The Physical Nature of Sound

The commonest source of sound waves in the air is a vibrating solid body. As the air molecules fly about and collide with one another in their random dance, they are pushed back by the solid body when it starts to vibrate, just as a jostling crowd of spectators awaiting a parade is pushed back by a cordon of police. The molecules, or spectators, in the front ranks collide more powerfully with their neighbors and push them back; and so the wave spreads through the crowd. Then each molecule (or spectator), bumping and jostling, takes advantage of the reverse movement of the solid body (or a relaxation of the cordon), and surges back to or beyond the original position, only to be pushed away once more. Among the molecules, as in the crowd, there are zones of denser pressure which move away from the source of the disturbance. These are the *sound waves.* The waves of pressure travel slowly in a New Year's Eve crowd, but they go at about a thousand feet a second in air. (The velocity of sound in air or "mach 1" is about 760 miles an hour at sea level and is now familiar as a unit of speed of jet planes and rockets.) Each molecule moves only a very short distance, however, and then returns to or beyond its original position. The air movement does not become a wind. The crowd is still in Times Square, not charging down Broadway. And anyone who has been a "molecule" in a large crowd will recall the "pressure waves" that made him surge back and forth.

Most solid objects vibrate when they are suddenly set in motion or suddenly stopped. Their *inertia* keeps them from starting all at once. Their *momentum* keeps parts moving even after one portion has met an obstacle. The momentum makes the wood, metal, or whatever it may be stretch until the attractions that hold the molecules together finally stop the forward movement. Now, if the object has only stretched out of shape and not shattered to bits, the elastic forces restore it to shape. Usually they restore the shape so rapidly, however, that it overshoots in the opposite direction, like the swing of a pendulum, and it may take many swings before the energy of vibration is dissipated, and the vibration ceases. Each movement pushes out a sound wave in the surrounding air. The vibration may be kept going by some continuing force, like wind flapping a flag; or the original event may be repeated, like a clock striking twelve. Air itself becomes turbulent when it moves rapidly, and its eddies and surges generate the sound waves that we hear as the wind whistles through a crack, around an airplane, or in our own ears.

Nature is as full of sound as it is of wind, of splashing water, and of hard, vibrating objects. It is a rarity to find a really silent event, except for those that take place so slowly that we can hardly even see them happen. Few objects are so soft and spongy as to be noiseless, although skin, flesh, and fur qualify as well as any. Nature, particularly inanimate nature, is noisy.

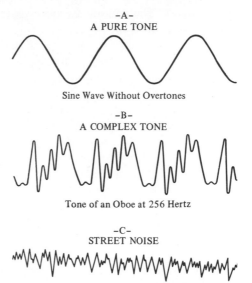

Figure 2-1. See text for explanation. Curve *B* is redrawn after D. C. Miller, *The Science of Musical Sounds* (*by permission of The Macmillan Company, publishers*). Curve *C* is a draftsman's copy of an original illustration by Fletcher. The fine detail of the original is not reproduced. The drawing serves, by contrast with *A* and *B* above, to show the mixed, irregular, random, and nonrepetitive character of noise. (*After Fletcher, Speech and Hearing, D. Van Nostrand Company, Inc.*)

## Wave Form and Frequency: Pure and Complex Tones

The simplest form of acoustic, vibratory, or electromagnetic wave is the *sine wave,* or sinusoid (see Figure 2-1). It is a smooth wave that has the interesting mathematical property that its first derivative (or slope or rate of change) follows a cosine curve that has the same form as the sine wave but is a quarter of a cycle in advance of it. The sinusoid is also related to circular motion. Imagine a rotating cam shaft that carries a circular eccentric cam. A vertical rod like the valve shaft of an automobile engine is moved up and down by the cam. On it is mounted a pen that writes on a vertical sheet of paper beside it. The sheet of paper moves horizontally at a constant speed. The pen on the valve shaft writes a sine wave on the paper.

It is a fundamental fact of physics that many natural free oscillations, such as electromagnetic oscillations, the swing of pendulums, mechanical oscillation of loaded springs like watch springs or tuning forks, and certain simple acoustic oscillations are sinusoidal. A simple sinusoidal acoustic signal is known as a *pure tone.*

Two kinds of measurement are enough to define a pure tone completely. One is *frequency,* usually measured in cycles (complete swings or double vibrations) per second. In these days of radio and its kilocycles we should all be accustomed to the idea of frequency. The other measurement is *magnitude* or *intensity,* and may be measured as the alternating *pressure* of sound waves or as the *velocity* with which air particles move to and fro. We may also think of an alternating rate of *flow of energy* in horsepower or watts.

Frequency refers to the recurrence of similar events per unit of time. Usually the recurrence is regular, and each of the equal intervals of time is known as a cycle. The course of events within each cycle, whether the simple swing of a pendulum to and fro or the sequence of puffs from the exhaust during one turn of the crankshaft of a motor, is similar. For sound waves and mechanical vibrations the second is the most convenient unit of time, and for many years acoustic frequencies have been expressed in *cycles per second* (abbreviated as cps or c/s) or for higher frequencies as *kilocycles per second* or kc.

In 1960, however, the Eleventh General Conference on Weights and Measures at Paris recommended that this unit of frequency, one cycle per second, be known as a *hertz,* abbreviated Hz, in honor of the German physicist, Heinrich Hertz, who studied electromagnetic radiation and discovered the hertzian waves. This usage, established for many years in Germany, has been adopted widely in many other countries and will probably become universal. We have adopted it in the present (1970) edition of this book. The hertz is thus the exact equivalent of cycles per second and a 1000 cps tone becomes a 1000 Hz tone. We may reasonably expect kHz to replace kc so that 1000 cycles per second will be 1 kHz. It has been suggested that when two different cycles of different events are both involved simultaneously, it will reduce ambiguity if "cycles per second" is retained for the slower sequence. Thus we may have a signal that consists of periodic bursts of a 1000 Hz tone at the frequency of three bursts per second. One burst and the silent period that follows it constitutes one cycle of the signal, and there are three such cycles per second. We prefer here to speak of 1000 Hz tone bursts at a repetition rate of 3 cps.

Many acoustic and mechanical systems, including most musical instruments, vibrate in more complicated although recurring patterns (see Figure 2-1). Such a *complex tone* can be analyzed by acoustic (or electrical) filters into a set of component pure tones, each with a definite frequency and intensity. The wave form of the complex tone depends also on the time relations, technically known as the *phase relations,* among the component pure tones. The graphic record of a complex tone can be resolved into its sinusoidal components by a mathematical procedure known as *Fourier analysis.* The application of the Fourier analysis in practice usually fails to preserve information on phase relations.

In a complex musical tone the various additional higher frequencies are known as *overtones* or *harmonics,* and their frequencies are simple, integral multiples of the frequency of the lowest tone, or *fundamental.* The frequencies and intensities of the harmonics are represented in the form of a *line spectrum* of the sound, as in Figure 2-2. It is called a line spectrum because the graphic representation of this distribution of energy is a series of vertical lines, not a continuous curve. The higher harmonics give a *quality* to the tone that is characteristic of the particular instrument. For the human voice the relative strengths of the components of higher frequency are responsible for the differences between the different vowel sounds which allow us to distinguish them even when they are sung or spoken at the same fundamental pitch.

*Noise.* Most of the sounds we hear are neither pure single-frequency tones nor even musical tones containing only one fundamental frequency and its higher harmonics. Instead, they are a scramble of many frequencies that may or may not stand in any simple numerical relation to one another. In fact, one very familiar noise, the hiss of an air jet or escaping steam, is completely random in its wave form. If we analyze such a random noise, we find equal amounts of energy in a given bandwidth (range of frequencies), whatever part of the spectrum we examine. High, low, and middle frequencies are equally represented. The spectrum is continuous with equal intensity per cycle of bandwidth. Since there is here an obvious analogy to white light, such a noise is often called *white noise*. It is a useful tool for the acoustic physicist, and fortunately it is easily generated by merely amplifying the

background hiss produced in certain electronic devices. Other noises have a predominance of high or low frequencies, and, although their pitches may be very vague, we can recognize that one such noise is pitched higher than another. The noises may be thought of as more or less "colored." The pure tone, with its spectrum consisting of a single line, corresponds to a pure color. A noise may be a mixture of a line spectrum, like the hum of an airplane

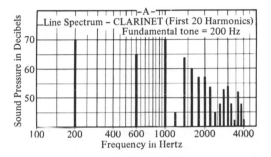

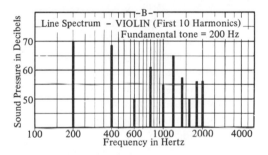

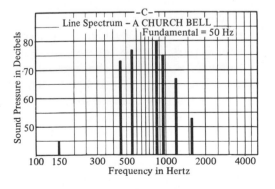

Figure 2-2. In the clarinet spectrum (*A*) the second and fourth harmonics (400 and 800 Hz) are more than 30 dB below the intensity of the fundamental tone. The sixth harmonic is also very weak. In the violin spectrum (*B*) the second, fourth, and sixth harmonics are the strongest and the odd-numbered harmonics are weak. The "overtone structure" gives the characteristic quality of each instrument. The strength of each harmonic is easily measured with the help of electrical filters that allow only a very narrow band of frequencies (a constant number of cycles per second) to pass through. The sound of a bell also has a line spectrum (*C*), but the energy is very irregularly distributed among a few of the higher harmonics. In the sounds of many bells, inharmonic frequencies are also strongly present. (*All from H. Fletcher, American Journal of Physics, 14:215–225 [1946].*)

motor, and a more or less uniform band spectrum, like the wind noise around the wings of the plane. Of course, unless the line spectrum (of the motor or from any other source) is more intense than the band spectrum at that particular frequency, the pure tone will be submerged in the noise, and the ear will be unable to detect it. The pure tone is then said to be "masked" by the noise. The masking of speech by traffic noise is very familiar to all of us.

### Measure of Sound: Intensity

We are all accustomed to steady pressure, such as 30 pounds per square inch in a tire, and to steady velocities, such as 1000 feet per second, approximately the velocity of sound in air. Alternating pressures and velocities are less familiar. They bear the same relation to steady pressures and velocities that an alternating electric current bears to direct current. Both kinds can do work, but the alternating current is continually reversing its direction. The concept of power, illustrated by the horsepower of our automobiles or the watts of electric power consumed by our electric light bulbs, is familiar to us. Acoustic power, although the quantities are extremely small, can be measured in the same units. Thus the physicist says that the acoustic power of the faintest 1000-Hz tone that can be heard by a good ear is about 0.000 000 000 000 000 1 watt per square centimeter or, in a more familiar unit, 0.000 000 000 000 000 000 13 horsepower per square centimeter. Noise becomes uncomfortable, as in a boiler shop, at 0.0001 watt and sharply painful at 0.01 watt per square centimeter.

Numbers of this sort, consisting chiefly of a decimal point followed by a string of nothingness, are more impressive than convenient. Moreover, the range that is covered between the faintest audible and the sharply painful sounds is tremendous. The latter are 10 million times as powerful as the former. It helps a little, but only a lit-tle, if we talk about the pressure (which is what the acoustics engineer actually measures with his sound-level meter) instead of the power, because the pressure is proportional to the square root of the power, and fewer zeros are required. (The faintest audible 1000-Hz tone has an acoustic pressure of about 0.0002 dyne per square centimeter; the painful tone, 2000 dynes per square centimeter.) Even so, our calculations consist chiefly of locating the decimal point correctly.

To deal conveniently with such an unwieldy range of values, a logarithmic system has been universally adopted in acoustics and in electrical engineering. The system has no fixed unit, like the pound or the centimeter, but deals only in ratios, like double, tenfold, or hundred fold. One logarithmic unit (to the base 10) of the ratio (of one acoustic power to another) is known as a *bel,* in honor of Alexander Graham Bell, who invented the telephone. Thus one bel means tenfold the power, two bels means tenfold and tenfold again, that is, a hundred fold the power. The bels count the number of steps the decimal point takes along the chain of zeros.

To avoid inconvenient fractional values of the bel, the *decibel,* which is one-tenth of a bel, is usually employed instead. It is abbreviated dB. (The capital B follows the rule of capitalizing abbreviations that are derived from proper names such as Bell or Hertz.)

Unfortunately there is the slight additional complication that we usually deal with *pressures,* whereas the decibel is defined as a ratio of two *energies* or powers. Acoustic pressures are proportional to the square root of the corresponding power. The ratio of the *squares* of the acoustic pressures corresponds to the simple ratio of the acoustic powers, and therefore the logarithm of the pressure ratio is *double* the logarithm of the power ratio. Thus tenfold (for acoustic pressures) is 20 dB, a hundred fold is 40 dB, and double pressure turns out to be almost exactly 6 dB.

The decibel scale is logarithmic. This means, among other things, that when we add decibels we *multiply*. If we wish to add sound pressures, as when sounds from two sources are present at the same time, we must first translate the decibels to actual intensities in watts per square centimeter. We then add the watts arithmetically and translate back into decibels relative to the reference level. For example, suppose that two different sounds measure 74 and 77 dB (relative to 0.0002 dyne per square centimeter), respectively. Their combined sound pressure is *not* 151 dB. As shown by the scales in Figure 2-4, 74 dB correspond to 1 dyne per square centimeter or $2.5 \times 10^{-9}$ watt per square centimeter; 77 dB correspond to $5.0 \times 10^{-9}$ watt per square centimeter. Their sum is $7.5 \times 10^{-9}$ watt per square centimeter. On the decibel scale this is about 78.8 dB relative to 0.0002 dyne per square centimeter. (Such calculations are readily made with the help of tables which resemble the familiar tables of logarithms.)

A decibel has no fixed absolute value or any units. It is simply a ratio, telling by what proportion one value is greater or less than another. To give the decibel scale an anchor, so to speak, we conventionally assume certain reference levels that are understood unless otherwise specified. For acoustic pressures the *standard reference level* is 0.0002 dyne per square centimeter or $2 \times 10^{-5}$ newtons per square meter. This value is conveniently close to the intensity of the faintest sound that is heard on the average by normal young ears under the best listening conditions. Sound that is painful, at 140 dB, exerts a pressure $10^{14 \div 2} = 10^7 = 10,000,000$ times as great. And the increase in absolute pressure from 140 to 141 dB is 10 million times as great as the increase from 0 to 1 dB (see Figure 2-4).

It might seem inconvenient to have the absolute value of the decibel change as we go up and down the intensity scale, but actually it is a convenience because the just noticeable difference that the ear can detect in the intensity of a sound has been found to be a nearly constant ratio or percentage, and thus an approximately constant number of decibels. The just noticeable difference varies only from 3 or 4 dB for very faint sounds to about 0.3 dB for very intense sounds. We can easily hear a pin drop if the room is almost quiet; but if an airplane engine is warming up nearby, a 10-pound box of pins might fall unheard. But the ability of an additional decibel of sound intensity to attract our attention varies only a little. There is also another way in which the logarithmic decibel scale corresponds approximately to the way in which the ear hears sounds. A sound that is 10 dB more intense than another sound of the same frequency sounds about twice as loud. Thus if a sound 40 dB above the standard reference level is increased to 70 dB, it sounds $2 \times 2 \times 2$, or eight times as loud. This is a very convenient approximate rule. However, if two sounds are of different frequencies, the rules for predicting their combined loudness when they are sounded simultaneously are much more complicated, as we shall see.

### The Sound-Level Meter

We have mentioned the sound-level meter. This is a basic tool for the acoustic engineer. The sound is converted into a corresponding electrical signal, which is then amplified and measured with a meter. The meter is calibrated to give directly the *sound pressure level* (SPL) in decibels relative to the standard reference level. The ear, as we shall see, is more sensitive to sounds of some frequencies than to others; but the sound-level meter is so constructed as to be almost equally sensitive to all frequencies from 20 to 10,000 Hz. It is strictly "flat" from 100 to 2000 Hz and "rolls off" gradually to 6 dB less sensitive at 21 Hz and at 11 kHz.[1] This frequency characteristic is designated as the "C scale" of the meter.

For special purposes two "weighting networks" are provided to give the "A scale" and the "B scale," respectively. These scales and their use will be described near the end of this chapter. When more than one frequency is present, the meter reads the total acoustic pressure as an *over-all sound level*. This over-all sound level is understood when we say, for example, that the noise in a weaving room is 100 dB and on a busy street is 70 dB (see Figure 2-3), but it is helpful to be explicit and write 100 dB(C).

Another basic acoustic instrument is the electrical filter which rejects signals that are above or below a desired *pass band*. If desired, the pass band can be made very narrow, only a few hertz in width. The filter is then said to be sharply "tuned" to a desired frequency. With such a filter the engineer can measure separately the components of a complex tone such as a musical chord. (The line spectra illustrated in Figure 2-2 were obtained in this way.) Or the pass band can be made wider, say a third of an octave or half an octave or a full octave in width. With such an *octave band filter* the sound-pressure level of each octave band of a complex noise, such as street noise or airplane noise, can be measured separately. In this way the *band spectra* illustrated in Figure 2-3 were obtained. The band spectrum is a very useful way of describing a complex noise and gives the acoustic engineer part of his fundamental data if he needs to design, for example, an audiometric booth to exclude the noise in question. High frequencies are, in general, easier to exclude than low frequencies; hence it is important for him to know not only the over-all level, but also how much energy is present in each octave band.

[1] IEC recommendation 179 (1965).

In Figure 2-3 the frequencies that divide one octave band from the next are 75, 150, 300, 600, 1200, 2400 and 4800 Hz. These and the corresponding series of half-octave and third-octave bands have long been conventional for the electrical band-pass filters employed by acoustic engineers. In 1967, however, the USA Standards Institute issued a standard for preferred frequencies and band numbers for acoustical measurement (USAS S 1.6-1967). The entire series of frequencies is based on 1000 Hz as its central point and is symmetrical with respect to it. One thousand hertz is the geometric midfrequency of one of the bands. The dividing cut-off frequencies for the octave bands in the preferred system are 45, 90, 180, 355, 710, 1400, 2800, and 5600 Hz. The corresponding midfrequencies are 63, 125, 250, 500, 1000, 2000, and 4000 Hz. We may expect that the preferred values will gradually replace the original values that appear in Figure 2-3.

### Sound Power

The acoustic engineer finds it very convenient to calculate the total acoustic power output of sound sources, such as jet engines, automobiles on the highway, ventilating fans, or the human voice. The sound power is expressed in watts, but here again it is convenient to use the decibel scale and to talk about the "power level" (PWL). Unfortunately, this additional use of the decibel leads to much confusion. The *power levels* are, of course, always much higher than the *intensity levels* (IL) that the same sources produce at the ears of the listeners. The power level is a measure of all of the watts of acoustic energy radiated in all directions by the source. The intensity level is only the number of watts that flows through one square centimeter at the position of the sound level meter. Thus a full symphony orchestra may generate 140 dB PWL (relative to $10^{-12}$ watt), but the listener may receive only 90 dB IL (rela-

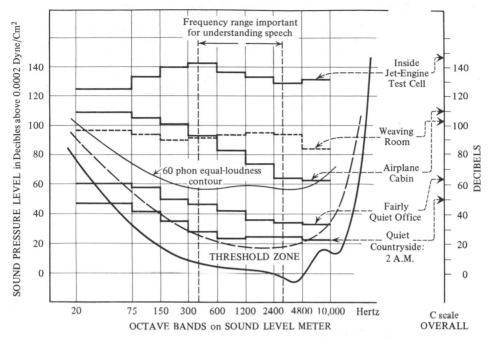

Figure 2-3. *The auditory area and octave band spectra of five steady background noises.* The threshold zone is the same as in Figure 2-4. It is not strictly logical to plot data based on pure tones, such as thresholds and equal-loudness contours, on the same scale of sound-pressure levels that is used for octave band analyses. The error is not large, however, in relation to the large dynamic range of the sounds represented here, and it does not affect the comparisons of one noise with another. The 60-phon equal-loudness contour is at a comfortable listening level. It lies entirely above the spectrum of the quiet office but below the spectrum in the airplane cabin.

The top spectrum was measured inside a typical jet-engine test cell, with the engine operating at military power. The peak of acoustic energy is in the 300 to 600 Hz band. The weaving room had mechanical looms; the floor was wooden. These two spectra are fairly "flat." The airplane spectrum was taken at the last window seat while the piston-engine plane was climbing. It is a sharply sloping spectrum. Notice that its over-all sound pressure level (right) is higher than that for the weaving room because of the large contribution of the lowest, 20 to 75 Hz, band. Speech is better understood in the airplane noise, however, because in the 600 to 1200 and 1200 to 2400 Hz bands the sound levels are lower than those in the weaving room. (The levels are nearly equal in the 300 to 600 band.)

In the "fairly quiet office" there were no business machines. Its over-all sound level of 64 dB is deceptively high because of the sloping spectrum. The "C scale" of the sound-level meter, used for these measurements, was "flat" from 100 to 2000 Hz and only 6 dB less sensitive and 40 and 10,000 Hz. The spectrum of the quiet countryside at 2 A.M. lies almost entirely within the threshold zone, that is, some people with hearing within the range of normal would hear only a very faint rustle (600 to 4800 Hz), although the over-all sound level is 50 dB. The noise in the jet-engine test cell is above the threshold for pain. (*Adapted from a figure by J. R. Cox, Jr., in Industrial Hygiene and Toxicology, Vol. I. New York: Interscience Publishers, 1958.*)

tive to $10^{-16}$ watt per square centimeter) at his seat in the balcony.

The usual reference for power level is the same as for sound level. For power it is usually expressed as $10^{-12}$ watt per square *meter,* which is the same physically as $10^{-16}$ watt per square *centimeter.* The sound power level is conceived as a flow of acoustic energy through an area of one square meter that forms the surface of an imaginary spherical source. Only a tiny fraction of this power reaches a distant listener. Our principal present concern with sound power is to avoid being misled when we encounter this other use of the decibel scale.

### Resonance

In describing the electrical filter, we referred to "tuning" the filter to a desired frequency. This idea of a tuned circuit should be familiar to everyone who "tunes" his radio or television circuit to a desired broadcast frequency or who tunes acoustical devices such as musical instruments. We know that a violin or piano string vibrates at a higher frequency when it is pulled tighter as in "tuning up," or when, on the violin, the vibrating part is shortened by the player's finger. And we have probably noticed that the bass strings of these instruments are thicker and heavier than those in the treble.

In general, any mechanical system that is free to vibrate tends to vibrate at a *natural frequency* that is determined by the mass of the vibrating parts and their stiffness. It is easier to set the system vibrating or *oscillating* at this frequency than at any other, in the sense that at a given amount of alternating pressure the vibrating system will build up a greater amplitude of movement. The system tends to move of itself or "oscillate" exactly in step with the driving force and does not tend to either lag behind or creep ahead. This relation of tending to move exactly in step with the driving force and to fall off in amplitude if the driving frequency is either increased or diminished is called *resonance*.

Energy tends to be stored in a resonant system, whether it be acoustic or electric. This energy is continually being changed back and forth from kinetic energy to potential energy. In a typical mechanical system these forms of energy are represented by the momentum of a moving mass and the elongation of a spring, respectively. Energy is removed from the system by doing work elsewhere or by being dissipated into heat by friction. Acoustic radiation of energy is a step toward frictional loss. Frictional dissipation of energy is called *damping*. "Damping" means to reduce the amplitude of mechanical vibration, and should not be confused with "dampening," meaning to moisten. It is better to "damp" the oscillation of a tuning fork than to "dampen" it, even though some dictionaries sanction the latter usage. If a system is too heavily damped it will not vibrate at all, but when displaced will simply creep back slowly to its position of rest without overshoot. Imagine a violin string vibrating in molasses!

For our purposes it is important to recognize that air in a container that has one or more openings is a resonant system. Air has mass, and it acquires momentum as it moves in and out of the container. The air is also compressible, so that it acts as both the mass and the spring. The natural frequency or frequencies of an air-filled system depend on the volume of the container, on the size of the openings, and, in more complicated ways, on the shape of the cavity. We know that the trombone player lengthens his "pipe" to reach a low note and that if we blow across the mouth of an empty bottle, it resonates at a lower frequency (lower pitch) than if it is half full, and so on. We shall see that the resonances of air-filled cavities enable them to store energy at certain frequencies and also to transmit these frequencies more effectively than others from one end to the other. This principle was utilized in the construction of nonelectrical hearing aids. The same principle in electrical circuits is the basis of most electrical filters.

### The Time-Pattern of Sounds

To describe music or speech, the physicist tells how the frequencies and the corresponding intensities vary from moment to moment. The rhythm (*stress pattern*) and the tempo, whether regular or irregular, are essential features that we learn to recognize as well as we do the sequence of different pitches. Speech and music are not static but are patterns that change from moment to moment.

### Biological and Psychological Aspects of Hearing

Sound is produced incidentally by almost all events in nature that involve the rapid motion of air or water or even moderate movement, particularly the impacts of solid objects. It is very difficult to make any sort of machine run without some noise. Sound is one of nature's surest signs of activity, and therein lies its primitive biological significance. Hearing keeps us *informed* of activities going on at some distance from us and *gives us warning* if that activity becomes more powerful or approaches very close. The important psychological consequences of loss of the primitive awareness and warnings of hearing are discussed in detail in a later chapter. Sight, to be sure, also informs us of distant events, but hearing is the true "watchdog" of the senses. (A watchdog should really be called a "harkdog," for he hears the stranger approach by night before he sees him.) The sun never sets for hearing, and sound waves come to us around corners and reach our ears whichever way our heads are turned. No "earlid" covers the ear in sleep. Experiments on the electrical activity of the brain show that the sleeping brain is at least partially aroused by sounds, even by rather faint sounds if they are unusual or if we have learned that they are warning signals for us.

When we recognize a warning sound, we usually also have some sense of the direction whence it comes. The sense of direction, *auditory localization,* is usually good enough to cause us to look in more or less the right direction. Both ears are necessary for this localization (or better lateralization) or *stereophonic effect,* and we must admit that we are often misled by the curved path of sound around corners and by its reflection as an echo from any large flat surface. It is interesting, however, that bats, dolphins, and some other birds and animals have developed to an extraordinary degree the power of locating distant objects by the reflection of high-pitched chirps that they themselves emit. Nature developed this sonar principle (like radar, but using sound) long before World War II! The blind can learn to make practical use of it, just as the deaf learn speechreading to replace a lost auditory function.

The highest level of audition lies in the recognition of the nature of distant activity. We know what is going on when we hear footsteps, traffic noise, barking dogs, and the like. And, above all, man, by his ability to distinguish and recognize the meaning of sounds, together with his ability to produce a great variety of them with his voice, has developed a system of communication with his fellows that far outdoes the communication between any other animals. The practical and social importance of speech and the hearing of speech need no elaboration. Two of man's greatest biological endowments are, first, his erect posture and his opposable thumb, which give him hands suited to the use of tools and, second, the capacity and organization of a brain suitable for the development of *language.* Language gave man not only the ability to share experience but a tool for abstract thinking.

### Frequency Limits of Audible Sound

The range of audible frequencies extends from about 20 to 20,000 Hz. Neither limit is at all precise. Not only the frequency but the intensity of a sound determine whether or not we can hear it (see Figure 2-4). The ear is limited, like a radio receiver, to a band of frequencies.

For the ear the most sensitive range is from 500 to 5000 Hz, approximately the same range of frequencies that is most important for understanding speech. Above 5000 Hz the sensitivity of the ear declines more and more rapidly, but the tones can still be heard at moderate intensities by most young ears. An uncertainty about the limits arises from individual differences in ears, particularly with increasing age. The child may be able to hear the "inaudible" dog whistle at about 20,000 Hz, whereas the old man may no longer hear even the overtones of the human voice at about 5000 Hz. These changes with age will be considered in detail in a later section (Chapter 4). We begin to *feel* very low tones through the nerves of touch as well as to *hear* them through the auditory nerve, but the smooth tonal character of the sound is lost and is replaced by a "flutter" at about 18 Hz (see Figure 2-5).

Below and above the range of frequencies that the ear can detect lie the *subsonic* (vibration) and the *ultrasonic* frequencies, respectively. The ultrasonic frequencies used to be called *supersonic,* but present usage is to speak of "ultrasonic frequencies" (by analogy with ultraviolet light) and "supersonic speeds." The ultrasonic waves can be compared to the short-wave radio broadcasts which cannot be picked up by an ordinary radio receiver. The physicist with his instruments cares little for the arbitrary limits imposed by human ears. The limits of hearing are certainly higher for dogs, cats, rats, and probably all small mammals. The physicist's instruments carry him on up into the ultrasonic region of high frequencies where blasts of air, crackling of twigs, the chirping of many insects, the cries of bats all produce pressure waves in air of the same kind as ordinary sound, but they are inaudible to us because of their high frequency. Actually, these ultrasonics in nature are rarely very intense and would probably not be very important to animals of our size, even if we could hear them. They do give fairly accurate information of the direction of their sources, for they travel in straighter lines, bend less around corners, and consequently cast deeper "sound shadows" than do the lower frequencies. However, as a general rule, ultrasonics are generated by *small* objects and are not transmitted so well through the air as are the longer wavelengths. The air is partially opaque to the ultrasonics, and, even if fairly intense at their source, they can be detected only at relatively short distances. The near ultrasonics in the first octave or so above the human limit may be important for small animals, but not for us. We need not fear them as possibly injurious, as some people have suggested, for they are feeble. Theory and experience agree that they are practically quite harmless.

### The Sensitivity of the Ear

When we said in a previous section that nature is noisy, we did not mean that nature's sounds are unpleasantly loud; we merely meant that they are audible. The sound waves have enough energy to stimulate the ear, and if nature is noisy, it is partly because our ears are so sensitive within the frequency range of best hearing. The human ear is actually so sensitive that at its best it can almost hear the individual air molecules bump against the eardrum in their random thermal flight. The distance that the eardrum moves in and out with each wave when we just hear the faintest audible tone at the most favorable frequency is less than 1 percent of the diameter of a single hydrogen molecule. This distance is, of course, far less than anything that we can see under the best microscope. As a matter of fact, it is about one ten-thousandth of the wave length of light. We cannot easily think of it in terms of inches, for it is less than a hundred-millionth of an inch. If the capital I at the beginning of this sentence were enlarged to the height of the Empire State Building, a hundred-millionth of an inch would correspond to about the thickness of a piece of cigarette paper.

The extraordinary sensitivity is due to the highly specialized structure of the ear. The outer ear of man, to be sure, is not as efficient as the ear of the dog or the rabbit in collecting sound energy coming from a particular direction. Cupping the hand behind the ear or inserting an ear trumpet causes an appreciable over-all gain in sensitivity, but the inner ear, where the delicate sensory cells lie protected in their special chamber within the hardest bone in the body, is just about as sensitive as it could usefully be. If the cells were stimulated by the random thermal motion of molecules, we would hear a continuous meaningless rattle or hiss and could not distinguish sounds any fainter than the best human ears can now detect. Nature has apparently gone the limit in developing an organ that is senstive to the telltale sound waves given off by most events around us. Small wonder, then, that so delicate an organ may sometimes be injured by very intense blasts of sound or degenerate when affected by disease. The wonder is not that our ears sometimes fail us, but rather that they stand the racket as well as they do.

Intense sounds can be felt, either as a single blast or as vibration, by the sense of touch. Our hairs may be set in vibration by the sound waves of the air and tickle the *touch corpuscles* at their roots. (A hair and its touch corpuscle is, as we shall see, a crude large-scale model of the actual sense organ in the inner ear.) Or with the tips of our fingers we may feel a piano case vibrate. We may even distinguish with our fingers, although crudely, whether the piano is vibrating rapidly (when a medium or high note is struck) or slowly (when one of the lowest notes is sounded). The sense of vibration, which is one aspect of the sense of touch, and the sense of hearing merge into one another in two ways.

From the point of view of evolutionary development, the inner sense organ of hearing is a highly specialized organ of touch, specialized to be "touched" only by vibrations of the air and never by a solid object. Secondly, when we "hear" the very lowest notes of a pipe organ, we are probably *feeling* the vibration quite as much as we are *hearing* it. As tones get lower and lower in frequency, the ear is less and less sensitive to them, and the tones must be stronger, with larger vibrations, in order to be heard. Finally, the point is reached at which the pressure waves begin to stimulate the skin of our hands, the linings of our noses and throats, the hairs of our heads, and even our bones, joints, and inner organs. The sense of hearing and touch merge as imperceptibly as do smell and taste. But touch, like taste, cannot distinguish the fine differences for which hearing (like smell) is specialized. Therefore, although we may, for example, perceive the *rhythm* of a piece of music as accurately by touch as by ear, we cannot feel the *tune*, because touch is so poor at discriminating the frequencies that give us our sense of musical pitch. Likewise, the tempo and stress of very loud speech can be felt, but only in the most favorable *context* can words ever be understood through touch alone.

### Minimum Audible Field

The psychophysicist is interested in the relations between our sensations and the dimensions and magnitudes of the changes in the external world (the stimuli) that arouse them. We know that the dimensions of physical sound are frequency and intensity, measured, respectively, in hertz and in decibels. On a chart scaled off in these two dimensions we can map the *area of audible tones* (Figure 2-4). It is bounded at the bottom by the *threshold of hearing*. The "threshold" is the faintest sound of a given frequency that a person can detect on 50 percent of a number of trials. The threshold curve expresses the

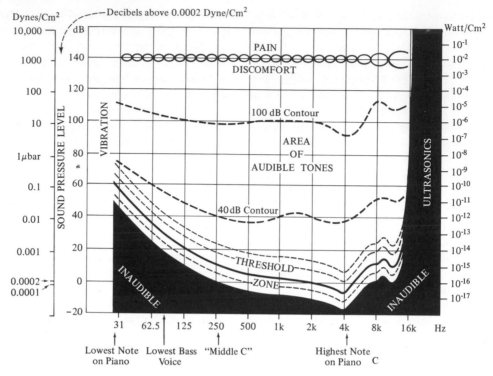

Figure 2-4. *The area of audible tones* was determined for a group of otologically normal men listening with both ears, facing the source, in a free acoustic field. The heavy lower contour represents their median hearing thresholds: the shaded zones show one and two standard deviations ($\sigma$) above and below it. Dips at 4000 and 12000 Hz are due largely to resonance in the ear canal and diffraction patterns around the head. The area of audibility at low frequencies merges into vibration. On the high-frequency side lie the inaudible ultrasonics. The practical upper limit is the threshold for pain, at about 140 dB SPL.

Two equal-loudness contours are shown for tones judged to sound as loud as 1000-Hz tones at 40 dB and at 100 dB SPL, respectively. (*Adapted from D. W. Robinson and R. S. Dadson, Journal of the Acoustical Society of America, 29:1284–1288 [1957]; and Britsh Journal of Applied Physics, 7:166–181 [1956].*)

*acuity* of human hearing, although the term "acuity" is ambiguous and is sometimes understood as referring instead to the ability to *discriminate* between two tones that are nearly the same. It is, therefore, safer to say that the curve in question represents the *threshold of sensitivity* of human hearing or the "threshold of detectability" of pure tones. Tones above threshold are audible, those below are inaudible.

In Figures 2-4 and 2-5 we have represented the threshold by a heavy solid line and four other shaded bands or lighter lines nearly parallel to it. We have done so because, in addition to differences related to age, people have different thresholds. Furthermore, one person's threshold varies somewhat from day to day and even from trial to trial. We must therefore think of a *threshold zone* rather than a sharp fixed boundary. Fortunately, for a given class of persons, such as males between 18 and 25 years of age whose ears show no abnormality when examined with an otoscope, the distribution of threshold turns out to be a random scatter above and below a median value with a strong "central tendency." The heavy "threshold" line in Figure 2-4 actually represents the median values for such an 18- to 25-year group tested at the National Physical Laboratory in England. These men were healthy and otherwise average individuals. The lighter flanking lines show the dispersion of the thresholds. The lines are one and two standard deviations, respectively, above and below the median. The heavy line, the median, is, of course, the 50 percentile contour. The zone between the two one-standard-deviation lines includes about 68 percent of the total group and the two-standard-deviation zone includes about 95 percent of the group.

This sort of scatter is perfectly normal. Individuals differ with respect to their sensitivity of hearing just as they do with respect to other measurable characteristics such as height and weight. To avoid confusion on this point we do not speak of a standard of normal hearing but instead of a *range of normal hearing.*

It is not easy to determine the threshold of hearing of normal listeners because great care must be taken to exclude all echoes and all unwanted background noises, from both the environment and the source of the test sounds. Also the subjects must be well motivated to listen carefully and consistently. Only under the best listening conditions can these extremely low thresholds be measured. The data obtained at the National Physical Laboratory actually agree well with earlier but less extensive studies performed at the Bell Telephone Laboratories.

The intensity of the sound field in such tests as these is measured, before the listener enters it, at the position corresponding to the center of the listener's head. The listener faces the source of the sound and listens with both ears. The threshold of hearing, measured under these conditions is called the *minimum audible field* (MAF). The dips in the threshold curve at 4000 and 12,000 hertz (Figure 2-4) are due partly to the acoustic resonance of the ear canals of the listeners and even more to the pattern of reflection and refraction of sound waves around their heads and ears. The thresholds vary, depending on the angle of direction (azimuth) of the source of sound with respect to the listener's head, and are different for a so-called "plane wave" advancing from a single direction as opposed to random incidence from all directions.

As we have noted, the frequency at which sounds become inaudible depends not only on the intensity of the sound but on the age of the listener. For low frequencies the threshold rises more gradually, and age is not a factor. The difficulties for very low frequencies are, first, to distinguish hearing from feeling and, second, to generate really pure low tones. The higher harmonics can be heard easily even though they may have less than one ten-thousandth of the acoustic energy of the fundamental.

The auditory area is bounded at its upper edge, for practical purposes, by the thresholds of discomfort, of tickle, and, finally, of pain. These thresholds vary from person to person and with the attitude of the listener toward these very loud sounds and toward the tests. There are also problems of just what the words "discomfort," "tickle," and "pain" mean. Many listeners are likely at first to report pain for a sensation that they later call merely "tickle" after they have once felt the sharp stab of true auditory pain. If prolonged, such very intense sounds are dangerous to hearing as well as painful, so the practical upper limit of the auditory area at about 135 dB sound pressure level is real. As it happens, these thresholds of discomfort, tickle, and pain are pretty nearly constant, regardless of frequency. Only the first unpleasantness, the *discomfort,* is a truly auditory sensation. Actually the *loudness* of the sounds keeps on increasing as the intensity is increased, regardless of discomfort, tickle in the ear, or pain.

### Minimum Audible Pressure and Hearing-Threshold Level

Some tests for impaired hearing are conducted binaurally in a free acoustic field, particularly with young children (as described in Chapter 8), but in most tests the two ears are studied separately, using a pair of earphones. The earphones have the great practical advantage of fitting snugly against the side of the head and excluding much of the ambient background noise. It is far easier and cheaper to build a booth that is quiet enough for such audiometry than a room that is quiet enough and adequately sound-treated for measuring minimum audible field. Less sound exclusion is needed for the conventional audiometric booth and, although some internal sound absorption is desirable, it is not necessary to prevent echoes entirely. Details of audiometric booths, audiometers, and the calibration of audiometers are given in Chapter 7, but the relations between monaural and binaural listening and between field listening and earphone listening will be examined here. These relations are important because we use our ears chiefly as a pair in an open auditory field, but our ears are usually tested separately, using the acoustic pressure developed in the very restricted volume of air under an earphone. These two situations are quite different.

The difference between hearing with one ear instead of two is not difficult to state if we are concerned only with the measurement of thresholds. Careful tests, both in an acoustic field and with earphones, have shown that two ears are more sensitive than one. The gain is about 3 dB. This gain in sensitivity is, however, a very minor advantage for binaural hearing compared with other major advantages, namely, the ability to recognize the direction of the source of a sound, the better detection of signals, and better discrimination of speech in the presence of noise. These three other advantages will be considered later, and we do not need to be concerned here with the way in which the greater sensitivity of hearing is achieved. It is not, as was once supposed, simply a matter of scooping up twice as much acoustic energy. It involves complicated interactions between the inputs from the two ears within the central nervous system.

The matter of measuring the acoustic pressure developed under the earphone is more difficult. It is possible to make such measurements by means of a probe-tube microphone. The plastic tube attached to the microphone is long and flexible enough to pass under the cushion of the earphone to almost any desired position except one. It is not practical to measure acoustic pressure deep in the ear canal, just in front of the drum membrane, while the subject is wearing earphones, although this can be done readily enough in an acoustic field. The usual choice is to measure the acoustic pressure just at the outer entrance of the ear canal. This position must be closely specified on account of acoustic resonances within the ear canal and in the small airspace under the earphone.

In addition to the problem of defining the standard position at which to measure the pressure, it now appears that the efficiency of the ear in detecting a faint sound is modified by the volume of air contained under the earphone and also, if this volume is small, on certain acoustic characteristics known technically as the "acoustic impedance" of the source of the sound. Even worse, the interaction between the ear and the source depends, in turn, on the anatomy and on the acoustic impedance of the ear that is under the earphone. The impedance and the resonances vary significantly from one ear to another. One way out of this difficulty is to make the volume of air under the earphone very large, of the order of a liter or so. Unfortunately, such an audiometer is clumsy. Its large ear chambers, too heavy for a headband, require firm independent support. It has never been popular in the United States as a clinical instrument.

The differences and uncertainties that we are discussing are not large enough to be of great practical significance, but they make very difficult the standardization and calibration of audiometers. Nevertheless, it would seem that if we could measure the acoustic pressure in the field and also at the entrance to the ear canal under the earphone, the threshold pressures should be the same. Unfortunately there is still a rather large discrepancy, about 6 dB, for which there is still no complete and satisfactory explanation. It probably involves effects like resonances, acoustic impedances, directional effects, and perhaps others. The discrepancy is known as "the missing 6 dB."

This unexplained discrepancy was pointed out by Fletcher and his collaborators at the Bell Telephone Laboratories more than 30 years ago. It was confirmed 20 years later by the studies at the National Physical Laboratory in England to which we have already referred. The curve for minimum audible pressure (monaural earphone listening) lies about 6 dB above the minimum audible field (monaural listening) and does not have such large peaks and troughs above 3000 Hz (compare Figures 2-4 and 2-5).

For completeness we should also mention here the standard of pressure used for the calibration of audiometers. This is the acoustic pressure measured in a carefully standardized *coupler* or *artificial ear* when the earphone that is placed on it is driven by a voltage that corresponds to the hearing threshold of an appropriate sample of otologically normal ears. Details are given in Chapter 7. The point here is that the standard artificial ear has a volume (6 cc) corresponding to the air-

space under an ordinary audiometric earphone, including the external and middle ear, but it has its own set of resonances and its own acoustic impedance. Its advantage lies in its simplicity and its reproducibility. The coupler pressures are of the same order of magnitude as the minimum audible pressures, but they are not identical with them. They differ slightly for different models of earphone. In particular these standard threshold coupler pressures must not be confused with the sound pressure of the minimum audible field.

A set of standard reference levels for pure-tone audiometers has been recommended by the International Organization for Standardization (ISO) on the basis of a number of studies of the hearing of healthy young adults. (Details will be given in Chapter 7.) These reference zero levels are given as coupler pressures. They represent median values for many listeners. In this respect they are similar to the median minimum audible field, which is also based on the hearing of a similar population of young adults. The minimum audible pressure, from 500 to 8000 Hz, is of the same order of magnitude as the physicist's reference level of 0.0002 dyne per cm², but it lies a few decibels above the physicist's level because of (1) the binaural advantage (about 3 dB), (2) the missing 6 dB, and (3) an arbitrary decision which put the physical reference level at the level of "good" rather than "average" hearing. This last difference is about 3 or 4 dB according to Robinson and Dadson.

The upshot of all this is that an ear that is, for example, 10 dB less sensitive than the median will require a level 10 dB above the reference level (ISO) of the audiometer to reach threshold. In an open auditory field the threshold (binaural) for a man with two such ears will likewise lie 10 dB above the median minimum audible field. Across the range of frequencies from 500 to 3000 Hz this median minimum audible field is approx-

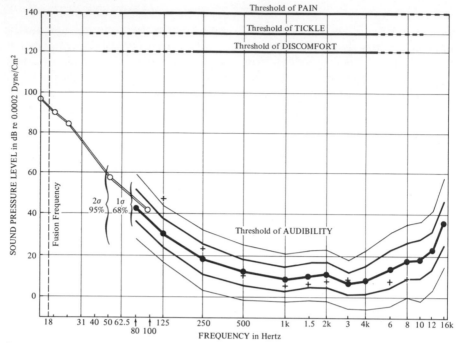

Figure 2-5. *"Area of Audiometry."* *Threshold sound pressure levels under an earphone, or minimum audible pressure (MAP)*, as determined at the National Physical Laboratory (British). The heavy solid line and filled circles show the median values for 99 men (198 ears) otologically normal and 18 to 25 years of age. The distributions of the thresholds are normal, and the modes, the medians, and the means are almost identical. The lighter lines show one and two standard deviations ($\sigma$) above and below the medians.

The pressures were measured with a probe-tube microphone "at the entrance to the ear canal," the average of two positions: one 7 mm outside, the other 3 mm inside the meatus. (The values at the latter position are slightly modified above 1 kHz by resonance effects of the ear canal.)

Coupler measurements were made for the same earphone (4026-A) using a British standard coupler (B.S.2042). At 250 Hz and above they all lie within $1\sigma$ of the probe-tube data plotted in the figure. These coupler measurements entered into the calculation of the ISO reference zero levels for pure-tone audiometers. The ISO values, for the USA earphone and coupler (WE 705-A and NAS 9A, respectively), are shown in the figure by the crosses (+). (*Adapted from R. S. Dadson and J. H. King, Journal of Laryngology and Otology, 66:366– 378 [1952].*)

The thresholds for the very low frequencies (open circles and double lines) and the fusion frequency were determined in a separate study on 10 subjects, using different, specially designed equipment. (*N. S. Yeowart, M. E. Bryan, and W. Tempest, Journal of Sound and Vibration, 6:335–342 [1967].*) They are included here to extend the area of audiometry to its logical limit at the "fusion frequency" of 18 Hz, below which the smooth tonal quality is lost. Actually audiometric measurements are rarely made below 125 Hz.

The thresholds of pain, tickle, and discomfort shown here were measured at Central Institute for the Deaf in 1945–1946. (*S. R. Silverman, Annals of Otology, Rhinology, and Laryngology, 56:658–677 [1947].*) They are coupler pressures (PDR-10 earphone and NBS 9-A coupler), comparable to the ISO reference levels. They were determined by increasing the sound-pressure level, starting at 100 dB, by 1 or 2 dB every 1.5 seconds until the subjects reported first discomfort, then tickle, then pain. This method allowed some habituation to the high-level sound and ensured that the intra-aural reflex was active throughout the test. Sounds of sudden onset from a low background level show somewhat lower thresholds of pain, tickle, and discomfort. These three upper thresholds were the same for subjects with normal hearing and for those hard of hearing. They are the approximate median values for the group. The dashed portions of the lines are extrapolations beyond the experimental data.

imately 4 dB above 0.0002 dyne per cm². The man in question should therefore be able to hear a tone in this frequency range at about $10 + 4 = 14$ dB sound pressure level (SPL).

## The Audiogram

Figure 2-5 shows the minimum audible pressure measured under an earphone, as determined at the National Physical Laboratory. The corresponding coupler pressures were determined also, and later they entered into the averages that constitute the international reference zero levels for audiometers. The crosses represent the international reference zero values, now given as coupler pressures for the WE 705-A earphone in MX-41 cushions measured in a National Bureau of Standards (USA) NBS-9A coupler. The thresholds of pain, tickle, and discomfort at the top of the figure were also measured under nearly similar earphones and are also given as coupler pressures. The three upper thresholds are therefore directly comparable to the crosses representing the zero of the audiometer.

A pure-tone audiometer is calibrated so that its zero reading at each frequency corresponds to the median hearing level for healthy young adults (the international standard). The average reference value is different for different frequencies. The audiometer measures the number of decibels that the threshold of the subject lies above each median value. The difference is the *hearing-threshold level*. The graph of hearing-threshold levels, illustrated in Figures 7-6 and 7-7, is known as the *audiogram*. Here the reference zero levels are drawn as a straight horizontal line across frequencies. Positive hearing-threshold levels, representing additional pressure needed to be heard by ears less sensitive than the average, are conventionally plotted *downward* to express the idea of reduced sensitivity of the ear. This convention was established by otologists who thought in terms of the sensitivity of the ear. It is opposite to that of the physicist who plots sound pressures as increasing upward (as in the figures in Chapter 4). The physicist thinks in terms of the *sound* which is the *stimulus* to the ear. The measuring instrument for the physicist is the sound-level meter, but for the audiologist it is the hearing-level meter or audiometer.

## The Speech Area

A particularly important part of the auditory area is the range of frequencies most important for the understanding of speech. This range extends roughly from 400 to 3000 Hz. Speech contains frequencies above 3000 Hz and below 400 Hz, but they are not necessary for almost perfect intelligibility of everyday conversational speech. The importance of the speech range will appear later in relation to the design of hearing aids and to the problem of auditory handicap. The part of the auditory area that is important for speech is bounded at the top by the thresholds of tolerance and, at the bottom, for practical purposes, by the background sound level against which we are likely to hear faint everyday speech. Practically, this is at an octave-band level of approximately 30 to 40 dB SPL in this part of the frequency spectrum. Figure 2-6 shows the range of frequencies most important for good understanding of everyday speech. It also shows the approximate distribution with respect to frequency and intensity of the actual sounds of conversational speech.

The extent to which a background noise will interfere with ordinary conversational speech depends on the relations of the spectrum of the noise (see Figure 2-3) and its intensity. An index for noise, known as the *Speech Interference Level* (SIL), consists of the arithmetic average of the three octave-band levels 600 to 1200 Hz,

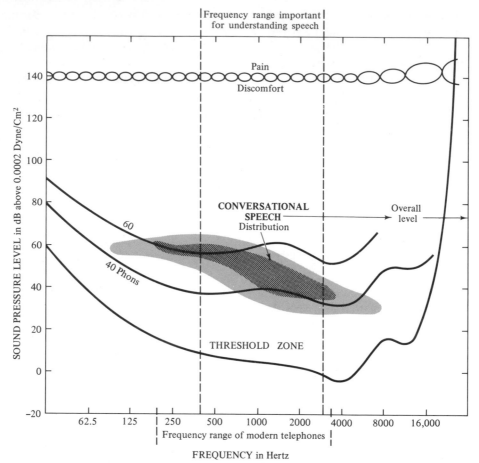

Figure. 2-6. The speech area. Speech is a mixture of complex tones, wide-band noise, and transients. Both the intensities and the frequencies of speech sounds change continually and rapidly. It is difficult to measure them and logically impossible to plot them precisely in terms of sound pressure levels at particular frequencies. This figure shows the approximate distribution of sound-pressure levels with respect to frequency that would occur if brief but characteristic bits of phonemes of conversational speech were actually sustained like pure tones. The density of the shaded area represents roughly the probability of finding in a sample of speech the particular combinations of intensity and frequency. Individual voices differ, however, and obviously the boundaries of the speech area are not sharp.

The over-all sound-pressure level of the stronger vowels in conversational speech at 1 meter is about 72 dB. The fundamental frequency of a deep bass voice is about 100 Hz, but the fundamental frequencies of most women's and children's voices are about 250 Hz. The strongest individual sounds in the frequency range below 100 Hz are louder than 60 phons, and the weakest significant elements are about 30 dB below the strongest. The weaker elements are very often masked by background noises. For good understanding of everyday speech the range from 400 to 3000 Hz is sufficient. This range includes almost all of the "formant" frequency bands of speech which distinguish the vowels and many consonants. (See *Man's World of Sound* by Pierce and David for a good acoustic description of speech.)

1200 Hz, and 2400 to 4800 Hz. This index is very useful to the acoustical engineer in predicting whether speech will be intelligible in certain noisy situations.

## Psychoacoustics

*Psychoacoustics* is concerned with what we hear. It describes the relations of our auditory sensations to the physical properties of the acoustic stimulus, such as its frequency spectrum, its wave form, its intensity, and its temporal relations. Psychoacoustics deals with attributes of sensation such as pitch and loudness and the apparent location of the source and also with judgments as to how loud a noise is, either relative to another noise or on an absolute scale. It is concerned with the ability of listeners to distinguish differences between stimuli. It is not concerned directly with the physiological mechanisms that underlie the detection or the differentiation of sounds but with the judgments and reports of human listeners. Most tests of hearing used to describe and measure impairments of hearing are actually psychoacoustic tests.

We shall not undertake a complete exploration of psychoacoustics, but we shall mention some of its important principles and define a few terms that may be encountered in relation to some of the more elaborate tests of hearing, particularly those designed to assess central rather than peripheral impairments. In the next chapter we shall examine the intermediate anatomical and physiological mechanisms and consider how anatomy, biophysics, and neurophysiology set certain limits on the psychoacoustic performance of human listeners.

### Pitch

*Pitch* is a quality of the sensation of sound that is most clearly recognized for pure tones. It is a quality by which we can arrange sounds on a scale from *low* or bass to *high* or treble. It is the quality that enables us to recognize a tune. The musical pitch of a note depends chiefly on the physical frequency of the sound waves and also, to a very limited extent, on their intensity. The positions of the lowest and the highest notes of the piano and its middle C (261.6 Hz) are shown in Figure 2-4. The relation of the *musical scale* to simple numerical ratios of the frequencies of the sound waves should be familiar. There is a particularly close musical relation between two frequencies that are an octave apart. The higher frequency is exactly double the lower frequency. The musical scale is thus related simply and directly to the *logarithm* of frequency.

The higher harmonics of musical tones, the human voice, and many other sounds are related in frequency to the fundamental and to one another in simple numerical ratios, such as 3 to 2, 5 to 3, and so on. These relations are implicit in the line spectra shown in Figure 2-2. The overtones are said to be *harmonically related* to one another. These simple relations are the basis of musical harmony and of musical scales.

Individuals differ considerably in their ability to recognize, remember, and reproduce musical *intervals,* either in sequence (melody) or in combination (harmony). Training and practice improve performance. Some people can "carry a tune" easily and accurately after only one or two hearings, and the ability to recognize and to mimic dialects in speech is closely related. Other people have very poor *musical memories*. A few gifted individuals have the faculty of *absolute pitch* and can identify a note (on the musical scale) as A or C sharp or E flat, for example, or sing such a note on demand. The relative contributions of endowment and training to absolute pitch are still debated.

*The mel scale.* In addition to the musical scale, there is another *psychological scale* of pitch. It is demonstrated (and defined operationally) by asking listeners to find, by adjusting an oscillator, a tone whose pitch is "half as high" or perhaps "twice high" as that of a standard tone, without regard to musical interval. Or we may present a tone of medium pitch, say at 500 Hz, and tell the listener that it stands at 10 on the pitch scale. Then we present other tones of various frequencies in random order and ask the listener to give to the pitch of each tone an appropriate number on the pitch scale. Variations of these methods are to ask the subject to bisect the pitch interval between two tones or to judge whether intervals between two pairs of tones are the same or different. These various psychophysical methods agree in producing a subjective scale of pitch that is quite different from the musical scale. Octaves in different parts of the scale have different subjective magnitudes. They are much smaller below 500 Hz than above it. For this subjective scale, a unit has been defined: the *mel*. The pitch of a tone of 1000 Hz at 40 dB above threshold is 1000 mels. The pitch curve is shown in Figure 2-7 as a solid line. The dashed line shows how it would be if each semitone, or each octave, were equal in subjective magnitude.

The smallest difference in pitch that a listener can detect on 50 percent of a series of trials is known as his *differential threshold* or *difference limen* (DL) for

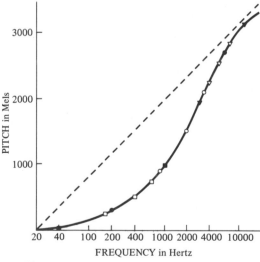

Figure 2-7. The solid curve shows the pitch scale in mels as a function of frequency. The dashed line shows the relation which would apply if all octaves were equal in subjective magnitude. (*Data from S. S. Stevens and J. Volkmann, American Journal of Psychology, 53:329–353 [1940].*)

pitch. ("Limen" is the Latin word for threshold.) We usually present a random series of pairs of successive tones that differ only slightly in frequency and ask the subject to tell us whether the members of each pair sounded the same or different. With these data we construct the *psychophysical curve* that relates percentage correct to the frequency difference between the tones. The curve is typically an "ogive," rising slowly, then steeply, then slowly to 100 percent correct. The difference limen, at 50 percent correct, is about 2 or 3 Hz for 1000 Hz at moderate intensities. The DL turns out to be very nearly constant with frequency if it is expressed in mels. *One just noticeable difference (j.n.d.) turns out, quite by coincidence, to be about one mel.* This is not an exact rule because the size of the DL (or j.n.d.) depends significantly on just how the tones are presented to the listener and also on individual differences among listeners in their ability to discriminate pitch differences.

A corollary of the approximate equivalence of the mel and the j.n.d. is that all j.n.d.s for pitch are of the same subjective magnitude. This is not surprising, and for many years this equality was simply assumed without proof. We mention it, however, because we shall soon see that for loudness the just noticeable differences are *not* all subjectively equal.

*The pitch of complex sounds.* The pitch of a continuing pure tone is clear and definite. The situation is more complicated when the tone is very brief or when more than one tone reaches the ear at once. Let us consider the second case first. The simplest and most common combination of frequencies is a fundamental and its series of higher harmonics (Figure 2-2). We hear the pitch as the same as that of the fundamental, although its musical quality is different. This is true even when the fundamental is very weak and most of the loudness is carried by the higher harmonics. It is still true when the fundamental itself is eliminated, leaving only the equally spaced overtones. This is known as "the case of the missing fundamental," and it explains why the bass notes of music are heard as well as they are through hearing aids and many small loudspeakers.

A musical chord does not, in general, have the simple harmonic series of frequencies, and modern music may contain almost any combination of frequencies, consonant or dissonant. The pitch of chords may be hard to specify. Sometimes they sound single, with a pitch somewhere between the extremes of the tones that are combined. Sometimes the components are heard separately, each with its own pitch and loudness. Even noises with continuous spectra, if they have a large part of their energy concentrated in one part of the spectrum, have more or less pitch.

*Ohm's law and periodicity pitch.* If two tones have frequencies that are not harmonically related, that is, in simple numerical ratio to one another, or if their frequencies are very different, it is usually easy to distinguish them and "hear them out" separately. The ability of the ear to analyze such a mixture, like a set of physical acoustic filters, is known as *Ohm's acoustical law.* (This law must not be confused with Ohm's electrical law, which relates the voltage, the current, and the resistance in an electrical circuit.) Ohm's law is one of the classical laws of psychoacoustics, but it is only a first-order approximation.

The ear does indeed act like a set of filters, but the filters are not very sharp. Furthermore, what we hear in a complex mixture depends significantly on whether we try, by an effort of attention, to separate the components or whether we accept the mixture as a single auditory sensation. However, the ear is more than a simple set of acoustic filters. It is sensitive to the periodic recurrence of peaks of acoustic pressure that may be produced by the interaction of tones that are not harmon-

ically related, or perhaps by a series of clicks or brief bursts of high-frequency noise. In other words, the ear can hear certain pitches that are *not* detected as acoustic frequencies by a set of physical acoustic filters. Unlike the acoustic filters, the ear is sensitive, to a limited extent, to wave form as such and thus to the phase relations in a mixture of pure tones. We shall return to this phenomenon of *periodicity pitch* in connection with the temporal pattern of nerve impulses in the auditory nerve. It is of practical significance in relation to the possibility of hearing by direct electrical stimulation of the nerve without the intervention of the ear.

*The pitch of brief tones: transients.* The tonality or definiteness of pitch of a sound depends also on the abruptness of onset and on the duration of the tone. A sinusoidal electrical signal can be started or stopped instantaneously and at any phase of its cycle, but such an abrupt onset must contain, mathematically and physically, other frequencies than that of the continuing pure sinusoid. Acoustic energy is "scattered," as we say, into other parts of the acoustic spectrum. This energy at other frequencies is known as the *starting transient.* Mathematically a tone is pure and has a single frequency only if it is of infinite duration. In addition, any physical transducer, such as a loudspeaker that has inertia, will be "excited" to vibrate or "ring," as we say, at its own resonant frequency unless it is sufficiently (critically) damped. The ear itself is one such transducer, and it is not critically damped. For all of these reasons, a spurious click is heard at the sudden onset (or termination) of an otherwise pure tone. To avoid such starting and stopping transients, we must make the onset and offset of a tone gradual over several cycles at least. Only then will we hear the tone as pure. Incidentally, such a gradual onset is required in standard pure-tone audiometers (see Chapter 7).

Quite apart from the starting and stopping transients, a tone must last for an appreciable time if it is to have a completely definite pitch. Some pitch quality is present even for stimuli of only one or two cycles, but the subjective pitch is not clear unless the tone lasts for something like a twentieth or even a tenth of a second. The necessary duration depends greatly on just how we define *clear* pitch. One reason that impulsive sounds like knocking on wood are indefinite in pitch is that they start abruptly and die out very rapidly, and they may also ring at more than one frequency simultaneously. A knock on wood may seem to have no pitch at all, but if it is followed by another knock on a different piece of wood, the pitch difference is easily recognized. We can play a tune with a set of well-chosen sticks of wood.

Very brief acoustic stimuli with a single dominant frequency may be produced by ringing an electrical filter with a brief electrical pulse. Such "filtered clicks" or "tone pips" are useful tools in psychoacoustic and physiological research, but their pitch is rather vague, like clicks, knocks, or thumps. "Pitchness" grades without boundaries from the definite pitch of a pure tone to the indeterminate pitch of unfiltered clicks or white noise.

We may comment here that, although some listeners have more "acute" hearing than others in the sense that their difference limens for pitch are smaller, we never encounter a person with any useful degree of hearing who is completely *tone deaf*. This term should be avoided. If it means anything, it should mean inability to distinguish differences in pitch. It is often misused in popular language to mean poor musical memory or poor ability to identify the components of a complex tone.

*Beats, aural harmonics, and combination tones.* Let us return to the question of how we hear two tones of approximately the same intensity but with frequencies that are very nearly the same. If the tones differ by only one cycle per second, the peaks of the waves will coincide and physically reenforce one another at one moment, but half a second later the slower will lag behind the other by half a cycle, and the two waves will cancel one another more or less completely. After another half second, they will be in phase again and again reenforce one another. This periodic waxing and waning or "amplitude modulation" will be heard as a waxing and waning of loudness at a frequency of one per second. These changes in loudness are known as "beats." They are the basis of a delicate method, used by piano tuners, to determine when two sound sources are exactly in tune. If the beats are slow, less than about six or seven a second, the effect is not unpleasant. A little faster and the effect becomes a "vibrato." If the difference in frequency is more than 20 per second or thereabouts, the sound is rough and unpleasant. Two such piano strings would be definitely out of tune. This detection of beats is another way in which the ear differs from a set of perfect acoustic filters. The two frequencies "overlap" and affect some of the same detector elements.

If the difference in frequency is made wider still, we can begin to hear the sound as a mixture of two tones. The necessary difference for separate identification is one way of defining a *critical band* of frequency within which the sensation is fused or single. We shall return to this important property of the ear and define it more carefully in relation to loudness and to the phenomenon of the "masking" of one sound by another.

A final aspect of pitch is the phenomenon of combination tones and of "aural harmonics," which refers to our hearing of new frequencies that correspond to the sums or the differences of the frequencies of two clearly separated tones that are presented simultaneously. Suffice it to say that these effects are produced physically in the inner or middle ear because the ear is not a perfect linear transmitting system. In fact we shall see in the next chapter that the mechanical nonlinearity of the ear begins at about the middle of the area of audible tones (Figure 2-4). There are increasing protective restraints of an elastic sort on the amplitude of movement in the inner ear as those movements tend to become large. Asymmetries and nonlinearity of the system introduce higher harmonics and also the sum and difference tones, including interaction among the higher harmonics of the two original tones. The same effect is produced in nonlinear or "overloaded" physical systems, and is the basis of troublesome harmonic distortion in hearing aids that are working near the limit of their capacity.

### Other Qualities of Sounds

We have discussed the pitch of pure tones and the different quality that is introduced by the presence of strong higher harmonics. We have mentioned also the quality of roughness that results from rapid beats or amplitude modulation. Several other psychological attributes of sound such as "timbre," "brightness," "brilliance," "density," and "volume" have been described. They seem to depend on various combinations of frequencies and intensities in the physical pattern of the stimulating sound. With one exception the details need not concern us in the present survey.

The exception is the particular and characteristic quality of a musical instrument or the human voice that is given by the reinforcement, by the principle of resonance, of all frequencies, whether fundamental or harmonics, that fall within a certain broad band or bands of frequency. The range of frequencies that is reinforced is called a *formant,* and it gives a very distinctive character or quality to the sound. The pitches of the tones may change, but those of the formants remain fixed. The vowels of speech differ from one another in the formants that are imposed by the resonant cavities of the mouth and pharynx. The formants change with different positions of lips, tongue, and jaw; but they are independent of the fundamental frequency of the voice. The latter is determined by the vibration of the vocal bands that periodically interrupt the stream of air through the larynx.

*Binaural hearing of pitch.* A sound of a given frequency does not, in general, have exactly the same pitch when heard in the right ear as it does in the left ear, yet most people are not aware of such differences between their ears. The discrepancies pass unnoticed for several reasons. First, the differences are usually small. The frequency in the right ear need be changed by only 1 or 2 percent to make the pitches equal. Second, the differences are not systematic. A difference of as much as 1 percent may extend over only a fraction of an octave, and the right ear may hear some tones sharper, others flatter, than the left; but systematic search almost always reveals noticeable differences at some frequencies. Third, we usually hear the same external sound in both ears simultaneously, and do not make the necessary successive comparisons. When the pitches and the loudnesses are nearly the same, we hear a single pitch that is the average of the right pitch and the left pitch. Only when the difference exceeds some critical amount do we hear two discordant pitches and complain of *diplacusis* or double hearing (see Chapter 4). When the sound is much louder in one ear, the pitch of that ear is dominant.

### Loudness

Loudness is the aspect of auditory sensation that relates most directly to the physical intensity or energy of the sound waves. It extends from "barely audible" through "comfortably loud" to "uncomfortably loud" and finally to "barely tolerable" and painful, as indicated in Figure 2-4. It happens that all audible sounds become intolerably loud at about the same physical intensity, about 135 dB sound pressure level, regardless of their frequency.

At low physical intensities, say 30 dB SPL, some frequencies are inaudible, others barely audible, and still others, in the range from 1000 to 4000 Hz, are clearly audible.

It is not difficult, with a little practice, for listeners to match quite reliably tones or noises of different frequencies or frequency spectra with respect to their loudness. In fact, as we shall see in Chapter 7, such *loudness balances* between tones of different frequency presented alternately are an important clinical diagnostic test of hearing. On the basis of a series of such loudness balances, we can construct a series of *equal loudness contours* such as those shown in Figures 2-3, 2-4, and 2-6. Each of these contours is identified by the physical intensity of the 1000 Hz tone through which it passes. The 100 dB and the 40 dB contours for free-field binaural listening are shown in Figure 2-4.

*Phon.* The loudness of a 1000-Hz tone defines a *loudness level*. The name of the unit of loudness level is the *phon*. Thus if a tone or a noise of any frequency spectrum is judged to be just as loud as a reference tone of 1000 Hz at 40 dB SPL (binaural field listening facing the source), it has a loudness level of 40 phons. The phon scale is a decibel scale which corresponds to the sound pressure level of the reference tone. It helps to describe the stimulus. It is not, however, a unit of subjective loudness. To generate a loudness scale we must go to the methods of magnitude estimation, half-loudness, double-loudness, and so on, exactly as we did for the pitch scale of mels.

*Loudness difference limens.* The difference limen (DL) for loudness is approximately one decibel. It has sometimes been stated, quite wrongly, that this is the basis for the choice of the decibel as a unit of measurement in acoustics. Actually, the difference limen varies from about 4 dB near threshold to less than 0.5 dB at high intensities, and it is larger for very high and very low tones than for tones in the middle range.

An old and familiar law of psychophysics, Weber's law, stated that the just noticeable difference in sensation (the difference limen) is a constant fraction of the total stimulus. This law would require that the DL for loudness should be a constant number of decibels. Weber's law is, therefore, only an approximation, and it breaks down rather badly at the ends of the scales of both frequency and intensity.

Weber's law was extended by Fechner to the question of psychological magnitudes. Fechner's "law" states that the psychological magnitude grows as the logarithm of the magnitude of the stimulus. But in spite of the nearly universal acceptance of this law for a hundred years, it is actually, like Weber's law, only a first approximation to the facts. Furthermore, it is founded on the *assumption* that all just noticeable differences are equal in subjective magnitude. This proposition, as we have noted, is true for pitch, but it is definitely false for loudness.

During the last 20 years, much attention has been given to loudness and loudness scales and more recently to other scales of subjective magnitudes also. One of the foremost investigators has been S. S. Stevens at Harvard University. Let us quote from a semipopular article written by him in 1957. He discusses loudness level and the phon, much as we have done above, and then emphasizes that "loudness level and loudness are really quite different concepts." He elaborates as follows:

Loudness level in phons is an arbitrary yardstick, and one that is nonlinearly related to loudness. What we need to know is how loudness itself depends upon loudness level. By this we mean: What do people say when they try to describe loudness in quantitative terms? In asking this question we are merely looking for the empirical answer to a very empirical question: How do people describe the apparent strength of a 1000-Hz tone when we present it at different levels and the listener describes its loudness in a numerical language instead of adjectives.

The practical side of this question had its origin in the fact that after the decibel scale was adopted, the acoustical engineers noted that equal steps on the decibel scale do not *sound* like equal steps and that a level of 50 dB does not sound like half of 100 dB. Since the engineer often faces the problem of communicating with a customer, it was soon realized that there was a need for a loudness scale whose numbers would make more sense to the customer than do the numbers of the decibel scale.

The generation of a loudness scale is in principle quite simple. All we need to do is produce an array of sounds and ask a group of listeners to assign numbers to them in such a way that the numbers reflect the perceived loudness of the sounds. In practice, of course, it turns out that many alternative techniques are possible and that subtle differences in experimental procedure sometimes influence what the listener says or does. The measurement of a subjective experience like loudness is difficult—so much so that many have argued that it is impossible. But results obtained in several laboratories in at least four different countries make it plain that people can make quantitative estimates of loudness. . . .

Four classes of methods have been used. They all concur in showing that loudness, as estimated by the median listener, approximates a power function of the intensity of 1000-Hz tone. *Loudness is proportional to the 0.3 power of the intensity (energy flux density)*. Or, if we define a unit of loudness, the sone, as the loudness heard by the typical listener confronted with 1000-Hz tone at an SPL of 40 dB (40 phons), we can write the equation as

$$\log_{10} S = 0.03P - 1.2$$

where $S$ is loudness in sones and $P$ is loudness level in phons. . . . Since people's judgments are variable, an equation of this sort must be regarded as only a first-order approximation. What the formula tells us is that in order to produce a 2:1 change in loudness we must change the stimulus by about 10 dB.

*The power law*. The power law for loudness as stated in the foregoing quota-

tion relates loudness to the acoustic "energy flux density." The data fall close to a straight line in a log-log plot, and the slope of this line is about 0.3. We encounter here an unfortunate ambiguity that turns on the double meaning of "power." Stevens employed the term in its mathematical sense in the phrase "loudness is proportional to the 0.3 power of the intensity." That is why he refers to "the power law." But sound intensity, the basis of the acoustic decibel scale, is closely related to sound "power" (explained above). So far there is no real confusion, but it is often more convenient to express the relation of loudness to sound pressure rather than to sound intensity. The pressure is proportional to the square root of the intensity, and therefore the slope of the line, which is the exponent in the "power law" equation, is twice as large, about 0.6. To avoid this possible ambiguity we shall call this relation the "sound-pressure law" or the power law (sound pressure). The full relation between loudness ($L$) and sound pressure ($p$) is given by the equation

$$L = k(p - p_o)^{0.6}$$

where $k$ is a constant that depends on units and $p_o$ is the threshold value.

The mathematical relation expressed by the power law has applications far wider than merely loudness. It appears to be the general "psychophysical law" for all "sensory continua" that relate to subjective intensity such as loudness, brightness, lifted weights, and so on: that is, *equal stimulus ratios produce equal sensation ratios*.

The various sensations, when studied by the methods of fractionation or direct estimation of magnitude, all yield power functions, but the value of the exponent (the slope of the line in a log-log plot) is characteristic of the particular sensation. The steepest that has been measured is electric shock (4.5), and brightness is the most gradual (0.33). Several sensations, such as temperature (cold on the arm), duration (of a white noise), and pressure (on the palm) have exponents very close to 1.0. The exponent for the apparent force of handgrip is 1.7.

Since the intensity of each sensation is described by a power law, it follows mathematically that when one sensation is compared directly with another, the relation will be another power law with its exponent equal to the difference between the two original exponents. A subject can match intensity across different sense modalities, just as he can match the loudness of two tones of different pitch, and he can squeeze a dynamometer in his hand and thus express his judgment of the loudness of a sound. This procedure generates a power law without requiring the subject to make a numerical judgment. This point has some theoretical significance. Also the instructions to the subject and the procedure are simple. It lends itself to possible clinical application in tests of hearing in which the rate of increase of loudness is abnormal (see Chapter 8).

The exponent of the power law is not completely fixed and definite, however. Even for a single modality, such as hearing, individuals differ rather widely from one another. In one experiment, for example, the average increase in sound pressure for 11 subjects required to double the loudness was 8.2 dB. One subject, however, was satisfied by 5.5 dB although another, at the other extreme, required 15 dB. These subjects also produced rather different slopes in the second session as compared with the first. It is important, however, that the power law does apply to individuals and is not merely an artifact of averaging.

*Binaural loudness.* It was assumed for many years that a sound heard with both ears sounds twice as loud as it does with one ear alone. This statement, like several others we have mentioned, is only approximately true. It is true at one particular loudness level, namely at 90 dB. The threshold for binaural listening is, as we have noted, some 3 dB lower than for monaural listening, and loudness increases a little more rapidly for binaural hearing. The exponent of the sound pressure law is about 0.60 for binaural and 0.54 for monaural. The power law is a very convenient way in which to describe these differences between monaural and binaural listening. The differences also emphasize the important part played by the central nervous system in integrating the input from the two ears and in determining the power law itself.

*Loudness at different frequencies.* We have described the equal-loudness contours in an earlier section. We now call attention to the narrowing of the auditory area in the low-tone and in the very high-tone range in which the threshold zone rises to meet a nearly horizontal threshold of discomfort (Figure 2-4). In these ranges the equal-loudness contours are spaced more closely, and the power law for sound pressure has larger exponents. It is in the middle of the frequency range, in which the dynamic range of hearing is greatest, that the exponent for loudness averages 0.6 or perhaps 0.66.

*Masking.* The loudness of a sound heard in the presence of another (background) sound is a matter of special interest. We all know from personal experience that faint sounds cannot be heard in the presence of background ("ambient") noise. The faint sound is said to be *masked*. The extent of the masking depends on the frequency and intensity of the test tone and the spectrum and intensity of the masker. We can determine the *masked threshold* for our test tones in a noise just as we determine the *absolute threshold* in quiet.

If the masking sound is a pure tone, its masking effect is greatest for tones near it in frequency, although the beats between test tone and masker when they are at nearly the same frequency confuse the issue. If a narrow band of noise is used, the beats are eliminated, and we find that masking is greatest in the frequency band of the masker. The elevation of threshold of the test tone becomes less and less as the frequency of the test tone recedes from that of the masker, but the curve of masked threshold is not symmetrical, except perhaps at very low sensation levels. At high levels, it falls off rather sharply toward the lower frequencies and much less rapidly toward frequencies higher than that of the masker.

The phenomena of masking have been explored in great detail. Complications arise when high intensity levels are tested, due in part to physical nonlinear effects and harmonic distortion within the ear. The shape of the masked threshold curves is of theoretical interest in relation to the mechanism of the inner ear. So is the problem of the signal-to-noise ratio between test tone and masker, and the ability of the ear to "dig the signal out of the noise" as compared with acoustic or electrical filters, but we shall be content here with this bare outline.

When a tone is just heard in a background of masking noise, it sounds, of course, very faint. A small increase in its intensity increases its loudness considerably. Finally, a tone 30 dB above its masked threshhold sounds as loud as if the masking noise were absent. The power law applies in this situation in which the noise partially masks the test tone (see Figure 2-8). For the first 30 dB above threshold the slope (exponent) is greater than for a free unmasked or, as Stevens puts it, "uninhibited" tone in the quiet. (The concept of inhibition is very useful here, as we shall see when we consider, in Chapter 3, the neural mechanisms that are involved in these interactions.) In vision there is an analogous inhibition of brightness of a test light by the glare of the background, and here too the slope of the power law for brightness is increased.

In more detail Stevens and his co-workers tell us that the slope of the power law

for an inhibited tone is constant from the masked threshold up to a level 30 dB above the masked threshold. Beyond this level the loudness increases more slowly, following the same function as a free uninhibited tone. The complete function is a broken line with a "knee" in it. If the masking noise is fairly narow in bandwidth, about 2 critical bands (see below) or less, and the tone lies within its frequency range, then the noise and the tone have about the same sound pressure level at the "knee," and they sound about equally loud. Probably at this point the noise and the tone are each inhibiting the other equally. If the tone is made less intense, it becomes more inhibited by the noise. If it is made more intense, it begins to inhibit the noise more than the noise inhibits the tone.

There are many second-order effects that have been described, related to the bandwidth of the noise, to matching inhibited tones to free tones, to the increasing steepness of slope as the SPL of the noise is increased, and so on. The relation that we wish to emphasize is the emergence of the tone from "inhibition" as schematically diagrammed in Figure 2-8.

*Recruitment.* A phenomenon very similar to the masking or inhibition of a tone by a surrounding band of noise is encountered in ears with certain types of sense-organ impairment that involve an elevation of threshold. The loudness of a tone grows more rapidly with increase in physical intensity than it does in the normal ear. This corresponds to the steeper slope of the power law for the partially masked tone, but in this case there is no masking noise to provide the "inhibition." This effect, first described by E. P. Fowler, Sr., is known as *recruitment of loudness,* and it will be discussed at greater length in Chapter 4. It is not yet clear how accurately the power law holds for these abnormal ears, but there is reason to think that it gives a good approximate description and that recruitment is usually substantially complete

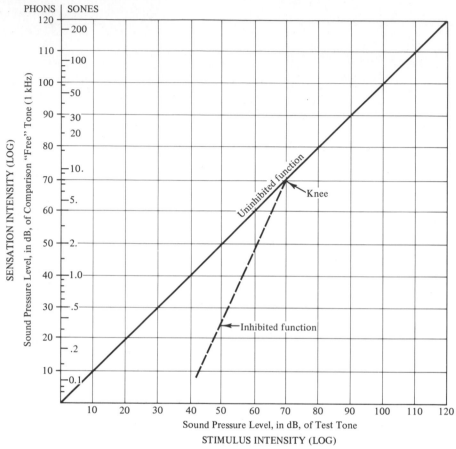

Figure 2-8. Schematic diagram to show the power-law function for loudness (solid line) and how masking increases the slope (exponent) of the lower portion of this function (dashed line). A given inhibiting sound (masker) affects only sounds weaker than itself. The over-all psychophysical function consists of two straight lines that intersect to form a "knee." The knee is usually 30 dB above the masked threshold. (*After S. S. Stevens, and M. Guirao, "Loudness Functions under Inhibition," Perception and Psychophysiology, 2:459–465 [1967].*)

The scale of stimulus intensity is logarithmic, in decibels. The scale of sensation magnitude (sones), based on magnitude estimation, is also logarithmic. An alternate scale is the physical intensity of another equally strong sensation such as loudness, brightness, strength of hand-grip, and so on, also on a logarithmic scale. The particular alternate scale in this figure is phons, that is, the sound-pressure level of a comparison free tone of 1000 Hz. The relation between sones and phons was determined experimentally. The relation between sones and sound pressure of other tones or bands of noise differs, depending on frequency and bandwidth.

at 30 dB above the (abnormally elevated) threshold.

*Addition of loudness.* When two tones or noises are heard at the same time, the combination sounds louder than either one alone. The laws of addition or "integration" of loudness have been studied inten-sively, but full agreement has not yet been reached on the rule or formula that is most satisfactory. The question is more impor-tant for the evaluation of loud noises that are disturbing or annoying than it is for the analysis of impairments of hearing, and for this reason we shall not go into detail but shall merely state a few useful generalizations which have emerged and which give us some idea of how the auditory system deals with complex sounds. The question is difficult because individuals differ in their judgments when matching the loudness of sounds that differ widely in their frequency spectra. Also, when two quite different sounds are heard at the same time, some subjects, according to their own statements, tend to hear them separately and judge the loudness of one or the other; but other subjects "integrate" them and hear the combined loudness as greater than that of either component.

There is no doubt, however, that sounds of nearly the same frequency or relatively narrow bands of noise are heard singly, and one of the basic concepts is that of a *critical band* of frequencies within which interaction or integration of loudness is quite complete for everyone. The over-all sound-pressure level within the critical band is all that really matters for loudness or for masking. The width of this band is related also to the pitch or mel scale. One rule is that the critical band for loudness is about 100 mels wide (over most of the frequency range), which is a very convenient coincidence. A critical band is approximately one-third of an octave in the middle frequency range, and it does not vary greatly with loudness level, except perhaps near threshold or at very high intensities. The bandwidth in hertz varies from about 90 Hz at the low end to 2000 Hz near 10,000 Hz. The range from 20 to 9300 Hz comprises 22 critical bands.

The concept of the critical band was introduced by Fletcher in 1940, but Fletcher was forced to make one plausible assumption in order to calculate the widths of his bands. Fletcher's bands, now often called "critical ratios," were narrower than our present bands by a factor of two and a half, but they were similarly related to frequency and to the pitch scale.

The critical band for loudness can be measured in several ways. One way is to sound several tones, equally spaced, at nearly the same frequency and then to increase the spacing between them. Listeners compare the loudness of the complex mixture to that of a single tone at the center frequency of the complex. When the overall spacing of the tones exceeds a certain amount, the complex begins to sound louder. (The complex may also be a band of noise of variable bandwidth.)

Another method is to measure the threshold, either the absolute threshold or the masked threshold, for two closely spaced tones or for a band of noise of variable width. The threshold for two such tones is lower than for a single tone, but as more tones are added, or as the band of noise is made wider, a critical bandwith is reached beyond which the threshold remains constant.

Another test is to determine the masked threshold for a narrow band of noise centered between two pure tones. As the separation of the tones is increased, the masked threshold of the noise remains constant until the separation reaches a critical value, after which the masked threshold decreases rather abruptly. Still another rather similar test is based on the sensitivity of the ear to phase differences.

These various measures of the critical band may not all yield quite the same numerical values, but they are all of the same order of magnitude, and all of them bear very much the same relation to frequency and to the mel scale. The critical band for masking is of practical importance in audiology in relation to the masking of a tone in one ear when testing the threshold of the opposite ear, as in tests of the bone-conduction threshold. Masking is fully efficient, and the loudness of the masker is the least when a critical band of noise, centered on the tone to be masked, is employed. The critical band is also of theoretical importance in relation to the action of the inner ear in the detection and analysis of sounds and of the central auditory system also.

## Formulas for Addition of Loudness

If two or more sounds of rather different frequencies are heard simultaneously, they do not seem as loud as the total sum of the loudness of each of them heard separately. On the other hand, the total loudness is greater than that of the loudest single component. Several empirical formulas have been proposed for calculating the total loudness. In general, we are more concerned with the loudness of noises with continuous spectra, like traffic noise or aircraft noise, and not with a collection of pure tones like a symphony orchestra, and it is convenient to measure the sound pressure of the noise in octave bands (as in Figure 2-2), or perhaps in third-octave bands. Tabulations are available of the loudness (in sones) of each of the octave bands at various loudness levels (in phons). The simplest formula, that of Stevens, states that

$$S_t = S_m + 0.3 \, (\Sigma S - S_m).$$

That is to say, the over-all loudness ($S_t$) is equal to the loudness of the loudest octave band ($S_m$) plus three-tenths of the sum of the loudnesses of all the remaining bands. The factor of three-tenths is strictly empirical. If third-octave bands are used, the factor is 0.15.

Various tabulations, charts, and nomograms to facilitate the calculations by this (and by other) methods have been published, but we shall not go into detail. For us it is enough to know that the loudness of a noise with a complex spectrum is dominated by, but not wholly determined by, the loudest part of its spectrum, and that addition is nonlinear in that the whole is less than the sum of the parts. There are interactions, probably of the nature of mutual inhibition or something analogous to partial masking, among the different octave bands of a noise.

*Examples of loudness.* When the sound-level meter was first devised it was called a noise-level meter, and its designers tried to make it deal with sounds in approximately the same way the ear does, so that its readings (in decibels) would correspond to the loudness (sones) that we hear. Two sets of filters (the so-called A network and the B network) were provided. Their pass bands corresponded roughly to the shapes of the human equal-loudness contours for faint and for moderate sounds, respectively. For example, the ear is much less sensitive to the 60-Hz hum that is usually present to some extent in the music that comes from our radios than it is to frequencies from 800 to 4000 Hz in the upper part of the musical range. If the music is soft, we may hear only the music, even though the hum is physically more intense than the music. If this is the case, the over-all level in decibels measured by the sound-level meter with the "flat" or "C" setting (no filter) will be determined chiefly by the hum. In this situation there is simply no practical relation between the loudness that we hear and the decibel reading on the meter.

For loud sounds like factory noise or heavy traffic, the C setting was to be used. For a number of years the meter was used consistently according to the original rules, and many characteristic "noise levels" in decibels were published. Some of these were cited in Figure 6 (page 45) of the first edition of this book. But after 1940, when octave-band filters came into general use, the A and B networks were used less and less, and the early noise levels measured with them are now usually confused with over-all sound levels measured without any network at the C setting. The result is that the old levels given for "quiet dwellings," "rustling of leaves," "whisper," and the like, look ridiculously low. We have therefore omitted any tabulation of such decibel levels from the 1960 and the present editions. Instead, we give in Figure 2-3 the octave band analyses of five noises, all relatively steady and easy to measure. The corresponding over-all levels are also given.

The following approximate rules, in terms of over-all sound level, are helpful for orientation:

A broad-band noise like most aircraft or factory noise is very loud at 90 dB and is definitely uncomfortable at 120 dB.

A shout at 1 ft from the ear is about 100 dB, but the highest voice level that can be maintained for long is 90 dB.

Conversational speech at 1 yd averages about 65 dB. The strong vowels reach 72 dB.

Faint but intelligible speech in a quiet room is about 40 to 45 dB.

In the above rules we have put some numbers on the sound level of speech (see Figure 2-6), but this introduces a new difficulty. The sound-pressure level of speech varies from instant to instant, from one word to the next, and from sound to sound within the word. The momentary instantaneous peaks of pressure are 10 to as much as 20 dB above the over-all long-time average. The needle of the sound-level meter dances up and down, and we must be content to settle for its "average maximum swing." A rather vague rule indeed! Abrupt brief sounds like a pistol shot or a hammer blow give particular difficulty. Certain special meters called "impact meters" deal with them better than does the simpler sound-level meter, but even these are not yet fully satisfactory, and the measurements made with them are not easy to interpret. For all of these reasons it requires some special instruction and training to use even the ordinary sound-level meter properly and to interpret the measurements made with it.

*Short-term summation of loudness.*

In the previous section we have referred to brief sounds like those of speech and also transients like pistol shots, hammer blows, and other "impulsive" sounds. The reading of a meter in response to an impulsive sound depends largely on the ballistic characteristics of the meter, including its damping and overshoot. The human ear, somewhat like a meter, integrates the energy of brief sounds to some extent. For example, as faint tones are made very brief, less than a fifth of a second, their thresholds rise. If they last for only a few cycles, the threshold may be 10 dB or more higher than for a prolonged tone of the same sound-pressure level. It requires about 200 msec for a steady tone to reach its full loudness. The ear actually behaves as though some quantity that we can call "excitation" is produced in proportion to the intensity of the sound and decays exponentially with a characteristic time constant. Such situations are familiar in neurophysiology. The integration and decay probably occur in the central nervous system and not in the ear.

### Threshold Shift, Fatigue, and Adaptation

There are several quite distinct changes in the sensitivity of the ear that are produced by exposure to sound and that can be detected either during the exposure or after it ends. The nature of the effect and the time it lasts depend greatly on the intensity of the exposure tone or noise. Because of the variety of conditions and effects, many terms have been employed, including *adaptation,* which implies a simple physiological adjustment, like dark adaptation in vision; *fatigue,* which implies a temporary exhaustion of a reserve of some sort; *residual masking,* which is confusing; and *acoustic trauma,* which clearly implies injury. A more neutral and less confusing term is *threshold shift.* We shall have more to say about threshold shifts, both permanent and temporary, in Chapter 4 when we consider the effects of exposure to high-intensity industrial noises.

To emphasize the complexity of the situation, we point out that at least three or four quite different mechanisms have been identified that can, and presumably do, contribute to the reduced sensitivity or reduced output of the ear. Unfortunately, the part played by each in various situations is not clear. One of these mechanisms is a reflex contraction of the muscles of the middle ear (the intraaural or stapedius reflex), rather like the constriction of the pupil or an eyeblink. Another is the action of efferent nerve fibers from the brain to the inner ear. Another is the physiological decrease in rate of discharge (the "adaptation") of nerve fibers to steady levels of stimulation. Another is an unspecified change, either physical, chemical, or both, in the sensory cells of the ear. Another is outright physical rupture and destruction of nerves, sensory cells, or supporting structures. Another is adaptation or "habituation" in the central nervous system.

"Per-stimulatory adaptation" refers to a diminution in loudness that occurs rather rapidly after the onset of a tone. It is demonstrated by making loudness balances between a stimulated ear and the opposite unstimulated ear. (This experiment is not quite as simple as it sounds.) The reduction in loudness level is rather considerable for a tone of moderate intensity.

The temporary threshold shift in certain pathological conditions may be so great that the tone simply becomes inaudible with an exposure of less than 30 seconds. In normal ears a short-lasting elevation of threshold for a test pulse usually develops rapidly, and recovery also takes place rapidly. Sometimes, however, the complete recovery takes place in two or three phases. The elevated threshold falls, then it rises or "bounces" to a second maximum at about 2 minutes after the end of the exposure tone, and then settles down to its stable level.

In general, threshold shifts following moderate exposures are rather quick adjustments, not always clearly related in extent to the strength and duration of exposure. The effect is greatest at the frequency of the exposure tone. At sound-pressure levels of about 90 dB and higher, however, a curious effect occurs. Threshold shift develops more rapidly, with increasing intensity and duration of exposure, as we would expect; but the frequency at which the shift is greatest is no longer than that of the exposure tone but now lies about half an octave above it. Lesser amounts of shift occur far into the frequency range above the exposure frequency, but little or no shift occurs more than about half an octave below it. This unexplained distribution in frequency and a slower rate of recovery should help us to distinguish this high-intensity variety of threshold shift from the quick shifts and adaptations that occur at lower sound-pressure levels. The former is more suggestive of a severe fatigue in the usual sense and possibly the beginning of injury, although followed by repair.

## Backward Masking

Another effect in the time domain is known as "backward masking." A brief test tone is followed after a short interval by a louder and longer burst of noise. Even though it may start as much as 50 to 100 msec later, the louder sound makes the earlier fainter sound inaudible. Clearly this effect takes place in the central nervous system where the excitation from the strong stimulus somehow overtakes and masks the earlier input. Masking involves much more than the basic physical interaction of sound waves at the physical level.

## Binaural Hearing: Directionality

We have already noted that two ears are better than one in detecting faint signals, either in a background of noise or in quiet, and that sounds are heard louder with two ears than with one. But by far the most important contribution of binaural hearing is to allow us to hear sounds from different sources as coming from different directions. Of course we are sometimes confused by echoes, and our sense of direction is confined to the horizontal plane, assuming the head to be upright; but in the primitive biological function of warning and identification, the sense of direction of the source is very important information.

We can learn something about the direction of a sound source with only one ear, if we search, and scan, and notice at which orientation of our head the sound is loudest. In this case we take advantage of the directionality of the ear, set as it is in the large acoustic baffle formed by the side of the head. But stereophonic hearing is far better than this. The sense of direction is immediate, and two sound sources are heard as clearly separate in space.

Two sets of clues provide the directionality. One of these is the relative intensity of corresponding sound waves entering the two ears. The differences in intensity, due to the "sound shadow" of the head, are considerable for high frequencies, and for frequencies above 2000 or 3000 Hz this loudness difference is the chief clue. At very low frequencies, however, the intensity differences are small, and the other clue, difference in time of arrival of corresponding sound waves, becomes dominant. The length of acoustic path around the head is great enough to provide for something approaching a millisecond of time delay. The two ears are sensitive to time differences of the order of a hundredth of a millisecond, enough to determine the direction (azimuth) within a few degrees of arc. The time differences are less effective above 1000 Hz, partly because at 1000 Hz the time difference between waves is 1 msec, and one sine wave is just like the one before and the one following. Thus the time differences above 1000 Hz become ambiguous.

Time differences and intensity differences usually reinforce one another, but if we present the sounds through earphones we can manipulate them independently. Time differences can be traded for decibels in the task of keeping the apparent source of the sound "centered." A curious effect occurs with earphones, however. The sound does not seem to come from straight ahead, even when timing and intensity are both equal, but to be *inside* the head at the midline. A little imbalance shifts the apparent source to right or to left, and if the difference is considerable, the source seems to be at one ear canal or the other. (Sometimes the sound seems to move around the back of the head or neck, but usually it stays inside.)

The centering of the image of a sound source in the midline of the head when the sound waves are simultaneous and equally intense in the two ears has been used as a delicate test for equal loudness. Centering the sound image is an easier, quicker, and more reliable judgment than listening to two tones alternately and adjusting them to equal loudness. Unfortunately, however, the processes in the central nervous system that lead to the sensation of "center image" are not the same as those for "equal loudness." Both are related to the intensity of the inputs of the two ears, but in different ways. This has led to difficulties in certain audiological tests in which it was assumed that the operations were identical.

When a sound from a discrete nearby source, such as a friend talking to us, is heard in a background of noise such as traffic noise or many other voices competing loudly in the "cocktail-party effect," we have some difficulty understanding our friend's words, and we hear them much more clearly with two ears than with one. One of our ears is likely to have some relative advantage of being turned more or less toward him, but in addition we notice that the sound to which we are listening comes from one place, and the noise comes from some other place or from many places. Somehow this makes the voice easier to "track," and the noise less confusing. These advantages of binaural hearing become very important in relation to the use of hearing aids when the inability to hear voices clearly in noisy places is a major complaint. We shall return to this problem and the use of binaural hearing aids in Chapters 10 and 11. The disadvantage of monaural listening, particularly due to the sound shadow of the head which amounts to a less favorable signal-to-noise ratio, contributes to the impairment of practical hearing.

There are many interesting effects that can be produced by delivering sounds in opposite phase to the two ears or by reversing in one ear the phase of the voice but not that of the noise, and so on. A useful rule that is usually true is that the more clearly the source of the voice seems to be separated in space from the source of the noise, the easier it is to hear the voice clearly and follow what it says.

## Detection of Signals in Noise

Much attention has been given recently to the problem of detecting signals that are very nearly masked in noise. Noise is a random affair and is best described in statistical terms. It appears that the performance of an observer should be described in the same way, perhaps because his nervous system is full of "physiological noise." His "threshold" varies at random from moment to moment. Typically, he is asked to state whether he did or did not detect a signal in a given interval of time during which it might or might not have been presented. For a given signal-to-noise ratio, he will correctly report the signal as

present in a certain percentage of trials and as absent in others. He will also, however, give a few "false alarms," stating that he heard the signal when it was not there, and he will make some "misses" in failing to report some signals that were present. The listener can deliberately change or be induced by proper instruction to change his criterion from a cautious conservative attitude to a liberal take-a-chance point of view, or vice versa. The instructions and the basis of reward or "pay-off" are important. With a liberal attitude, the observer will score many more hits but at the expense of more false alarms. Thirty years ago we argued about the "maybe-maybe" threshold of the psychologist and the "honest-to-goodness" threshold of the engineer. Now we know that the relation among hits, misses, and false positives is quite lawful. A graphic representation of the relation is known as the "receiver operating characteristic" (ROC) curve. We shall not go into detail, but merely emphasize that here another variable in psychophysics, namely the attitude of the listener, has been brought under experimental control and mathematical description. The analysis allows us to measure separately two elements that determine the response of the listener. One is his *strategy,* liberal or conservative; the other is his basic *sensitivity.*

It is also possible to record and make use of the degree of confidence that the observer feels with respect to each particular judgment. The "detection theory" has already made significant contributions to our theoretical understanding of the nature of the psychophysical threshold and the processes of detection and discrimination, and it is likely to influence the design and conduct of many audiological tests of the future.

## SUGGESTED READINGS AND REFERENCES

van Bergeijk, W. A., J. R. Pierce, and E. E. David, Jr. *Waves and the Ear*. New York: Doubleday & Company, Inc., 1960.
A very readable little paperback.

Cox, J. R., Jr. "The Measurement of Industrial Noise," Vol. III, Chap. 8, in *Industrial Hygiene and Toxicology,* Leslie Silverman (ed.). 2nd ed. New York: Interscience Publishers, 1959.
This chapter describes fully the use of the octave-band filter from the point of view of an acoustic engineer.

Fletcher, H. *Speech and Hearing*. Princeton, N.J.: D. Van Nostrand Company, Inc., 1929.
A classic, now out of print.

————. *Speech and Hearing in Communication*. Princeton, N.J.: D. Van Nostrand Company, Inc., 1953.
A rather extensive revision of his earlier monograph.

Pierce, J. R., and E. E. David, Jr. *Man's World of Sound*. New York: Doubleday & Company, Inc., 1958.
A very readable and informative introductory treatment.

Rao, V. V. L. *The Decibel Notation*. New York: The Chemical Publishing Company, Inc., 1946.
Mathematically oriented but relatively simple.

Stevens, S. S. (ed.). *Handbook of Experimental Psychology*. New York: John Wiley & Sons, Inc., 1951.
Chapter 25 ("Basic Correlates of the Auditory Stimulus," by J. C. R. Licklider) and Chapter 26 ("The Perception of Speech," by J. C. R. Licklider and G. A. Miller) are especially pertinent.

Stevens, S. S. "Calculating Loudness," *Noise Control,* 3:11–22 (1957).
A semipopular article with useful graphs.

————. "The Psychophysics of Sensory Function," Chap. 1, in *Sensory Communication,* Walter A. Rosenblith (ed.). Cambridge: M.I.T. Press, and New York: John Wiley & Sons, Inc., 1961. An authoritative discussion.

————, and H. Davis. *Hearing: Its Psychology and Physiology*. New York: John Wiley & Sons, Inc., 1938.

This is a monograph for advanced students. The second part, physiology, is now seriously out of date.

————, **F. Warshofsky, and the Editors of LIFE.** *Sound and Hearing.* New York: Time, Inc., 1965.

A wide popular survey, beautifully illustrated.

USA Standards Institute, 10 East 40th St., New York, N.Y. 10016.

*Test Code for Apparatus Noise Measurement* (Z24.7–1950).

*Acoustical Terminology* (*Including Mechanical Shock and Vibration*) (S1.1–1960)

*Preferred Frequencies and Band Numbers for Acoustical Measurements* (S1.6–1967)

New name and address:

American National Standards Institute, Inc.

1430 Broadway, New York, N.Y., 10018.

*Procedure for the Computation of Loudness of Noise* (S3.4–1968)

# CHAPTER 3

# ANATOMY
# AND PHYSIOLOGY OF THE
# AUDITORY SYSTEM

## HALLOWELL DAVIS, M.D.

Concerning the structure of the ear and how it gathers sound waves and brings them to the sensory cells we can be rather definite. Some understanding of both the structure and the function of the various parts of the ear is needed to understand the different types of deafness and the means of preventing or circumventing them.

## THE OUTER EAR AND
## THE CANAL

We need not describe the outer ear. Look at your neighbor or get a mirror and you will do as well as we can do with words or diagrams. The external ear, the *pinna* or *auricle,* is not very important acoustically. Man has lost or never acquired the three main functions of the external ear of most animals: (1) to collect and focus the energy of a large cross section of sound waves from a particular direction; (2) to make possible precise judgments of the direction of sound by turning the ears (instead of the whole head) until the sound becomes loudest; and (3) to keep water and dirt out of the ear canal, as seals and moles do, by special valvelike movements of some of the external parts that for us are rudimentary rigid structures.

The human ear canal is irregularly oval in cross section and varies from man to man in details of size and shape quite as much as does the external ear—to the distress of those whose task it was during World War II to devise a simple ear plug for all ears to protect them against the blasts of heavy artillery and antiaircraft batteries. Sometimes the canal is nearly round; sometimes it is little more than a vertical slit. The canal runs nearly horizontally toward the center of the head for a little less than an inch (2.5 cm) as shown in Figure 3-1, and there it dead-ends at the drum membrane or *tympanic membrane.* The skin of the outer portion of the canal bears stiff hairs and secretes a dark, bitter-tasting wax (*cerumen*) that as a rule discourages the entry of insects and keeps the skin of the canal and drum membrane from drying out.

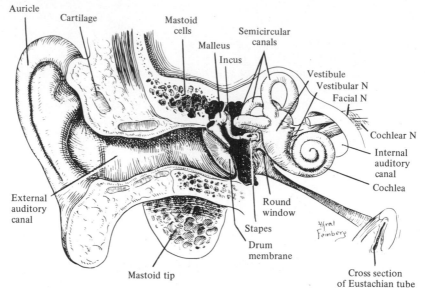

Fig. 3-1. In this semidiagrammatic drawing of the ear, the inner ear is shown with the temporal bone cut away to reveal the semicircular canals, the vestibule, and the cochlea. The cochlea has been turned slightly from its normal orientation to show its coils more clearly. The opening for nerves through the bone to the brain cavity of the skull is quite diagrammatic. The Eustachian tube actually runs forward as well as downward and inward. The muscles of the middle ear, shown in Figures 3-2 and 3-3, are omitted.

## THE MIDDLE EAR

The middle ear includes the tympanic membrane and the air-filled cavity behind it as well as its contents, including the set of tiny bones, the *ossicles.* The entire structure is known as the eardrum from its resemblance to the familiar musical instrument. In popular usage the drum membrane that terminates the external canal is called the "eardrum" but it is only one surface of a three-dimensional structure. It is more accurate to call it the *drumhead* or *drum membrane.*

With proper illumination and when the canal is straightened by pulling the pinna gently backward and upward, the drumhead can be seen as a pearl-gray wall at the end of the canal. The thin, tough, flexible fibrous membrane is attached to the bony wall of the canal by a tough ring of fibrous tissue, the *annulus,* and forms a diagonal partition as shown in the diagram in Figure 3-2. It is not stretched flat across

but is conical in shape like the cone of a loudspeaker. It points upward and inward into the middle-ear cavity behind it. The angle of the cone, about 135 degrees, is very favorable for stiffness.

The stiff central portion moves as a whole when driven by waves of sound pressure, except for frequencies above 2000 Hz. It can do so because the outer edge is slack or folded, again like the cone of a loudspeaker (see Figures 3-2, 3-5). Its area is about 0.67 cm² or a tenth of a square inch on the average. Through the translucent membrane can sometimes be seen, like the hour hand of a clock at 11 o'clock (in the right ear), the "handle" of the hammer, the *malleus,* the first of the chain of ossicles that transmit the vibrations of the drumhead to the inner ear. The malleus serves also to keep the membrane stretched tight and cone-shaped under the influence of a small muscle, the *tensor tympani,* that attaches to it near the base of the handle.

The enlarged round head of the malleus nestles into a well-fitting socket in the anvil or *incus,* the second of the ossicles, and for sounds of ordinary intensities the two move together as a single unit. They execute a rocking motion as the drumhead vibrates, turning around a horizontal axis just behind the upper edge of the drumhead and perpendicular to the external canal (see Figure 3-4). The axis on which they turn is formed by a short axlelike projection of the malleus and another from the incus. The projections are attached by firm but flexible ligaments to the walls of the middle-ear cavity. The bony mass of the ossicles is delicately balanced around the axis so that the inertia (or, more accurately, the *turning moment*) of the system is small, and the ossicles do not tend to strain and rattle when they vibrate. The incus ends in a long slender curved tip near the center of the middle-ear cavity and in contact with

the tiny head of the stirrup (*stapes*), the last of the three ossicles.

The stirrup is well named from its shape, and its oval footplate is sealed by the *annular ligament* into the *oval window* that looks into the inner ear. The stapes moves in and out like a piston at low and moderate amplitudes of movement. At high amplitudes, such as are reached by really loud low-frequency sounds, the movement of the stapes is restrained by the annular ligament. The ligament is thicker and narrower at the posterior than at the anterior end of the oval window, and as a consequence the footplate of the stapes swings like a door with its hinge at the posterior end. The classical descriptions of the movements of the ossicles are based on observations of movements of sufficient amplitude to be clearly visible. These movements are nonlinear, but the smaller linear oscillations are actually more typical. The restraint of

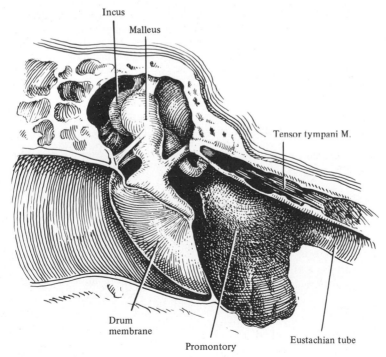

Fig. 3-2. This view of the drum membrane (partly cut away) and the middle ear is from a slightly more lateral angle than that in Figure 3-1. The tensor tympani muscle lies in a separate canal (partly cut away) just above the Eustachian tube. Its tendon turns at nearly a right angle in the tendinous sheath from which it emerges.

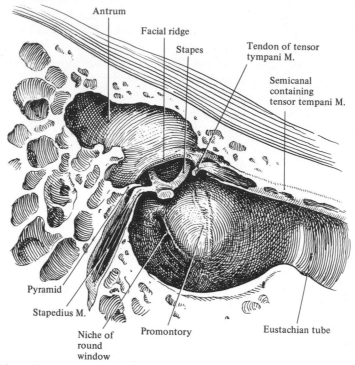

Fig. 3-3. The middle ear is here viewed from the external canal, with the drum membrane, the malleus, the incus, and some of the surrounding temporal bone cut away. The tendon of the stapedius muscle turns at an angle as it emerges from the tip of the "pyramid." When the stapedius contracts, the stapes rocks on the posterior (left in this figure) end of its footplate so that the footplate swings outward like a door into the cavity of the middle ear. The facial nerve runs in a bony canal in the facial ridge just above the stapes.

movement by the annular ligament is one of a series of mechanical restraints in the

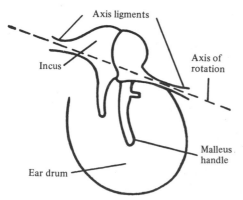

Fig. 3-4. Diagram of the axis of rotation of malleus and incus. (*From Békésy and Rosenblith in Introduction to Experimental Psychology, John Wiley & Sons, Inc.*)

middle and inner ear that protect the sense organ from rupture at high amplitudes. They do this at the expense of more or less harmonic distortion.

The tendon of another tiny muscle, the *stapedius*, attaches to the neck of the stapes. It pulls the stapes outward and backward, thus counteracting the opposite pull of the tensor tympani. The two muscles work together to take up any slack in the ossicular chain and to stiffen the whole system. The balance between them is so good that the drum membrane itself scarcely moves at all when they contract.

The middle-ear cavity is a narrow cleft between the slanting eardrum and the irregular bony wall opposite it, and is nearly filled by the ossicles. Its capacity varies from 1 to 2 cm³. However, it opens directly into the air cells of the temporal bone behind, and the *Eustachian tube* opens into its anterior wall about midway between floor and roof. The two muscles that we have mentioned are not located in the middle-ear cavity itself. The tensor tympani lies alongside the Eustachian tube, and the stapedius in a little bony tunnel all its own. The longest dimension of the middle ear—the vertical dimension—is about 1.25 cm or half an inch, and a magnifying glass is required to appreciate the fine mechanical architecture of the ossicles with balanced suspensions and their adjusting muscles.

Another opening between the middle ear and the inner ear is the *round window*, located just under the oval window. It is closed by an elastic membrane rather like the tympanic membrane, but thinner, much smaller, and stretched flat. This opening serves as an elastic termination of the acoustic pathway in the inner ear, as shown in Figure 3-5. If the walls of the inner ear were completely rigid, the stapes could not move in the oval window, because the fluid within is practically incompressible. Pressure could be transmitted, but the mechanical movements would be negligible, and it is mechanical movement that ultimately stimulates the sensory cells.

The air-filled cavity of the middle ear and the mastoid air cells that lead from it as a blind alley are ventilated periodically through the Eustachian tube. The tube connects the middle ear with the back of the nasal cavity, called the *nasopharynx*. The first portion runs through the temporal bone. It is permanently open, like a funnel, in contrast to the longer wider portion toward the pharynx, whose walls are composed of cartilage and flexible membrane, and which is normally collapsed. The Eustachian tube enters the nasopharynx diagonally under a valvelike flap of tissue that closes the orifice except during certain

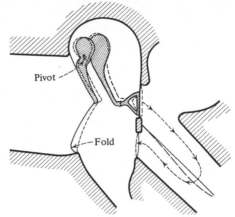

Pivot

Fold

Fig. 3-5. Schematic diagram of the tympanic membrane, the ossicles, and the basilar membrane. The solid figures of the ossicles and the solid lines for the tympanic, the basilar, and the round-window membranes show the positions of these structures at rest. The broken outlines of the ossicles and the broken lines for the membranes show their directions of movement during inward displacement of the tympanic membrane by a sound wave. The cross shows the axis around which the ossicles rotate. The dot shows their center of gravity. The stapes is drawn at right angles to its true position in order to show its motion clearly. At high intensities it rocks around an axis through the posterior edge of the round window. The movement of the stapes, for moderate tones, is almost certainly like a piston, not a door. The "fold" in the tympanic membrane and the amplitude of movement are exaggerated. (*Modified from Stevens and Davis, Hearing: Its Psychology and Physiology, John Wiley and Sons, Inc. 1938.*)

movements, such as swallowing and yawning. Sometimes, also, the tube opens during a sneeze or a cough or when the air pressure is increased by blowing the nose.

The function of the Eustachian tube in equalizing the air pressure inside and outside the eardrum is described more fully later. Immediate equalization of small changes, such as are caused by contraction of the tensor tympani muscle, is provided by a small slack segment of the eardrum itself, at its top and above the axis of rotation of the malleus. Equalization for a longer term is needed, however, because any air bubble left in the tissues of the body is gradually dissolved and absorbed by the blood: first the oxygen and then, slowly, the nitrogen. The air in the middle ear must therefore be replenished periodically.

The middle ear with its drum and ossicles increases the sensitivity of hearing for airborne sound. The drum receives energy from a relatively large cross section of light, tenuous, highly compressible air. The energy is delivered through the ossicles to the smaller footplate of the stapes, about one-thirtieth the area of the drum. This reduction of area favors the efficient transfer of the energy to the dense, watery, almost incompressible fluid that fills the inner ear. From the technical point of view the membrane and ossicles are a very efficient impedance-matching device between the two media, air and water. The total force is the same, the pressure is increased, the volume displacement is reduced. Thereby the drum and ossicles appreciably increase the sensitivity of the ear. Loss of drum and ossicles causes some hearing loss, but not a very serious one. Simple interruption of the train of ossicles reduces the sensitivity by about 25 dB. A simple hole in the drum may cause only a 5- or 10-dB loss.

The ear and its drum membrane and ossicles probably serve also to protect the inner ear from injury by loud sounds. The air enclosed in the rather small middle ear must exert some cushioning effect for low tones, because loud tones of low frequency have a very appreciable amplitude of movement. Just how important this effect may be has not yet been determined. The joint between the malleus and the incus also yields elastically when the sound waves become very powerful, and at very high amplitudes the stapes begins to rock in a different and less efficient direction, sideways instead of lengthwise of the footplate.

## INTRA-AURAL REFLEXES

The contractions of the muscles of the middle ear stiffen the drum membrane and the ossicular chain and thereby reduce the transmission of low tones. Contraction in response to loud sound is set off by reflex action from the lower centers of the brain a few hundredths of a second after a loud sound first reaches the eardrum. The increased tension of the membrane also raises the "natural period" of vibration of drum and ossicles. The net result is a rather considerable loss of sensitivity for low and for high tones and a rather slight loss for the middle range. The most important practical result is probably the protection the intra-aural muscles give to both the middle and the inner ear against possible damage by large amplitudes of movement. We have used the general term *intra-aural reflex* for the reflex contraction of one or both of the intra-aural muscles in response to sound. It is sometimes called the *acoustic reflex*. Also, because the stapedius muscle seems to be the more active of the two, it may be called the *stapedius reflex*. The contractions may also be evoked by tickling the skin near the entrance to the ear canal or by a tiny puff of air directed into the corner of the eye. The tensor tympani may be the more active in these reflexes to touch. Probably they both participate more or less in both reflexes. The reflex response is bilateral even when stimulation is unilateral.

The amplitude of movement of the tympanic membrane in the acoustic reflex is extremely small and difficult to measure. The reflex has been studied extensively, however, by detecting changes in the *acoustic impedance of the ear*. The method depends on measuring the proportion of the energy of a test tone that is reflected back from the drumhead. The changes in impedance can be analyzed into changes in stiffness and in resistance, respectively. When a tone of 90 dB or so is first turned on, the reflex contraction is brisk, but apparently it is not well maintained. It is much better maintained if the stimulating sound is an irregular noise. There is still considerable question as to the threshold sound level for the reflex. It is certainly well above the threshold for hearing, somewhere in the middle range of intensities. The measurements of acoustic impedance and the intra-aural reflexes are useful tools for several audiological tests described in Chapter 8.

Another method for study of the action of the stapedius and tensor tympani muscles is to implant electrodes in them in chronic animal experiments. The electrical output of each muscle (its electromyogram) signals each contraction and its relative intensity. Apparently these muscles are very active, at least in cats, and participate in almost all patterns of movement that involve much of the musculature of the head and neck.

In human psychoacoustics it is still a question how much in the way of adaptation or other changes of threshold (or loudness) should be attributed to the activity of the intra-aural muscles. They are certainly involved more or less directly and probably significantly in all experiments at 90 dB SPL and above—and perhaps below as well.

## THE INNER EAR

The inner ear is a series of channels and chambers in the temporal bone that are so complicated in shape that they are known as the labyrinth (Figure 3-6). In these bony canals, filled with clear watery fluid, lies a corresponding series of delicate membranous tubes and sacs, filled also with a watery fluid and containing sensory cells and their supporting structures. The central portion, the *vestibule*, of the labyrinth joins the snail-like coil of the organ of hearing, the *cochlea*, and the loops of the three *semicircular canals* that form the sense organ for turning in space. In the vestibule itself lie the *utricle*, sensitive to the pull of gravity and to acceleration (as in an elevator or automobile), and the *saccule*. The latter apparently shares the

functions of the utricle, although in fish, which have no cochlea, it seems to be the sense organ for vibration and whatever true hearing the fish may have.

These different mechanical senses, responsive to sound and to acceleration, have very similar sensory cells that are specialized organs of touch. The cochlea "feels" the alternating mechanical movements caused by sound waves. Gravity is felt by the utricle as it pulls on tiny grains of calcium carbonate attached to microscopic hairlike extensions of the sensory cells. The cells at the enlarged ends of the semicircular canals feel the pressure of the fluid within the canals as it tends to lag behind, because of its inertia, when we turn our heads.

Three practical consequences of the close anatomical association between the nonauditory labyrinthine sense organs and the cochlea are: first, that the symptom of dizziness (vertigo) is often associated with certain forms of deafness; second, that the surgeon can make the bony channels of the vestibule and semicircular canals alternative pathways for sound; and third, tests of the function of the nonauditory labyrinth are very helpful in the differential diagnosis of certain forms of hearing loss. Other details of this part of the labyrinth need not concern us here. The opening of a new oval window by the fenestration operation for the restoration of hearing in otosclerosis will be described in Chapter 6 and the tests in Chapter 8.

The cochlea is coiled like a snail in a flat spiral of two and a half turns (Figure 3-7). The canal within is a little over an inch (35 mm long) and ends blindly at the apex. The canal is partly divided into upper (*vestibular*) and lower (*tympanic*) galleries (*scalae*) by a spiral shelf of bone protruding outward from the inner wall of the passage like a shelf along the inner wall of a circular staircase. The division of the two galleries is completed by a fibrous flexible membrane, the *basilar membrane*,

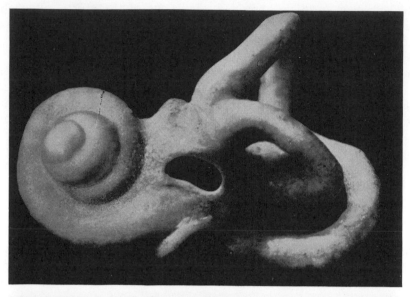

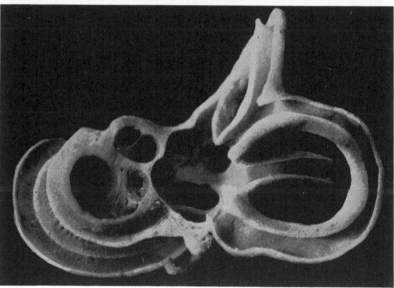

Fig. 3-6. In the top photograph the left bony labyrinth of an infant has been removed from the substance of the temporal bone. The oval window appears clearly in the center. Below it, seen obliquely, is the protruding rim of bone around the opening of the round window.

In the bottom photograph the right bony labyrinth, viewed from within the head, has been opened to show the hollow vestibule and canals. Notice the spiral shelf of bone that partly subdivides the canal of the cochlea (lower left). The hollow central core of the cochlea, through which the nerve emerges, is clearly shown, and also the round window, with rim partly cut away, opening into the canal of the cochlea (lower center). (*Rudinger*)

that stretches across from the lower edge of the bony shelf to the spiral ligament that attaches it to the outer wall. The basilar membrane and the shelf both terminate a millimeter or two short of the end of the galleries so that the two galleries join at the apex of the cochlea. On the vestibular surface of the basilar membrane lies the

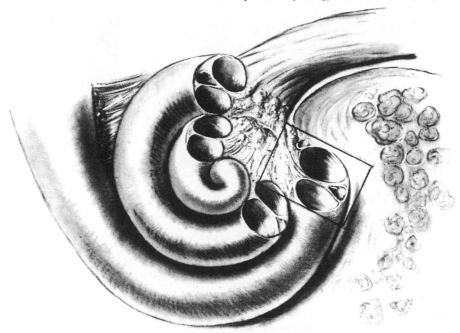

Fig. 3-7. The cochlea has been opened to show cross sections of its turns and also the distribution of the nerve to the turns. The area in the rectangle is shown enlarged in Figure 4-10.

membranous tube that contains the sensory cells and their supporting structures, known as the *organ of Corti.* The basilar membrane is just over an inch long (32 mm) and tapers in width from about 0.5 mm near the apex down to 0.05 mm at the base of the cochlea near the oval window. The oval window opens into the vestibule near the end of the vestibular gallery, and the round window opens into the tympanic gallery beneath at the base of the cochlea.

We have mentioned the membranous tube that contains the sensory cells of the cochlea. This is part of the *membranous labyrinth* that follows the general pattern of the channels of the *bony labyrinth* (Figure 3-6), rather like a partly inflated inner tube in an automobile tire, and encloses all of the sense organs. The membranous labyrinth is a closed system. It contains a watery fluid, *endolymph*, which differs significantly in chemical composition from the *perilymph*, which surrounds it and fills the remainder of the bony labyrinth. The perilymph has very nearly the same composition as the cerebrospinal fluid that bathes the brain and spinal cord, and in fact there is a small channel, the *perilymphatic duct*, that connects the perilymphatic space with the cranial cavity.

The endolymph of the cochlea is apparently secreted and perhaps reabsorbed also by a very vascular glandular structure, the *stria vascularis*, that lies along the outer wall of the endolymphatic space or *scala media*. The scala media is triangular in cross section. Its bottom, in the conventional view of Figure 3-8, is the basilar membrane and the special structures of the organ of Corti attached to it; the outer wall is largely the stria vascularis, and the third side is a very thin membrane, *Reissner's membrane*, that separates the endolymph of scala media from the perilymph of scala vestibuli. The basilar membrane and the structures attached to it plus Reissner's membrane are sometimes called the "cochlear partition" because, with the bony spiral lamina, they divide scala vestibuli from scala tympani. This over-all term is a con-

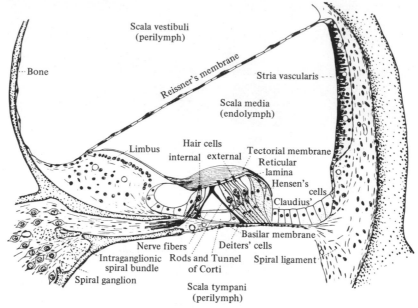

Fig. 3-8. Cross-sectional drawing of the canal in the second turn of a guinea pig's cochlea. The human cochlea is very similar to this. The position corresponding to this section can be identified in Figure 3-7 by the triangular cross section of scala media within the guide rectangle. Note the nerve cell bodies in the spiral ganglion at the left.

venient simplification when we are talking about mechanical movements and acoustic properties. We shall simplify even further and usually speak only of the basilar membrane. This is legitimate because the basilar membrane provides nearly all the stiffness, mass, and acoustic resistance of the partition, and thus determines its acoustic properties. Reissner's membrane is acoustically "transparent" although it is a good chemical and electrical barrier.

The organ of Corti, which contains and supports the sensory cells, is rather complicated in structure. It is stiff mechanically, and it protects the sensory cells from movement and deformation except at the precise place on their upper surface where the minute acoustic vibrations cause the first step in the physiological excitation which leads to setting up nerve impulses. Figure 3-8 shows a typical cross section of the organ of Corti in a guinea pig.

The heavy *pillars of Corti*, which are cells stiffened by intracellular filaments, join at their tops to form a series of tri-

angular arches. The basilar membrane forms the base. The space within is the *tunnel of Corti*. The knobs or plates at the upper ends of the pillars form part of a stiff upper surface of the organ of Corti, the *reticular lamina*. This surface includes also the platelike upper ends of specialized supporting cells, *Deiters' cells*, and of the sensory cells. The latter are set into the reticular lamina much like rows of small manhole covers in a tile pavement. The supporting structure is completed by the somewhat softer outer wall of *Hensen's cells* and the inner supporting cells near the inner pillars of Corti. A solid ridge of fibrous tissue, the *limbus*, is firmly attached to the upper surface of the bony spiral lamina. The limbus provides attachment for one edge of Reissner's membrane and also for the *tectorial membrane*. The tectorial membrane lies on the reticular lamina and is attached at its outer edge to Hensen's cells.

The tectorial membrane is a viscous slow-flowing jelly stiffened by a system of fibers that arise from the outer edge of the limbus. The tectorial membrane is thus a long ribbon attached firmly along one edge to the limbus and more flexibly at its outer edge to the organ of Corti. The tectorial membrane can swing up and down, rather stiffly, like the cover of a book. Within the restriction of its double attachment to the organ of Corti, it can also slide across the reticular lamina as the two structures move up and down together, as illustrated in Figure 3-10. This sliding, shearing action stimulates the sensory cells by bending the fine hairs or *cilia*, which project up from the sensory cells or *hair cells* and are imbedded in or attached to the lower surface of the tectorial membrane, or perhaps by tilting or bending the surface from which the cilia arise.

Many of the older descriptions and pictures of the tectorial membrane show it floating free from the organ of Corti, waving like a leaf on a stem attached to the limbus. The reason is that the chemical fixation necessary to preserve tissue for the usual microscopic study shrinks the tectorial membrane very badly and pulls loose its attachments to Hensen's cells, the inner supporting cells, and the hair cells. Our description is based on studies of fresh specimens seen under the dissecting microscope. The relation between the tectorial membrane and the hair cells is similar to the relation in the utricle, saccule, and semicircular canals where the cilia of hair cells are embedded in gelatinous accessory structures that are acted upon by fluid pressure, gravity, or inertial forces.

Under the dissecting microscope the physical properties of the basilar membrane have been explored by probing, pulling, and cutting. The organ of Corti and the tectorial membrane tend to move together as a single relatively stiff section of the cochlear partition. Most of the bending takes place in the remaining flexible portion of the basilar membrane, as shown in Figure 3-9. The basilar membrane is not under lateral tension, as was once supposed. If it is cut, the edges do not draw apart. The narrow portion in the basal turn

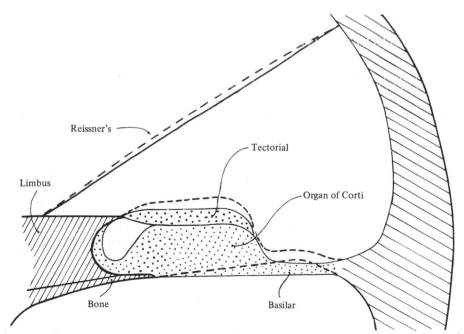

Fig. 3-9. The organ of Corti and the tectorial membrane form a relatively stiff section of the cochlear partition. Most of the bending takes place in the more flexible portion of the basilar membrane between the organ of Corti and the spiral ligament.

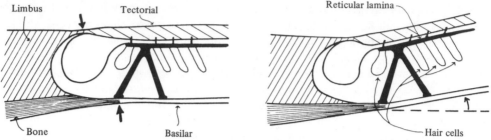

Fig. 3-10. At the left the organ of Corti and tectorial membrane are in the position of rest. Their respective "hinge points" where they attach to the limbus and the bony lamina are shown by the heavy arrows. At the right the partition has moved "upward." Because of its different hinge point the tectorial membrane must slide past the reticular lamina and bend the hairs.

is much stiffer than the broader portion near the apex by a factor of at least 100 when measured in terms of the volume displacement of fluid that is produced by a given force.

From observations such as these it is practically certain that when the organ of Corti is moved up and down by sound waves, as described in the next section, the tectorial membrane must slide past the reticular lamina as shown in Figure 3-10. This is a mechanical necessity because these two rather stiff structures have different hinge points on limbus and bony lamina, respectively. Thus the final mechanical action of which we are sure is a lateral bending or shearing of the cilia, in and out with each sound wave.

Before considering the fine anatomy of the sensory cells and the nerve fibers that innervate them, let us consider in more detail the movement of the cochlear partition as a whole when driven by sound.

### Analysis of Sound by the Ear

When the stapes is forced like a piston into the oval window, it presses on the perilymph in the vestibule. The perilymph is nearly incompressible, like water, and the walls of the bony labyrinth are rigid except for the flexible round-window membrane. The pressure wave spreads very rapidly throughout the labyrinth, and the round window bulges outward into the air-filled middle ear. This allows the stapes to move inward more freely, and fluid is displaced toward the round window. The cochlear partition is in the path of this movement of fluid and, being flexible, it is displaced toward the round window, as shown in Figure 3-5. If the movement is slow, or if the position is maintained, there is time for fluid to flow up scala vestibuli through the helicotrema and down the scala tympani. For sounds of more than about 60 Hz, the basilar membrane is flexible enough and the inertia of the fluid great enough for the fluid near the helicotrema to remain stationary while the cochlear partition and also the round-window membrane bulge back and forth.

The basilar membrane has some stiffness, as we have mentioned. It is elastic enough to return to its original shape and position after it has been deformed or displaced, and it has appreciable mass. It therefore has a natural period or resonant frequency at which it will move most easily and at greatest amplitude when driven by an alternating force like a sound wave. The basilar membrane is graded in width, widest at the apex and narrowest at the base of the cochlea. The stiffness is closely related to the width. Thus the membrane is stiffest at the base and most flexible at the apex. The resonant frequency is highest in the basal turn and lowest at the apex. In accordance with the principles of resonance, the basilar membrane does, indeed, show maximum amplitude of vibration for high tones near the base, for medium tones in the second turn, and for low tones near the apex.

This relation was proposed as a hypothesis by Helmholtz, but we are indebted to Georg von Békésy for the most complete experimental analysis of the acoustics of the ear and the details of how it acts as a frequency analyzer. Georg von Békésy was a physicist by training, and his methods primarily acoustical and optical. The experiments were difficult to perform and are rather complicated in detail. He actually measured, under the microscope, the amplitudes of movement at different positions along the membrane in relation to different frequencies and intensities of driving

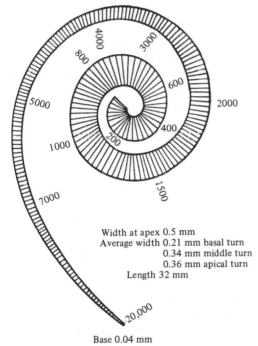

Width at apex 0.5 mm
Average width 0.21 mm basal turn
0.34 mm middle turn
0.36 mm apical turn
Length 32 mm

Base 0.04 mm

Fig. 3-11. In this diagram the width of the basilar membrane is exaggerated relative to its length to show more clearly its progressive widening as it approaches the apex. The approximate positions of maximum amplitude of vibration in response to tones of different frequency are also indicated. (*From O. Stuhlman, Jr., An Introduction to Biophysics, John Wiley & Sons, Inc.*)

sound. For these and other studies of the ear, extending over 25 years, he was awarded the Nobel Prize in Physiology and Medicine in 1961.

The pattern of mechanical activity described by von Békésy has been confirmed by other workers and in other ways. The electrical output of the hair cells, for example, has been used to detect and measure movements of the organ of Corti instead of observing the movements under a microscope. And it is gratifying that the map relating frequency to position along the basilar membrane, as derived from direct physiological experiments, agrees with inferences drawn from psychoacoustics, notably the relation of the mel scale to frequency (see Chapter 2). In Figure 3-11, the approximate positions of maximum movement are given, as compiled by Stuhlman in 1943. This map is still satisfactory. We now feel justified in speaking of the *place principle* of frequency analysis in the cochlea to denote this well-established relation between frequency of sound waves and position of maximum mechanical movement.

### Place Principle, Cochlear Map, and Psychoacoustic Correlates

Several features of the cochlea map are worth noting. First, the highest audible frequency, about 20,000 Hz, is associated with the extreme basal end of the membrane just behind the round window. The frequency of 2000 Hz lies at the midpoint along the basilar membrane between base and apex. From the upper limit down to 1000 Hz or perhaps 500 Hz each octave occupies about the same distance along the membrane, approximately 5 mm. Below 1000 Hz, the spacing is equal distance for equal bandwidth instead of for equal ratio of frequencies. This results in a progressive compression of the lower musical octaves into shorter and shorter distances. The apical end of the membrane at the helicotrema is reached at about 60 Hz. A curious result of the compression of the lower octaves is the position of middle C of the piano (262 Hz), which is much nearer to 90 percent than to 50 percent of the distance between the two ends. We should recall from Chapter 2, however, that the mel scale of pitch shows a very similar compression of subjective pitch in the low frequencies, and so do the difference limens, each of which is equal to about one mel. From this correspondence we arrive at the generalization that one just noticeable difference in pitch corresponds to a constant difference in position of maximum amplitude of about 0.02 mm. The relation of critical bandwidth to frequency follows a similar trend, and we find a rough equivalence of one critical band to one millimeter of length and to about 100 mels.

The reader is reminded that a certain amount of pitch information seems to be carried, for low frequencies, by the periodicity of wave form, whether sinusoidal or complex. We shall return to this point, but the *periodicity principle* of pitch should be mentioned here as an important supplement to the basic place principle outlined above.

### Damping and Frequency Discrimination

The frequency analysis in the cochlea depends directly on the principle of resonance (see Chapter 2). If a system such as a portion of the basilar membrane is to be selective with respect to frequency, it must be free to continue vibrating for at least one or two oscillations after the driving force ceases. In other words, the system must be less than critically damped and not "dead beat." For the finest discrimination, it should be only lightly damped. On the other hand, a lightly damped system builds up only slowly to its maximum amplitude, and is a poor instrument for detecting time differences between signals. The ear actually represents a good compromise between frequency resolution and time resolution. Experiments by von Békésy showed that at large amplitudes of movement the ear is a little less than critically damped. Actually it is difficult to understand how the auditory system does as well as it does in frequency discrimination *and* in its sensitivity to time differences. The reason is that the auditory system is more than a simple set of independent acoustic resonators. Perhaps damping varies with amplitude. The sense organ is complex, and it is powerfully assisted by the central nervous system.

### The Traveling Wave Pattern of the Basilar Membrane

The time pattern of the movement of the basilar membrane when driven by a continuous tone is quite complicated. The various parts do not move in step (in phase) with one another. The natural periods of different segments differ, as we have noted, and, according to the principles of resonance, the portions of the membrane that are tuned to frequencies higher than the driving force tend to move ahead of the force while the parts with lower natural periods tend to lag behind. But the membrane is a continuous structure, not a set of independent resonators. No segment can get very far ahead of or lag far behind the adjacent portion. The final pattern of movement in any system in which the stiffness, and consequently the tuning, is graded continuously, as they are in the basilar membrane, is a series of *traveling waves*. The waves arise at the stiffer end and travel toward the more flexible region. At the stiff end the movement is very nearly in phase with the driving force. As the waves travel they increase in amplitude, but they lag more and more behind the driving force. At the position of maximum amplitude they lag by nearly a full cycle. The details of the pattern are shown in Figure 3-12.

The behavior of the membrane in re-

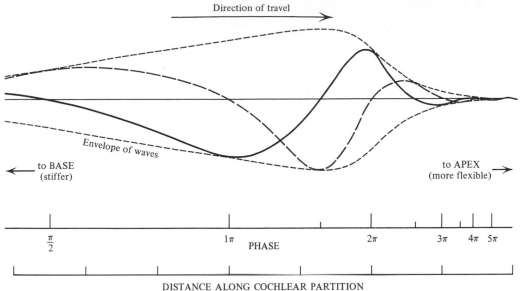

Fig. 3-12. The waves in the basilar, membrane move from base toward apex. Their velocity becomes progressively slower and their wavelength shorter. The solid curve shows the pattern of discplacement at the instant that the upward displacement at the basal end is maximal. The dashed curve shows the pattern a quarter of a cycle ($\pi/2$) later. The phase differences are relative to the extreme basal end. The dotted lines are the envelopes of the displacement patterns. The envelope increases slowly, goes through a maximum between $3\pi/2$ and $2\pi$ and then falls off rapidly. The position of the maximum along the membrane is a function of frequency, as shown in Figure 3-10, but the relation of maximum to phase lag is constant. The small short waves beyond about $3\pi$ are probably of no physiological importance. In this diagram the vertical dimension of displacement is exaggerated to show the patterns more clearly. The formation of traveling waves depends on the gradient of stiffness along the cochlear partition. (*After Békésy*)

sponse to a single wave, or pulse, or transient is quite similar. A traveling wave starts at the basal end and moves up the cochlea. The point at which it reaches its maximum amplitude depends on the duration of the original (unidirectional) pulse. If the wave arrives at the apical turn, it does so only after a delay (travel time) of more than a millisecond. The mechanism of transmission of such a pulse is *not* like the travel of a wave down a rope when we shake one end, in which the energy is passed from segment to segment along the rope. The pressure wave in the fluids spreads very rapidly throughout the cochlea. The movement of the membrane under the influence of the pressure differences across it requires time, more in the apical

than in the basal turn, although, as we have noted, the movement of each segment is modified by its coupling to its neighbors.

In summary, the *envelope* of the traveling wave pattern is located at a position that depends on frequency, as shown in Figure 3-11. The envelope is not symmetrical. All of the membrane basal to the position of the maximum moves somewhat. A short distance apical to the maximum there is no movement. At the maximum there is a considerable phase lag in the instantaneous displacement, but the basal region moves nearly in phase with itself and also with the driving force. The basal region is therefore capable of giving accurate time information, both for steady tones and for transients.

## Bone Conduction

Any vibration of the basilar membrane will stimulate the sensory cells and give rise to the sensation of sound. It makes no difference how the vibrations in the cochlea may have been set going. Ordinarily the pathway for sound is through the external ear and across the chain of ossicles, but sound waves may also be transmitted directly through the bones of the skull. A vibrating tuning fork may be heard by air conduction if it is held opposite the open ear, or by bone conduction if its stem is applied to the top of the head, to a tooth, or to the mastoid bone behind the ear. Transmission is not so efficient across the skin and through the bone as it is by the normal route, but if the normal route is obstructed, as in certain forms of deafness, bone conduction may be put to great practical use. Its diagnostic importance will also be discussed in later chapters.

The sound waves traveling in the skull probably set up mechanical movement of the fluid relative to the bone in several ways. For one thing, the membrane of the round window is more flexible and yielding than is the footplate of the stapes, so that when the labyrinth as a whole is compressed by a sound wave reaching it through the bone, the round window is the most yielding of the various outlets. The fluid from the vestibule and the semicircular canals, as well as that within the cochlea, is therefore driven toward the round window. This fluid movement is exactly like that normally set up by the vibrations of the footplate of the stapes and is analyzed by the cochlea and heard in the brain exactly like airborne sound. For another thing, the head is vibrated as a whole by sounds below about 800 cps. The ossicles tend to lag behind because of their inertia. The resulting relative movement of skull and ossicles is exactly equivalent to vibrations set up by airborne sound. Fortunately, this effect is minimized by the dynamic balance of the malleus and incus around their axis of rotation described earlier in this chapter.

These are two of the most important but by no means all of the mechanisms and pathways of bone conduction. Of course, any very intense sound in the air will set the skull vibrating to some extent; a telephone receiver held tightly against the ear may do so even more effectively. Our own voices generated inside our heads reach our ears by bone conduction as well as by air conduction. But it is air conduction that gives the ear its great sensitivity, particularly for the higher audible frequencies.

## The Hair Cells and Their Nerves

In the description of the organ of Corti we mentioned briefly the sensory cells, known as hair cells, and their orderly arrangement in one row of "inner" or internal hair cells on the side of the tunnel of Corti nearer to the modiolus and three rows (with sometimes parts of a fourth row) of "outer" or external hair cells on the opposite side. The inner and outer cells differ somewhat in shape and size, as shown in Figure 3-13, and also in the shapes of the nerve endings that attach to their lower ends, and in their relations to their supporting cells. Inner and outer are alike, however, in the set of "hairs" or *cilia* (stereocilia) that project from their cuticular surfaces into the endolymphatic space. There are as many as 80 cilia on each hair cell, and they are arranged in rows in the same over-all pattern, like a W with its narrow double-pointed base turned away from the modiolus.

An electron microscope is needed to see the hairs clearly. They are about a micron (0.001 mm) in diameter and perhaps ten times as long. A "root" can be traced well down into the cuticular layer, but the electron microscope does not tell us whether the cilia are primarily chemical, electrical, or mechanical devices. Their outer ends are

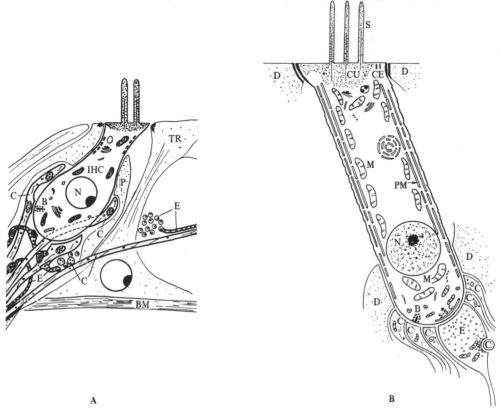

Fig. 3-13. *A*. Diagram of an inner hair cell and its innervation. *B*, synaptic bar; *BM*, basilar membrane; *C*, afferent cochlear nerve fibers; *E*, efferent nerve fibers of the olivo-cochlear bundle; *N*, nucleus; *P*, phalangeal supporting cell; *TR*, tunnel rod. Note the nerve fibers cut in cross section, forming the inner spiral bundle and the tunnel bundle. Note how the efferent fibers to the inner hair cells form synaptic junctions on the afferent nerve fibers and endings as well as on the hair cell.

*B*. Diagram of an outer hair cell. *B*, synaptic bar; *C*, afferent cochlear nerve fiber; *CE*, centriole; *CU*, cuticular plate; *D*, Deiters' cells; *E*, efferent nerve terminal; *M*, mitochondria; *N*, nucleus; *S*, stereocilia; *S-SC*, subsynaptic cisterna. This (*B*) part of the figure is drawn at at higher magnification than the left (*A*) part. (*Courtesy of C. A. Smith. Reproduced, by permission, from the Advancement of Science, Vol. 24, No. 122 (June 1968).*

imbedded in, or at least attached to, the tectorial membrane. Apparently in the cochlea, as well as in other related organs, when the cilia are bent toward the base of the W, nerve impulses are triggered off in the nerve fiber that connects with the hair cell. When they are bent the other way, the nerve impulses are inhibited; and when bent sideways, there is no effect.

The inner hair cells are snugly packed among the supporting cells. The "upper" cuticular surfaces of both inner and outer hair cells form part of the stiff reticular lamina. The lower end of each outer hair cell rests in a cup provided by a specialized supporting cell (Deiters'). The remainder of the hair cell is bathed by a fluid, probably much like perilymph, that fills the tunnel of Corti and other intracellular spaces in the organ of Corti. Many nerve endings, in intimate contact with one another as well as with the hair cells, cover the end of the cell opposite to the hair-bearing end (see Figure 3-13).

The electron microscope shows two different types of nerve endings clustered around the lower end of each hair cell. Some are large with many vesicles; others are smaller and clearer. Each nerve fiber usually branches and has several such terminals, but all the terminals on any one fiber are of one type or the other. The details of innervation vary as between inner and outer hair cells, as between cochlear and vestibular hair cells, and as between ears of different animal species; but there are always the two kinds of endings. One variety, usually the smaller, clearer ones, are the endings of the well-known auditory nerve fibers that carry impulses from the cochlea to the brain (*afferent* fibers). The cell bodies of these afferent neurons, which contain the nucleus and other vital structures, are located in the spiral ganglion in the modiolus of the cochlea, close to the hair cells with which their nerve endings are in contact (see Figures 3-7 and 3-8).

The larger variety of nerve ending contains many vesicles. The cell bodies of these nerve fibers are located in the brain stem, in the superior olivary nucleus. The *efferent* fibers carry nerve impulses from the brain to the cochlea, and their effect is to raise the threshold of the afferent endings and their fibers. Some type of efferent control of sensitivity such as this seems to be characteristic of many sensory systems.

### Number of Hair Cells and Their Innervation

The total number of hair cells in a human ear is about 12,000. About 3000 of them are inner hair cells; the remainder are outer cells. Each inner hair cell is about 10 microns in diameter; the outer hair cells, about 8 microns. The basilar membrane is about 32 mm long. There are, therefore, about 400 hair cells per millimeter. Another approximate relation is that one octave in the middle range of frequencies occupies some 5 mm, and one just noticeable

difference in pitch corresponds to about 10 microns or the diameter of a single inner hair cell.

The number of nerve fibers is about double the total number of hair cells. There are about 25,000 to 30,000 cell bodies in the spiral ganglion of Corti (see Figures 3-7 and 3-8) within the modiolus. Each cell body sends a short receptor fiber to the organ of Corti and a long nerve trunk, an axon, to the cochlear nucleus. There are, in addition, about 500 efferent fibers coming from the superior olivary nucleus. These fibers run in the *olivo-cochlear bundle*, or "bundle of Rasmussen." Of the efferent fibers to each ear, 70 to 80 percent have their cell bodies in the opposite side of the brain stem.

The efferent fibers run up and down the cochlea in the intraganglionic bundle (Figures 3-8 and 3-14), or as the internal spiral fibers beneath the inner hair cells, or the external spiral fibers among the external hair cells. They branch freely, as they obviously must, since there are 50 times as many hair cells as there are efferent fibers.

The ratio of afferent nerve fibers to hair cells is approximately two to one. The connections are not simple, as each neuron may innervate at least two or three neighboring hair cells, and each hair cell is reached by two or more afferent fibers. This overlap provides some redundancy and also a factor of safety in case of death of either a neuron or a hair cell. (Both neurons and hair cells are highly specialized cells, and if one of them dies others do not regenerate to take its place. The loss is permanent.)

Before the nature of the efferent fibers was recognized, the spiral fibers in the organ of Corti were all assumed to be afferent. The wide branching and distribution of the efferent fibers contributed strongly to the interpretation that one afferent fiber innervates external hair cells over a wide extent, perhaps 2 or 3 mm, of the organ of Corti. Now, from experiments that in-

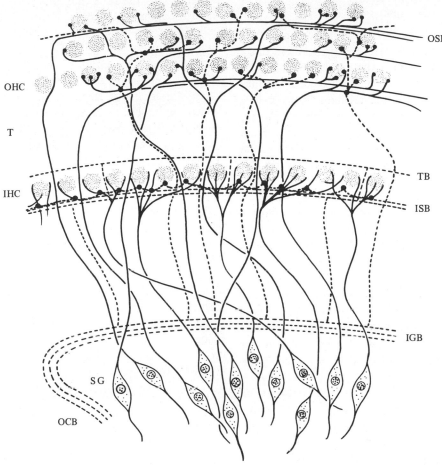

Fig. 3-14. The plan of innervation of the hair cells is shown here. The details are based on studies of the cochleas of animals, particularly cat, guinea pig, and chinchilla, but the human ear follows the same general pattern as far as we know. The spiral ganglion cells of the cochlear nerve and their dendritic processes are shown by solid black lines. The efferent olivo-cochlear nerve fibers are shown by the dashed lines.

*OSB* = outer spiral bundle; *OHC* = outer hair cells (stippled); *T* = tunnel of Corti; *TB* = tunnel bundle; *IHC* = inner hair cells; *ISB* = inner spiral bundle; *IGB* = intraganglionic (spiral) bundle; *SG* = spiral ganglion; *OCB* = olivo-cochlear bundle. (*From C. A. Smith. Reproduced, by permission, from The Advancement of Science, Vol. 24, No. 122 (June 1968).*

volve cutting the efferent fibers in the brain of guinea pigs or other small animals, allowing the fibers to degenerate, and then studying the nerve endings under the electron microscope, we are practically sure that the intraganglionic and internal spiral fibers are efferent. The exact status of the external spiral fibers is not yet clear. Some are efferent, but the afferent fibers also run for some distance along the cochlea before

making contact with hair cells. The critical point which is uncertain is the distribution along the organ of Corti of the group of hair cells innervated by a single afferent external nerve fiber. The present writer believes that the distribution is quite limited. This opinion is based largely on the excellent frequency discrimination of the human ear and the sharp "tuning" of the afferent fibers that will be described in a later section.

## Nerve Impulses:
## the All-or-None Law

We have described the organs of the inner ear, their physical properties, and how they move under the influence of sound waves. The movements are graded continuously in amplitude, and they all occur in a single sound-conducting system or "channel," whether it be the air of the external canal, the ossicles in the middle ear, the fluids, or the cochlear partition of the inner ear. At the cochlear partition, the single channel begins to subdivide. The frequency analysis performed by the basilar membrane means that some sensory cells are moved more than others according to their position and the frequency of the sound.

At the sensory cell a very different kind of action occurs. The input to the cell is a bending of its "hairs" or cilia. The final result is an output of nerve impulses in the sensory nerve that innervates it. The relation of this output to the mechanical input is highly nonlinear; it is discontinuous in both intensity and time, and it involves the contribution of energy by both the sensory cell and the nerve fiber to support this new form of activity. We often refer to the "triggering" of nerve impulses. The action is analogous to pulling the trigger of a machine gun and thereby firing one or a series of shots. We will consider first the action of a typical nerve cell or neuron and then the process of excitation in a sensory cell.

The nerve impulse is the unit of action in a nerve fiber. It is a wave of electrochemical activity that travels in the auditory nerve fibers at about 25 m per second. (Some nerve fibers of larger diameter conduct more rapidly, about 100 m per second, while small nonmyelinated fibers in the autonomic nervous system conduct at about 1 m per second). The nerve impulse can be compared to the burning of a fuse of gunpowder. The heat of the burning ignites the next adjoining section of the fuse,

which ignites the next one, and so on in a chain reaction. The energy of the nerve impulse, like the heat of the burning fuse, comes from the fiber itself, not from the initial stimulus (the match) that triggers it off. The impulse is not graded in intensity according to the strength of the stimulus. Its strength depends only on the state of the fiber at that particular point. The fuse burns or it does not burn. The impulse, like the burning, is "all or none."

There is an important difference between the nerve impulse and the fuse. The nerve automatically recharges itself after each impulse and is ready to conduct another impulse after an interval of 1 to 2 or 3 msec. This recharging interval is known as the *refractory period*. Another difference is that the excitation of the impulse from segment to segment of nerve is electrical, not thermal as in the fuse. We can place an electrode on the nerve fiber and record the electrical change or "action potential" (see Figure 3-17). This allows us to *measure the activity of a nerve fiber in terms of the number of impulses per second*.

The typical *neuron* consists of four major parts. One is the *cell body* that contains the nucleus and other vital structures necessary for the continued life of the cell. Special chemical substances are formed here and are distributed down the nerve fibers by a slow outward flow of protoplasm. The second part of a neuron is its receptor or *dendritic portion,* which receives stimuli, usually chemical, from other neurons or sensory cells. It responds, as we shall see, by generating a local graded electric current. A third part is a set of effector *terminals,* which form synapses with other neurons and secrete a particular *chemical mediator*. These junctional or synaptic actions will be described in more detail in the next section. The fourth major part of most neurons is absent in some small nerve cells in the central nervous system, but it constitutes most of what we know as a peripheral "nerve." It is the nerve fiber or *axon*. It is long and threadlike, and it connects the input (dendritic) with the output (secretory) endings. The larger axons, including those of the auditory nerve, are covered with a thin insulating sheath of a white fatty substance known as *myelin*. The axon is specialized for rapid, economical, and reliable transmission of very simple all-or-none messages, the *nerve impulses*.

The discontinuous all-or-none activity is carried out very economically. It provides very reliable transmission of signals over long lengths of nerve, as from the foot or hand to the brain, and the transmission is very rapid. On the other hand, the code of the nerve fiber is very limited. The impulses are not graded in intensity like electric currents in a telephone wire. They are merely dots in a very simple telegraphic code, more like those of a digital computer. The only significant gradations are (1) the average number of impulses per second and (2) the time relations between impulses in the same and in neighboring fibers. Each fiber is effectively insulated from its neighbors. The maximum frequency of impulses is 1000 per second for the first two or three impulses, falling rapidly to an average maximum rate of about 200 to 300 per second.

A major problem of auditory neurophysiology is to understand how all of the auditory information that reaches the brain passes through the bottleneck of the auditory nerve. How is it coded in sequences of dot-dot-dot impulses in the individual nerve fibers? We may add that the same problem appears again and again in the central nervous system wherever information is coded for transmission by the axons that make up the "tracts" of white matter.

### Synapses and Synaptic Action

Within the neurons and hair cells we will not be concerned with the nucleus, the mitochondria, and many other details of internal structure that are revealed by the electron microscope. With the exception of the cilia of the hair cells, they are common to most cells throughout the body. The surfaces of contact between cells themselves are of special interest to us, however. These specialized junctional structures are known as the *synaptic junctions* or *synapses*. Nearly all synapses are chemical mechanisms. By this we mean that a particular "neurohumor" or *chemical transmitter* is liberated from a ready state and diffuses rapidly across the very narrow "synaptic cleft" and reacts with a specialized receptor surface on the receiving neuron.

Certain charged particles (ions) then become free to move, and an electric current begins to flow. In many nerve cells we can, with very fine intracellular electrodes, detect and measure the associated "postsynaptic potentials." The postsynaptic potentials from many nerve endings combine with one another. The excitatory effect is related to the total number of excitatory impulses reaching a particular neuron. When an adequate integrated postsynaptic potential is reached, it triggers off a nerve impulse in the axon. There are a number of different chemical transmitters. Acetylcholine and norepinephrine are two of the best known, but the transmitters in the cochlea have not yet been identified.

Not all synaptic action is excitatory. Some nerve fibers and their terminals are specialized to secrete *inhibitory transmitters*. Inhibition in this context means a process that opposes or makes more difficult the triggering of nerve impulses in a neuron. This is the action of the efferent fibers to the cochlea. There are several mechanisms of inhibition, but the most common is a change in the electrochemical properties of the postsynaptic surface of the "receiving" neuron, specifically to reduce the electrical impedance, so that the excitatory postsynaptic potentials are short-circuited and do not combine so effectively with one another.

## From Sound Waves
## to Nerve Impulses

One step in the chain of transmission of auditory signals to the brain is not fully understood, namely, how the mechanical bending of the cilia of the hair cells controls the release of the chemical transmitter at the opposite end of the hair cell. We do know that in various sense organs the receptor cells are specialized to be extremely and selectively sensitive to one particular form of incoming energy, whether it be chemical (taste and smell), thermal (temperature sense), light (vision), electrical (electrical organs in certain fish), or mechanical (touch, acceleration and hearing). The hair cells of the ear with their cilia are the most sensitive of the *mechano-receptors*. They are sensitive to deformations of atomic dimensions and at energy levels only just above that of thermal agitation of molecules. Because of this extreme sensitivity we can be quite sure that at the critical point of deformation, whether it be in the cilia or in the cuticular plate in which they are imbedded, there must be a release of energy by the hair cell like the first step in the triggering of a nerve impulse—in other words, an amplifying or "booster" action.

The hair cells do actually respond with an electrical output. The response is not an explosive all-or-none reaction like a nerve impulse, but instead it is graded, like a local postsynaptic potential, according to the amplitude of the mechanical displacement. It follows the wave form faithfully without discontinuities or refractory periods. It can be detected readily by placing a pair of electrodes, either one on the round window and another elsewhere near the cochlea, or, better, both within the cochlea, one on each side of the cochlear partition. This electrical response of the hair cells has been used extensively to study the action of both normal and injured ears. It is known as the *cochlear mi-*

*crophonic,* because the transduction of the signal from an acoustic to an electrical form resembles the action of a microphone. We may add, however, that the action is not a passive piezoelectric effect as in a crystal microphone. It resembles more closely a resistance microphone in which the mechanical movement modulates or valves the flow of electric current from a battery. The battery in this case is the hair cell itself, which maintains an electrical potential between its inner and outer surface in the same way that a nerve fiber recharges itself after transmitting an impulse. This concept of the action of the hair cell is somewhat theoretical, but it seems to be our best working hypothesis at present. It is illustrated in Figure 3-15.

The second step in the action of the hair cell is the liberation of its chemical transmitter. The liberation of chemical transmitter is presumably controlled by the current flow of the cochlear microphonic through the cell, just as the liberation of transmitter from axon terminals at synapses is controlled by the action potentials of the nerve impulses arriving over the axons. The hair cell is rather like a neuron without any axon.

In this summary account we have bypassed certain interesting specializations in the cochlea such as the unique high potassium content of the endolymph and the strong electrical polarization of the endolymphatic space of scala media. The polarization and presumably the chemical composition also are maintained by the stria vascularis (see Figure 3-15). These specializations probably make the cochlea more sensitive or more efficient, but one or both are absent in other simpler mechano-receptor organs.

This hypothesis of mechano-electrical excitation meets the requirement of providing a "biological amplifier" in the receptor cell and it is in harmony with both experimental observations of the cochlear microphonic and analogous electrical action

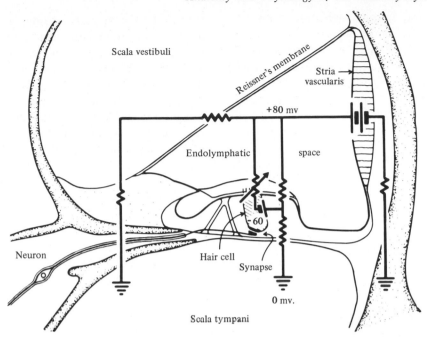

Fig. 3-15. Model for mechanoelectrical excitation in the cochlea. Only one (external) hair cell is shown, to represent all hair cells. The endolymph in scala media is polarized 80 mv positive, and the interior of the hair cells 60 mv negative relative to scala tympani. These polarizations are maintained by biological "batteries" shown in the stria vascularis and the (lateral) cell membrane of the hair cell, respectively. The electrical pathways through Hensen's cells and basilar membrane and through Reissner's membrane and limbus represent all of the shunting pathways from scala media to scala tympani. A variable resistance, sensitive to mechanical deformation, is represented at the cuticular surface of the hair cell. It is probably located near the centriole (see Figure 3-13). Changes in the resistance modulate the leakage current through the hair cell and thus the level of polarization at the synaptic surface at the lower end of the hair cell. The level of polarization here controls the rate of liberation of the chemical mediator which excites the afferent nerve ending. The cochlear microphonic, that is, the potential difference between scala media and scala tympani, is the result of the IR drop across the variable resistance in the cuticular layer.

in other receptor organs. Fortunately our over-all understanding of the action of the ear does not rest on this particular model of the excitatory action of the hair cells. We know that some excitatory process does operate, even at threshold levels of input, and we can study the output of nerve impulses in the fibers of the auditory nerve and relate this output directly to the acoustic input to the ear.

### The Sensory Unit and Its Response Area

At this point we introduce the concept of the *auditory sensory unit,* meaning *one afferent auditory neuron and the hair cell or cells which it innervates.* This concept is very helpful in understanding many forms of auditory impairment. We make the assumption, noted in the previous section, that the cells innervated by any one fiber form a reasonably compact group, and we disregard the overlap that results from the innervation of one hair cell by two or more afferent neurons.

The definition of the auditory unit centers on the afferent nerve fiber and its responses to auditory stimuli. This is realistic because in animal experiments we can place a very fine electrode on or in a single fiber in the auditory nerve and both count and time the nerve impulses of the particular sensory unit. We can determine its threshold of response at various frequencies and thus describe its "tuning." We find, as a matter of fact, that each unit is sensitive to only a limited band of frequencies. The band is broader for intense than for weak tones. Each unit is most sensitive for one particular frequency, which is called its *characteristic frequency* or "best frequency."

The *response area* refers to the entire group of tones to which the unit responds. Plotted in the dimensions of frequency and intensity, as in Figure 3-16, the response

area is a triangle pointing downward with its vertex at the best frequency. In general, the response areas are very steep on their high-frequency side, but they extend rather widely toward the lower frequencies at high intensities. Without going into detail, we can say that this asymmetrical shape is just what would be expected from the asymmetrical shape of the envelope of the traveling waves (see Figure 3-12) and the harmonic distortion produced by the nonlinear action of the ear at high intensities.

The most surprising feature of the response areas is their steepness and narrowness, that is, their sharpness of tuning, particularly for the higher frequencies. The

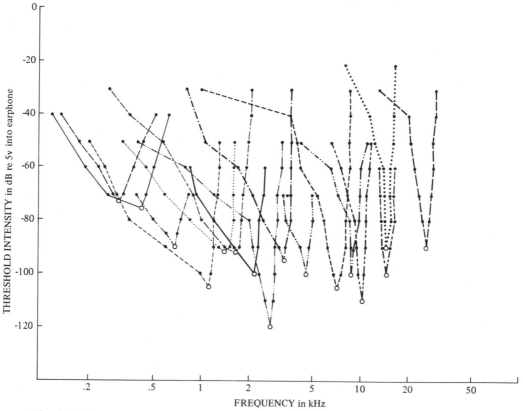

Fig. 3-16. Response areas (tuning curves) of 16 auditory sensory units of a cat. All tones within each response area caused an increased rate of discharge in that unit. The lowest point in each area represents the threshold at the "best frequency" of the unit. Note the steep upper boundaries of the response areas and the extensive overlap of the areas. Each area was determined by systematically increasing the frequency at successive (increasing) sound levels. (*Data from N. Y. Kiang et al., Stimulus Coding in the Cat's Auditory Nerve, Annals of Otology, Rhinology and Laryngology, 71:1009–1026 [1962].*)

narrow response areas are a confirmation of our interpretations (1) that the cochlea acts as an acoustic filter and (2) that each afferent fiber innervates only a very short segment of the organ of Corti.

Some of the sensory units are very sensitive at their best frequencies. Here their thresholds may be as low as the behavioral thresholds of the animal. Other units, even though they may have exactly the same best frequency, have higher thresholds. It is tempting to speculate that the different threshold levels are somehow associated with the location of the hair cell(s) of that unit, either in the inner or in one of the outer rows. The inner hair-cell units *probably* have the higher thresholds, but there is no direct evidence.

Actually the recent studies by Nelson Kiang and his associates show that much of this spread of threshold levels was illusory, and suggest a rather uniform high sensitivity of all units, at least in the cat. It seems unlikely that inner and outer hair cells have the same threshold, but for the present we must accept a paradox. On the other hand, if we consider a group of *neighboring* sensory units with *somewhat different best frequencies,* we see that because of the steep response areas there is still considerable gradation of threshold for any one particular frequency. In Figure 3-16 almost any vertical line, representing a pure tone, will cross three or more response areas. There are actually some 25,000 sensory units in a human ear, and their response areas overlap richly. This overlap, with consequent gradation of threshold, is very important for understanding the increase of neural activity in response to increasing sound intensity.

Nearly every sensory unit is spontaneously active, even when every effort is made to ensure perfect quiet. The impulses do not come at regular intervals like the heartbeat, but the long-term rate, averaged over half a second or even less, is quite stable and does not fluctuate with the animal's pulse or respiration. The spontaneous background activity is a fine example of "physiological noise." When we speak of the "threshold" of a unit we mean the sound level that causes a reliable, significant increase in average rate, say by 20 percent, above the spontaneous activity. A stronger tone causes a higher average rate of discharge of nerve impulses. A rather modest increase to perhaps 25 dB above threshold drives the sensory unit at its maximum rate, something of the order of 500 impulses a second. Such a high rate cannot be maintained for more than a fraction of a second, however. The average rate settles down in a second or two to about 200 impulses per second. This rate can continue for many minutes. The initial slowdown is the physiological adaptation which was mentioned in Chapter 2.

### Summary of Peripheral Auditory Physiology

A diagram in the next chapter, Figure 4-1, summarizes the sequence of actions in the ear from the external air to the axon terminals of the sensory units in the cochlear nucleus. It shows how the transition from sound conduction and frequency analysis to nerve impulses is located in the cochlea. There the excitation of the sensory units occurs, and the auditory nerve transmits all-or-none impulses to the brain stem. The diagram also illustrates how the bone-conduction pathway through the skull bypasses the middle ear, with its drum membrane and ossicular chain, but joins the primary air-conduction pathway in the fluids of the inner ear before the frequency analysis is performed by the basilar membrane. The arrangement of the hair cells in the figure is completely diagrammatic. Each cell in the diagram represents a group of cells in a short segment of the organ of Corti. The arrangement of units lengthwise of the organ of Corti expresses the tuning of the units, each with its best frequency.

The gradation of thresholds among sensory units is also indicated.

The general pattern represented here is very useful in helping to understand the various forms of auditory impairment that will be described in Chapter 4, notably the distinction between conductive impairment, sense organ or sensory impairment (referring to the organ of Corti), neural impairment (referring to the neurons of the auditory nerve), and central impairment in and beyond the cochlear nucleus. In the cochlear nucleus, each sensory unit is represented as dividing to terminate in three different regions in the cochlear nucleus. (Three is probably a minimum number.) The different areas probably initiate different forms of "information processing." In and beyond the cochlear nucleus, the connections and processes become very complicated, and we refer to them as neurological and, in another frame of reference, as psychological, as we will explain shortly.

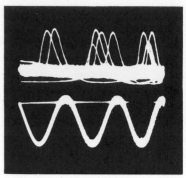

Fig. 3-17. Action potentials (upper tracing) recorded from a microelectrode in a nerve fiber of the auditory nerve of a guinea pig. The lower trace shows the sound stimulus, a 1000 Hz pure tone, recorded by a microphone. Approximately 170 sweeps were superimposed. Ten nerve impulses appeared. The action potentials are all-or-none transients, but three of them appear smaller here because of the electrical background noise, shown by the broad base line. Note that the action potentials all are approximately, but not exactly, in the same time relation to the sound waves. (*From I. Tasaki, J. Neurophysiol., 16:97–122 [1954] by permission.*)

### The Volley Principle and Periodicity Pitch

If the ear is stimulated by a low tone, say 500 Hz or less, the nerve impulses in the sensory units that respond are grouped together in successive bursts or "volleys." There is a preferred phase or portion of the cycle in which impulses tend to be excited, and actually they are more or less *inhibited* during the opposite half of the cycle. Each axon does not fire at exactly the same phase of every cycle, and it may skip one or several cycles. When it does fire, there is a random distribution in the timing, sometimes earlier, sometimes later, as shown in Figure 3-17. Impulses in different sensory units that are excited by the same sound wave thus differ a little in their times of arrival, partly because of this random variability and partly because of the delay of the Békésy traveling wave, which may differ somewhat for different neurons. Nevertheless when we record, in animal experiments, from the auditory nerve as a whole, the grouping of nerve impulses is very clear at 500 Hz. Volleys are definite at 1000 Hz, clearly detectable at 2000 Hz, but barely demonstrable at 4000 Hz. Above 4000 Hz the timing of the impulses is truly random. Below 1000 Hz, however, the grouping represents a significant mechanism by which frequency information is conveyed to the brain.

This information is the basis of the psychoacoustic phenomenon of periodicity pitch described in Chapter 2, but the frequency principle makes only a limited contribution, for low frequencies only, and it is not the major or sole mechanism for conveying frequency information as Rutherford originally (1886) and Wever and Bray later (1930) suggested.

### Electrical Stimulation of Hearing

If an alternating electrical current of a frequency in the audible range is passed through the head in the neighborhood of the inner ear and adjusted to a suitable intensity, it is sometimes possible to hear a tone or at least a noise. This is known as the "electrophonic effect." The current is most effectively applied by filling the external ear canal with salt solution and immersing the end of one wire in it. The circuit is completed through a metal plate on the forearm. The strength of the current must be carefully adjusted, because at only a few decibels above the threshold of hearing the current may begin to be felt as a tickling, burning, prickling, and finally, painful sensation. The effect may also be obtained when an amplitude-modulated carrier wave in the ultrasonic frequency range is applied with both electrodes on skin outside the ear canal.

There are several different mechanisms of the electrophonic effect. Most of them depend on the conversion of the alternating electrical current into mechanical movement of the tympanic membrane, the ossicles, or the skin. It is in this way that pure tones can be heard, either corresponding to the frequency of the electric current or one octave above it. The fundamental action is like that of a condenser microphone operated in reverse as a loudspeaker. It takes advantage of the alternating attractions between two oppositely charged conducting structures, such as the tympanic membrane and the bony wall of the middle ear, separated by a dielectric, such as the air in the middle ear. When a high-frequency carrier is used, a rectifying action in the tissues precedes the transduction into mechanical movement, and the movement, usually of the skin, may be carried to the cochlea by bone conduction.

These mechanisms are all basically electrostatic effects of one sort or another, even though they have been mistaken for electrical stimulation of the ear or even of the brain itself! If a pure tone is heard, we can be quite sure that some cochlear function remains.

A quite different form of the electro-phonic effect is the actual electrical stimulation of the auditory nerve. Sometimes this can be achieved before muscular twitching or pain, or both, become intolerable. Electrodes have actually been introduced experimentally into (damaged) human cochleas to stimulate the nerve or parts of the nerve selectively and to test the possibility of developing a hearing aid on this principle.

Unfortunately the sensation produced by such direct electrical stimulation of the auditory nerve is not a pure tone. It is either a noise or at best a sort of buzz. The sensation corresponds to the periodicity pitch discussed in the previous section and in Chapter 2, and, as might be expected, the buzzlike "tone" is heard at only rather low frequencies. One subject in such an experiment did learn, with practice, to distinguish a few spoken words, but could do so only when the choice, that is, the vocabulary, was very small.

Useful communication by speech was not achieved, nor is there any prospect that it will be in the future, even if the very formidable surgical and biological problems of developing electrodes that would be tolerated for years by the nerve tissue and of placing the electrodes effectively in cochlea or nerve are overcome. The point is that the normal frequency analysis of the cochlea is lost. Attempts to substitute for it by elaborate electronic devices will suffer from our inability to stimulate the proper nerve fiber when a particular audio frequency reaches the device. Actually the attempts to produce useful hearing by direct electrical stimulation have confirmed very well indeed the theoretical predictions made on the basis of the place principle and the volley principle as to the quality and extent of hearing that could be expected from this approach.

### Psychophysiological Relations

The physical and physiological properties of the ear help us to understand the boundaries of the auditory area. The behavioral threshold is at roughly the same level as the threshold of physiological stimulation of the most sensitive auditory units. Discomfort and pain occur when the mechanical restraints on amplitude of movement become severe and injury is imminent. The upper frequency limits in behavioral animal experiments correspond roughly to the highest frequencies for which good electrical responses are obtained from the cochlea. In pitch discrimination, the difference limen seems to correspond to about the same distance on the basilar membrane as the width of a hair cell. These order-of-magnitude agreements give somehow a comfortable feeling of confidence that we "understand" the detection of faint sounds, the discrimination of pitch, and so on. But this feeling is legitimate only as long as we remember that we have only a bare outline and an order-of-magnitude approximation of a few aspects of the auditory mechanism. For other aspects, such as loudness and particularly the auditory qualities and the ability to pick a particular signal or voice out of a confused mixture of sound, we have only very poor models or, in the anatomical or physiological sense, no model or "understanding" at all.

## THE CENTRAL AUDITORY SYSTEM

As we proceed inward from the sense organ into the central nervous system, both the anatomy and the physiology suddenly become much more complicated. The system is composed of nerve cells or *neurons* and a special supporting tissue, the *glial* cells. Most of the neurons have axons, many of them covered with myelin sheaths as in peripheral nerves, which conduct the familiar all-or-none nerve impulses. In many places these myelinated axons are grouped together, as in peripheral nerves, and form definite *tracts* (white matter) that connect one area of the brain with another. But there are other areas (gray

matter) where the cell bodies and the dendrites of the neurons are concentrated in vaguely defined masses or *nuclei*.

The gray matter is where specialized axon terminations make contact (*synapses*) with the widely branching *dendrites* or with the cell bodies of other neurons. We can study the cell bodies with fine microelectrodes. Their all-or-none discharges resemble those of their axons, but they also show graded modifications of their resting electrical polarization which are produced by synaptic action (*postsynaptic potentials*). Another feature not seen in peripheral nerves is a tendency to synchronized electrical activity. The resulting slow waves can be detected by large electrodes placed in or near the areas of gray matter. Another difference in the gray matter is a very much higher rate of metabolism, which in turn requires a much richer blood supply. Chemical events, including chemical transmission from axon to dendrite at the synapses, become very important, and the action of nuclei or "nerve centers" can easily be modified by anesthetics, by stimulants, and by other drugs. Many of these synaptic properties are represented in the periphery in the junctions between sensory cells and nerve fibers or between axon terminations and muscle cells, but in the gray matter they are dominant. The greatest complexity of the central nervous system, however, arises from the sheer number of neurons (billions) and the extraordinary richness of their branching, their distribution, and their interconnections. The interconnections include many feedback loops.

In a general way the central nervous system is organized around four major sensory input systems and two major motor output systems. The major sensory systems are: (1) the chemical senses of smell and taste, (2) the somatosensory system from skin and skeletal muscles, (3) the visual system, and (4) the auditory system. In addition there is the vestibular system for orientation to gravity and for acceleration, but this is closely integrated with the feedback kinesthetic system from the muscles and also with the visual system. The control system for the skeletal muscles is one of the motor outputs. It is sometimes called the "voluntary" muscle system, but a better term is *somatic*. The other motor system is the "involuntary" or *autonomic* system. With the endocrine glands of internal secretion, the autonomic nervous system is concerned with the internal regulation of the body.

The structure of nervous tissue, from the various classes of neurons and glia down to the microstructure revealed by the electron microscope, is still under study. The larger anatomical tracts and nuclei that constitute each of the sensory and motor systems are well known, but additional subdivisions and also numerous cross connections among the various systems are continually being discovered. In addition there are large areas of gray matter, with interconnecting tracts of white matter, that are not clearly related to any one of the primary sensory or motor systems. They form a large part of the *cerebral cortex* (see Figure 3-18) and are usually known as the "association areas."

Much is known about the function of the nervous system in terms of reflex motor responses to well-defined sensory stimuli and to combinations or sequences of stimuli. Behavior is related to bodily needs and their associated "drives" and to physiological states such as waking and sleeping.

Electrical "evoked responses" from particular areas within the brain help to relate neurophysiology to neuroanatomy. Still more is learned by direct stimulation, usually electrical but sometimes chemical, of central nervous structures and from simply observing the patterns of spontaneous electrical activity (the "electroencephalogram") in various physiological states such as waking and sleeping. The disrup-

tive effects of lesions, either as they occur naturally by disease or accident, or deliberately as in experimental investigations in animals, or as they relieve symptoms of disease in humans, are also very informative.

The purpose of this topical review is to emphasize the complexity of the central nervous system and the variety of different kinds of information that contribute to our knowledge of it. One of the difficulties in the study of the central nervous system is to integrate these different classes of information.

The integration of neuroanatomy, neurochemistry, and neurophysiology is fairly satisfactory, although it is by no means complete. We do *not* understand, for example, the forces that guide growth and development or the intimate relations at the molecular level among chemistry, microstructure, and physiological activity. We have no conception of the physical substrate of memory or learning. There is no need for a longer catalogue of our ignorance.

On the positive side a rough parallelism has been established between successive anatomical areas or "levels" along the sensory input pathways. This relation is outlined for the auditory system in Figure 3-18. In this diagram the assignment of particular functions to particular "levels" or nuclei in the midbrain is purposely vague. The functions undoubtedly overlap greatly. The diagram does not include the efferent or feedback relations from the "higher" levels, remote from the sense organ, to the "lower" or more peripheral levels. In fact, one of the problems of sensory neurophysiology is to determine the contribution made by each tract and nucleus to the over-all function of the whole system, both when the system is intact and when it is modified, either by lesions or by drugs.

In the diagram the physiological functions are arranged in sequence from bot-

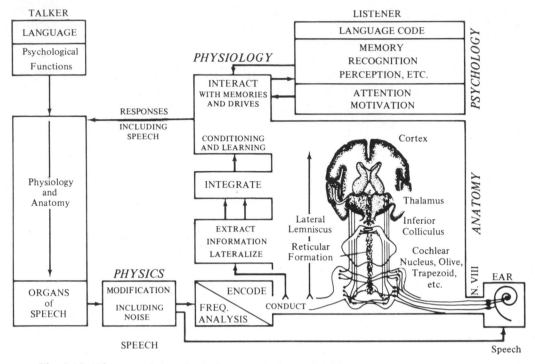

Fig. 3-18. Diagram of the physical, anatomical, physiological, and psychological aspects of speech communication, from talker (left) to listener (right). The simplified anatomical diagram shows the ear, the eighth nerve, the major auditory tracts and nuclei of the medulla, the inferior colliculus of the midbrain, the medial geniculate body in the thalamus, and the primary auditory projection area in the superior convolution of the temporal lobe of the cortex. The centrally located reticular formation is also indicated. The cerebral hemispheres and the thalamus are cut in frontal section, the medulla and midbrain in cross section. Note the crossing of many but not all of the auditory pathways to the opposite side of the medulla and brain stem, and input to the reticular formation. Many other connections, for example, to the cerebellum, and the efferent pathways, are omitted.

   The physiological processes that correspond very roughly to the successive anatomical levels appear in the central column. The psychological processes (at the top) are not assigned to any particular level, but in general they require the participation of the cerebral cortex. (*Modified from H. Davis in International Audiology, 3:209–215 [1964].*)

tom upward in order of their apparent complexity. So too the anatomical structures increase in complexity, both in terms of the absolute number of neurons and in terms of interconnections, as we go from auditory nerve to cerebral cortex. The psychological functions, such as perception, memory and motivation, abstract ideas, and the language code, are located in the diagram at the very top of the scale of complexity and are vaguely assigned by inference to the thalamocortical anatomical area. In fact it can be argued plausibly that such very complex activities as speech, language, abstract thinking, and planning for the future require a certain minimum gross amount of available nervous tissue available for the task. As a matter of comparative anatomy only the larger whales and some dolphins have brains that are as large as, or larger than, the human brain.

   An "understanding" of the anatomical and physiological substrate of perception, memory, thinking, and so on, is a difficult but fascinating long-term goal. It bridges the chasm between the subjective (and strictly psychological) inner world of each of us and the objective physiological, anatomical, chemical, and physical world of our bodies and their environment. The two worlds coexist in *time,* but the only thing that is able to cross the bridge between them is *information.* Both worlds are real, but the methods of observation and the concepts derived from them are different, and logically we must keep them separate.

Psychology studies behavior of the whole animal or person without concern for anatomy or physiological mechanisms, and constructs its own laws of learning, memory, drives, and so forth. Psychology also studies the modification of behavior by lesions, disease, and drugs. Physiology and psychology meet, so to speak, in that they study the same man or animal, and often they use the same words, such as memory, learning, and drive. But the physiologist and the psychologist cannot "explain" one another's observations or concepts. They can only seek parallelisms that may suggest further experiments and observations, each in its proper frame of reference. And when the physiologist talks and thinks about psychology, he is usually guilty of outrageous oversimplification, and vice versa.

A useful aphorism concerning the central nervous system is: *Remember that everything is more complicated than you think.* Perhaps this is an understatement, and we should say "Everything is very much more complicated than we can readily conceive."

As implied in the foregoing discussion, the neurophysiology and the neurology of the auditory system are far too complex to be summarized usefully in this textbook of audiology. The point of view of audiology is fundamentally that of psychology with special emphasis on psychophysics. It might even be misleading to present here an oversimplified systematic outline of neuroanatomy and neurophysiology. We shall therefore present only a few generaliza-tions that the present writer has found useful in his teaching.

### Excitation, Inhibition, and Summation: Integration

In the central nervous system, *inhibition,* meaning reduction of ongoing activity or raising the threshold for new activity, is as important and widespread as excitation. Many neurons secrete an inhibitory instead of an excitatory chemical transmitter at their axonal synaptic endings. The inhibitory transmitter increases the electrical conductance of the surface membrane of the dendrite or cell body and thus short-circuits and makes ineffective the excitatory postsynaptic potentials. The dendrites and the neuronal cell bodies sum algebraically the simultaneous inhibitory and excitatory inputs that reach them from different sources. This is known as *spatial summation.* The neuron discharges all-or-none impulses along its axon when a critical level of electrical depolarization is reached at a particular region, usually the "axon hillock," where the axon originates. The frequency of discharge depends on the degree of depolarization. A slow "spontaneous" or "tonic" discharge may continue indefinitely. The postsynaptic electrical potentials that are summed outlast the individual incoming nerve impulses so that *temporal summation* takes place over times up to a tenth of a second. This amounts to a very short-term memory. In general either temporal or spatial summation or both are required to modify the output of a neuron.

The summation of excitatory and inhibitory inputs, over space and time, are characteristic of the dendrites of neurons and thus of the gray matter in the nervous system. They are called neural "integration." Only through the balancing of excitation and inhibition, combined with negative feedback, is close motor control and coordination possible. In sensory systems inhibition is essential for fine discrimination. The principle of organization here is a *mutual inhibitory action,* based on anatomical cross connections between neighboring sensory units or between the second-order neurons that they activate. The interaction is strongest between the units that are closest to one another. The result is that a unit that is more strongly stimulated tends to inhibit its neighbors and thereby to be released from their inhibitory influence. This is a sort of positive (or double negative) feedback that serves to enhance contrast at boundaries. The mechanism is often called "lateral inhibition" because it was first described in the visual system between sensory units that lie side by side. "Mutual inhibition" is a more general term. In the mammalian auditory system this mutual inhibition is very clear in the first synaptic integrating area, namely, the cochlear nucleus in the medulla oblongata, and clearly assists in sharpening the response areas of its second-order neurons.

### Successive Integrating Stations, Multiple Pathways, and Parallel Processing

Various nuclei in the brain stem that are linked by clear tracts or "bundles" of white matter constitute the auditory system. The more important of them are indicated in Figure 3-18. The system branches repeatedly, first in the cochlear nucleus where the incoming sensory neurons divide and distribute to two major subdivisions (see also Figure 4-1). There are several output pathways from this nucleus.

There is always a delay of the order of a millisecond between the arrival of a volley (a nearly synchronous group) of impulses in incoming fibers and the appearance of a corresponding output volley. The cumulative delay measured at successive stations gives an estimate of the minimum number of synapses that must have been crossed. The term "second-order neuron" in the previous section means a neuron

that lies beyond at least one synapse, not counting the junction, if any, between specialized receptor and the first or primary neuron. The minimum number of synapses between the primary neuron and the cerebral cortex is probably three. This minimum number, and also the minimum delay along the shortest route to the cortex, can be established by observing the evoked responses at various points along the pathway. The first volley, which is the easiest to observe, has probably been overemphasized in the past. The later volleys of impulses (or asynchronous impulses) in the same or other pathways are equally important. There is at least one major pathway to the cortex in addition to the one shown in Figure 3-18, probably through the reticular formation. Other pathway(s) may be anatomically quite diffuse.

The classical term "relay station" for the successive nuclei misses a most important point. *Integrating station (or area)* is much better. Output to motor mechanisms, to other sensory systems, or feedback to more peripheral parts of the auditory system occur at all anatomical levels. The auditory cortex is only one of many final "destinations" of the incoming information. Auditory input is distributed widely. Different aspects of information contained in it are extracted in different ways (for example, by mutual inhibition as opposed to spatial summation), in different places, and for different purposes. We must think of simultaneous multiple and parallel processing of information.

### Tonotopic Organization

In the auditory pathways, as in other sensory systems, the spatial relations within the original sensory surface, whether organ of Corti, retina, skin, or somatic musculature, tend to be retained. This orderly arrangement is clear in each of the two major divisions of the cochlear nucleus. Since position along the organ of Corti is related to acoustic frequency, the arrangement is said to be "tonotopic." The tonotopic organization becomes less clear in successive integrating areas, and may be almost absent in the auditory cortex of many animals, including the cat.

Electrical activity in response to the onset of a pure tone is very widespread throughout the auditory area. Furthermore the primary auditory area, defined by the distribution of fibers from the medial geniculate body in the thalamus, is probably not the only auditory gateway to the cortex.

In the human brain the "primary projection area" of the medial geniculate body is located in the temporal lobe, on its superior surface deep in the Sylvian fissure. It is oriented perpendicular to the surface of the skull, and its electrical activity is not effectively recorded by a scalp electrode placed over the Sylvian fissure. Other neighboring area(s), called secondary auditory area(s), seem also to be part of the auditory system, both in man and animals, but the difference in function of these secondary areas, which are present in all of the sensory systems, is not known. Between the major sensory or motor areas lie the less clearly assigned "association areas" that are essential for certain very complex functions such as language, or the meaning of visual symbols, or memory of spatial relations, or the ability to plan effectively for the future.

### Homolateral versus Contralateral Representation: Dominance

In the somatosensory system (skin and somatic muscles) the topological representation is clear and systematic. The representation of each organ (hand, foot, mouth, torso, and so on) is roughly proportional to its sensory use in exploring the environment. (The manual skills of man and monkey are probably an outgrowth of this exploratory use of the hand as opposed to locomotion.) The right side of the body is represented in the left thalamus and cortex, and vice versa; that is, representation is contralateral.

In the motor control and the somatosensory representation of the limbs, the separation of right and left is complete and representation is strictly contralateral. In man, one side or the other, usually the right hand and its left cortex, are preferred or "dominant" for the learning and execution of motor skills. The visual system is organized in man with the left half of each retina projecting to the left cortex and the right halves to the right cortex. Lateral dominance or preference of right or left eye as a whole may be demonstrable but it is not particularly important. In the auditory system both ears seem to share each auditory cortex to a large extent, although the contralateral ear is more strongly represented. The extent of the homolateral representation is uncertain.

The partial crossing of the afferent auditory pathways to the opposite side takes place in the medulla in the tracts from the cochlear nucleus to the trapezoid bodies and to the superior olivary complex and the other midbrain auditory integrating areas (Figure 3-18). Each area receives some innervation from each cochlear nucleus. The first area, in time sequence and anatomical directness, in which interaction between right and left input occurs is apparently the superior olivary complex. Here some sort of priority or dominance is established in favor of the *earlier* or the *stronger* auditory input, right or left. The subjective counterpart is a perception of the sound in a spatial frame of reference, usually external, but under conditions of receiver listening inside or at the surface of the head. Another integrating area, the inferior colliculi, where there are clear pathways across the midline, seems to be related to reflex turning of head, eyes, or both toward the source of a new sound. There are feedback connections to the cochlear nuclei from anatomically "higher" centers, and also from the superior olivary complex to the cochlea (bundle of Rasmussen).

The relative simplicity and directness of

the first interaction between right and left suggests that its function is both primitive and important biologically. Apparently it is the orientation of ears (or head) to the direction of the source. This response appears early in human infancy.

There are very few indications of a dominant ear if neither one is impaired. There is, however, a strong dominance of one cerebral cortex, usually the left, for the learning of speech, both its receptive and its motor aspects. (The hemisphere not dominant for speech is probably dominant for learning spatial relations.) The dominant hemisphere for speech is not necessarily the dominant hemisphere for manual skill. Dominance for any of these functions may be altered, or develop differently, if there is early injury (before two years). The uninjured side becomes dominant. This so-called "plasticity" in the developing human brain wears off gradually after two years of age. Sensory input certainly and probably some sort of motor feedback also seem to be involved in establishing the initial patterns of sensory organization and motor skill which later appear as dominance.

## Midbrain Functions and Cortical Functions

Contrary to earlier opinion, the basic auditory discriminations of pitch and loudness and perhaps other qualities as well *can* be relearned or even learned originally by an animal that has been completely deprived of its auditory cortex. Original learning in the normal animal does involve the cortex, as shown by loss of the learned response following removal. The ablation must be complete, primary and secondary areas bilaterally. Any small part of the auditory area is sufficient for retention of the learned discrimination. This is evidence of a broad type of cortical "localization" or organization, and also of an extraordinary degree of "equipotentiality" within the major area. In the cortically deprived animal,

however, there are limitations of another sort. Broadly, the animal cannot use auditory information effectively in either the temporal or the spatial frame of reference. It can learn to discriminate tones but not to recognize *sequences* of tones, that is, even the simplest of tunes. Also it is handicapped in correct *lateralization of the source* on the basis of the cues of relative loudness or temporal precedence. The human loses his ability to understand speech after injury to certain "speech areas." One interpretation of these deficiencies related to cortical injury is that a short-term auditory memory, which is necessary for the recognition of temporal patterns, has been lost.

## Anatomical Equipotentiality and Speed of Execution

The principle of equipotentiality, meaning that any part can perform the function of the whole, apparently operates within large subdivisions of the brain. This power of "substitution," or "alternate pathways," or "cortical reserve" may extend beyond the cortex, although it is less and less clear as we approach the periphery, either on the sensory or the motor side. Certainly the nervous system is extremely adaptable in many ways. Equipotentiality is very puzzling, however, when we ask where memories are stored. The answer seems to be "everywhere and therefore nowhere." Somehow it seems to be the wrong question. The memory file in the nervous system is not item by item, spatially organized as in a filing cabinet. Memory seems to be diffuse. The clearest handicap that is related in general to the loss of central nervous tissue, either locally or diffusely (if it is less than an entire auditory or motor or somatosensory area) is a loss of speed. The job can be done but more slowly. Also learning is more difficult. It is as if a certain number of neuron-microseconds are required for complicated tasks of pattern recognition, and so on, but that a considerable amount of trading of neurons for microseconds is possible. Perhaps some neural operations that formerly could be performed in parallel must now be carried out serially by the remaining available neurons.

### Other Aspects of Neurophysiology

These disjointed comments do little more than sample the complexities of the nervous system and how it operates. For example, we will not even comment on the effects of electrical stimulation of the cerebral cortex. Further detail on some topics will be provided in appropriate contexts in other chapters, notably in Chapter 4 in relation to central dysacusis; in Chapter 8 in relation to some of the more complicated audiometric tests; and in Chapter 16, in consideration of the early development of the auditory system.

## SUGGESTED READINGS AND REFERENCES

**von Békésy, G.** *Experiments in Hearing.* (E. G. Wever, ed.) New York: McGraw-Hill Book Company, 1960.
> A collection of all of von Békésy's papers on the ear, beautifully edited, arranged, and indexed. The earlier papers, written in German, have been translated into English.

Békésy Commemorative Issue of the *Journal of the Acoustical Society of America,* Vol. 34, No. 9—part 2, 1962.
> Twenty-five papers dealing with auditory anatomy, physiology, or psychophysics. Some are reviews, others are original contributions. They include electron microscopy, the efferent olivo-cochlear bundle, the impedance of the middle ear, and the acoustic reflex.

**Davis, H.** "A Model for Transducer Action in the Cochlea," *Cold Spring Harbor Symposia on Quantitative Biology,* 30: (Sensory Receptors), 181–190. Published by Cold Spring Laboratory of Quantitative Biology, Cold Spring Harbor, L.I., New York, 1965.
> This is the author's most recent discussion of his model for cochlear excitation.

**Field, J., H. W. Magoun, and V. E. Hall (eds.).** *Handbook of Physiology, Section 1: Neurophysiology.* American Physiological Society, Washington, D.C., 1959. (Especially Chapter 23, "Excitation of Auditory Receptors," by H. Davis, and Chapter 24, "Central Auditory Mechanisms," by H. W. Ades.)
> This is the standard reference book for neurophysiologists.

**Polyak, S. L., G. McHugh, and D. K. Judd.** *The Human Ear in Anatomical Transparencies.* Elmsford, N.Y.: Sonotone Corporation, 1946. (Distributed by T. H. McKenna, Inc., New York).

A unique and very effective presentation of the anatomy of the ear accompanied by an excellent text.

"Proceedings of the International Conference on Audiology, St. Louis, May, 1957." *Laryngoscope,* 68:209–682 (1958).
This volume contains a planned symposium on the physiology of the auditory system and also many contributed papers. It is probably the best summary of several aspects of audiology in the English language as of 1957.

**Rasmussen, G. L., and W. W. Windle (eds.).** *Neural Mechanisms of the Auditory and Vestibular Systems.* Springfield, Ill., Charles C Thomas, 1960.
This volume is based on the proceedings of a conference sponsored by the National Institute for Neurological Diseases and Blindness in 1959.

**Simmons, F. B.** "Electrical Stimulation of the Auditory Nerve in Man," *Arch. Otolaryng.* (Chicago) 84:2–54 (1966).
An excellent review and a full account of the operation, and also the results of an 18 month study of a single case.

**Stevens, S. S. (ed.).** *Handbook of Experimental Psychology.* New York: John Wiley & Sons, Inc., 1951.
Chapter 27 ("The Mechanical Properties of the Ear," by G. von Békésy and W. A. Rosenblith) and Chapter 28 ("Psychophysiology of Hearing and Deafness," by H. Davis) are particularly pertinent.

**Wever, E. G. and M. Lawrence.** *Physiological Acoustics.* Princeton, N.J.: Princeton University Press, 1954.
This book deals authoritatively with sound conduction in the middle ear.

# CHAPTER 4

# ABNORMAL HEARING AND DEAFNESS

## HALLOWELL DAVIS, M.D.

## DEFINITIONS AND DISTINCTIONS

The word "deafness" has been used to mean either partial or total loss of hearing. In French the word "surdité" and in Spanish the word "sordera" have just this broad meaning. In English, however, the term "hard of hearing" has been introduced to replace the phrase "partially deaf." Unfortunately we have no corresponding noun, "hardness of hearing," equivalent to the German "Schwerhörigkeit," to replace "partial deafness." Our nearest equivalents are "impairment of hearing" and "hearing loss."

The medical and social problems of hard-of-hearing patients are quite different from those of the totally deaf, and therefore the two should not be grouped together indiscriminately. The psychological value of this point is discussed at some length in later chapters, but there is still some confusion resulting from old habits of speech and from the necessity of distinguishing between two or three terms.

The introduction of new terms and the change in the meaning of old ones depend on the gathering of new information, the development of new insights, and the formulation of new purposes. We therefore repeat some old definitions, carefully worded and phrased, and introduce certain new or nearly new additional terms. A change in terminology involves, of course, the rejection of some old terms and the restriction of the meaning of others.

### Deafness, Hearing Loss, and Dysacusis

The simple, everyday concept of "deafness" is a total or severe impairment of hearing, and in this book we shall continue to use "deafness" to include total loss of hearing, whatever the cause. Impairment of hearing of the sort that simply requires the other person to talk louder we shall call a "hearing loss," and we shall avoid the term "partial deafness." Hearing loss and deafness both imply a loss of sensitivity of hearing, presumably in the peripheral hearing mechanisms. Both lie along the same

83

dimension, and the question is where to draw the line between hard of hearing and deaf.

The usefulness of a criterion depends on our purposes, and the important purposes for which these terms are useful are social, educational, and medical. We shall adopt a *social criterion for deafness,* namely, that *everyday auditory communication is impossible or very nearly so.* In terms of hearing levels we find a zone of uncertainty from 70 to 90 dB (ISO) averaged over the frequencies 500, 1000, and 2000 Hz. Within this zone some individuals are socially deaf, but more of them are merely very hard of hearing. The frequent successful use of hearing aids makes it undesirable to include this "gray area" automatically under the term "deaf," as has often been the custom in the past. *We propose to confine the term deafness to hearing-threshold levels for speech greater than 92 dB (ISO).* A good reason for selecting this particular boundary is that the most authoritative medical rule for estimating the handicap imposed by hearing loss (see Chapter 9) reads "if the average hearing threshold level at 500, 1000, and 2000 Hz is over 92 dB (ISO), the handicap for hearing everyday speech should be considered total." Our criterion thus has a medical sanction in a social and economic context.

We point out that in the previous paragraphs we have given "hearing-threshold levels for speech" that are actually inferred from ISO hearing levels for pure tones. As explained in Chapter 7 there has been, ever since speech audiometry was introduced, a discrepancy between the hearing-threshold level for speech as measured directly by a speech audiometer, calibrated according to the American Standard for speech audiometers of 1952, and the hearing-threshold level for speech as inferred from the average levels for the pure tones 500, 1000, and 2000 Hz when the latter are measured with a pure-tone audiometer calibrated to the ASA-1951 reference zero levels. This discrepancy

has been clearly recognized only recently. Fortunately it practically disappears if the pure-tone audiometer is calibrated to the new "ISO" reference levels.

In the previous edition of this book (1960) the "hearing level for speech" which was used to define the lower limit of "deafness" was given as 82 dB. This is the value which was recommended by the Committee on Conservation of Hearing as corresponding to "total handicap" for hearing everyday speech. The context here was explicitly the average of the three pure-tone hearing-threshold levels and not a directly measured hearing-threshold level for speech. In the present edition we have therefore changed the number of decibels to 93 dB (ISO), and we introduce the convention of specifying it as "hearing-threshold level for speech (ISO)" as a short-hand way of reminding the reader that we refer to the average pure-tone hearing-threshold level and not to the level determined by speech audiometry. (The International Standards Organization has not issued any recommendation for a reference zero level for speech audiometers.)

We do not here propose any educational criterion for deafness. Whether a child is judged to be "educable" or not may involve his visual skills, his intelligence, his emotional stability, and so on, perhaps in addition to handicaps other than deafness. Most deaf children, as well as hard-of-hearing children, can be educated, although the methods may differ, as we shall see in Chapters 16 and 17.

The successful use of a hearing aid may make the difference between being socially deaf or being merely hard of hearing even for some persons whose hearing-threshold levels for speech are 93 dB (ISO) or higher. For them hard of hearing is a better practical designation than deaf. This is true even though in the context of accidental injury or industrial hearing loss their handicap for hearing everyday speech is considered total. In assessment of handicap for purposes of compensation the evaluation is made without the use of a hearing aid.

So far we have considered only the dimension of sensitivity of hearing. On this dimension the zone of normal includes hearing-threshold levels for speech from 0 to 25 dB (ISO). The condition known as hard of hearing begins at 27 db (ISO) and that for deaf begins at 93 db (ISO) (see Chapters 2 and 9). There is, however, another dimension or, rather, several other dimensions of hearing which may be impaired. For example, a person may say "Don't shout. I hear you, but I can't make out the words." Then it is his "discrimination for speech" that is faulty. Or he may be unable to attach meaning to auditory signals because of a failure of understanding of the type we call "auditory agnosia." And there are other kinds of impairment which we shall consider in more detail later in this chapter. All of these other types of impairment of hearing have one feature in common which makes it desirable to have a single term to include all of them. The common feature is that *they are not simple losses of sensitivity of hearing.* These impairments cannot be measured properly in decibels. *The inclusive term that we shall use for all of these other impairments of hearing is dysacusis.*

Dysacusis is not a new word in the medical vocabulary, but it is not yet widely used. It means, however, just what we want to say: "faulty hearing." "Acusis" (or acousis) refers to hearing, as in the more familiar terms "presbycusis," "diplacusis." "Dys-" as a prefix may mean "ill" or "painful," but it also means "difficult," "faulty," "impaired," or "abnormal."

Dysacusis (also spelled "dysacusia" and "dysacousia") may be due to malfunction of the sense organ, or it may be due to abnormal function of the brain. Thus certain forms of diplacusis, presbycusis, and discrimination loss we will call "peripheral dysacusis," and we will use the term "central dysacusis" for such conditions as psychogenic or hysterical block of hearing, auditory agnosia, phonemic regression, and so on.

A point that must be emphasized immediately is that *deafness or hearing loss* on the one hand and *dysacusis,* both peripheral and central, on the other hand, *are not mutually exclusive.* A patient may have both a hearing loss, measurable in decibels, and also a dysacusis in the form of a loss of discrimination or some phonemic regression or the like. In case of doubt, dysacusis should be considered the broader term equivalent to impairment of hearing of all kinds, two or three of which may be present at the same time. Hard of hearing *implies specifically one kind of impairment,* the one that is best understood and most readily measured, namely, *simple loss of sensitivity,* presumably in the ear itself or in its nerve. Deafness will remain the general term for the symptom of total or nearly total loss of hearing, but we shall avoid the term "central deafness." Of course, before a diagnosis is made we may use the terms "deaf" and "dysacusic," or "hard of hearing" and "dysacusic" pretty much interchangeably. Dysacusis is the word to use when we wish to emphasize either (1) that the symptom is not merely reduced sensitivity of hearing, or (2) that the trouble may lie in the central nervous system rather than in the ear.

For those who enjoy complete, well-rounded systems of nomenclature there are the terms *anacusia* (or "anacousia") and *hypoacusia* (or "hypoacousia"), which can be used as exact synonyms for deafness and hearing loss, respectively.

## Varieties of Auditory Impairment

From the medical and anatomical point of view there are three major types of impairment of hearing: poor conduction of sound to the sense organ, abnormality of the sense organ or its nerve, and impairments that result from some injury to or failure of function in the central nervous system. These broad divisions are illustrated in Figure 4-1. One problem of otological and audiological diagnosis is to assess correctly the part played by each *type of impairment* for each particular patient. Another is to determine just *where the impairment is located*, whether in the external ear, the middle ear, the cochlea, the organ of Corti, the auditory nerve, or within the central nervous system. Another problem, of course, is to determine the probable *cause* of the difficulty. Unfortunately the dividing lines between types of difficulty, such as impairment of physical sound conduction versus failure of excitation of nerve impulses, do not always coincide with obvious anatomical boundaries such as the tympanic membrane or the oval window. This has led to considerable difficulty in the choice and consistent use of appropriate terms.

The common mild or moderate impairments that are due to failure of normal physical conduction of sound to the cochlea are hearing losses, and the people who suffer from them are hard of hearing. If it is only physical conduction that is impaired, the hearing threshold level cannot be worse than about 70 dB (ISO) because at this level bone conduction takes over, and the sound is heard, provided the sense organ is still intact. Really loud speech can still be understood, and the successful use of a hearing aid is relatively easy. We shall therefore speak of *conductive hearing loss* and give up the old term conductive deafness. As we shall see, conductive hearing loss includes but is not quite equivalent to "middle-ear impairment."

Auditory agnosia, phonemic regression, and hysterical or psychogenic dysacusis are very clearly the result of some abnormal functioning of the central nervous system. The patient may or may not respond to a test with an audiometer, and he may give very different results on different trials. He is, however, unable to understand speech, or does so only in a very limited way, even though he may "hear" something on the audiometer.

Greater difficulties of definition appear when the trouble lies anatomically within the cochlea or in the central auditory connections, or both. For this group of disorders we shall use either dysacusis or hearing loss, depending on whether we wish to emphasize loss of discrimination or loss of sensitivity. We shall lean toward the medical tradition in our basic classification and usually speak of *sensory-neural hearing loss*.[1] Sometimes we want to distinguish between disorders of the sense organ and impairment of the auditory nerve. Modern diagnostic tests are making this distinction possible and, as we shall see, the accurate diagnosis of the site and type of the trouble is of great importance for prognosis and, above all, for treatment. We shall then speak of "sense-organ dysacusis" or "sense-organ hearing loss," on the one hand, and "neural hearing loss" (or sometimes "neural dysacusis"), on the other. We shall avoid the familiar but less grammatical form "nerve deafness," and particularly the pernicious term "perceptive deafness." The latter is a wastebasket term once much used by otologists to catch everything that is not conductive. This usage disregards the prior use of the terms "perception" and "perceptive" by psychologists. If the term ever had a proper logical meaning, it should have meant approximately what we now call "auditory agnosia" or "central perceptive dysacusis," but for a long time it was a synonym for "nerve deafness."

Still another term is necessary to describe the common combination of conductive and sensory-neural hearing losses. For this we shall use the familiar term "mixed

[1] (The American Academy of Ophthalmology and Otolaryngology favors the spelling "sensorineural." We shall continue to use "sensory-neural," however, to emphasize that we mean "sensory and/or neural."

hearing loss," but it will not include impairments that lie central to the auditory nerve.

When, as also may happen, a person has some conductive, or sensory-neural, or mixed hearing loss, and also some *central* difficulties of the central perceptive or of the psychogenic variety, we shall speak of a "combined dysacusis" or perhaps of a "peripheral hearing loss with a psychogenic (or central or agnosic) overlay."

The proper antonym for "central" is "peripheral." "Peripheral" hearing loss means "conductive, or sensory-neural, or mixed" hearing loss. The otologist may sometimes use the word "retrocochlear" to cover the anatomical areas beyond the cochlea, that is, auditory nerve, brain stem and beyond, or, practically speaking, everything outside the primary domain and responsibility of otology. "Retrocochlear" or "retrolabyrinthine" includes tumors of the auditory nerve but excludes sense-organ impairment.

A pair of contrasting terms in common use are "organic" and "functional." Organic implies that the difficulty is caused by an anatomical injury or abnormality which a pathologist could identify if he looked in the right place. Functional may mean either "nonorganic," or "physiological," or "with no visible pathology" or "better understood on a psychological than on an anatomical basis." An objection to these terms, in addition to the vagueness of functional, is the implication that they usually carry that a difficulty is exclusively organic *or* functional, whereas, more often than not, anatomical, physiological, and psychological factors are all significant.

*Hearing loss and hearing level.* The term "hearing loss" has carried a heavy burden for the last three decades. In the medical and social senses in which we have used it here it has served to mean "an impairment of hearing that does not entirely prevent practical communication by speech." But hearing loss has also been used to mean the number of decibels by which the threshold of hearing is elevated above the zero level to which an audiometer is calibrated. Hearing loss has also been used to mean a change for the worse or shift of threshold from one level to another. Thus, the term can be very confusing, as in the following statements which might have been made in a court or before an industrial commission.

This employee suffered a hearing loss of 40 dB from exposure to noise. He had a hearing loss of 25 dB before employment, which, however, is just within normal limits. His actual hearing loss was 65 dB when he was examined the day after stopping work. Of this loss, 10 dB later proved to be a temporary hearing loss, so his permanent hearing loss now appears to be 55 dB. This is not conductive. It is a pure sensory-neural hearing loss.

In Chapter 2 we introduced the relatively new term "hearing-threshold level" to take some of the load off hearing loss. Hearing-threshold level is the number of decibels that a person's threshold of hearing lies above the reference zero of the audiometer for that particular frequency (or for that particular speech test). The U.S.A. Standards for Audiometers of 1951 and 1952 required that the intensity dial be labeled "hearing loss," and most audiogram charts were marked the same way; but in the next revision (after 1968) the term will undoubtedly be "hearing level" instead. The sound pressure levels produced by an audiometer, measured in an appropriate coupler and referred to standard audiometric reference zero level are "hearing levels." The audiometer reading which corresponds to the faintest tone that a person can hear is his "hearing-threshold level" for that frequency.

Furthermore, when there is any possibility of ambiguity, we shall call a shift or change of threshold a *threshold shift* and not a hearing loss. The least one can do to avoid confusion when referring to a change of level is to speak of a "loss of hearing" and not a "hearing loss."

In sum, we shall use (1) *hearing level* to designate the output of an audiometer referred to an audiometric zero level, (2) *hearing-threshold level* to designate the sensitivity of an individual's hearing, and (3) *threshold shift* for any change in his hearing-threshold level; and we shall reserve (4) *hearing loss* for the general condition of impaired hearing or the process that causes it. The implications of "hearing loss" are of a partial handicap or of an abnormality of structure or function. "Hearing-threshold level," however, carries no implication of handicap or even abnormality. It simply states the result of an objective psychophysical measurement. The calibration or reference zero level of the audiometer should always be specified (ASA-1951 or ISO), as noted in Chapter 7. A practical rule to keep the usage of these terms straight is: "If decibels are involved, the proper term isn't 'hearing loss'; it is either 'hearing level' or 'threshold shift.'"

Another rule to which we shall return in Chapter 9 is: "There is no such thing as percentage of hearing level or even percentage of hearing loss." Occasionally we talk of percentage of handicap, and a lawyer may talk about percentage of disability, but these values are calculated by arbitrary rules and only for particular purposes such as compensation.

Now with our new terms to help us, let us try again that statement made in court by the examining physician. He now says:

This employee suffered a loss of hearing from exposure to noise. The threshold shift was 40 dB. His hearing-threshold level before employment was 25 dB (ISO), which is just within normal limits. His actual hearing-threshold level the day after he stopped work was 65 dB (ISO). Of this, 10 dB proved to be a temporary threshold shift, so his final and presumably permanent hearing-threshold level now appears to be 55 dB (ISO). He

does not have any conductive hearing loss; his impairment is purely sensory-neural.

## PERIPHERAL HEARING LOSS

A few moments' study of the anatomy of the ear, described in Chapter 3 and summarized in a diagram in Figure 4-1, will make clear the distinctions between middle-ear impairment and cochlear impairment. The distinction is important because the prognosis and the treatment, as well as the causes of the two types, differ considerably. It is sometimes very simple to distinguish between the two by tests of hearing, but it is always possible and even probable that any case is really a mixture or combination of the two impairments. Figure 4-1 also shows that the division between the conductive process and the sensory-neural processes lies within the cochlea at the hair cells. Conductive hearing loss includes middle-ear impairment but extends beyond it.

Conductive hearing loss may be caused by plugging the external canal, damping the free movement of the drum, or restricting the movements of the ossicles. Any of these will reduce the intensity of the airborne sound that finally reaches the inner ear. Wax impacted in the canal is the commonest form of plug, and wax in contact with the drum or the scars of old healed perforations of the drum may restrict its vibrations. Adhesions of scar tissue on the ossicles or a bony new growth of otosclerosis around the edge of the stapes in the oval window may restrict the normal movements of the ossicles even more severely.

### Middle-ear Hearing Loss

The classical test to distinguish middle-ear from cochlear or sensory-neural impairment is the difference between air-conduction hearing levels and bone-conduction hearing levels. With severe impairment of conduction in the middle ear, as from adhesions or otosclerosis, the audiometer may show a hearing-threshold level for airborne sound as high as 60 or possibly 70 dB (ISO). The patient may be quite unable to hear a vibrating tuning fork held close beside his ear. Thus, his "air conduction" is said to be "reduced." But if the shaft of the vibrating fork is now applied to his skull, or the bone-conduction vibrator of the audiometer is placed on the mastoid bone just behind his ear, he may be able to hear the sound as well as a normal person does in the same test. There is no reduction in his "bone conduction."

If he can hear normally by bone conduction, we infer that his inner ear and auditory nerve must be normal and that his difficulty in hearing depends only on some obstacle in the external or middle ear to the conduction of airborne sound. Audiograms showing hearing-threshold levels by air conduction and by bone conduction in sensory-neural loss and in middle-ear conductive loss are shown in Chapter 7, where the audiogram is explained in detail.

It is tempting to assume that if *bone* conduction is reduced, there must be a corresponding degree of sensory-neural hearing loss. However there are practical pitfalls. Some skulls and the skin and soft tissues over them do not conduct sound as well as others. As another example, when the footplate of the stapes is firmly fixed in the oval window by otosclerosis, the fluids in the inner ear can no longer move so freely under the influence of bone-conducted acoustic energy. This makes the hearing-threshold level at 2000 Hz for bone conduction 10 to 15 dB poorer than it would otherwise be. At 500, 1000, and 4000 Hz the threshold shift is usually only 5 to 10 dB. The resulting dip in the bone-conduction audiogram is sometimes called the "Carhart notch." Following successful fenestration or stapes surgery the bone-conduction threshold shifts back toward zero by this amount.

In addition, there are special technical difficulties in obtaining accurate measurements of hearing-threshold levels by bone conduction, such as the presence of too much background noise in the test room. These will also be considered in Chapter 7, but in general the audiologist or otologist hesitates to conclude that he is dealing with sensory-neural hearing loss simply on the basis of finding poor hearing by bone conduction without supporting evidence.

Conductive hearing loss is not much of a handicap to hearing in a noisy place. In fact, a man with pure conductive hearing loss of moderate degree can hear conversation just as well as the average person can (and better than a great many) in traffic, in airplanes, and in similar noisy surroundings. Under these conditions he simply does not hear, or hears only faintly, the noise that disturbs his companion with normal hearing and masks speech at ordinary conversational levels. But in noise all of us automatically talk louder—loud enough so that we can hear ourselves above the noise. The loud speech overrides a moderate conductive hearing loss. The problem for our hard-of-hearing listener is no longer that of *hearing* the speech but only of *distinguishing* it from as much of the noise as also succeeds in reaching his sense organ. Since he does not hear much of the noise and his sense organ is normal, he can distinguish and understand the loud speech as well as anyone. Furthermore, the training in understanding speech that has been forced on him by his hearing loss is likely to give him an actual advantage over a person with normal hearing. This ability to hear in noisy places as well as, or better than, normal persons has been given the impressive name of *paracusis Willisii* and is characteristic of conductive hearing loss.

### Inner-ear Conductive Hearing Loss

Until recently all inner-ear impairments were automatically classed as sensory-neural. It now appears useful to recognize that physical changes can occur in the basilar membrane and the tectorial membrane, or both, and that they may reduce the efficiency with which acoustic energy is

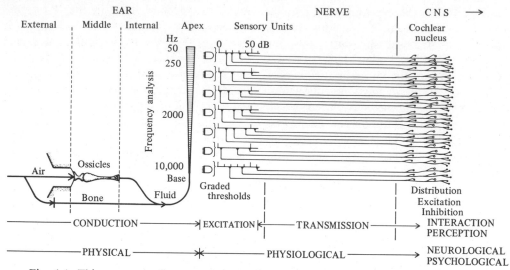

Fig. 4-1. This summary diagram of the peripheral auditory mechanism is semianatomical. The air-conduction pathway shows the ossicles simplified to a subdivided columella, disregarding their lever action. The single bone-conduction pathway combines all of the pathways that bypass the ossicular chain. The air and bone pathways unite beyond the ossicles in the fluids of the inner ear. The tapering basilar membrane is represented as straight. Here acoustic frequency analysis takes place, as indicated. All of this is part of the physical process of sound conduction.

The sensory units are represented by nerve fibers (with cell bodies omitted), running from the hair cells arranged along the basilar membrane to the cochlear nucleus where they branch to several (here three) distinct regions, each of which preserves the tonotopic organization of the basilar membrane. Each of the hair cells shown in the diagram represents the group of cells in a short segment of the organ of Corti. In such a segment there is partial overlapping of innervation (See Figure 3-14). The sensory units from any small segment, represented arbitrarily here by groups of 3 or 4, have different thresholds for any given tone. The gradation of thresholds is represented here by an arbitrary scale of decibels, 0 to 50, for each small segment. The actual range of gradation is not known, nor is its relation to anatomical distribution, such as inner versus outer hair cells. (Further discussion in text in Chapter 3.) The efferent auditory nerves are omitted from this diagram.

delivered to the hair cells. In this chapter we define the sense organ and sensory hearing loss as beginning at the hair cells, as indicated in Figure 4-1. This provides a more logical set of definitions with (1) proper distinctions between anatomical areas and physiological processes, (2) recognition of the tissues of the basilar and tectorial membranes as the potential site of significant physical changes, notably as the result of aging, (3) a more plausible explanation of the results of certain tests of hearing, notably the "recruitment of loudness," which will be discussed below, and (4) a conceptual framework adequate for

our rapidly increasing knowledge of the pathology of the inner ear.

Some useful generalizations about conductive hearing loss and its alleviation are as follows.

1. A conductive abnormality always causes more or less attenuation of the acoustic energy that reaches the sense organ. The normal young ear is about as efficient physically as it can possibly be, and can only get worse. Nature does not introduce new amplifiers into the system.

2. The attenuation is usually, although not always, different for different frequen-

cies. Sometimes the attenuation is greater the lower the frequency. This gives the so-called "rising audiogram," which was once thought to be characteristic of conductive hearing loss or middle-ear impairment. Quite often, however, the audiogram falls toward the high frequencies. This is particularly true of the types of inner- and middle-ear conductive impairment associated with aging. Theoretically we may also expect small increases of acoustic transmission in one part of the spectrum associated with attenuation in neighboring parts. This would be the result of a shift in the resonant frequency or natural period of one of the components of the transmission system due to changes in its mass or stiffness, or both, but such increases in transmission are small and rather rare.

3. Conductive impairments may occur in different parts of the system simultaneously, and their effects will be additive.

4. Conductive impairments may make the system more nonlinear in its action and thus increase the distortion of the acoustic wave forms that reach the sense organ.

5. The attenuation of conductive impairment can be imitated by electrical or acoustic filters and, subject to limitations imposed by nonlinearity, it can be offset by amplification, provided also that the frequency characteristics of the amplifier are properly chosen.

6. Any nonlinear distortion associated with the impairment will not be corrected, but is likely to become worse when the input signal is increased in order to deliver more acoustic energy to the sense organ—and the amplifier may introduce additional distortion of its own.

### Sensory-neural Hearing Loss

Sensory-neural impairment is best understood in anatomical and physiological terms. The concept of the sensory unit (see Chapter 3) is helpful. It will be recalled that a sensory unit is an auditory nerve fiber plus the hair cell or cells that excite it. There is actually a slight overlap among units, with one fiber innervating two to several hair cells while one hair cell may be innervated by two to a dozen or so nerve fibers. We shall center attention on the nerve fibers rather than on the cells, because the nerve is the bottleneck for transmission of auditory information and also because the traffic of impulses in single fibers has been studied experimentally.

As a simplification, Figure 4-1 shows several groups of fibers running to different segments of the organ of Corti on the basilar membrane. The hair cells of that segment are indicated schematically by a single hair cell and by an intensity scale for each segment. The nerve fibers attach to the scale at different points. This is a graphic representation of the differences in threshold of different sensory units in a given small segment of the organ of Corti. Such differences, particularly as between inner and outer sensory units presumably exist. The range of 60 dB, used arbitrarily in Figure 4-1, may prove to be somewhat too large. Note also in Figure 4-1 the scale of frequency along the basilar membrane, which expresses the place principle. Recall also that the threshold of hearing lies at an extremely low energy level and that, in animal experiments, most if not all units are actually firing spontaneously at low rates even in the quiet.

In such a system as this we can expect several types of impairment, including (1) absence of units, (2) abnormal thresholds for some or all units, (3) increase in spontaneous activity, (4) abnormally rapid fatigue, (5) abnormal effects or lack of any effect at all from the efferent nerve supply (not shown in the diagram), and possibly (6) abnormal peripheral interactions among neighboring sensory units. Each of these impairments might affect all units equally, its effect might be graded uniformly in some way, or it might be distributed at random. The different impairments can combine with one another and also with conductive impairment in either middle or inner ear or both. It is not surprising that there are many auditory signs and symptoms or that a single cause may produce a variety of effects. Nevertheless the concept of sensory units allows us to construct a series of models approximating the major clinical types and etiological groups of impairments. These models are tentative explanations which may help us to understand the nature of each impairment and the possibilities for its therapy or rehabilitation.

Three additional characteristics of the sensory units, in addition to their anatomical distribution and graded thresholds, are important. One is the "all-or-none" character of the nerve impulses which they carry. Another is the small dynamic range for each unit of acoustic intensity between threshold level and saturation level, that is, the level of stimulation at which the sensory unit reaches its maximum number of impulses per second. With a steady stimulus the long-term rate is normally maintained indefinitely, but the long-term rate is considerably below the initial transient maximum output. Still another characteristic of a unit is its rather narrow "response area" or frequency range (see Figure 3-16). The threshold rises rapidly, although unsymmetrically, both above and below the best or characteristic frequency. The steepness of the boundary helps to explain frequency discrimination. The overlap of response areas explains the wide dynamic (intensity) range over which the total output of impulses from all units increases with increase in the stimulus level. Units that are "tuned" above the stimulating frequency, and also some tuned slightly below it, are progressively activated as the intensity increases.

## Particular Sensory-neural and Mixed Hearing Impairments

*Abrupt high-tone hearing loss.* The word "abrupt" refers here to the shape of the audiogram, not to any suddenness in time of the onset of the condition. As a matter of fact this type of impairment is very stable and probably has a congenital hereditary basis. It is much more common in males than in females, and it has long been confused with noise-induced hearing loss. The sensitivity of hearing is normal or nearly so for low tones but falls off abruptly at a rate of as much as 80 dB per octave or steeper. Sometimes the loss is total above the abrupt drop. Sometimes the audiogram continues to fall toward the very high frequencies, but less steeply. Very rarely does it rise toward higher frequencies. The loss is usually bilateral and at nearly the same frequency in each ear. The hearing for high tones is so poor that it is usually appropriate to call the condition "abrupt high-tone deafness," meaning deafness for high tones with an abrupt transition.

The handicap in terms of understanding speech depends critically on the frequency at which the drop in sensitivity occurs. If it is at 3000 Hz or above, the practical handicap is very slight. If it is at 1000 Hz or below, the handicap is great. The high-frequency components that give character to the plosive and fricative consonants and even to some vowels are lost, and the listener is dependent on recognizing very small differences among the sounds that he is able to hear. His discrimination score for word lists (see Chapter 7) is reduced, although not to zero. He may be able, perhaps with some effort, to understand speech in quiet surroundings, but if much noise is mixed with the speech, he has more difficulty than a person with normal hearing.

The audiogram of one ear of an individual with abrupt high-tone loss is shown in Figure 4-2, together with a "map" of the

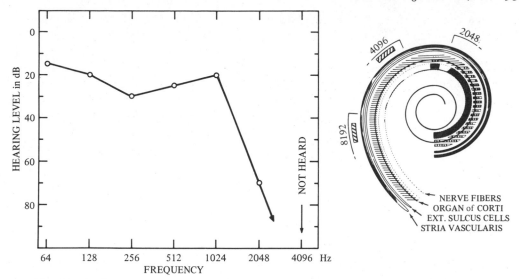

Fig. 4-2. Audiogram and chart of postmortem findings in an ear with abrupt high-tone loss. The actual fall in sensitivity of hearing may have been even more abrupt (steeper) than shown because no measurements were made between 1024 and 2048 Hz.

Inner spiral, nerve fibers; black = normal, white = degenerated.

Second spiral, organ of Corti; rectangle with large dots = organ of Corti with normal hair cells, plain line = organ of Corti degenerated.

Third and fourth spirals; black = normal, and white = abnormal external sulcus cells and stria vascularis, respectively.

Outside the spiral on the right are indicated the zones required for the normal reception of frequencies 2048, 4096 and 8192 Hz, based on correlation of audiograms and locations of abnormalities of 79 human ears. The shaded rectangles show the most probable locations for 4096 and 8192 Hz. (*Data and chart from Crowe, Guild, and Polvogt. Bull. Hopkins Hosp., 54:315–739 [1934]* © The Johns Hopkins Press.)

abnormalities found at postmortem examination of that ear. The sensory units, both the nerve fibers and the hair cells, are missing from the basal (high-frequency) portion of the first turn. The transition from normal to complete absence of sensory units is very abrupt. This is a clear case of what we may call *subtractive hearing loss,* meaning a loss of sensory units, in contrast to "conductive hearing loss."

*Gradual high-tone hearing loss.* This term also refers to the slope of the audiogram, but as a rule the impairment does develop gradually over a period of months or a few years, as in some forms of otitis media; or over many years, as in chronic suppurative otitis media or in presbycusis. Typically the audiogram is

fairly flat up to 1000 Hz but then slopes steadily downward toward the higher frequencies at a rate of 10 to 30 dB per octave. Sometimes the downward slope begins at 500 or 250 Hz. The bone-conduction audiogram may or may not show a similar but perhaps less pronounced slope. These gradually sloping audiograms are frequently associated with conductive impairment of the middle ear and (probably) of the inner ear also, that is, with "mixed" hearing loss.

At postmortem, some loss of sensory units, either the nerve fibers or the hair cells or both, has been shown in some cases, particularly in individuals who were 65 years or older at death. The loss of units is usually most severe in the basal turn and progressively greater toward the extreme basal end. But in at least half of the ears examined in the classical study by Crowe, Guild, and Polvogt in 1934 no loss of sensory units could be demonstrated to be sufficient to account for the known hearing loss, particularly when due regard was given to the location in the basal turn of the areas critical for hearing particular frequencies such as 4096 and 8192 Hz (see Figure 4-2). Neither was there in these ears any fixation of the stapes by otosclerosis or any gross adhesion in the middle ear that could account for the hearing loss. In short, no basis in pathology could be found for the hearing impairment.

On the basis of this and other studies we conclude that in gradual high-tone hearing loss without middle-ear disease a loss of sensory units *may* contribute significantly to the impairment in many cases, but loss of units is rarely a complete explanation, and often not even a partial explanation. We must invoke as the primary cause more subtle and sometimes hypothetical factors such as elevated thresholds (sensory impairment) or inner-ear conductive changes which cannot be detected under the microscope. Partial loss of units, even if it is most severe in the basal turn, does not explain why the audiogram should slope systematically downward or even why it should be affected at all. In fact in some experimental situations of partial injury of the auditory nerve the loss of units may be considerable although behavioral thresholds remain normal. This is to be expected from our model. If the loss of units is random, provided some very sensitive units remain and are well distributed along the basilar membrane, the threshold should not be affected. There is no necessary relation between the density of sensory units and the threshold of the most sensitive units.

The gradual steady slope of the audiogram in typical "gradual high-tone hearing loss" is in sharp contrast to the "4000 Hz notch" that is very characteristic of *noise-induced hearing loss*. In this condition the threshold shift, relative to audiometric zero, is greater for 4000 Hz, and usually for 6000 Hz also, than for 8000 Hz. The origin and certain other characteristics of this type of high-tone sensory-neural loss will be described below. We still do not have enough good postmortem information on noise-induced hearing loss to say whether some sensory units are actually destroyed or whether, as seems quite probable, they suffer only an elevation of threshold, or both.

*Congenital and Toxic Impairments.* Congenital and toxic impairments will be considered later from the etiologic point of view and with respect to prospects of rehabilitation. They include many very severe hearing losses. In terms of our model we can say that definite abnormalities such as the complete absence of hair cells, can frequently account for the impairment. In some congenital conditions, however, although the organ of Corti seems to be deformed, the hair cells still are present. Sometimes the tectorial membrane is detached, rolled up in the inner sulcus, and covered with a layer of epithelial cells; or perhaps Reissner's membrane is adherent to the organ of Corti, or both. These obvious anatomical defects can logically be classed as "inner-ear conductive impairments." Some may argue that the sense organ as a whole is abnormal even though the hair cells and nerves are present and that it is therefore a "sensory" impairment. Whichever term is used, however, it is reassuring to know that in some of these conditions many sensory units seem to be present although it may be difficult to stimulate them.

*Loudness recruitment* is a symptom which seems to be clearly related to abnormality of the sense organ and which cannot be caused by a conductive impairment. The phenomenon, observed by Dr. Edmund P. Fowler in 1928 and named by him in 1939, is an abnormally rapid growth of the sensation of loudness as the intensity of a sound is increased. In terms of the power law, discussed in Chapter 2, the exponent in the power law equation is larger than normal, and therefore the slope of the graph is steeper. In everyday experience we are aware that a fairly intense sound in a normal ear may be masked by background noise and be inaudible until its "masked threshold" is reached. When it emerges from the masking, it quite rapidly becomes louder, and at about 30 dB above the masked threshold it sounds as loud as it does without any noise in the background. This is a perfectly normal form of loudness recruitment. The abnormal form occurs without any masking noise. It can only occur, however, if the threshold is elevated by a sensory impairment. The measurement of loudness recruitment by "loudness balance" is described in Chapter 8.

Loudness recruitment in sensory hearing loss is usually but not necessarily complete at about 90 dB hearing level (ISO). Sometimes the loudness overshoots (overrecruitment) and a particular tone sounds louder to the abnormal ear than to the normal ear. Sometimes at high hearing levels the growth of loudness becomes less rapid than normal (decruitment), but in the absence of other symptoms the net result of pure recruitment is that the function of the abnormal ear is *less* impaired at high hearing levels than at low levels. In fact not only loudness balances but discrimination tests for intensity, for frequency, and for words are within normal limits.

The condition in which pure loudness recruitment is most clearly and regularly seen is a moderate but permanent noise-induced hearing loss or threshold shift. The only clear impairment is elevation of threshold over part or all of the spectrum. The recruitment definitely offsets part of this impairment and can be considered a "benign recruitment."

We emphasize the benign character of pure recruitment because recruitment is often associated with various forms of dysacusis that will be described below. These may be quite distressing and prevent the understanding of speech. Unfortunately the term recruitment was often used to include all of these other impairments, and it became at one time almost synonymous with what we now call "peripheral dysacusis." This misuse of the term should be carefully avoided.

As a diagnostic sign recruitment is very helpful if the patient is able to make the necessary loudness balances reliably. Recruitment is very characteristic of what we call sense-organ impairment, but not of conductive or neural impairment. It is produced by a retrocochlear neural lesion such as an eighth nerve tumor in only about 25 percent of cases. Here partial recruitment is more common, however.

In terms of sensory units, we know that the dynamic range of intensity of the ear is compressed in sensory hearing loss. This could be brought about by a systematic elevation of the thresholds of the more sensitive units. It is reasonable to suppose that in the case of habitual noise-exposure it is the units to which acoustic energy is delivered most efficiently that have the lowest thresholds and also are exposed to the greater mechanical stresses at high sound levels. Permanent elevation of threshold might be brought about by physical change in macrostructure of the hair cells or by chemical changes in microstructure. Here we can only speculate, but the hypothesis of a systematic elevation of thresholds without destruction provides a plausible and adequate model for recruitment of loudness. In other conditions other explanations of recruitment (all of them hypothetical) are more probable.

*Peripheral dysacusis.* The impairments that we have considered so far are quite well grouped together as "hypoacusia," meaning loss of sensitivity of hearing. Elevation of the threshold is the general characteristic.

In conductive hearing loss the equal-loudness contours, described in Chapter 2, are elevated. Their form, like that of the threshold curve, may be changed, but their spacing remains constant. In sensory hearing loss, recruitment usually partially offsets the threshold hypoacusia: the spacing of the equal loudness contours is compressed, usually more at some frequencies than at others. All of this lies in the intensity-loudness domain.

*Diplacusis.* Diplacusis, or "hearing double," is an impairment in the frequency-pitch domain. One symptom is that a given pure tone has different pitches in the two ears. This is *diplacusis binauralis.* Careful comparisons show that most people have a little diplacusis for some parts of the frequency scale most of the time; but unless the condition becomes rather considerable, amounting to differences of a quarter of a tone or more, they are quite unaware of the inequalities. As pointed out in Chapter 2, the brain can average small pitch differences between the ears just as it averages small differences in color vision between the two eyes. There is a limit to this integrative ability, however, and if the tones are heard separately and differently, the symptom may be quite disturbing and distressing, particularly to musicians and music lovers.

Another kind of diplacusis is a loss of the clear musical tonal quality of the sound of a pure tone. The tone becomes "rough," "impure," "noisy," or "buzzing," or may sound like a complex inharmonious mixture of tones. In extreme cases two or more distinct tones may be heard simultaneously. In diplacusis binauralis one ear may hear the tone normally while the other hears it as noisy and impure as well as at a different pitch. The hearing of two tones or a tone and noise simultaneously in one ear is called "diplacusis monauralis." It is clearly a form of dysacusis, and in its presence the ability to discriminate spoken words is reduced or even lost entirely.

*Tinnitus.* Tinnitus means "head noises" or "ringing in the ears." The subject hears sound or sounds more or less continuously, without any related acoustic stimulus. Most people have some weak high-pitched tinnitus most of the time, although they may not notice it except in very quiet surroundings. The loudness is likely to be matched to that of a tone some 20 dB above threshold. Other people have head noises that they describe as rushing or roaring, and they may compare them to wind in the trees or to an air blast, or sometimes a low-pitched roar. Such a roar is common in Menière's disease. Sometimes it is related to and therefore "beats" with the pulse. In tense, emotional people tinnitus becomes very annoying and may even interfere with sleep.

There seems to be a close relation between some varieties of tinnitus and the extra noises and "impurities" of diplacusis monauralis. In tinnitus the noise is spontaneous and comes and goes unpredictably. But, as we all know from experience, tinnitus is regularly one of the aftereffects of exposure to a very loud noise, whether a single explosion, a very loud whistle, or the continuing din of a boiler shop. In diplacusis the tinnitus is evoked by speech or other external sounds and is heard at the same time with them. Mild spontaneous tinnitus may be inhibited or masked by speech; strong tinnitus may interfere with speech reception.

In terms of our model with its sensory units, the common, mild tinnitus obviously corresponds to the spontaneous discharge which has been found in most if not all auditory nerve fibers. It should probably be regarded as normal or "physiological." A little hyperexcitability would drive a unit to a faster rate of discharge, and a more severe "irritation" would cause a still faster discharge and perhaps involve more units. This might be heard subjectively as sound. The discharges of the more sensitive units are accelerated by very small additional mechanical disturbance and could be triggered easily in other ways also, just as burning, tingling, or itching may follow after mechanical bruising of skin. It is not entirely facetious to speak of ringing tinnitus as "an itch in the organ of Corti."

It is often assumed that tinnitus may be associated with the early stages of a progressive degenerative process that will impair hearing. There is no need for concern. A strong tinnitus may continue for years without any change in the audiogram. It is true that irritation within the ear, mechanical as in noise-exposure, or biochemical (probably) as in Menière's disease, has an associated tinnitus. Tinnitus *may* be caused by wax impacted against the drum membrane and completely filling the external auditory canal, and it is a constant symptom in otosclerosis. It is often assumed to be caused by the mechanical or chemical irritation of a developing otosclerotic process, but perhaps it is only physiological tinnitus that is heard because a conductive impairment keeps out the external sounds that would ordinarily mask it in most environments.

*Temporary threshold shift with dysacusis.* In one set of wartime experiments (1943) normal human ears were exposed to loud, pure tones for many minutes. The chief object of study was the temporary elevation of threshold (threshold shift) that is produced for a restricted range of frequencies above the exposure tone. Frequently continuous tinnitus, tinnitus evoked by speech, and also tonal diplacusis were all produced. Only one ear of each subject was exposed, so that the distortion of pitch could be measured by pitch matching. Pitch shifts up to nearly an octave were produced. The shifts were less for loud test tones than for weak ones. Recruitment of loudness was demonstrated by loudness balancing. The threshold was considerably elevated for a restricted range of frequencies a little above the frequency of the exposure tone, producing a partial

"tonal gap." (Fortunately the threshold shift, the tinnitus, and the diplacusis were all temporary.) When two tones were heard in response to a single test tone their pitches usually corresponded to frequencies on each side of the "tonal gap."

Apparently the normal pattern of a continuously graded excitation (the traveling wave pattern) and correspondingly graded outputs of the sensory units had been temporarily disrupted by the local elevation of thresholds. Some sensory units were depressed, and others, less affected but nevertheless irritated, caused tinnitus. The normal, integrated pattern of neural activity was broken into two (or more) parts, and two (or more) tones or bands of noise were heard. This experiment gives a fairly firm basis for some of our "explanations," and it also points very strongly to an integrating function in the central nervous system that makes a widespread excitation normally sound like a single pure tone. Perhaps this function too can sometimes go wrong and produce a different class of distortions or head noises that do not depend on abnormal or spontaneous patterns of action in or among the sensory units, but which arise more centrally.

*Menière's syndrome.* In previous sections we have referred, in passing, to "Menière's disease." It is more accurate, although a bit pedantic, to call it "Menière's syndrome," because it is a set of symptoms that tend to occur together. We do not know the cause, and we cannot be sure that there is a single dominant cause of a single "disease." We shall return, in Chapters 5 and 6, to the possible causes and the treatment of the condition, but the group of symptoms must be mentioned here as a fine illustration of "peripheral dysacusis." The disturbance seems to be a mixture of elevated thresholds of hearing (depression of activity) and hyperexcitability, expressed by tinnitus (cochlear) and by vertigo (vestibular).

The symptoms occur typically in sudden

attacks during which the vertigo is the most distressing and disabling feature. The attacks may persist for hours or days, fluctuating in intensity. In addition to the vertigo there are usually cochlear symptoms consisting of loud, roaring tinnitus, inability to understand speech, elevation of hearing thresholds by as much as 30 to 60 dB, loss of tonal quality, gross distortion of sounds, and often a lowered threshold of discomfort from loud sounds. Recruitment is a very prominent feature, often including overrecruitment. The elevation of hearing thresholds may not appear in the early stages. Some patients have attacks of the cochlear dysacusis without the vertigo. For many others the attacks are purely vertiginous without much impairment of hearing. At first the cochlear symptoms are almost always unilateral. The course of the "disease" is capricious. The symptoms fluctuate from day to day and subside ultimately, with or without medical treatment, usually leaving a residue of cochlear hearing loss. Also, unfortunately, the symptoms tend to return at a later date.

One anatomical abnormality has been clearly associated with Menière's syndrome. The membranous labyrinth is distended like a toy balloon as if the endolymph were under increased pressure. Reissner's membrane may bulge so that scala media entirely fills scala vestibuli. Other features of the pathology are not certain as the attacks are not fatal and opportunities for good postmortem study of ears obtained during or soon after an attack have been rare. The known abnormality has led to the name *endolymphatic hydrops* as an alternative to Menière's disease. It is not easy, however, to understand why the increased pressure in the membranous labyrinth should cause the dysacusis and the vertigo. The elevated threshold of hearing might be attributed to a mechanical conductive impairment analagous to that caused by increased pressure of air or fluid in the middle ear, but this will not account for the recruitment of loudness.

The hyperexcitability of sensory units and their spontaneous overactivity in both cochlea (tinnitus) and vestibular apparatus (vertigo) strongly suggest a chemical or metabolic abnormality. The onset and also the cessation of the vertigo may be either abrupt or gradual. The dysacusis usually comes and goes gradually. An abrupt onset suggests to some a mechanical disturbance. Perhaps the mechanisms are not always the same in the two parts of the labyrinth. The excessive formation of endolymph might well be another result of an irritative condition. One theory relates the attacks to fluctuations of the salt and water balance of the body and a postulated inability of the stria vascularis to cope with it.

*Dysacousia: painful hearing.* The primary meaning for dysacousia (or its short form, dysacusis) in many medical dictionaries is *painful hearing*, namely, pain produced by loud or even by moderate sounds, although we use the term more broadly. Painful hearing may be an isolated symptom, one of the symptoms in Menière's syndrome, or it may occur in other combinations. The condition may be wrongly attributed to neurosis. There are probably several causes or varieties. For example, if the middle ear is tender from inflammation and the tympanic membrane is tense with pus, the additional mechanical stress of loud sound can be painful. Also sound can induce mechanical movement reflexly by the contraction of the stapedius or the tensor tympani muscle or both, and this could be painful in an inflamed ear. Pain is felt even in the toughest normal ear if sound is loud enough, above 140 dB SPL, and there are wide individual variations. A sudden sound, whether an explosion, a crash, or a whistle, is more painful than sound at the same level reached in successive small steps. (Incidentally, the thresholds of pain and of discomfort shown in Figure 2-4 were determined by the method of successive small increments of a steady tone. The ears had the advantage that the intra-aural muscles were already contracting reflexly when the last increment of sound pressure level was added.) People complain quite legitimately of uncomfortable loudness at levels well below 120 dB SPL, and some may experience true pain at what are ordinarily quite tolerable levels. In some of these conditions it is possible that there is a failure of the normal protective feedback mechanisms such as the intra-aural or stapedius reflex, the efferent inhibitory mechanism, and perhaps loudness adaptation also.

A practical aspect of painful hearing is the very sharp limit which it may impose at a rather low sound pressure level on the dynamic range of sound available for communication. If, as is often the case, the threshold is elevated by a sensory-neural impairment, and loudness recruitment is present in addition to the painful hearing, the dynamic range between threshold of hearing and threshold of severe discomfort may be no greater than the dynamic range of speech itself. The situation is just the reverse of automatic volume control in a radio transmission system. This difficulty is considered again in Chapters 10 and 11 on hearing aids.

*Fast Auditory Fatigue.* One more abnormality in the category of abnormal auditory signs and symptoms is *fast auditory fatigue.* This phenomenon is the basis for auditory tests (see Chapter 8) that distinguish quite well between sense organ dysacusis of the Menière's syndrome family and neural hearing loss, such as is produced by compression of the auditory nerve by a tumor. This distinction is very important from the neurosurgical point of view because the tumor, if allowed to grow, may become a threat to life. The differential diagnosis is often difficult, partly because the tumor may compress the cochlear ar-

tery as well as the nerve and thus cause some cochlear symptoms in addition to the neural injury. The effects of nerve compression on the audiogram and on speech discrimination may be indistinguishable from sensory dysacusis, but as a matter of clinical experience the presence of recruitment points strongly to the sense organ, and fast auditory fatigue points strongly to the auditory nerve.

The fast fatigue appears when a continuous tone is sounded. A normal listener hears the tone loudly at first, then less loudly, due to "per-stimulatory auditory fatigue" or "adaptation" (see Chapter 3), but the tone remains audible and at a fairly steady loudness after the first 15 or 20 seconds. If the nerve is partially compressed by a tumor, however, the loudness continues to fall, and finally the tone becomes inaudible. If its intensity is increased by a few decibels, it becomes audible again, but it then fades out. On the other hand, a tone that is interrupted, for example on for half a second then off for half a second, can be heard indefinitely, as it is by a normal ear.

The exact site of the failure of neural transmission in fast auditory fatigue is not known. The nerve fiber seems to be involved, although it is just possible that restricted blood supply to the sense organ is somehow responsible. The failure might be either at the dendritic terminations, at the point of compression, or at the axon terminals, which must all receive essential chemical material from the cell bodies in the spiral ganglion. The phenomenon strongly suggests that there is a metabolic bottleneck somewhere, beyond which only a limited supply of necessary material can be stored during periods of low activity. This supply is exhausted by high or moderate activity, it can be partially restored during a brief rest, but then can be quickly exhausted again. Continued stimulation, even if there is no evidence of successful transmission, continues to use up the necessary material as fast as it is formed but without ever reaching the threshold necessary to initiate (or conduct) the all-or-none nerve impulses.

Effects very much like this can be produced experimentally in peripheral nerves, and we can consider this hypothetical mechanism to be plausible although unproved. Whatever the details may be, the defect seems to be a failure of sustained transmission of impulses in the neural part of the sensory unit. The defect may be more evident in some groups of sensory units than in others. It is more likely to appear in response to high-frequency tones than to tones of low frequency. The phenomenon is useful diagnostically on a strictly empirical basis, but it may be unnoticed until the test is made because most sounds of interest in everyday life are not long continued but, as in speech, are continually interrupted or else changing in frequency. In the presence of a rapidly growing tumor, however, speech discrimination is usually very bad.

*Decruitment.* In retrocochlear lesions, and perhaps in some sensory impairments also, a careful loudness-balance test may reveal the opposite of recruitment, namely a failure of the sense of loudness to grow as rapidly as it normally does. This effect is known as "decruitment." It may be confined to one or two audiometric frequencies. It is not likely to cause much practical handicap and is not yet of proved diagnostic significance, but it is of theoretical interest in relation to the model of sensory units.

In the model diagrammed in Figure 4-1 the sense of loudness is assumed to depend largely on the *total number* of sensory units that are driven well above their resting rates of discharge. This includes units "tuned" to frequencies above that of the stimulus, even though the tone is heard as single in pitch. Now if there is a reduction in total number of units available, there should be a limit to the maximum loudness

that can be heard. The loss might be complete, as in abrupt high-tone loss (compare Figure 4-2), or partial with a random distribution. Such a random or partially random distribution of the blocking of sensory units is just what we might expect in the case of compression of the auditory nerve by a retrocochlear tumor.

## Prognosis, Treatment, and Management

The presence of a hearing loss immediately raises a series of practical questions. Will the hearing deteriorate still further? Can progressive deterioration be prevented? Can the hearing be improved by surgery, by medical treatment, or otherwise? Is the hearing loss caused by some infection or tumor which, if untreated, may threaten health in other ways? Is a hearing aid indicated? The answers depend on the nature and on the location of the impairment.

In general the conductive impairments of the external and middle ear are easily accessible for treatment, and by their nature they are amenable to control: some by drugs, others by surgery, and for the most part by surgical repair as well. Nature often assists the surgeon by forming new connective tissue, skin, or mucous membrane as needed. Preventive measures are often quite effective, although we cannot prevent the progressive changes in the tissues associated with advancing age.

The inner ear, on the other hand, is beyond the reach of surgical repair. It is almost impossible of access, and its parts are far too small and delicate to repair. Nature does not assist by forming new neurons, or hair cells, or specialized supporting structures to replace those that may have degenerated or become misshapen. Even in the control of the irritative processes of Menière's syndrome, medicine and surgery have little to offer after the disease has become chronic.

The one impairment of neural hearing

loss that can be assisted surgically is compression of the auditory nerve by a tumor.
The location of the tumor is retrocochlear
in the internal auditory meatus or within
the cranial cavity. The problem of diagnosis lies in the area of neuro-otology and
neurosurgery, and it usually involves signs
and symptoms related to the nonauditory
vestibular portion of the labyrinth or to
other nearby neural structures such as the
facial nerve. The chief objective is to find
and remove the tumor to protect life. If
done in time, however, there may be at
least partial improvement of the hearing
loss caused by compression block of the
nerve fibers.

*Use of a hearing aid.* Conductive
impairment offers the best opportunity for
the successful use of a hearing aid. Actual
success depends on many factors, as we
shall see in Chapters 10 and 11, but at least
the sense organ is still intact and can respond if stimulated. The prospects for successful use of a hearing aid in sensory-
neural impairment, as we have defined it,
are less favorable. The function of a sensory unit that has degenerated cannot be
replaced. In general, a dysacusis that involves distortions such as diplacusis or
tinnitus cannot be improved by a hearing
aid, and the discomfort and confusion are
likely to be made worse rather than better.
On the other hand, there has been in the
past a tendency to dismiss all too easily the
possibility of significant assistance and to
say simply, "You have nerve deafness, and
a hearing aid won't help. Save your
money." We believe that the distinction
between conductive and sensory impairment within the cochlea is important. A
conductive component in the inner ear, as
well as one in the middle ear, can be offset
by amplification. Many cases of inner-ear
impairment are really cases of *mixed* hearing loss, and should be evaluated as such.
A hearing aid may help considerably if
the wearer does not expect too much and
can adapt to it.

# CAUSES OF HEARING LOSS AND DYSACUSIS

In this section we shall review the causes
of various types of impairment of hearing.
The nature of the medical and surgical
problems of prevention and cure will become apparent, but the details of programs
of conservation of hearing and of medical
and surgical treatment will be reserved for
the two following chapters.

## Hearing Loss in the External and Middle Ear

*Congenital malformations.* Although
cupping the hand behind the ear may amplify speech sounds reaching the eardrum
by as much as 10 dB, the pinna or auricle
is not very important acoustically. Congenital malformation or absence of the external ear is likely, however, to be associated
with malformations in deeper structures,
and these may cause a severe loss of hearing. One such malformation is closure or
*atresia* of the external canal. If normal
hearing by bone conduction shows that the
inner ear is intact, an operation to relieve
atresia of the external canal is occasionally
successful. Usually, however, it is found
at operation or by X ray that there are also
malformations of the middle ear, and then
the best result that can be attained is
a hearing-threshold level for speech of
about 45 dB (ISO).

*Impacted wax.* Except for congenital
malformations, diseases of the external
canal rarely produce permanent hearing
loss. The most common cause of hearing
loss from within the external canal is wax
(cerumen), which may harden in the canal
and become *impacted* so that it prevents
the sound waves from reaching the drum
and the middle ear. Blockage of this type
is often first noticed after swimming, washing the hair, or bathing. A droplet of water
suddenly closes the last tiny channel which
was sufficient for the effective reception of
ordinary sounds, and only then does the
victim know that something is amiss.

*External otitis*. Occasionally changes occur in the skin of the external canal which permit the growth of bacteria and fungi. Infection of the skin and inflammatory changes involving other structures produce a condition called *external otitis*. This occurs most commonly in hot, wet climates. One type of external otitis is like a pimple or boil in the skin of the external canal, usually near the outer end. It may be produced by scratching the skin of the canal with a fingernail or some instrument such as a hairpin or toothpick. It is usually caused by one of the organisms that are commonly found on human skin and which cause no harm unless they invade one or more hair follicles.

External otitis may cause symptoms that suggest middle-ear infection (otitis media) and mastoiditis, but it differs from otitis media in often producing no hearing loss unless the swelling of the skin or the trapped secretions completely close the ear canal. The most prominent symptom is pain on manipulation of the auricle.

*Otitis media*. The middle ear is an air chamber containing the mechanism that conducts sound from the air in the external ear to the fluid in the inner ear. This includes the drum membrane, the ossicles (malleus, incus, and stapes), and their ligaments. Diseases of the middle ear may involve one or more of these structures and produce a conductive hearing loss.

*Inflammation in the middle ear is the most common cause of conductive hearing loss.* This inflammation is called *otitis media* and usually develops from a cold in the head. The nasal secretions pass backward and infect the Eustachian tube, as shown in Figure 4-3. The infection then travels along the tube itself or along the lymphatic vessels surrounding it until the middle ear is reached. When the lining of the Eusta-

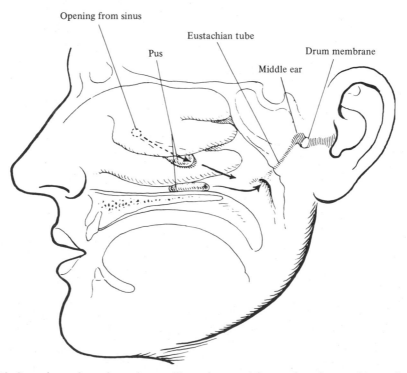

Opening from sinus

Eustachian tube

Pus

Drum membrane

Middle ear

Fig. 4-3. Secretions of pus from the maxillary sinus, and from other sinuses also, easily travel along the floor of the nasal cavity to the mouth of the Eustachian tube and can infect the middle ear.

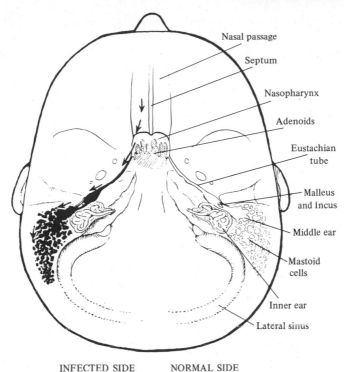

Nasal passage

Septum

Nasopharynx

Adenoids

Eustachian tube

Malleus and Incus

Middle ear

Mastoid cells

Inner ear

Lateral sinus

INFECTED SIDE      NORMAL SIDE

Fig. 4-4. In this diagram the head is viewed from above. The dark shading on the left indicates the extent of the air-filled system of middle ear and mastoid cells that is ventilated by the Eustachian tube. Notice also how close these cavities, which may become infected, come to the brain cavity and large blood-filled channels, such as the lateral sinus.

chian tube is inflamed, the tube cannot be opened by swallowing, and the air pressure in the middle ear is no longer equalized. The oxygen in the air of the middle ear is absorbed by the blood that nourishes its mucous lining, and a partial vacuum is produced. The drum membrane is pressed inward and the ossicular chain is forced near to its limit of movement, with all of its ligaments tense. In this situation the conduction of sound is impaired. Furthermore the reduced air pressure in the middle ear sucks, so to speak, clear tissue fluid from the mucous lining. If much fluid accumulates it further impairs sound conduction. The condition is called *nonsuppurative* otitis media as long as bacteria do not invade the cavity.

Occasionally otitis media is produced by puncturing the drum membrane from the outside with a dirty instrument, such as a toothpick or a hairpin, and introducing infection in this way. With few exceptions, however, otitis media starts with a common cold. Indeed, since the middle ear is actually another air cavity leading from the nose, otitis media can be considered as a cold in the ear. Furthermore, the middle ear is directly connected in turn with the mastoid air cells, as illustrated in Figure 4-4. Middle-ear and mastoid cells form a single air-filled cavity that is only partly subdivided. Each chamber, large or small, is lined with mucous membrane and is connected with the others. With every otitis media there is bound to be some inflammation of the lining of the adjoining mastoid air cells. It is the tremendous surface of the mastoid cells that accounts for most of the secretion of fluid present when the middle ear becomes infected.

It will be remembered that in the early

stage of a cold the secretion from the nose is watery. In the ear, this stage is properly called *nonsuppurative, or serous, otitis media.* As the disease progresses, the watery secretion thickens into pus. Now, when the material in the middle ear has become infected, the disease is said to be in the *suppurative, or purulent,* stage. There is usually excruciating pain until the drumhead breaks or is opened by a surgeon, or until the growth of bacteria is checked by medication. Often there is pain and tenderness behind the ear over the mastoid.

When properly treated, these conditions usually subside, with or without transient hearing loss, and should then be designated as *healed.* A mild but long-standing otitis media is occasionally called *subacute.* (It is hard for people to think of the word "acute" without considering it as "severe," but severity is not implied in the medical meaning of the word. Nevertheless, a popular misunderstanding persists.)

If an ear discharges pus for more than two or three months, and especially if it has a bad odor, the condition is called *chronic otitis media.* There is another misunderstanding concerning the term *chronic catarrhal otitis media.* The words distinctly mean a long-standing watery secretion in the middle ear, but the term is often wrongly applied to a "healed" otitis media that has the scars and adhesions which produce hearing loss. In an effort to avoid this error, some authors have made matters even worse by calling healed otitis media a "dry catarrh"—a direct contradiction in terms. Many such inconsistencies occur in medical terminology. This discussion of terms has been included because these old terminologies persist and unfortunately can still be found in modern classifications of disease for purposes of record and also in popular parlance.

AERO-OTITIS MEDIA. A fine example of uninfected watery effusion into the middle ear occurs during airplane flight if the Eustachian tube is not opened frequently during descent. At the reduced barometric pressure of the higher altitude the middle ear contains less air than at sea level, where the atmospheric pressure is greater and the air is consequently more dense. Normally as the barometric pressure increases during descent, more air enters the middle ear through the Eustachian tube, a bubble at each swallow, and equalizes the air pressure between inside and outside. If air does not enter, the differential pressure between the outside air and the middle ear builds up and forces the drum membrane inward. Uncomfortable pressure and fi-

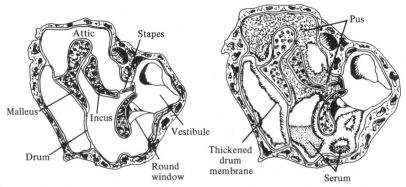

Fig. 4-5. At the left is an enlarged drawing of an actual section through a normal middle ear. At the right is a corresponding section through an infected middle ear. The drumhead is thickened, and the middle ear is filled with pus and serum, which restrict the movement of the ossicles. Pus in the middle ear is a more frequent cause of hearing loss than any other except perhaps senility.

nally acute pain is felt, deep in the ear canal. Clear watery fluid gradually collects in the middle ear and partly relieves the difference in pressure. This fluid comes ultimately from the tiny blood vessels (capillaries) of the mucous membrane lining of the middle ear.

There is normally a delicate balance between the mechanical force of the blood pressure, which tends to drive the watery portion of the blood (serum) out into the tissue spaces, and the physicochemical osmotic force, due to the dissolved proteins in the blood, which tends to hold the serum within the capillaries. The mechanical pressure in the tissue, supported by the air pressure in the middle ear, tends also to resist the outward movement of fluid. When the air pressure in the middle ear is reduced, some fluid moves out into the tissue and ultimately into the middle-ear cavity. The action is literally a suction of serum into the cavity from the blood. The resulting condition is called *aero-otitis media*, or otitis media due to *barotrauma* (injury from change in barometric pressure). Similar nonsuppurative otitis often occurs among caisson workers and submarine crews. Diving, especially high diving and skin diving, may also produce effusions of fluid.

SEROUS AND MUCOUS OTITIS. A subacute form of nonsuppurative otitis media has recently become very prevalent throughout the world. Why it was previously rare no one knows. When the fluid in the middle ear is thin and watery, the disease is called *serous otitis* or middle-ear effusion or (formerly) catarrhal otitis media. When the effusion is thick, the condition is called *mucoid* or *mucous otitis* or even "glue ear." Some otologists deny that there is any inflammation involved. They therefore object to the suffix "-itis" and prefer to speak of "otic transudates." However, the cellular and chemical content of the fluids of the middle ear in such cases both indicate that there is inflammation and closure of the Eustachian tube, so we shall class this condition as a nonsuppurative otitis.

The cause or causes of serous and mucous otitis are not clear. The most common appears to be the treatment of suppurative otitis with antibiotics or other biochemicals but without adequate drainage. The bacteria are destroyed or held inactive, but the fluid in the middle ear remains. Another cause is allergy. Some cases are certainly allergic in origin, but it is impossible to explain all cases on this basis. Another suggested cause is a virus infection of the middle ear.

The fluid that collects in the middle ear causes a hearing loss. The loss may vary all the way from a mild gradual high-tone loss to a very considerable loss for all tones. When thick mucus is present, the hearing loss is most severe and may resemble that seen with otosclerosis. Some surgeons have actually performed fenestration surgery in such cases. Actually, of course, it is quite sufficient to remove the effusion from the middle ear by puncture or incision of the drumhead. The consequent relief of hearing loss is one of the most dramatic affairs in otology.

Since the use of antibiotics for treatment of acute otitis media has become so popular, many physicians not in the specialty of otology have felt complacent when the pain and other symptoms of otitis media disappear following the use of antibiotics. They may have neglected to inspect the ear carefully or may have failed to incise the drumhead in spite of the possibility that some fluid remained in the middle ear. The only remaining symptom is the hearing loss, which may be noticed by the parent or detected by routine testing of hearing in schools. The diagnosis is not always easy, but characteristically the drumhead has a creamy, thick appearance with some slight bulging in the posterior half, and it does not move when positive and negative pressures are applied through a pneumatic otoscope.

In these cases a wide incision should be made in the drumhead because it is sometimes peculiarly difficult to evacuate the thick gluelike material from the middle ear. If this mucoid material is not removed by the surgeon, it will remain, as it is obviously impossible for it to drain spontaneously through the Eustachian tube. The conductive hearing loss will persist, and the condition may in time lead to the formation of adhesions in the middle ear which firmly fix the ossicular chain with bands of fibrous tissue.

*Cholesteatoma.* Another important cause of hearing loss, and an important cause of more serious complications as well, is cholesteatoma. This is simply a cyst that is lined internally with skin. This cyst grows from the upper part of the drumhead as a pouch within the middle ear (see Figure 4-6). It seems to originate from chronic wetting of the deep parts of the external canal or from inflammation of the middle ear. In any case, a pouch forms, and then the lining desquamates into the pouch. It will be remembered that the outer layers of the human skin come off in thin, tiny sheets. As these cornified layers of skin come off in the pouch, the cyst becomes larger and larger. Eventually such a soft-tissue cyst may erode away the ossicles or other bony structures and cause symptoms. It constitutes a foreign body in the middle ear and favors suppuration.

The degenerative products formed in such a cyst include a fatty substance called cholesterol. This is the basis of the name cholesteatoma. Usually the patient complains of an intermittent discharge from the ear that has a peculiarly foul odor. The hearing level may be quite good, either within normal limits or perhaps 25 or 30 dB (ISO). Examination of the ear usually shows a small perforation at the margin of the drumhead, usually at the flaccid upper part.

*Allergy.* Hypersensitivity of the tissues of the middle ear, the Eustachian tube, and the inner ear to various foreign proteins in the air or blood stream has been described. Perhaps the most common is the sensitivity to bacteria called "bacterial allergy." Occasionally, a patient has tinnitus or a hearing loss whenever he or she eats particular foods, such as wheat, milk, eggs, chocolate, nuts, or citrus fruits. Cer-

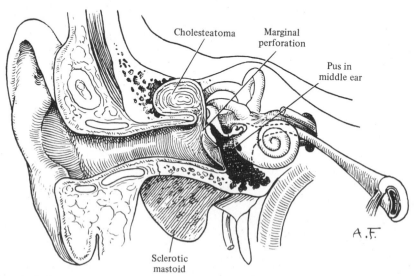

Fig. 4-6. A cholesteatoma forms an inpocketing of skin at the margin of the drum membrane.

tainly severe pollen allergies contribute to blockage of the tubes and may make an individual more susceptible to the various types of otitis media.

*Other abnormalities of the middle ear.* It is not necessary for us to include in this general discussion of medical problems the numerous rare conditions which may involve either the external, the middle, or the inner ear. Tumors, syphilis, tuberculosis, bullet wounds, fractures of the skull, and a variety of other medical and surgical conditions may involve the ear as well as other parts of the body. It is not the problem of the audiologist but of the otologist to diagnose these conditions, and a description of them would be out of place here. By far the most important causes of conductive hearing loss in order of numerical occurrence are (a) inadequate attention to normal function of the Eustachian tube and inadequate treatment of infections of the middle ear and (b) the special disease of the middle and inner ear known as *otosclerosis.*

*Otosclerosis.* Otosclerosis is a unique bone disease that affects the bony capsule surrounding the inner ear. This bone, normally the hardest in the body, becomes invaded by a different kind of softer bone which grows intermittently and then becomes hard again, that is, "sclerotic." The most common site for the growth of this new bone is in the region just in front of and below the oval window. The most common effect of the new bony growth, if it does anything at all, is to fix the footplate of the stapes firmly in the oval window so that the stapes no longer moves freely. The effect is much like that of some forms of arthritis which limit the movements of fingers, the knee, or the spine; in fact, the two diseases have many points in common. When the stapes becomes fixed, the vibrations carried to it from the drumhead through the malleus and the incus are not effectively transmitted to

the fluid of the inner ear. Fortunately, *otosclerosis causes fixation of the stapes and hearing loss in only about 10 percent of the cases in which it occurs.*

Otosclerosis is a hereditary disease. It is frequent among the Caucasoids (whites and East Indians) but extremely rare among the Mongoloids (Japanese, Chinese, Indonesians, American Indians) and among Negroids. The distribution suggests that the disease very likely arose as a single genetic mutation. Its rare appearance amongst Mongoloids and its presence among American but not among African Negroes are well explained as the result of restricted interbreeding. In the incidence there is a slight but definite unexplained predominance of the female sex. These statements are based on a recent (1967) careful survey, entitled "The Incidence of Otosclerosis as Related to Race and Sex" by Altmann, Glasgold, and MacDuff. The authors point out that "the data on the racial distribution of otosclerosis are amazingly scarce for all races, even for negroes living in the U.S.A. The above statements must therefore be regarded as still subject to future modification."

Part of the data on the incidence of otosclerosis expresses the relation between the number of cases of otosclerosis confirmed at operation and the size of the entire population of the hospital clinics. Another large part of the data comes from examination of temporal bones for evidence of fixation of the stapes in the oval window. Here we must make a distinction between *clinical otosclerosis,* in which fixation of the stapes actually occurs, and *histological otosclerosis,* in which the presence of the otosclerotic process is demonstrated postmortem somewhere in the otic capsule. From the point of view of heredity all of the persons with histological otosclerosis are carriers of the trait. Those with clinical otosclerosis are simply the less fortunate members of the much larger group of carriers. It is thus easy to understand why, although the disease is hereditary, the hearing loss very frequently skips one or more generations.

More precisely the survey of Altmann, Glasgold, and MacDuff gives the incidence of histological otosclerosis among whites as 8.3 percent and for stapedial fixation as 0.99 percent. The female predominance in both classes is about seven to six. Histological otosclerosis among Negroes in the United States (chiefly in New York) is about one-seventh as common as among whites.

Otosclerosis begins in youth. There have been cases presenting the clinical picture of otosclerosis in young children four, five, and six years of age, and fixation of the stapes has been observed at operation as early as the seventh year; but these fixations are probably congenital, not otosclerotic. The hearing loss of otosclerosis is *usually* first noticed at adolescence or in the early twenties. Nearly always the hearing loss is evident before the thirtieth year, although in a few cases it makes its appearance when the patient is still older. Otosclerosis may become worse during pregnancy, but since the disease is often progressive during early adulthood in any case, until the hearing loss reaches the 50 or 60 dB (ISO) level, and since pregnancy by no means always accelerates the process, *otosclerosis should not be considered a deterrent to the bearing of children.*

The fixation of the stapes occurs only gradually over a period of years. As the hearing loss comes on, more and more powerful sound is required to overcome the increasing resistance to movement, but with the help of a good hearing aid speech may be understood almost perfectly. Ultimately, however, in most cases of otosclerosis in which the hearing loss is severe, there is, in addition to the conductive hearing loss, some sensory-neural loss as well. It is not clear whether this sensory-neural loss is really due to the otosclerosis or is

merely coincidental. Sometimes, however, the loss of hearing becomes very severe.

The otosclerotic process may invade the niche of the round window as well as the area near the oval window. In rare cases the round window may be closed by the bony overgrowth while the stapes remains mobile. Hearing is impaired because fixation of the round-window membrane deprives the cochlea of its "elastic release." The cochlear fluids can no longer move freely in response to the push and pull of the stapes, and the sensitivity of hearing is reduced accordingly. The immobilization of the fluids reduces hearing for bone conduction as well as for air conduction.

Erosion of the hard bony wall of the cochlea by the abnormal, spongy vascular tissue can be demonstrated by x-ray, using the technique known as "tomography" or "polytomography." This method blurs the details of the x-ray shadow of structures that are nearer to or farther away than the desired depth of focus. By reducing the confusing overlay it reveals changes in the bony structures that do remain in focus. The decalcification caused by otosclerosis can be detected readily in a tomogram taken at the proper depth and angle. "Tomography" or "planigraphy" is also the best method for identifying small acoustic neuromas in the internal auditory meatus.

Otosclerotic invasion of the cochlea itself is more common than was formerly supposed, and opinion differs concerning the extent to which hearing may be impaired by it. The stapes is often involved also, and the cochlear component is then likely to be blamed for any associated sensory-neural loss of whatever sort that may be present. The audiogram of pure "cochlear otosclerosis" is said to be flat or U-shaped. Just how or why the hearing should be affected if there is no mechanical fixation of either window is not clear. It is usually assumed to be some unspecified chemical or "toxic" effect. It is worth remembering that certain forms of congenital impairment, including maternal rubella, also frequently show U-shaped audiograms. Fixation of the stapes does not. Stapes surgery can restore normal hearing if only the stapes is affected; it cannot relieve a cochlear sensory-neural component.

When the hearing loss first appears, the patient is often much troubled by *tinnitus* or ringing in the ears. This ringing may be like a high-pitched whistle or like the sound of a bell. It is much more troublesome at night or when the surroundings are quiet. Sometimes the sound may resemble a rushing of air or water and be synchronous with the pulse. A few patients may also have brief spells of mild dizziness.

*In its early stages, the hearing loss of otosclerosis is purely conductive.* The bone conduction is normal, or nearly so, but air conduction is impaired. At first the middle range of tones, 1000 and 2000 Hz, are often less affected than the lower tones. As a rule, the highest tones, 4000 Hz and above, are still less affected at first. As the disease progresses, however—and in a few cases it progresses very rapidly—there is a greater and greater hearing loss for the higher tones by air conduction, and the loss of sensitivity by bone conduction centering at 2000 Hz begins to appear. It is when these hearing losses for the higher tones appear that the tinnitus is likely to become severe. Its high-pitched, musical character is evidence of a localized irritation in the sense organ.

We have also mentioned the symptom of *paracusis Willisii,* which is characteristic of conductive hearing loss in general. The patient with otosclerosis seems to hear better in a noisy place, for example in an airplane, in an automobile, or in a factory. The reason is that people with normal hearing naturally raise their voices to overcome the surrounding noise. The man who has only a partial conductive hearing loss can discriminate the voice from the noise as well as anyone else, if only the voice is loud enough to reach his inner ear. He also hears fairly well over the telephone. But as the otosclerosis progresses and perhaps if sensory-neural difficulties are added to the mechanical obstruction at the stapes, the patient can no longer so easily distinguish conversation, and he is much handicapped at a party where more than one person is speaking. The more he tries to hear, the less he hears. When he becomes fatigued or nervous, his hearing becomes appreciably worse.

DIAGNOSIS OF OTOSCLEROSIS. The chief points on which a diagnosis of otosclerosis is made are (1) a progressive but moderate loss of hearing, particularly in a young person; (2) a history of hearing loss in the family; (3) no previous infections of the ear that might account for the hearing loss; and (4) normal eardrums. The drum membrane may perhaps show a pink glow (Schwartz's sign) during the active period, or there may be several small atrophic areas like healed perforations, but nothing more.

The hearing levels by air conduction are about equal for all frequencies, or, in the early stages, a little worse for the low frequencies. By bone conduction hearing is substantially normal or a little depressed from 1000 to 4000 Hz. Otosclerosis may, of course, be combined with other types of conductive hearing loss, such as those due to chronic infection of the middle ear. In such cases it may be very difficult to decide how much of the hearing loss may be due to the otosclerosis and how much to the chronic otitis media. Otosclerosis may also be combined in later years with some degree of presbycusis, in which case the audiometric tests show worse hearing for the high frequencies.

THE COURSE OF OTOSCLEROSIS. Otosclerosis rarely progresses to very severe hearing loss. To call otosclerosis "progressive deafness," as it was once known, is therefore misleading. Many patients believe that this diagnosis means that they will soon be totally deaf. For this reason the term should never be used. Usually there is very little, if any, further loss after the hearing has reached a level of 50 to 60 dB (ISO). The hearing may stay the same for 20 years or more, with a gradual additional loss when the high-tone neural hearing loss of old age adds itself to the conductive hearing loss of otosclerosis.

For many years it was believed that inflation of the Eustachian tubes and pneumatic massage of the drum would loosen the bony fixation of the stapes and improve the hearing in otosclerosis. This has been proved false. The improvement reported by some patients was apparently purely illusory or psychic in origin.

Since the hearing loss of otosclerosis in its early stages is a conductive loss, the patient can anticipate good results with a hearing aid. If the inner ear is still intact, one should consider also the possibility of overcoming the mechanical barrier at the entrance to the inner ear by means of surgery, employing the "fenestration operation" or the "stapes surgery" described in Chapter 6.

### Inner Ear Impairments

*Presbycusis* (*presbyacusis, presbyacousis*). By far the most common cause of inner-ear hearing loss, and probably of all hearing loss, is advancing age. Actually aging also affects the middle ear, and it affects the inner ear in several ways. We shall here consider presbycusis as a whole.

The possibility that aging may cause *conductive impairment in the middle ear* has been generally overlooked for many years. Of course the older a person grows, the more opportunity does he have for episodes of otitis media, either acute or as recurrence of a chronic condition. If there is a history of chronic otitis media with discharge from the ear and other symptoms, this point of view is reasonable. It is also true that the older a person becomes, the more exposure to noise, with its effects on

hearing, does he accumulate. It now seems, however, that even without severe noise-exposure or recurrent otitis media elderly people, particularly those beyond 80 years of age, do develop a middle-ear conductive hearing loss. The impairment is greater for high than for low frequencies. Also it is greater for air conduction than for bone conduction. The presence of an "air-bone gap" in the audiogram clearly establishes *this part* of the hearing impairment to be due to changes in the middle ear.

The nature of the changes in the middle ear with age have not been clearly established, but it is well known that in elderly people connective tissue loses much of its elasticity. Their skin becomes flabby and wrinkled. If such changes occur in the ligaments of the joints between the ossicles so that the bones are not held snugly together, or if the drum membrane loses its stiffness and becomes flabby, there should be just such conductive impairments.

The characteristic audiogram in elderly people is a gradual high-tone loss, as described in the previous section. The slope is very gradual below 1000 Hz, although the sensitivity may be depressed at all frequencies. The slope is steepest above 2000 Hz. There may be an air-bone gap in more advanced age or if the presbycusis is added to a previous middle-ear impairment, but the cochlea is clearly the area chiefly involved. There is little or no recruitment of loudness in this condition unless there is a noise-induced component.

Actually changes in the sensitivity of hearing begin in adolescence. Children not only have a wider frequency range than adults, but throughout the entire range their thresholds tend to be lower. This fact was not clearly appreciated until the results of a systematic survey of the hearing of children in certain public schools in Pittsburgh were published in 1963. In this study it was necessary at the very start to modify the audiometers to provide test tones 20 dB below the usual lower limit

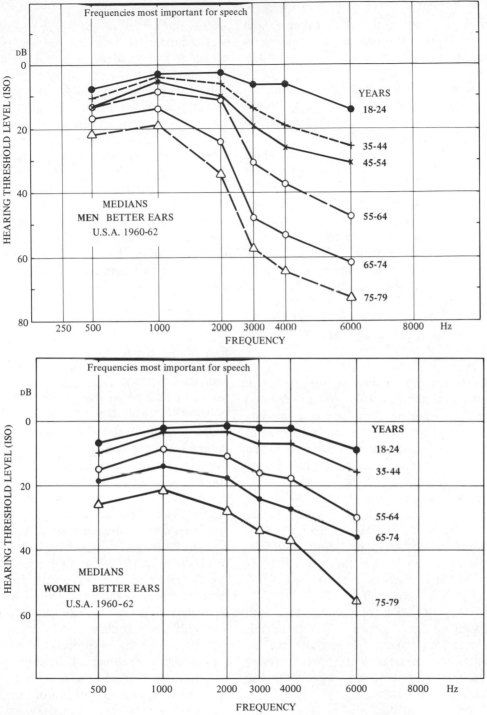

Fig. 4-7. Composite audiograms for the better ear in men (*A*) and women (*B*), by age groups. The values plotted are the medians or 50-percentile values. Some of these data are shown in another form in Figure 9-2. There the 25-percentile and 75-percentile values are also shown. (*These data of the National Health Survey are taken from Hearing Levels of Adults by Age and Sex. United States 1960–1962. Public Health Service Publication, No. 1000, Series 11, No. 11.* They have been recalculated to the ISO zero reference level.)

111

of clinical audiometers of that date (about 0 dB ISO). Of course additional precautions to provide sufficiently quiet test booths were also needed.

A few years later a survey of adult hearing was carried out by the U.S. Public Health Service, also using modern audiometric instruments, methods, and test booths. More details concerning this survey of 1960–1962 will be found in Chapters 7 and 9, but the trends of the relations of hearing threshold to age and to frequency are shown in Figures 4-7a and 4-7b. The hearing of men for high frequencies falls off faster than that of women, but the general trends are the same: from the age of 18 years onward the median sensitivity of hearing falls. The fall is slight at and below 1000 Hz. The fall is greater the higher the frequency and the older the person.

In Figures 4-8a and 4-8b a series of curves are drawn showing the *change* in hearing thresholds with age, as deduced by Drs. Spoor and van Laar from a study of several surveys made in several countries. Here the curves have been smoothed and are drawn according to the mathematical equation that yielded the best fit for the median values. The trends suggest that the fall in sensitivity actually begins at birth, not at 18 years of age. The U.S. Public Health Service data were not available for inclusion, but the agreement between the two sets of data of Figures 7-7 and 7–8 is noteworthy.

The association of hearing loss with advancing age is proverbial. Actually this association accounts for much of the resistance to the use of hearing aids by young and middle-aged persons who could use them to good advantage.

Most clinical studies of presbycusis during the last 50 years were directed toward describing the impairment due to age alone and finding the specific pathological changes associated with age that would account for the hearing loss. In order to isolate the effects of the aging process it was customary to exclude from the studies all patients who had any significant conductive impairment as revealed by an air-bone gap. This arbitrary exclusion delayed the recognition of significant changes in the middle ear due to age. Also it was often tacitly assumed that there is a single "disease process" or pathological change responsible for presbycusis. When one such change, namely loss of sensory units in the basilar turn was found, this change was accepted as an adequate general explanation. This attitude was reflected in the previous edition of this book in which we dismissed presbycusis in a single cursory paragraph. In it we wrote:

> The structural change that is responsible is perfectly well known. The sensory cells in the part of the organ of Corti toward the base of the cochlea simply degenerate and vanish as do the nerve fibers that connect with them. . . . We can only wonder why the part of the organ sensitive to high tones is almost invariably first involved.

Our present view is that at least five different aging processes contribute to the over-all pattern of presbycusis. One is a conductive middle-ear impairment that develops late in life in the eighth decade and beyond. The second is the conductive cochlear component discussed in a previous section. Its nature is hypothetical, but loss of elasticity and increase of internal friction in the basilar membrane, that is, a more "leathery" character, would give the characteristic pattern of gradual high-tone loss. Other tissues show just such changes as part of the aging process. The third component is the loss of sensory units, which occurs chiefly in the basal turn. The decrease in the number of sensory units is not significant, however, in more than half of the ears with high-tone, sensory-neural impairment that have been studied. A fourth category should perhaps be reserved for possible chemical or metabolic abnormalities which may follow changes in blood

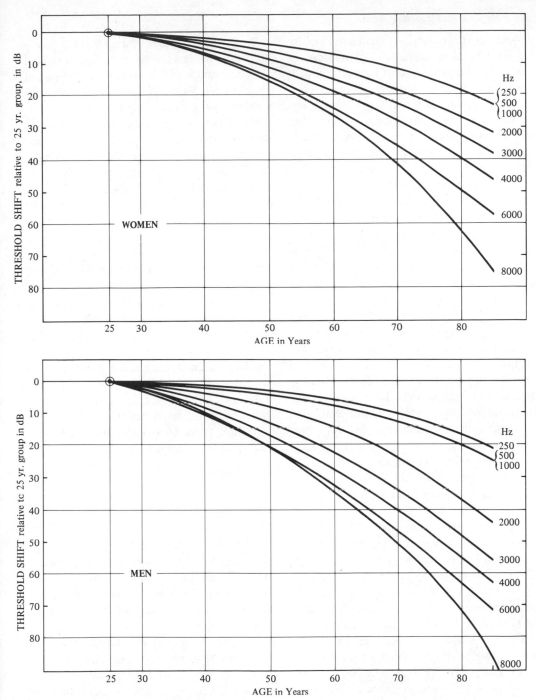

Fig. 4-8. The change of sensitivity of hearing with age for men (*A*) and for women (*B*). The parameter is frequency in Hz. Data for men and women from eight different publications from four different countries were combined, taking as reference in each study the hearing level of the age group centering at 25 years. In these studies individuals with histories of otological disease or severe noise exposure had been eliminated. A mathematical equation was found that describes the combined data well, with different values of its parameters for men and for women. The curves are smooth curves derived from the equation. (*Adapted from Spoor and van Laar, International Audiology, July 1967.*)

vessels or in the stria vascularis. Finally we must emphasize the loss of neurons in the central nervous system that occurs with aging, particularly if there is severe arteriosclerosis. In a later section we shall describe "phonemic regression" and other well-known symptoms of old age that contribute very importantly to the over-all clinical picture of presbycusis.

*Drugs, poisons, and allergens.* There has been much speculation in the past as to possible injury to hearing from excessive use of certain drugs, notably quinine and the salicylates (aspirin). It seems probable that both of these drugs *may* have caused some sensory-neural hearing loss in particularly hypersensitive or allergic individuals. Permanent injury will almost certainly be avoided, however, if the use of the drug is stopped as soon as tinnitus occurs. Excessive use of coffee, tobacco, or tea is thought by some to cause tinnitus, hearing loss, and vertigo. Rare toxic effects from carbon monoxide, arsenic, lead, and other poisons have been reported from time to time. Certain drugs taken during pregnancy may affect the hearing of the fetus. A quinine derivative, chloroquine, has apparently produced severe congenital deafness. The injurious effects of thalidomide taken during pregnancy are well known.

Recently a group of antibiotic drugs, notably *dihydrostreptomycin* and *kanamycin,* have been found to be definitely ototoxic. Apparently these drugs become concentrated in the endolymph, and they injure or kill hair cells. The process is slow, and the hearing loss may not appear for as long as two or three months after the medication is given. This is why for several years dihydrostreptomycin was not suspected as a cause of hearing loss. It was routinely used at one time, in mixtures with other antibiotics such as penicillin, for so-called prophylactic therapy. Now it is used only when there is a specific and compelling indication for it, as a matter of life or death, and then only as a calculated risk.

*Circulatory disturbances?* This group of causes is largely hypothetical, invoked as the most probable cause of the sudden attacks of Menière's syndrome and of sudden loss of hearing without other symptoms. Vascular spasm is often mentioned without proof and, as we shall see in Chapter 5, therapy is guided accordingly. "Sludging of the blood," a condition in which the red blood corpuscles adhere to one another to an abnormal degree, has also been implicated. There are suggestions of a strong psychogenic factor in Menière's syndrome, as in peptic ulcer, and this might operate by way of the blood supply.

Very puzzling indeed are the rare but well-documented cases of sudden loss of hearing, usually unilateral, without apparent adequate cause. There may or may not have been a precipitating event, such as exposure to cold. A vascular spasm, embolism, or other "accident" is as good a guess as any and better than most. The important point is to know that such sudden losses *can* happen.

**Noise**

*Temporary hearing loss.* Whoever has worked in a really noisy factory, driven a tractor on a farm, or indulged in much pistol or skeet shooting can recall how his ears rang for hours afterward, and voices sounded muffled and indistinct. Loud sounds could be heard as well as ever, but he was temporarily hard of hearing. After a few hours, or by the following day at least, his hearing had recovered. Recovery from this hearing loss is usually so complete that the hearing loss may properly be considered a fatigue rather than an injury. We call this a *temporary threshold shift*.

It is a curious fact that the temporary threshold shift produced by exposure to a loud tone or noise is confined almost entirely to frequencies *higher* than the frequency of the offending tone or noise. *The greatest shift is for tones about half an octave above the exposure tone,* but all of the higher frequencies may be more or less affected.

Hearing for lower tones, on the other hand, remains almost as good as ever. Furthermore, the high tones, in addition to being more annoying (although not more painful), also cause a more rapid shift of threshold. The greater susceptibility of the ear to fatigue by high tones offsets the greater intensity of the low components in most loud noises, both natural and man-made. For most noises, therefore, the temporary effect is usually a partial high-tone loss, *most severe for high frequencies above the range essential for speech.* Ears vary so much in their susceptibility, and noises vary so much in their spectra, that isolated numerical statements are not very meaningful, but an example may be given from some wartime experiments. Exposure to a 1000 Hz tone at 120 dB (about at the threshold of discomfort) for half an hour usually caused a temporary threshold shift of about 35 dB over the upper half of the speech range. Hearing was usually normal the next day, but the last part of auditory sensitivity to recover completely was almost always the band *between 3000 and 5000 Hz.* This band seems to represent a vulnerable spot in the sense organ of hearing that recovers more slowly, regardless of what tone or noise produces the threshold shift.

*Permanent injury from noise.* Temporary threshold shift may be called "fatigue," but somewhere injury begins. We know that the muzzle blast of a big gun or the explosion of a nearby shell may rupture the drum membrane or cause permanent sensory-neural hearing loss. (Curiously enough, if the membrane *does* rupture, there is likely to be less permanent sensory-neural loss of hearing than if it does not. Blast deafness is rarely total in any case.) In animal experiments it has been found that blasts may disorganize the organ of Corti or shake great pieces of it loose into the surrounding fluid. The injured part of the organ does not regenerate but instead is replaced by a layer of simple cells. The same sort of permanent injury is produced by a sufficiently intense noise or pure tone. The intensity required to cause such breaking of the organ of Corti depends in part on how long the noise lasts.

*Acoustic trauma.* Injury to the ear by a single brief exposure to sound, particularly to an explosion or gun blast, is called "acoustic trauma." This term has been, and in European countries still is, used to include loss of hearing from prolonged and repeated exposure to noise. It is useful to distinguish the two conditions, however, particularly for medicolegal reasons. In acoustic trauma, as we shall use the words, it is easy to identify the actual incident and the time that it happened, and usually the responsibility for it. From the audiological point of view the loss of hearing may be very severe at first, but much recovery can be expected, and improvement usually continues for several months. This degree of recovery is in sharp contrast to the chronic noise-induced hearing loss among industrial workers in very noisy trades. Their improvement in hearing after the first 48 hours off the job is very slight indeed.

Another form of acute injury to hearing is a loss resulting from a blow to the head. A blow on the external ear, the old-fashioned "boxing the ears" of children as a form of punishment, can cause not only severe pain in the middle ear and possible injury to the drum membrane or fracture or dislocation of the ossicles but even permanent injury to the inner ear. The injury is caused by a violent wave of air-conducted "sound." Similar damage to the inner ear may even be caused by a very sharp blow on the skull, such as may occur in an automobile accident. Here the injury is best described as acoustic trauma by bone conduction.

*Noise-induced hearing loss* is the preferred term for what was once called "boilermakers' deafness" or "industrial hearing loss." It is a loss of hearing that develops gradually over months and years. With most industrial noises the loss *almost always begins at 4000 or 6000 Hz*, where the recovery from temporary threshold shift is slowest, but this depends significantly on the spectrum of the noise.

*Noise exposure.* The ear can tolerate for a few seconds a painfully loud noise that would disrupt the organ of Corti or at least cause degeneration of some of its sensory cells if continued for minutes. In other words, the duration as well as the intensity of the exposure is important. Injury from noise exposure depends on decibels, on frequency, and also on duration

measured in seconds, hours, months, or years. The sound levels necessary to produce rapid injury, say 150 dB or more, rarely occur as sustained sound except near the exhaust of some jet engines and rockets. Those who work in such situations must take special precautions, and certain areas may be forbidden entirely as too hazardous for hearing. But for the more ordinary, less severe noise exposures, the usual practical question about injury is: "Will the temporary hearing loss produced day after day and week after week ultimately become permanent?" The answer is "Yes," *if* the noise is loud enough and if a long exposure is repeated often enough; but we do not know how loud and how often is "enough." Some ears are more

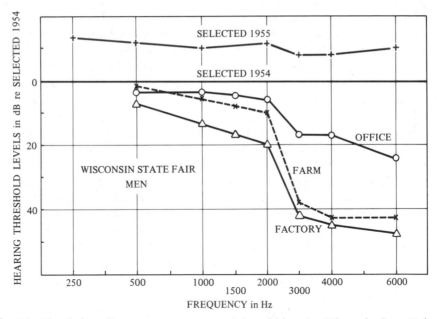

Fig. 4-9. The "selected" groups were young adults, visiting the Wisconsin State Fair, who were judged to be otologically normal and with no history of noise exposure or otic pathology. The other groups were self-selected from among visitors to the Wisconsin State Fair in 1954. The self-selection probably introduced some bias toward impaired hearing. Factory and farm workers showed more high-tone hearing loss than did office workers. The median hearing-threshold levels, relative to the selected 1954 group, for office workers, for farm workers, and for factory workers are shown separately. The divergences from the selected group express the combined effects of age, noise exposure, previous diseases of the ear, and the biases of self-selection. The difference between the "selected" levels of 1954 and 1955 is discussed in Chapter 7. The "Selected 1955" levels were included in the calculation of the ISO reference zero level.

susceptible to temporary threshold shift than are others, and there are probably similar differences in resistance to permanent injury. In the practical situations of the drop-forge worker or the skeet shooter who has suffered a permanent hearing loss, we rarely know how loud the sound was that finally caused the permanent injury. Rules, criteria, and methods for the prevention of noise-induced hearing loss are considered in the next chapter. It is comforting to know that the sound levels of sonic booms caused by supersonic aircraft are far below the pressure levels that can cause a permanent hearing loss, even with repeated exposures.

*Aggravation of hearing loss by noise.* It is a legitimate question whether exposure to noise that is not loud enough to damage a normal ear might nevertheless injure a hard-of-hearing ear. The question is most often raised with respect to the use of a hearing aid, which may deliver speech sounds at very high levels, as described in Chapter 11. Some people have been advised against the use of a hearing aid on this account by physicians who have made a diagnosis of sensory-neural hearing loss, for fear that the noise would accelerate the process of degeneration that was thought to be the cause of the hearing loss. In many cases this advice amounted to conservative cruelty. There are, indeed, certain types of hearing impairment in which such caution is proper, but they are few.

In the first place it should be obvious that if the impairment is conductive in nature there is no danger. The handicap of a hearing loss is not great enough to require an aid until the impairment amounts to 20 to 30 dB. This is about the equivalent of a good earplug, and the conductive impairment gives protection against the noise, like an earplug. It may do much better! Remember that all middle-ear impairment and also much inner-ear impairment is conductive.

The conservative view with respect to hearing aids was undoubtedly based in large part on the interpretation of presbycusis as a progressive degeneration of sensory units. We have pointed out that this is only a part—and probably the smaller part—of the story of presbycusis. Nearly all presbycusis probably has considerable built-in protection provided by its conductive components.

Noise will not accelerate the progressive conductive changes of presbycusis or otosclerosis, and neither will it delay them. If the user of a hearing aid finds that his hearing has continued to fail, this is no evidence that the hearing aid is responsible.

Caution concerning noise is legitimate in all cases of sensory-neural impairment that show signs of irritation, such as diplacusis and loud tinnitus. Often these conditions carry their own warning sign in the form of painful hearing. This type of pain or serious discomfort should be carefully respected.

An unfortunate condition without warning signs is a hereditary form of progressive degeneration of hearing in childhood. It is doubtful that noise influences this condition, and it is probably wiser to use a hearing aid to help the child learn as much language as possible before his hearing fails entirely rather than to withdraw the aid and make the child educationally deaf immediately.

A new problem lies in the application of hearing aids to congenitally deaf infants. To solve it we need to know, first, at what age a diagnosis of impairment of hearing can be made reliably and, second, at what age an infant with near-normal hearing will give reliable indication of auditory pain or discomfort from a hearing aid. Opinions on these points differ, but obviously some caution and common sense are in order here. The problem will be considered again in Chapter 16.

*Other possible effects of noise.* We

need not fear any mysterious general effects, such as fatigue, headache, neurosis, or sudden death, from any special sounds or combination of sounds. On careful investigation, the persistent rumors about such effects prove to be unfounded. The ears are much more sensitive to noise than is any other part of the body and are always injured first. To be injurious, sounds must be powerful, and usually long-lasting or repeated as well. *There is no magic in any strange disharmony or in any high-frequency "ultrasonic death ray" at any practical intensity.* Noise is unpleasant, but in a wartime experiment designed to imitate piloting an airplane a steady loud noise did not measurably impair the performance of men in any of a large variety of tests of coordination, steadiness, memory, puzzle solving, and the like. Those who *must* work in noise soon learn to disregard it. We may guess that those who dislike their work and are irritable tend to blame noise more than it really deserves for their ills.

With the increase in the noise from traffic and from airplanes there has been increased popular protest against the noise, and concern is expressed that the "nervous strain" of the noise of our industrial civilization may impair mental health. This problem goes beyond the limits set for this book. A more limited concern, however, is the proposition that the habitual noise-exposure of western civilization causes a significant impairment of hearing, not only in industrial workers but in all urban dwellers. The poorer hearing of high frequencies in men as compared to women, mentioned in an earlier section, is interpreted by many as due to more frequent, more prolonged, and more severe noise-exposure of men. Actually the noise-exposure of the average American male is well below the industrial warning level given in Chapter 5, particularly if he is an office worker. Some, however, have had dangerous exposures in military training, in driving a tractor, in skeet shooting, and

so on. It is possible, however, that lesser but more habitual exposures in subways, dance halls, airports, and so on may have a similar effect on men and women alike. In this connection the case of the Mabaans, studied by Dr. Samuel Rosen and his associates, is often cited.

The Mabaans are a primitive African tribe who live in a remote area near the border between Sudan and Ethiopia. Their agrarian culture is that of the Stone Age, and they live particularly quiet, peaceful, well-ordered lives, go nearly naked, and eat a simple vegetarian diet. They do not engage in warfare, beat drums, or even sing loudly. They apparently live to a considerable age, although they keep no records of births or deaths. It was actually much easier for Dr. Rosen to measure their hearing than to determine exact ages, but they do not seem to suffer from presbycusis. The point is that the hearing of these primitive people, who lived their entire lives in these quiet surroundings, is very sensitive, *even in old age and for high frequencies.*

Does this mean that *our* presbycusis is due to noise? Not necessarily. The Mabaans differ from us in more ways than one. They are notably free not only of social stress and turmoil but also of arteriosclerosis and cardiac disease. On the other hand, if a Mabaan moves to an Egyptian city such as Cairo and joins our world and eats our food, he does develop some presbycusis, and he becomes liable to cardiac and circulatory troubles, peptic ulcers, and so on. His life is no longer serene. It is troubled and it is noisy—and the Mabaan does not hear so well.

Other studies of other well-defined groups in different climates, with different dietary habits and cultures, for example, in Finland, Yugoslavia, and Germany, have confirmed the association of the retention of good high-frequency hearing with freedom from arteriosclerosis and coronary disease. Such studies should throw more light on the causal relations here and help us to evaluate the relative contributions of heredity, way of life, diet, and noise.

## CONGENITAL AND CHILDHOOD DEAFNESS

*Congenital* means strictly "existing at birth," but according to common usage we extend it to include those conditions that are caused by or associated with the birth process, such as birth trauma, or that develop in the first few days of life, such as icterus neonatorum. A condition that is congenital may or may not be hereditary.

In children and young people the most common "cause" of sensory-neural hearing loss, if we are to accept medical statistics at their face value, is "congenital," but the meaning of the term as it appears in medical records is not entirely clear. It is a sort of wastebasket classification in which are placed all cases of impaired hearing in children for which no likely cause can be found. The term "congenital" may be wrongly applied to cases in which the impairment is actually due to scarlet fever, meningitis, or some other disease of childhood which destroyed hearing before the child learned to talk. There is no doubt, however, that babies may sometimes be born deaf and also that there is a hereditary tendency, fortunately rare, for the sense organ of hearing and the auditory nerve to degenerate at an early age without apparent cause.

### Bacterial Infection

The inner ear may be the site of a bacterial pus-forming infection somewhat similar to infection in the middle ear. This is not a congenital condition, but it may occur during the first year or two and lead to very severe or total loss of hearing and its attendant handicap in the failure to develop speech. (Such infection may also occur later in life after speech has developed.) The infection usually reaches the inner ear through the endolymphatic and

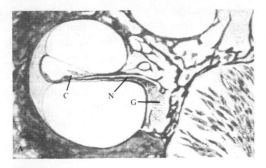

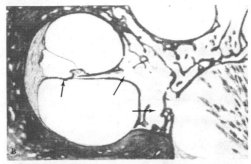

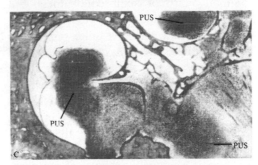

Fig. 4-10. Two types of sensory-neural impairment are represented in this figure. Section *A* represents a normal cochlea. The location of this section in relation to the inner ear as a whole is shown by the rectangle in Figure 3-7. The organ of Corti (*C*), the fibers of the auditory nerve (*N*), and the ganglion cells (*G*) are labeled in this section.

Section *B* shows the lower turn of a cochlea of a person with high-tone loss. The arrows show where the organ of Corti, the nerve fibers, and the ganglion (nerve) cells are absent. This is typical of abrupt high-tone loss (compare Figure 4-2).

Section *C* shows the destruction of the organ of Corti, basilar membrane, and nerve by pus, as in meningitis.

perilymphatic connections between the inner ear and the cranial cavity. Infection and inflammation of the coverings of the brain and spinal cord, the "meninges," is known as *meningitis*. The agent is most frequently the meningococcus which has a special predilection for the meninges. Sometimes it is a pneumococcus, a staphylococcus, the tubercle bacillus, or other variety. If the infection reaches the inner ear, it may destroy the auditory nerve, the organ of Corti, and most or all of the other delicate auditory structures. This is illustrated in Figure 4-10.

*Typhoid fever* and *diphtheria* are two bacterial diseases that probably affect the ear remotely by the *toxins* formed by the bacteria in the gastrointestinal tract or the respiratory tract, respectively. The result is more or less complete degeneration of the organ of Corti and associated structures. These diseases were formerly a relatively common cause of acquired deafness, but thanks to the widespread practice of immunization they are now quite rare in the United States. *Dihydrostreptomycin* and *kanamycin* are two antibiotic *drugs* which are effective against the tubercle bacillus, and they may be used in extreme cases in spite of the danger, mentioned in a previous section, that they may injure the ear directly.

There is obviously no hope of regeneration or repair of a missing organ of Corti, and no type of treatment, medication, or stimulation will improve the hearing of anyone whose deafness is due to meningitis or any similar bacterial infection. This proposition applies also to toxic degeneration and to viral infections such as mumps and measles, which also cause severe and permanent anatomical changes.

In the 1920s and 1930s meningitis was the most common, single, clearly identified cause of acquired total deafness in childhood. Since that time preventive innoculations have greatly reduced the prevalence of the disease, and antitoxins and antibiotics have saved the lives of a larger proportion of patients. But the life may be saved only after destruction of the inner ear, and bacterial infection still appears on our lists of causes of childhood deafness.

**Viral Infections**

Almost any of the common infectious diseases of childhood, which in general are viral rather than bacterial, may in severe cases affect the inner ear. Frequently, as is usual with mumps, only one ear is damaged, but all too often both ears suffer. A virus is submicroscopic in size, much smaller than a bacterium, and it usually reaches the ear directly from the blood stream instead of from the cerebrospinal fluid of the cranial cavity. As mentioned above, a virus does not stimulate the formation of pus, but it may severely injure delicate specialized structures such as the organ of Corti and the tectorial membrane. One type of end result is an intact basilar membrane with a formless mass of cells covering it, usually heaped up near the limbus. Many of the cells are endothelial cells that have replaced other dead cells. Sometimes remains of the tectorial membrane, all curled up and covered with endothelium, can be identified. Sometimes a few hair cells and nerve fibers remain, particularly at the extreme apical or the extreme basal end of the basilar membrane. If the sensory units do survive and function, there is a remnant of hearing which may be reached with a hearing aid. The hearing loss may be very severe, but it tends to be very stable.

In 1928 an extensive study was made, under the leadership of Dr. G. E. Shambaugh, Sr., of the causes of deafness and severe hearing loss in children enrolled in a number of public schools for the deaf. In more than half of the pupils, most of them studied in retrospect on the basis of their medical and family histories, no cause could be assigned, but "infectious diseases of childhood" including typhoid fever, diphtheria, and "high fever" (not otherwise identified) accounted for deafness in about 15 percent of the pupils. Some of these diseases, notably typhoid fever, diphtheria, and scarlet fever, have now been brought under control and cause few impairments, but other diseases are still very significant as causes. No precise recent statistics are available, however.

*Maternal rubella.* One particular viral disease, however, has now emerged as a major cause of congenital deafness. It is *rubella* or "German measles." Particular strains of this virus that are unusually virulent have appeared, and the disease has twice assumed epidemic proportions. The first recognized outbreak occurred in Australia about 1942. It was following this epidemic that it was recognized that rubella in the mother during early pregnancy could cause a congenital deafness. The largest and most recent epidemic was in 1963, 1964, and 1965. The northeastern seaboard of the United States suffered most severely, but the disease was quite widespread throughout the midwestern and Pacific coast states.

By good fortune a continuing cooperative long-term study of a large group of expectant mothers was in progress in Baltimore and other medical centers when the epidemic appeared. This study was sponsored by the United States National Institutes of Health. In it several important features of rubella and its effects on the developing embryo or fetus were discovered.

For the mother the disease is usually a mild infection. Actually about half of the Baltimore mothers who gave birth to infants in whom the virus or antibodies were detected by laboratory tests had had no clinical symptoms of rubella themselves. It is the developing embryo, not the mother, that suffers. In the Baltimore study there were 165 children with confirmed prenatal rubella. Of these, 73 failed to pass their hearing test. But congenital deafness is only one of the many developmental defects that may occur. Vision may be impaired. The heart may be defective, and

the nervous system may be abnormal in a variety of ways, from minor defects to complete idiocy.

The chances of developmental defects, including severe hearing loss, proved to be greatest when the maternal illness occurred during the first 3 months of pregnancy. Previously it was believed that the embryo was vulnerable *only* during the first trimester, but it is now clear that the virus may persist and injure an embryo that is conceived weeks or even a few months after the infection, and injury to a fetus can occur at least as late as the seventh month of pregnancy. Nineteen mothers in the Baltimore study contracted rubella during the second trimester of pregnancy. Two fetuses were stillborn, with positive viral cultures. Six viable infants showed abnormalities compatible with prenatal rubella. Only five of the infants failed to give laboratory evidence of rubella at birth.

It had been generally assumed that the mechanism of the injury was an interference with the control of development. Heart, nervous system, eyes, and ears go through important and complex stages of development in the first trimester. But the length of time that the child carries the virus is also significant. The children who carry it for long periods after birth tend to suffer more severely than those from whom it disappears after birth. Here inhibition of normal growth appears to be involved.

The anatomical appearance of the inner ears of a few infants with congenital rubella deafness that have been studied is rather like that seen following postnatal viral infection. There is severe but incomplete injury to the organ of Corti and what looks like a "healing" regrowth of epithelium. It is quite possible that the virus, as well as toxins, can pass through the placenta and that the embryo or fetus is damaged in utero. Very likely the protective mechanisms of the fetus are less effective than those of the mother. The ear and other developing organs may be directly infected, and some of their cells destroyed by the virus.

The rubella virus was isolated in the middle sixties and by 1968 a successful vaccine against it was announced. Programs for systematic innoculation are under way (1969) in several states of the U.S.A. One such program, in Massachusetts, administers the vaccine to children in the first two grades of school, with the expectation of extending it later to adolescent and post-adolescent females. A primary concern is to prevent if possible, another major epidemic which, without a program of extensive innoculation, should be expected in the early seventies. In addition, we can look forward with confidence to testing women for their immunity to rubella and to protecting prospective mothers who do not have a sufficient "titer" of antibodies.

Rubella is not the only viral infection that can cause congenital deafness or dysacusis. Almost any severe infection can do so, particularly during the first trimester when the embryo seems to be more vulnerable than later during fetal life. Influenza and mumps seem to be the most dangerous, after rubella, but at the other extreme the common cold creates no such hazard.

Rubella rarely causes total deafness. The children with this type of congenital impairment may be severely hard of hearing and educationally deaf in the sense that they do not hear speech sounds well enough to learn speech and language spontaneously. They need hearing aids. Very frequently they retain fairly good hearing for the very high frequencies (4000 Hz and above) or for low frequencies (250 and 125 Hz), or both. They respond to many environmental sounds, including the human voice, and it may be several years before it is realized that they actually have a serious hearing handicap. The consequences of such delay in diagnosis can be very unfortunate, as we shall point out in the discussion of central dysacusis. These children with serious but incomplete hearing losses have frequently been misdiagnosed as aphasic, mentally retarded, or "brain-damaged."

*Encephalitis.* Encephalitis or infection of the brain is a final member of our list of infections. It can cause a great variety of symptoms of "brain injury," including central dysacusis. The impairments are usually neurological, not audiological, but sometimes there is peripheral cochlear impairment, just as in so many viral infections, and the hearing loss or deafness may be the greatest handicap.

## Rh and Other Incompatibilities

Another cause of congenital dysacusis, either peripheral or central, is the incompatibility of certain blood proteins of the parents. More specifically, the rhesus or "Rh" factor may be present or absent. Other factors are "A," "B" and "O." The incompatibilities all operate according to the same pattern and cause their injury to the ears or to the nervous system either directly or by the condition known as "jaundice of the new-born" or *icterus neonatorum* or *kernicterus* during the first few days of life. The jaundice of kernicterus is caused by abnormal destruction of red blood cells when or before independent life begins at birth. One of the degradation products of the red blood pigment, hemoglobin, is bilirubin, one of the bile pigments. Its yellow color causes the jaundice, and its selective accumulation in certain areas or "nuclei" in the brain causes brain injury. The auditory system is one of the systems that is likely to be injured.

The dangerous parental combination is father Rh-positive and mother Rh-negative, or the corresponding ABO combination. The common feature is that the father's tissues contain a protein that the mother's lack. To her body it is a foreign protein, and if this hereditary characteristic is transmitted by the father to the embryo the mother's system may react against the embryo (or later the fetus) by the same mechanism that develops immunity against any foreign proteins, such as those of pathogenic bacteria. A critical condition is that enough of the "foreign" Rh (or A) factor cross the placental barrier. Then the mother's system forms "antibodies" against it. These antibodies in turn may cause a miscarriage or toxemia or, if they in turn cross the placental barrier, either injure the fetus immediately or through a postnatal kernicterus. Fortunately this biological accident is less likely in a first pregnancy, but it seems as if a first pregnancy may sensitize the mother's system and make difficulties more probable in any later pregnancies in which the heredity is Rh-positive. It may be possible in the future to protect an Rh-negative mother with an anti-Rh antibody that inactivates any Rh-positive fetal blood cells that may pass into her circulation.

The treatment for icterus neonatorum is massive blood transfusions for the infant. It must be done promptly and thoroughly, amounting to complete blood replacement. Too little or too late may still save the life but only after permanent injury has been done by the bilirubin. Infants who have had even a mild "bilirubinemia" (15 mg per cc or more bilirubin in the blood) for any reason should be considered "at risk" with respect to their hearing.

### Birth Injury, Anoxia, and Other Nonhereditary Causes of Dysacusis

For completeness and convenience we mention here a few other causes of congenital dysacusis, even though their usual area of injury is central rather than peripheral. Almost all of these relate to various complications of labor, such as prematurity (best defined as a birth weight of 2500 grams or less), either prolonged or precipitate labor, or difficult delivery involving the use of obstetrical forceps with traction on the neck, or birth injury from any cause. Such injuries are usually complicated by hemorrhage in or around the brain. Premature babies are particularly liable to intracranial hemorrhage. Toxemia of pregnancy from any cause, quite apart from Rh incompatibility, carries a risk of injury to hearing.

At birth a very common cause of injury is apnea or failure to breathe, particularly if it goes to the stage of cyanosis (blueness). Certain midbrain auditory centers are among those most susceptible to injury from such asphyxia.

A rather rare accident that deserves passing mention is the use for a premature infant of an incubator that is too noisy.

Injuries may occur at any age. We must remember that not only skull fractures that might crack the temporal bone but blows to the ears ("boxing the ears") and even blows to the skull can sometimes cause acoustic trauma.

### Metabolic and Endocrine Disorders

A completely different type of difficulty arises from certain metabolic or endocrine disorders in childhood. The clearest association of dysacusis is with hypothyroidism (cretinism). Impairment of hearing, very likely of a mechanical conductive sort, may accompany the slow skeletal and muscular development, the low metabolic rate, the sluggishness of movement, the mental retardation, the pudgy thickening of the skin, and other abnormalities.

### Hereditary Deafness

There are many forms of hereditary deafness. The deafness may occur as an isolated trait or it may occur in combination with other abnormalities of development in a variety of "syndromes." Each syndrome is probably caused by a single faulty or "mutant" gene.

*Genes* are the units of heredity, and are carried in the chromosomes. They acquire their individuality from the chemical details of the DNA (deoxyribonucleic acid) molecules of which they are composed. The action of genes upon the final characteristics of the body is very complex. The DNA molecules determine the detailed structure of the RNA (ribonucleic acid) molecules made in the cell; these specify the structure of protein molecules, which in turn take part in a very large number of chemical reactions of metabolism and development. It is therefore easy to understand that a single fault, or *mutation,* in the DNA of a particular chromosome in an ovum or a sperm cell may profoundly modify not only one but many characteristics of the adult derived from it.

The simple Mendelian rules of heredity concerning the assortment of genes and the probabilities of their various combinations in the offspring are probably familiar, but they will be recapitulated here in part. In the first place, every type of gene is represented twice in an individual, one member of the pair received from the father and the other from the mother. The genes of a pair may be different as a result of mutation. Mutations alter, impair, or even eliminate the function of a gene. Any of these differences may or may not be obvious, and this will depend in part upon the interaction of a mutant gene with its partner in the organism which carries them. The effects of most mutant genes can be seen most clearly when both of the genes in question in the organism are of the mutant type. When paired with its normal alternate, a mutant gene may be masked in its expression by the activity of the normal alternate. This is because most mutations merely eliminate a genetic function.

If the normal alternate alone performs as well as two normal genes would, the normal alternate completely masks the mutant, and it is called "dominant." The impaired mutant is called "recessive." But often a mutation is not masked completely in its expression by its normal partner. The mutation is then called "incompletely recessive" or its partner is "incompletely dominant." However, if the mutation is expressed as strongly when it is present in a single dose as when there are two doses, it is dominant, and in relation to such mutations the normal counterpart is recessive.

A parent passes on to his (or her) child one, but only one, member of each gene pair. The matter of which one is transmitted is wholly a matter of chance. This is the Mendelian principle of *segregation.* The segregation of each gene pair into its two members in the formation of ova and sperm is usually independent of the segregation of other gene pairs which control different functions, and thus different gene pairs are said to be *independently* (or randomly) *assorted.* The exception to this general rule is that different sets of genes which are located on the same chromosome tend to segregate as a group and are usually passed on together. Such genes are said to be "linked." In humans there are 43 pairs of chromosomes and thus 43 "linkage groups."

If one dominant mutant gene is received from either parent, the child will display the effect of the gene unless its expression is modified by other factors. When a child having one dominant mutation matures and has children, the chances of its being passed on to the next generation are 50 percent for each child. If an individual receives the same type of dominant mutation from both his parents, he will not only display the effect of the mutation, but he will transmit the mutant gene to all of his children.

If a mutant gene is recessive, it will be expressed only when it is received from *both* parents. If each parent carries two recessive genes, each of their children will automatically receive two recessive genes and will express them, other things being equal. If one parent carries a pair of recessive genes, but the other carries only their dominant counterparts, each of their children will get a dominant gene from the second parent, and will never express the recessive gene contributed by the first. If each parent carries one recessive mutant and one normal gene, the chances—in the case of every child born to them—are 25 percent for receiving two mutant genes (one from each parent), 50 percent for receiving one normal and one mutant gene (because either gene of the pair can be transmitted by either parent), and 25 percent for receiving a normal gene from both parents. The corresponding probabilities when one parent carries two mutant recessives and the other parent only one are 50 percent for each child receiving two mutant genes, and 50 percent for its receiving only one. These simple ratios are part of the familiar Mendelian laws of heredity. They emphasize the importance of avoiding consanguineous marriage (that is, marriage of cousins) in the case of rare recessive genes, because of the greatly increased chances that members of the same family carry a given gene.

The expression of mutant genes does not depend entirely on the alternate genes with which they are paired, as described above. The extent to which their effects are seen in an individual, or even the probability that a mutant gene will be detectable at all, depends on other influences. Thus, the gene in question may vary in its expression according to its interaction with other types of genes in the same person, and also according to the prenatal and postnatal environment in which the child develops. For instance, hemophilia, in which there is a tendency to bleed because the time required for the blood to clot is prolonged, may vary in severity in different individuals who carry the gene, although all of them will show some effect.

Mutant genes may vary in their expression in different individuals not only quantitatively but also in their so-called *penetrance*. By penetrance we mean the *proportion of individuals* carrying a mutant gene who actually display the characteristic effect of that gene. "Incomplete penetrance" implies that people who are identical in carrying a recessive mutant gene-pair, for instance, may nevertheless vary qualitatively in that some of them give no detectable sign of the gene at all. The degree of penetrance attributed to a gene will obviously depend on what we mean by "detectable." If we have a sensitive measuring instrument, for example, an audiometer as opposed to merely a family's detection of the practical handicap of someone's hearing loss, the penetrance of a mutant gene for sensory-neural hearing loss may be quite high. At the same time the quantitative degree to which the gene tends to be expressed may be rather small.

All individuals who carry a mutant gene can pass it on to their children, regardless of whether it is dominant or recessive, whether it has high or low (incomplete) penetrance, or whether its expression tends to be strong or slight. A mutant gene may be present in many individuals in whom it never reaches the threshold of expression and detectability. It should be clear that differences in "penetrance" and in "expressivity" are quite distinct from dominance and recessiveness and that they apply to dominant and to recessive genes alike.

To return to deafness, the term "familial deafness" expresses the tendency of the deafness to appear rather frequently in a family as an obvious trait, like red hair. This would be the behavior of a dominant gene of high penetrance. The contrasting term is "sporadic" deafness, which seems to appear in isolated instances. This would be the behavior of a dominant gene of very low penetrance, or of a rather rare recessive gene which gains expression through chance combination with an identical but equally rare partner, or possibly the occurrence of a new dominant mutation. Any type of hereditary deafness can vary in severity in decibels or in its range on the frequency scale.

Otologists and pathologists have been fascinated by various hereditary syndromes which include deafness in combination with other abnormalities. The other abnormalities include bizarre skeletal deformities, abnormal pigmentation, and defects of eyes and central nervous system. Each syndrome is known by the name of the doctor who first described it in the literature and they are well described in medical monographs. Examples are the *Waardenburg* syndrome, the *Klippel-Feil* syndrome, and the *Treacher-Collins* syndrome; and there are others. We also name certain types of abnormality of the labyrinth or of the middle or the external ear which may occur in isolation.

One of these, *Scheibe's* type (sacculocochlear type), is worth mentioning because Drs. Whetnall and Fry state in their monograph that it occurs in about 70 percent of cases of hereditary deafness. The abnormalities are confined to the cochlear duct and saccule. The organ of Corti shows the greatest change in the apical turn, where it may consist of only "a mound of undifferentiated cells." The stria vascularis is degenerate. The tectorial membrane is flattened over the organ of Corti, or rolled up in the internal sulcus, or attached to Reissner's membrane. The cochlear duct may be dilated, but more often it is collapsed. Reissner's membrane may be adherent directly to the organ of Corti. This description is strangely similar to our description in an earlier paragraph of the effects of viral infection.

Another type to recall, mentioned earlier, is the delayed degeneration of the organ of Corti that occurs during childhood. The immediate reason for and mechanism of the degeneration is not known, but the same kind of thing happens in waltzing guinea pigs, in albinotic cats, and probably in other kinds of hereditary deafness in animals.

An interesting suggestion made recently by Dr. E. Wedenberg of Stockholm is that the carriers of the gene for at least some form(s) of hereditary deafness may be identified by careful audiometry. They show dips in the high-frequency range of the audiogram which are not reasonably explained by noise-exposure, and their stapedius reflex is weak or absent. Wedenberg believes that these are incomplete expressions (associated with the low penetrance) of the gene in question. This is very interesting theoretically, but it does not point as yet to any practical application unless it be to alert parents to the possibility of sporadic deafness so that it will be detected early and managed appropriately.

With the recognition of the low penetrance of some genes that produce deafness *it becomes reasonable to suppose that the majority of cases of unexplained severe congenital hearing loss and deafness are actually sporadic hereditary deafness.* The incidence of most other forms of childhood deafness should be reduced progressively with better prevention and treatment of infectious diseases and better prenatal and postnatal care, but there is no cure and no effective prevention for sporadic hereditary deafness—only early detection and good management.

## CENTRAL DYSACUSIS

### Organic Impairments

In general, the more peripherally a lesion is located in the nervous system, the more clear-cut are the signs and symptoms and the easier it is to make a diagnosis and to locate the lesion anatomically. Lesions of the auditory system within the brain can rarely be localized or even clearly identified by their symptoms, except perhaps to say that the lesion is more probably on the right side or on the left. More often the questions asked will be whether there is *any* pathological condition that would be visible at postmortem and, if so, whether it has any clear localization like a tumor or is completely generalized like arteriosclerosis.

Among the numerous causes of central impairment are generalized infections such as encephalitis and meningitis, specific infections such as syphilis, degenerative diseases such as multiple sclerosis, the progressive death of individual neurons due to old age, "cerebral vascular accidents" of various sorts such as cerebral hemorrhage or the blocking of blood vessels by local clotting (thrombosis) or by a clot originally formed elsewhere (embolism), and clearly local injuries such as gunshot wounds, skull fractures, birth injuries, and the scars and adhesions resulting from these. Congenital abnormalities, either specific malformations or generalized conditions such as mongolism, should be mentioned also. A subtle general or partially localized injury may follow prolonged asphyxia, either at birth or from drowning (with delayed resuscitation) or carbon monoxide poisoning. Some areas of the sensory systems in the brain stem seem to be particularly susceptible to such asphyxial injury. Finally, and very important, there are brain tumors, cysts, and abscesses.

*Acoustic neurinoma.* In a previous section we have considered the type of impairment that is most commonly associated with a tumor of the eighth nerve—the so-called acoustic neurinoma or neuroma. From the audiological point of view it is logical to class the impairment as *neural,* although from the anatomical and surgical point of view these tumors are *central* lesions.

Acoustic tumors are not malignant, and they may grow very slowly over the years, but the earlier they are recognized and removed, the better the chance of preserving the facial nerve and possibly the eighth (auditory) nerve also. The symptoms of pressure on the eighth nerve are hearing loss, mild tinnitus, and vertigo, and sometimes there are also symptoms due to pressure on other cranial nerves or the brain stem. The position of these tumors at the base of the brain makes their removal a serious operation. Audiological tests, described in Chapter 8, and tests of vestibular function may be very helpful in establishing the diagnosis firmly.

The overlap between otology and neurology is well illustrated by the problems of diagnosis and surgical removal of acoustic neurinomas. The overlap includes also the lesions, disorders, and malfunctions of the central auditory system. The auditory dysacuses may be accompanied by equally or more important impairments of other systems, as in cerebral palsy. But, regardless of which specialist first recognizes the case or which one makes the final diagnosis or who handles the treatment, the audiologist can assist by performing the tests that are described in later chapters and by evaluating the results for the benefit of his medical and surgical colleagues. The audiologist does not make diagnoses, but his tests often indicate a strong probability of one diagnosis or anatomical localization as opposed to another. And it makes little difference whether the joint specialty that the audiologist serves is known as "neuro-otology" or "otoneurology."

The foregoing list of cerebral diseases, injuries, and impairments is not exhaustive, but it illustrates the variety of conditions that must be considered by the neurologist in making a diagnosis, and it also illustrates the specific localization of some lesions and the diffuseness of others. And even if a lesion like a tumor is perfectly definite and discrete, the symptoms that it causes may be very vague indeed, particularly if it is located in one of the "association areas" of the cerebral cortex. But sometimes the audiologist, by appropriate tests that involve the understanding of speech under difficult listening conditions, or presented at high speed, or requiring the fusion of information delivered to the two ears, may assist the neurologist to a diagnosis or a localization. The basis of such tests will be considered in Chapter 8.

An impairment of hearing associated

with any of the foregoing diseases or conditions is said to be an "organic" dysacusis.

### Functional Dysacusis

There is another major class of central auditory impairments which do not have any apparent organic basis but which relate instead to distortions of attention, motivation, and understanding, that is, to psychological factors. These are known as *nonorganic* or *functional dysacuses.*

We call attention here to what may be, for some, an extension of the concept of dysacusis to include psychological factors such as inattention, hysterical deafness, deliberate feigning, and so on. It seems useful to include them all, however, in the blanket term because it is often very difficult to distinguish one from another and from organic dysacuses. Some of the psychological factors will be considered specifically below.

It is particularly important to recognize that the functional impairments may be combined with, and to some extent arise from, organic impairments, particularly from peripheral hearing loss. We then speak of a *functional overlay.* It is often very difficult to determine the extent of the overlay, or even to distinguish between the organic and the functional components. Here three major questions must be considered.

First, what is the degree of motivation and cooperation of the subject? Is a child incompetent because of mental retardation or the psychiatric condition known as *autism* or *childhood schizophrenia?* Is an adult deliberately exaggerating a hearing loss, that is, feigning or simulating for reasons of his own? More technically, is it a case of *pseudohypoacusis?* Or does he fail to understand what he is expected to do? Is his *span of attention* too short? Obviously a test of peripheral hearing that does not require active cooperation by the subject can be of great help in answering such questions (see Chapter 8).

Second, what is the extent of any peripheral hearing loss, that is, true hypoacusis? A severe or even a moderate hearing loss, such as might be caused by a congenital defect, an infection, or acoustic trauma, may establish certain patterns of attention and behavior which become firmly established but which may nevertheless be reversible with proper management and training. In other words, how great is the functional overlay?

Finally, at what age did the impairment appear? If a child has had sufficient hearing in his first two or three years of life to learn speech and develop language spontaneously, his over-all prospect for rehabilitation will be very much better than that of the child who has never developed speech. On the other hand the "plasticity" of the nervous system of the young child, mentioned in Chapter 3, may make learning or relearning easier if he suffers a partial organic impairment early, rather than later in life. As we shall point out below, we simply do not yet know how much the development of the nervous system is influenced by early sensory deprivation, either partial or total. Here the distinction between organic and functional ceases to be very meaningful. We shall return to this question in Chapter 16.

### Audiometric Tests in Central Dysacusis

Central dysacusis does not cause elevation of the threshold of hearing, except for what may be attributed to failure of attention and cooperation, nor does it impair hearing for particular frequencies as in abrupt, high-tone hearing loss. The characteristic difficulty is *difficulty in understanding speech* or even the failure to recognize the meaning of simple acoustic signals. The term *central auditory imperception* is sometimes used to describe the difficulty. One of the best diagnostic clues to central dysacusis is a discrepancy between the ability to understand speech and the prediction based on pure-tone audiometry. A patient may say "I hear you, but I can't understand the words." Or he may just seem bewildered. Another major characteristic, particularly of certain functional impairments, is a variability of thresholds from one test to another.

Pure-tone audiometry may be very important for the recognition and assessment of a peripheral organic component, but it is practically useless for the description of a functional overlay. Central dysacusis is not measured in hertz or in decibels. Better dimensions are to be found in speed of perception, in synthesis, and in understanding. This point is illustrated in the following descriptions of several particular forms of central dysacusis.

### Phonemic Regression in Old Age

The term "phonemic regression" was coined by Dr. Raymond Carhart to describe a condition that he noticed fairly often in elderly people who came to his hearing clinic at Northwestern University. They complained of difficulty in understanding what other people said. By pure-tone audiometry these elderly people showed nearly normal hearing-threshold levels, at least up to 2000 Hz, if the tests were carried out carefully, deliberately, and sympathetically, and with adequate rest periods. But with speech audiometry, particularly with the recorded speech tests, described in Chapter 8, these people had great difficulty. They understood only a few words correctly and soon became discouraged.

It is easy to recognize in this the pattern of old age. The attention span becomes short, and the person will not and cannot be hurried. Given time, he may answer correctly, but seldom quickly. He has much more difficulty with the complicated acoustic patterns of speech than with simple pure tones. That is why Dr. Carhart calls it *phonemic* regression. These people usually have the high-tone sensory-neural hearing loss of presbycusis, but their failure to understand words is far greater than can be explained by this loss alone.

The cause of phonemic regression lies in the brain, not in the ear. Generalized cerebral arteriosclerosis is probably the most common cause. Many individual cells have died throughout the brain and there may be many bits and patches where the loss is more than just a thinning of the cell population. The brain still remembers old experiences and habits, but it learns or remembers little that is new. Attention is short. Naps become frequent. And even familiar performances, like recognizing the meaning of words or sentences, although often still possible, may require special motivation and plenty of time. These elderly people have particular difficulty understanding speech in a background of noise. For those with phonemic regression a hearing aid is of little help, nor does it help to shout at them. It is more important to speak *clearly, simply,* and, above all, *slowly.*

### Verbal Dysacusis (Sensory Aphasia)

Verbal dysacusis means specifically the failure to understand the *meanings* of words even though the sounds are presumed to be heard quite perfectly and correctly. "Word deafness" is a reasonable popular translation, but the term *aphasia* has been used more and more widely. Strictly, aphasia refers to the inability to say, or perhaps to find, the word one wants to express an idea. But understanding incoming words and finding the proper word to say are closely related to one another, and both functions are likely to be impaired by the same organic lesion, and it is reasonable to use the same term for both. We may, however, wish to distinguish *motor or expressive aphasia* from *sensory aphasia* in some circumstances.

Verbal dysacusis may be caused in adults by an injury, as in an automobile accident or a "cerebral vascular accident," to the parietal-temporal area of the hemisphere (usually the left) that is dominant for speech. This speech area and also another more anterior area (Broca's area) and a third supplementary speech area are shown in Figure 4-11, but we shall not go into the details of the anatomy of the areas. The management and rehabilitation of such patients and current issues and theories are considered in a later chapter.

The relearning of speech, both motor and sensory, may be slow and tedious, but

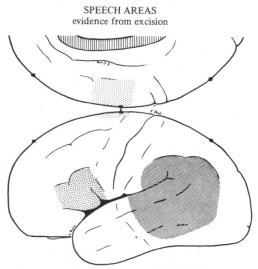

SPEECH AREAS
evidence from excision

Fig. 4-11. The three speech areas, shown in this diagram by Penfield and Roberts, are believed to be of different values. The posterior, or parietotemporal, area is the most important. The anterior, or Broca's, area is the next most important but is dispensable—in some patients at least. The superior, or supplementary motor, area is dispensable but probably is very important after damage to one of the other speech areas. This diagram is based on postoperative study of patients from whom known areas of the cortex had been removed to relieve them of epileptic seizures. Very similar speech areas can be deduced from the interference with speech that has been produced at operation by electrical stimulation of the exposed brain. Note that the speech areas are located only in the hemisphere that is dominant for speech, usually the left. (*From W. Penfield and L. Roberts. Speech and Brain-Mechanisms. Princeton, N. J.: Princeton University Press, 1959,* London: Oxford University Press.)

it is usually possible. Our understanding of the neurological and physiological basis of the aphasias, the "agnosias," and the related conditions of cerebral injury, epilepsy, and the like is advancing rapidly, but we must always approach the practical problems of the clinic on the basis of direct observation and experience and not rely on neurological or physiological theory.

## Congenital Aphasia Based on Birth Injury

Some children who do not learn to talk spontaneously resemble in many ways the aphasic adult. Their hearing is good to the extent that their attention can be attracted by sounds, including voice sounds, but the sounds seem to convey little or no meaning. They may imitate speech sounds and intonations, but they do not learn words. With patience, and by reducing speech to its elemental parts and gradually building up a series of associations with sounds and written symbols, they can be taught to understand and to speak, but an outstanding characteristic is a *difficulty in learning,* particularly in learning language. This condition has been given the name *congenital aphasia* or "childhood aphasia." (Aphasia here does not mean the *loss* of a function [speech] that was once learned but instead a *failure to develop* speech in the first place.) In addition there are some children who, after learning speech, do become truly aphasic following a severe illness such as encephalitis. This is an *acquired aphasia.* Then there is the final combination in which an injury occurs early in life and apparently prevents the normal learning of speech.

Following the analogy of aphasia in adults, the failure to develop speech has usually been attributed to a congenital defect or birth injury, or to a brain injury in early childhood before speech was learned, that has affected certain critical areas of the brain. Actually in only one such case, a boy with multiple congenital defects, has a postmortem examination been reported. This brain did indeed show extensive malformation and degeneration in both temporal lobes and in the medial geniculate bodies of the thalamus. In spite of the anatomical absence of the primary auditory projection areas of the cortex this boy had been taught with fair success at an oral school for deaf children, and at the time of his death (at 10 years of age) had a vocabulary of several hundred words. His use of language was best in structured lessons, but spontaneous speech was effective. He comprehended oral language best when it was spoken slowly. He understood only the most familiar expressions when they were spoken at a normal rate. His puretone audiogram was within normal limits. This case meets the criteria for congenital aphasia.

It now appears, however, that this type of case, with no significant hearing loss, is rare. Certainly the organic defect that must be assumed to account for congenital aphasia, namely, an extensive injury limited to both cortical auditory areas (like that in the case described above), is very improbable. This improbability has led many to question whether the implicit diagnosis of "brain injury," particularly when it is not supported by other neurological signs or symptoms, is a reasonable explanation for failure to learn speech. At least one alternative explanation is available for many cases.

### Congenital Aphasia Based on a Partial Hearing Loss

Careful audiometric study of one group of so-called "aphasic children" showed that nearly all of the children had a very significant loss of hearing for frequencies in the middle range, that is, for the frequencies important for the understanding of speech (Dr. L. L. Elliott at Central Institute for the Deaf). Often, however, they had fairly good hearing for either the very high or the very low fre-

quencies, or both. This pattern of hearing loss is actually rather common among children whose mothers have suffered from rubella early in their pregnancies. It was rather characteristic in the history of these children that the hearing loss was not recognized until the fourth or fifth years. They had often been wrongly diagnosed as mentally retarded, and they frequently had developed serious problems of behavior. This situation and its management will be considered more fully in Chapter 16.

The alternative hypothesis invoked to explain the difficulty in learning is essentially developmental. It is postulated that the auditory system requires sensory input during the early years, particularly during the second year when the normal infant begins to learn speech, in order to complete its development, and that if this normal organization does not occur, it is more difficult to bring it about later, even though sounds are then made audible by amplification. The failure to recognize the partial hearing loss leads to false expectations and inappropriate management. The child develops what may be called a "habitual disregard" for sound as a means of communication. It makes no difference whether the hearing loss is hereditary, congenital, or acquired, but it is important that the loss is present during the years when children normally learn to talk.

This interpretation is still a hypothesis, but it is supported by experiments on the visual system in kittens that are deprived of eyesight by suturing their eyelids closed for the first weeks or months of life. These kittens develop long-lasting visual defects that persist after their eyes are opened. Anatomical abnormalities of organization and even degenerative changes have been demonstrated by the work of Wiesel and Hubel. It is not appropriate here to describe these experiments in detail, but the analogy is very suggestive. Much more important, however, is the clinical experience that young children in whom the partial hearing loss is detected early and who are given the benefit of early and habitual exposure to loud speech, with a hearing aid as soon as they are old enough, do develop speech and effective use of their residual hearing much better than children with similar audiograms who have not had the advantage of early auditory exposure and training.

*The practical implication of this hypothesis is, of course, to recognize early the auditory defect and to initiate the proper management,* as described in Chapter 16. In any case the diverse usages of the term "congenital aphasia" and the connotations that have become attached to it have made it very confusing and almost useless. We recommend that it be used only when the diagnosis is unquestionable. Most of the children in our experience to whom it has been applied are now known to be hypoacusic, many of them quite severely so; but their really important impairment is their failure to have learned speech and a *difficulty in learning* in general. Above all, we, as audiologists or speech therapists, must not postulate a brain injury without a clear history of trauma or illness or supporting neurological signs or, preferably, both.

## Dyslogomathia: A New Term

*Dysmathia* is a more appropriate term than aphasia. Dysmathia is an old Greek word that means exactly what we want to say, namely, *difficulty or slowness in learning.* If we wish to be more specific and say *difficulty in learning speech and language,* we can form a new word, *dyslogomathia.*[2] The familiar root "logos" carries the connotation of both speech and language.

[2] The writer is indebted to Prof. W. M. Sale of the Department of Classics at Washington University for suggestions and advice concerning the new word dyslogomathia. Plato used *dysmathia* for "difficulty in learning." The root *math* survives in English in *mathematics.* *Logo-* is a familiar Greek combining form meaning *word, speech* or *discourse,* or *reason.*

In summary, true congenital aphasia based on an anatomical defect or birth injury does occur, but it is rare. Dyslogomathia, based on partial sensory deprivation, is a more probable explanation in a majority of the cases in which children show some reactions to fairly loud sounds but do not spontaneously develop speech, and often have great difficulty learning speech later. Further study should clarify the situation and allow us to accept, reject, or modify this working hypothesis.

## Psychogenic Dysacusis vs. Feigning (Pseudohypoacusis)

An extreme form of functional or nonorganic dysacusis is so-called *psychogenic dysacusis.* This condition is caused by psychological changes in the personality. By definition there is either partial or total inability to hear, either as an isolated condition or as a psychogenic overlay in addition to an organic dysacusis. Nerve impulses initiated in the ear by sound waves reach the brain, but *they are not consciously heard.*

Psychogenic deafness or a psychogenic overlay merges imperceptibly into *feigning* or *pseudohypoacusis.* The difference is that the person who feigns *knows* that he can hear, whereas the patient with psychogenic deafness does not know that his peripheral hearing is as good as it actually is. This is a very difficult distinction for the audiologist to make, and as a matter of fact the diagnosis can logically be made with confidence only in retrospect when either the patient has been cured by appropriate psychiatric treatment or has confessed to deliberate deception. As we shall see in Chapter 8, the detection of malingering is easy, with the help of special audiometric tests, but the measurement of actual threshold levels and the proof of motive usually depend on a battle of wits between the audiologist and the subject. The assessment of motivation becomes very important. In general the *diagnosis of psychogenic deaf-*

*ness or overlay is made only as a last resort and when it is in keeping with an overall pattern of behavior and medical history that suggests a particular pattern of emotional stress and conflict.*

In civilian life in the United States at the present time (1968) psychogenic deafness should be regarded as a rare condition. No case reports have appeared in the literature during the last 15 years. Nevertheless it was apparently fairly common among military personnel in World War II and also in certain other cultures. There are few descriptions of the condition, and for this reason we retain from the first edition of this book the following account, written in 1945.

Laymen in general have been unaware of the existence of psychogenic dysacusis, or functional deafness, and the medical profession has tended to underestimate its importance, in spite of occasional obvious cases of "miraculous" cures at shrines, by faith healers, or for no evident or reasonable cause. The experience of World War II showed, however, that psychological factors may be among the common causes of deafness and hearing loss in military service. Of course, hearing loss is not necessarily *either* organic *or* psychogenic. Very often it is both, in uncertain proportions. The best estimate we can find is based on a careful study of the last 500 cases admitted to the Hoff General Hospital (United States Army) at the end of World War II for auditory rehabilitation. Fifteen percent of these men were found to have indications of a psychogenic factor in their hearing loss. For some of them the history of the hearing loss did not coincide with the usual clinical history or with the results of the otological examination. For others the audiogram varied widely from day to day, or the hearing loss for speech was much more or much less than the audiogram suggested it should be. Perhaps a hearing aid gave no improvement at all or else a startlingly great improvement. These 15

percent, a total of 75 men, were treated by appropriate methods (which we shall not attempt to describe) for psychogenic dysacusis. The accuracy of the original estimate was substantial by the fact that 60 of the 75, or "12 percent of all patients admitted, had either a complete return of hearing to normal or a substantial improvement" at the time of separation from the Army.

This figure, high enough to make some otologists incredulous, does not mean that 12 to 15 percent of the cases of hearing loss were *purely* psychogenic, but it does mean that psychological factors accounted for at least a significant part of the hearing loss in approximately one in eight men whose hearing became inadequate in military service. The special stresses of combat service obviously increased the proportion of cases of psychogenic dysacusis. Psychogenic hearing loss was a prominent factor in the army cases studied, and in all probability it is more prevalent and important in civilian life than has previously been suspected, but the importance and prevalence in civilian life of psychogenic deafness, as distinct from a mild psychogenic overlay and from malingering is still an open question.

*Hysterical deafness.* The most common type of psychogenic deafness is called *hysterical deafness*. In this type, deep emotional conflicts within the personality structure involve the sense of hearing and manifest themselves in a total loss of hearing. Conflicts of which the individual is unconscious, rather than an impairment of the auditory mechanism, are the real cause. The disturbing emotional problem is converted into an impairment of hearing. Such substitution for the emotional problem is called *conversion*, and the resulting deafness is termed a *conversion hysteria*. Hysteria may involve senses other than hearing. A man may suffer from hysterical blindness or from anesthesia or paralysis of any part of the body without any physical impairment of the eye, or nerves, or muscles. But in any case of hysterical loss, the individual is unaware of the conflict which has found a substitute solution, or at least he does not understand its true nature.

It is impossible in this chapter to describe the different types of emotional disturbance which find their solution in hysterical symptoms. In every personality there are some emotional conflicts which do not present any problem in the ordinary course of living. In general, however, the more severe the emotional conflict, the less able is the individual to withstand strain of any kind. Actually, 38 percent of the cases of "blast deafness" (acoustic trauma) admitted to Hoff General Hospital were diagnosed either as purely psychogenic or else as organic hearing loss with a large functional overlay. For example, a soldier exposed at close range to the burst of a large shell or a land mine escaped with his life, but was temporarily deafened by the noise. Later his ears recovered, but his unconscious emotional forces prevented his regained "hearing" from becoming conscious. What was probably a true physiological deafness at first was continued as a psychogenic dysacusis. Some men who regained most of their hearing spontaneously after a temporary blast deafness have reported that their recovery of hearing was quite sudden, or that for a time their hearing fluctuated with their mood or condition. They heard poorly when tired or nervously tense and better than usual when relaxed by a convivial dose of alcohol. These stories clearly suggest a *temporary* psychogenic dysacusis that passed off without recognition or special treatment.

A particular kind of emotional conflict may be the basis of hysterical deafness in time of war. Since hearing serves to create, through language, a structure for the moral code, and since war liberates the basic aggression in human nature, conflict is inevitable. From childhood on, we have been taught not to kill. War reverses that moral prohibition as well as many others. It is

not surprising, therefore, that the conflict present in accepting this reversal should, in some persons, result in the rejection of hearing. To liberate his basic aggression, such a man must say, "I will not hear the voice of conscience." The hearing apparatus through which the moral code was formulated then becomes involved in a basic emotional conflict that is sometimes solved by a complete or partial rejection of the apparatus itself—with consequent deafness. This rejection is, of course, not conscious but takes place at the unconscious level. The soldier is utterly unaware that his deafness is *psychogenic* and was not caused by physical injury to his ears.

When a civilian becomes hysterically deaf (which apparently happens only rarely), we can infer that his inner conflict is correspondingly more severe, since the loss of hearing is precipitated by a milder stress. We must also infer that hearing has an unusual importance for such a person. There are, of course, great individual differences in the relative importance of the sense of hearing. In most of us one type of imagery plays a stronger part than do the others; vision, hearing, or the sense of motion may predominate in our relation to the world. When asked to recall the melody of a song, one person may *picture* the printed score, another may *hear* the melody, while a third may *feel the finger positions* required to play it.

In addition to these individual differences, however, auditory images generally affect most of us powerfully in the emotional field. This is particularly true in emotionalized memory. In terrifying situations, it is often the sounds involved in the experience, rather than the sight of it, that convey the horror. If one has witnessed an accident in which a man was hurt, his cries may persist in memory long after the visual image of the experience has faded.

This tendency of auditory imagery to persist in memory is strengthened in the man whose perceptive interests and imaginative capacities are integrated around hearing. If the experience which he is trying to forget is charged with emotional material, as it always is in war, it is possible for repression to blot out hearing and to make him deaf.

As for the civilian who becomes hysterically deaf, previous experience must contain incidents or situations that threaten him as deeply as combat does the soldier. An understanding of these incidents or situations can be gathered only through a careful case study of his development.

*Therapy of psychogenic dysacusis.* The prevention and the therapy for all other forms of dysacusis, deafness, and hearing loss will be found in the following chapter. It is appropriate, however, to consider the therapy of psychogenic dysacusis here because it illustrates very vividly the nature of the disorder. In fact, the diagnosis of psychogenic dysacusis usually rests almost entirely on the success, at least temporary, of some attempt at therapy.

The most effective treatment of hysterical deafness is based on the *positive suggestion* that the hearing loss is only temporary. To make the patient accept positive suggestion is difficult because in many of the hysterically deaf we see what Charcot, the great French psychiatrist, has called *la belle indifférence* to their conversion symptoms. Since they have achieved even a false resolution of their emotional conflict, they appear placid and quite undisturbed by the fact that they have given up their hearing. When they describe their deafness, they rarely emphasize their own feelings about the loss, but instead point out the objective or practical inconvenience of not being able to hear a car start, for example, or to hear directions. Even these practical difficulties are usually brushed aside by such a remark as, "But that is not important."

It is better to teach the patient how to *listen* than to teach him speechreading, for speechreading may only help to confirm the symptom of deafness and make it less accessible to treatment. By suggestive therapeutic methods the hysterically deaf may be encouraged to regain their hearing. But, unless some relief from the basic emotional conflict is achieved by the therapeutic process, the cause for the conflict remains, and the conversion symptom may merely shift over into another sensory field or take the form of a partial paralysis. A "cure" of psychogenic dysacusis may be only temporary, but this at least demonstrates that part or all of the deafness or hearing loss is functional. It does not mean that the cure is necessarily permanent or that the fundamental problem may not again appear in some other incapacitating symptom. If the hearing losses of the soldiers at Hoff General Hospital were purely the result of combat pressure, release from army service might have been sufficient to make their cure permanent. It is probable that a civilian who becomes functionally deaf from the pressures of living cannot be cured without psychiatric therapy deep enough to change the patient's personal concept of himself and his relationships with others.

### Depression Deafness

Hysterical deafness does not include all the cases of deafness or dysacusis that should be classified as psychogenic. Dr. D. A. Ramsdell (see Chapter 18) has differentiated a type, which he terms "depression deafness," in a schizophrenic personality structure. Personality tests, case histories, and the presence of recognized schizophrenic symptoms indicate that this type of dysacusis is not due to conversion, as has been previously supposed. (Schizophrenia is a type of mental disorder characterized by a progressive isolation of the individual from reality. Feeling unable to meet the practical demands of his environment, the patient escapes into an unreal world of phantasy.)

An intensive study of depression dysacusis reveals that there is a particular pattern in the case histories of such patients. The patients emphasize the subjective effects of their hearing loss and show definite hypochondriacal symptoms. They speak, not of the objective inconvenience of their impairment as does the hysteric, but of the change in their own feeling state. They are perplexed and frightened, and find the world about them incomprehensible and overwhelming. Failure of the sense of hearing to operate normally in such a patient is not due to conversion as a means of solving a basic conflict. The simulation of hearing loss or deafness acts as a protective defense against the precipitation of a schizophrenic episode. Hearing, more frequently than do the other senses, becomes involved in the schizophrenic's escape from reality.

It is a well-known fact that hearing may be accentuated in early schizophrenia to the point where the patient hears imaginary voices or has "auditory hallucinations." The reverse may also be true, and the patient may become deaf as part of the schizophrenic process. Such a patient is basically suicidal, but since he stops short of an actual biological death, the case may more properly be described as one of partial suicide. By giving up hearing, the patient succeeds in arriving at the state that one individual has described as "being buried alive." The patient restricts himself to a world that lacks the movement and flow so characteristic of the complete world of reality. He severs the auditory coupling, which is the chief link in maintaining an experience of aliveness and of identification with a moving world. In schizophrenic depression, the reward for the deafness, which corresponds to *la belle indifférence* in the hysteric, is the maintenance of only a visual orientation to the world around him.

In any case of psychogenic deafness or hearing loss, careful diagnosis should always be made before therapy is undertaken. Superficially the two types of psychogenic dysacusis appear much alike, but the treatment appropriate for depression deafness is quite different from that indicated in hysteria. For cases of depression deafness, therapy should be as painstaking and as careful as if one were dealing with threatened suicide because the wrong type of therapy may precipitate a psychotic episode.

It would be unwise to attempt here a detailed explanation of the therapy for either type of psychogenic dysacusis. If medical examination and tests of hearing indicate that the hearing loss is not due to impairment of the hearing apparatus, professional psychiatric aid should be obtained.

The variety of types of central dysacusis is illustrated by the experience of one particular clinic. Here 8 percent of the children referred for communication disorders were eventually diagnosed by psychiatrists as having autism or infantile schizophrenia, another 7 percent had severe emotional disturbances, 14 percent were mentally retarded, 15 percent had auditory agnosia or verbal dysacusis, and 19 percent had one or another type of central dysacusis as well as deafness or a hearing loss.

## SUGGESTED READINGS AND REFERENCES

Nearly all of the readings cited below are primary publications in the scientific literature which give evidence on which statements in the text are based. The titles are good guides to their subject matter.

**Altmann, F., A. Glasgold, and J. P. MacDuff.** "The Incidence of Otosclerosis as Related to Race and Sex," *Ann. Otol.,* 76:377–392 (1967).
This supersedes the 1944 study by S. R. Guild.

**Boies, L. R., J. A. Hilger, and R. E. Priest.** *Fundamentals of Otolaryngology, A Text Book of Ear, Nose & Throat Diseases,* Philadelphia, London: W. B. Saunders Company, 1964.

**Bordley, J. E., P. E. Brookhouse, J. Hardy, and W. G. Hardy.** "Prenatal Rubella," *Acta Otolaryng.* (Stockholm), 66:1–9 (1968).

**Clarke, C. A.** "The Prevention of 'Rhesus' Babies," *Scientific American,* 219:46–52 (1968).

**Davis, H.** "A Functional Classification of Auditory Defects," *Ann. Otol.,* 71:693–704 (1962).

————, **C. T. Morgan, J. E. Hawkins, Jr., R. Galambos, and F. W. Smith.** "Temporary Deafness Following Exposure to Loud Tones and Noise," *Acta Otolaryng.* (Stockholm), Supplement 88 (1950).
An experimental study of temporary threshold shift and peripheral dysacusis in man, carried out in 1941–1942.

**Elliott, L. L.** "Descriptive Analysis of Audiometric and Psychometric Scores of Students at a School for the Deaf," *J. Speech Hearing Res.,* 10:21–40 (1967).

————, **and V. Armbruster.** "Some Possible Effects of the Delay of Early Treatment of Deafness," *J. Speech Hearing Res.,* 10:209–224 (1967).

**Glorig, A., and H. Davis.** "Age, Noise and Hearing Loss," *Ann. Otol.,* 70:556 (1961).

**Goodhill, V.** "Pathology, Diagnosis and Therapy of Deafness," Chap. 9 in *Handbook of Speech Pathology,* L. E. Travis (ed.). New York: Appleton-Century-Crofts, Inc., 1957.

**Hopkins, L. A., and R. P. Guilder.** "Concerning the Heredity of Deafness. Pedigree Data 1930–1940." *Clarke School Studies:* Monograph I. Ann Arbor, Mich.: Edwards Brothers, Inc., 1949.

————, **and M. T. Macklin.** "Studies on the Inheritance of Deafness in the Pupils of the Clarke School for the Deaf," *Laryngoscope,* 56:570–601 (1946).

**Huizing, E. H., A. H. Van Bolhuis, and D. W. Odenthal.** "Studies on Progressive Hereditary Perceptive Deafness in a Family of 335 Members, I. Genetical and General Audiological Results. II. Characterstic Pattern of Hearing Deterioration." *Acta Otolaryng.* (Stockholm), 61:35–41; 161–167 (1966).

**Knapp, P. H.** "Emotional Aspects of Hearing Loss," *Psychosom. Med.,* 10:203–222 (1948).
A good discussion of psychogenic overlay.

**Landau, W. M., R. Goldstein, and F. R. Kleffner.** "Congenital Aphasia," *Neurology,* 10:915–921 (1960).
A case of true "congenital aphasia" with autopsy report.

**Lindenov, H.** *The Etiology of Deaf-Mutism with Special Reference to Heredity.* Copenhagen: Einar Munksgaard, 1945. (Translated from Danish by A. Anderson.) A fine historical summary and a source book of results. Interpretation is in Mendelian terms without the concept of penetrance.

**Martin, N. A.** "Psychogenic Deafness," *Ann. Otol.,* 55:81–89 (1946).
One of the rare clinical papers on this topic.

**Penfield, W., and T. Rasmussen.** *The Cerebral Cortex of Man.* New York: The Macmillan Company, 1950.
Based on studies of conscious patients during brain surgery.

———, **and L. Roberts.** *Speech and Brain-Mechanisms.* Princeton, N.J.: Princeton University Press, 1959.
An important book for speech pathologists.

**Princeton Conference on Brain Mechanisms Underlying Speech and Language.** Chm.: C. H. Millikan. F. L. Darley (ed.). New York: Grune and Stratton, Inc., 1967.
Proceedings of a conference held at Princeton, New Jersey, November 9–12, 1965.

**Rosen, S., M. Bergman, D. Plester, A. El-Mofty, and M. H. Satti.** "Presbycusis Study of a Relatively Noise-free Population in the Sudan," *Ann. Otol.,* 71:727–743 (1962).
This is the study of the Mabaan tribe.

**Schmidt, P. H.** "Presbycusis: The Present Status," *Int. Audiol.,* Supplement 1 (1967).
In our opinion this is the best summary of presbycusis to date.

**Senturia, B. H.** *Diseases of the External Ear.* Springfield, Ill.: Charles C Thomas, 1957.

**Van Egmond, A. A. J.** "Congenital Deafness," *J. Laryngol.,* 68:429–443 (1954).
An excellent survey lecture.

**Ventry, I. M., and J. B. Chaiklin (eds.).** "Multidiscipline Study of Functional Hearing Loss," *J. Aud. Res.,* 5:179–262 (1965).
Extensive studies carried out under the auspices of the Veterans Administration.

**Whetnall, E., and D. B. Fry.** *The Deaf Child.* London: William Heinemann Ltd., 1964.
This monograph contains some excellent descriptions of various syndromes of congenital deafness, and much more concerning assessment and management of deaf children.

**Wiesel, T. N., and D. H. Hubel.** "Extent of Recovery from the Effects of Visual Deprivation in Kittens," *J. Neurophysiol.,* 28:1060–1072 (1965).
A very important animal experiment.

**Williams, H. L.** *Ménière's Disease.* Springfield, Ill.: Charles C Thomas, 1952.
An authoritative monograph by an eminent otologist.

# CHAPTER 5

## THE MEDICAL TREATMENT OF HEARING LOSS AND THE CONSERVATION OF HEARING

**HALLOWELL DAVIS, M.D.**
**EDMUND PRINCE FOWLER, Jr., M.D.**

This chapter might have been entitled, as it was in the first edition, "Medical Aspects of Hearing Loss." The abnormalities of structure and function and the types and the causes of deafness and hearing loss have, however, already been described separately in Chapter 4, and the remaining "medical aspects" are essentially (1) the medical treatment of some few conditions that are amenable to it, (2) the hygiene of the ear, and (3) conservation of hearing. Actually, medical treatment has rather little to offer to restore lost hearing, but preventive medicine can and does contribute greatly to the conservation of hearing.

In the present chapter we shall first review the possibilities and principles of medical treatment of the conditions described in Chapter 4. We shall then see how these possibilities, coupled with appropriate systematic audiometry, provide conservation of hearing.

## MEDICAL TREATMENT OF HEARING LOSS

### External Ear

The blockage of the external ear canal by impacted wax is rather frequent, particularly in later adult life. When blockage occurs, there is little the patient himself can do except visit a doctor, who will remove the impacted wax without injury to the canal or the drumhead. Normally the wax works its way out unnoticed bit by bit; but there are some people whose wax simply does not come out of the canal in this way, and every six months or every year they should have the wax removed by a doctor before it "macerates" or otherwise injures the skin of the canal. Hydrogen peroxide is sometimes used to soften the wax, which may then be washed out by irrigation with warm water. If this is done, the canal should be thoroughly dried afterward. Actually, if the ears are kept clean, the average person does not develop impacted wax. The constant insertion of the earmold of a hearing aid or of matchsticks or hairpins often pushes the wax so deep into the canal that it must be removed by a doctor. Impacted wax sometimes makes, by reflex, an annoying dry cough. Persons fearing tuberculosis have even had X-rays taken when their only trouble was impacted wax.

## External Otitis

The skin of the external canal is in some areas very closely attached to the underlying cartilage and bone, so that any infection of it is very painful. It is unwise, as a rule, to open a limited external otitis with a knife, as is often done with similar abscesses elsewhere in the body, to let out the pus. Incision, and other types of manipulation as well, will often spread the infection and produce a diffuse external otitis.

The physician can treat external otitis quite effectively with a variety of local applications. The old-fashioned eardrops of alcohol and boric acid are sometimes effective, but often painful. For the patient, the important thing is to keep water out of the canal. Water softens the skin and spreads the infection more widely. If the canal has been wet, either from essential washing away of dead skin or wax, or inadvertently, from ill-advised use of any watery medication, such as hydrogen peroxide, the canal should be dried out with 95 percent ethyl alcohol. The alcohol will sting for a few minutes, but the ultimate benefits justify the temporary discomfort.

Another variety of external otitis (the "eczematoid" type) is a chronic scaling of the skin that is very difficult to treat successfully. Fortunately, this type rarely causes deafness, unless the canal is neglected and allowed to fill with wax and the cast-off scales of skin.

## Aero-otitis Media

Aero-otitis media depends entirely on failure to ventilate the middle ear through the Eustachian tube while descending from a high to a low altitude. *The best way to avoid aero-otitis is not to fly while suffering with a cold.* Colds inflame the tissue at the mouth of the Eustachian tube and prevent its proper function. If the tubes are partially blocked, continual swallowing on descent will help to equalize the pressure. This is helped by chewing gum, which produces enough saliva to allow for sufficient swallowing to open the tubes and equalize the pressure while the subject is making a normal descent. It is helpful to tilt the head back while swallowing. Airline pilots are instructed to descend or to depressurize a cabin at a rate of not more than 300 feet a minute. Occasional swallowing during such a slow descent will suffice for most people. Passengers who are asleep should be awakened before descent, and children and others who constantly have trouble with their Eustachian tubes during flight should be given water to drink. Inhalants such as benzedrine that tend to shrink swollen mucous membranes may also be very helpful.

Professional aviators and commercial travelers who must do a great deal of flying and who have recurrent aero-otitis should have their Eustachian tubes treated medically if they wish to continue flying without developing some permanent loss of hearing. In a similar category are submarine crews, deep-sea divers, skin divers, and caisson workers. If the tubes do not open with swallowing, yawning, or moving the jaws about, an attempt should be made to open the Eustachian tube by strong blowing of the nose. If this does not work, a doctor may employ a drug like ephedrine to shrink the mucous lining of the nose temporarily, or he may have to inflate the tube with various blowing or swallowing

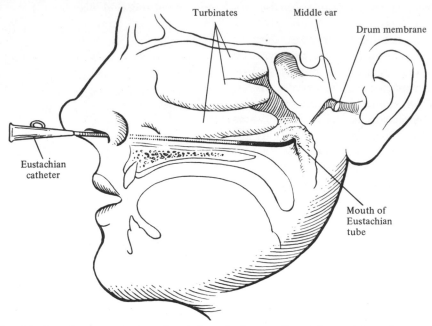

Fig. 5-1. A catheter can be introduced through the nostril and inserted into the opening of the Eustachian tube.

maneuvers (Valsalva or Politzer), or with a catheter passed through the nose (Figure 5-1). In rare instances of severe aero-otitis, incision of the drum may be necessary to remove the fluid.

### Acute and Chronic Otitis Media

*Chronic otitis media,* particuarly if it is recurrent or frequently reactivated, forms adhesions that impede the transmission of sound and may destroy the eardrum membrane, the ossicles, and other structures. It is a common and important cause of hearing loss. Of course, the first concern of an otologist confronted with a case of otitis media is with the general health and safety of the patient. If some loss of hearing must be risked or even deliberately produced by removal of the ossicles together with the pus and diseased tissue in order to be sure to check the infection, the otologist does not hesitate to remove them (see Chapter 6). Where possible, of course, he spares the hearing, but his first concerns are life and health. Treatment of otitis

media by drugs may help restore or save hearing, but unless the infection is very mild, it is best to provide drainage for it. Drainage is nature's most effective way of getting rid of infection and the products of infection.

For *acute otitis media,* and sometimes also for the chronic condition, the surgeon easily provides drainage by incising the lower back portion of the drum, where the incision has been found to cause no loss of hearing. If the drum is not opened, it will usually rupture spontaneously sooner or later. It has been found that more hearing loss and more mastoiditis requiring surgical attention occur after spontaneous rupture of the drum than after surgical incision.

The bacteria that usually cause acute infection of the middle ear can be killed by various antibiotics, notably penicillin. There are physicians who treat all otitis media with these drugs without surgery. This, however, is not good practice, because subacute, or chronic, otitis media is likely to recur in certain cases if drainage is not provided in addition to drug therapy. *Acute otitis media should not be treated by patients themselves or by druggists.* The tendency is to stop the drug as soon as the pain or the discharge subsides, and this is too soon. On the other hand, prolonged use of the drugs without medical supervision is dangerous. Inadequate dosage only extends the disease and makes the bacteria less susceptible to the drug being used. It is the recurrent, subacute, or chronic types of otitis media that cause hearing loss, and it is in these conditions, as a rule, that complications develop.

*Prevention of otitis media.* Also aimed at the prevention of recurrent and chronic otitis media are the *surgical removal of the adenoids* that block the Eustachian tubes and the *treatment of nasal infection.* Blockage of a tube and nasal infection both predispose to infection of the Eustachian tube and therefore to otitis media.

Unfortunately the surgical removal of the adenoids does not always enable the Eustachian tubes to open readily, particularly if chronic nasal or sinus infection is present. At one time radium or X rays were used to shrink the lymphoid tissue which makes up the adenoid and which is extremely sensitive to radiation. This form of treatment has been generally abandoned, however, because of the possibility of injury to other nearby tissues, notably the pituitary gland and mid-brain structures.

The details of medical treatment of chronic nasal infection are numerous and extend beyond the scope of this book.

*Blowing out the ear. Inflation,* whether performed by an instrument fitted to the nostril or by a silver catheter passed through the nose to the pharyngeal orifice of the tube, will improve the hearing, temporarily at least, if there is a plug of mucus blocking the tube. Often inflation is the only effective relief for temporary middle-ear hearing loss, but the method can be abused, and it is useless in cases of otosclerosis or of neural hearing loss. An old theory has been proved false: that wiggling the ossicles back and forth by blowing air up the Eustachian tubes will loosen them and improve the hearing. Inflation through a catheter is now reserved for diagnostic purposes and for patients who have a temporary blocking of the tubes by excessively thick secretions. Many people can clear their own tubes by yawning or blowing the nose. The self-inflation maneuver of Valsalva is familiar, that is, blowing while holding the nose. If this does not work, the Politzer maneuver may succeed. The otologist places the olive-shaped tip of an air-filled "Politzer bag" in the patient's nostril and squeezes the bag as the patient swallows. Too much strong inflation may produce a loose, floppy drumhead, however, and there is always the danger, too, of forcing infected material up the tube from the back of the nose.

## Treatment of Sensory-neural Hearing Loss

Physicians are on sure ground in objecting to the theories of those who say that manipulation, injections, or stimulation by sound can improve a hearing loss that has been clearly established as sensory-neural. If sensory cells or nerve fibers have once degenerated, they *cannot* be restored. Of course, the middle-ear conductive component of a mixed hearing loss might be improved by surgery, but not the inner ear sensory-neural component. Whatever effects may have been obtained in particular cases either must have resulted from the training that the patients received that enabled them better to understand speech with whatever residual hearing they may have had, or must have been pure self-delusion. Of course, nearly all deafened patients want to believe that their hearing is being improved by whatever is being done for them, and the therapist wants to believe that he is helping the patient. The powerful suggestion acting on both of them too often gives rise to a false belief that the new form of therapy, whatever it may be, has actually improved the hearing. Moreover, "nerve stimulants" cannot restore the missing fibers or cause degenerated sensory cells to resume their function. Nevertheless, patients are continually being dosed with vitamins, antihistamines, and many other types of medication, with the expectation that the function of their long-defunct auditory nerves will be improved. The suggestion that hearing may be restored by stimulation by sound is, of course, utterly fantastic. The only possible beneficial effects of drugs are the arrest of the disease process and perhaps, in some cases, the relief of tinnitus.

Incidentally, the cessation of a severe tinnitus not only eliminates a very distressing symptom but may improve the hearing to a certain extent by removing an interfering masking noise. The improvement, however, is never more than 10 or 15 dB. Unfortunately, the relief of tinnitus by any direct treatment is so rare that one wonders whether the disappearance is not always spontaneous when it does occur. Tinnitus, it must be remembered, is a subjective symptom and as such is susceptible to suggestion. Many a patient has been taught by a sympathetic and understanding physician to minimize the annoyance caused by his head noises.

### Menière's[1] Disease and Sudden Hearing Losses of Vascular Origin

There are two types of sensory-neural hearing loss which are sometimes amenable

[1] The spelling of Menière's name has given medical writers some difficulty. Apparently Dr. Menière himself was not consistent. The original form was apparently Ménière, with an acute accent on the first e, but on his last paper we find it spelled Menière. His son subsequently established the simpler form for the family name, and that spelling is recognized in France. In the present edition of this book we follow the French usage instead of the prevalent English-American form, Ménière, of our earlier editions.

to medical treatment: Menière's disease, that is, the sudden attacks of vertigo, deafness, and tinnitus described in Chapter 4; and certain sudden, severe hearing losses, with or without vertigo, which are presumably of vascular origin. Both conditions often have a strong psychogenic component in that they seem to occur most often in highly energetic, driving perfectionists when life stresses become excessive. Often the symptoms occur after a distressing, frustrating, emotionally disturbing event rather than during it. Also, the ear symptoms frequently occur in patients who have developed other recognized psychosomatic diseases, such as high blood pressure or gastric ulcer.

The collection of symptoms known as Menière's disease or Menière's syndrome takes its name from the French physician Prosper Menière, who first described the syndrome in 1861. His descriptions were remarkably complete and accurate. He correctly distinguished a group of cases characterized by sudden onset of vertigo, nausea, vomiting, and loss of hearing from "apoplectiform cerebral congestion," and he also correctly attributed the cause of his syndrome to a disturbance in the labyrinth.

Essentially, the treatments for Menière's disease and sudden vascular hearing losses are very similar, from the medical standpoint, to those used for other vascular diseases elsewhere in the body. If the disease is entirely in the ear, the otologist is likely to prescribe some vasodilator drug, such as nicotinic acid or injections of histamine. In the sudden catastrophic types of severe hearing loss, often designated as "sudden deafness," he may, in addition, prescribe anticoagulation drugs, such as those used for apoplexy, for venous thromboses, or for heart attacks. This treatment should be carried out in a hospital under the supervision of a man skilled in the use of anticoagulants. Some physicians also recommend procaine, given intravenously, again in a hospital under rigid supervision. The procaine increases the blood flow through the small blood vessels, but it increases the work that the heart must do, and the heart must be in good condition to take on this added load. These various treatments must be started at once to be effective, and unless they are accompanied by careful study of the patient's stress situations and the possibility of alleviating them, the hearing losses are likely to recur; each time they do recur they are more likely to remain permanent.

Some otologists emphasize the importance of the psychosomatic background of Menière's disease and find that immediate and emphatic reassurance and, if possible, relief of other emotional stresses are extremely helpful, especially in the earlier attacks. Beyond this, medical treatment has little to offer that has proved merit. Many drugs, special diets, and several bizarre forms of treatment have been tried, and encouraging results have been reported with some of them. The drug or regimen chosen depends on the theory of the cause of the disease that is favored by the physician, or it may be on a purely empirical basis. Nicotinic acid, to cause dilation of the small blood vessels, is a favorite drug; methantheline and propantheline are also popular. A full list would include atropine, histamine, Diamox, a salt-free diet, and many others.

In some patients some of these drugs have had clear and favorable effects. The symptoms have improved while the drug was being taken regularly, but became worse when the dosage was reduced or stopped. Other patients have shown little or no consistent benefit. It is very difficult, however, to establish a firm case for any drug or any theory: one of the major characteristics of Menière's disease is the fluctuation of symptoms—the spontaneous remissions and the return of "attacks" without obvious cause. The only sure relief from the symptoms of Menière's disease is the surgical destruction of the labryinth described in Chapter 6. The advantages of medical treatment are that it does no harm, it gives opportunity for spontaneous improvement, and it is of benefit in many cases.

### Prevention of Neural Hearing Loss and Dysacusis

As mentioned in Chapter 4, several drugs are specifically toxic for the inner ear. The most important of these are kanamycin, neomycin, and, especially, dihydrostreptomycin. These should be avoided unless essential for preservation of life. Certainly, they should never be used prophylactically. Large doses of other less toxic drugs, such as straight streptomycin, aspirin and other salicylates, and quinine and quinidine should be used with caution. Some individuals, especially those with poor kidney function, are very susceptible to these drugs. The onset of tinnitus or of slight vertigo will often herald the occurrence of an ototoxic reaction to them.

Some of the severe congenital hearing losses of childhood can be prevented by improved methods of resuscitation at birth and the more careful anesthetizing and medication of mothers in labor. Substitution transfusions in babies with Rh and AO incompatible blood may save some, but many of these measures, especially the saving of tiny premature babies, probably increase the number of children in the population who survive with communication disorders.

## CONSERVATION OF HEARING

The movement for conservation of hearing really began with preventive measures and screening audiometry in schools more than 30 years ago. The part played by the American Hearing Society is mentioned in Chapter 20. The development of the group-screening audiometer by the Bell Telephone Laboratories (the Western Electric 4C audiometer) was an epochal event for conservation of hearing, not only in children but, as we shall see, in adults also.

Another organization that has continued actively to promote conservation of hearing, particularly from the point of view of preventive medicine, has been the Committee on Conservation of Hearing of the American Academy of Ophthalmology and Otolaryngology. This committee, composed of leading otologists who are interested in problems of hearing and a few nonmedical consultants, encouraged the establishment of conservation of hearing programs, particularly in schools. Later, through its Subcommittee on Noise in Industry (later known simply as the Subcommittee on Noise), it extended its efforts to this wider field. Still more recently it established additional subcommittees on hearing in children, hearing in adults, audiometers, research in otolaryngology, and the like.

### Children

*Screening audiometry.* It is often not easy to identify an ear with chronic otitis media unless the ear is actually discharging pus. A fully trained otologist may not always be available to look at the eardrum membrane with his otoscope. Another method for picking out children who may need attention is to test their hearing. Tests of hearing, including pure-tone audiometry, are described in Chapter 7, but it is obvious immediately that it would be both time-consuming and wasteful to test every ear at all frequencies when most ears are perfectly normal. The answer has been "screening audiometry." All of the children in a school are tested briefly and quickly to identify or screen out, as by a sieve, those whose sensitivity of hearing is below some arbitrary hearing level. Those who are thus screened out are then given a full, careful, audiometric test and otologic examination. Of course, a good many of them turn out on the full test to be normal or very nearly so. The screening test is planned to screen out

the borderline cases so as not to let any really abnormal cases go undetected.

It must not be assumed that screening audiometry in schools will detect every child who has a mild or incipient otitis media or enlarged adenoids or even frank cholesteatoma. Children have such sensitive hearing that audiometers with extended dynamic range and correspondingly good quiet audiometric booths are required to determine their hearing thresholds. It is often difficult to provide quiet enough locations to carry out the screening test at a level low enough to detect all of those who should be screened out for further study.

Actually, a recent survey of the hearing of children in certain selected schools in Pittsburgh, continued over several years, showed a very disappointing correlation between the results of the hearing tests and direct otological examination of the ears of all of these same children. The tests were actual determinations of the hearing threshold levels, not merely screening tests. The children whose ears were judged abnormal otoscopically in one way or another did indeed average some 10 dB less sensitive by audiometry, but there was a large overlap between the groups. In the conclusions of the survey, published in 1963, we read the following:

It has been assumed in the past that conventional audiometric screening will reveal not only those children with "hearing loss," but also those with ear conditions needing medical care. The Pittsburgh data indicate that audiometric testing, however complete it may be, cannot identify all children with physical abnormalities which may have predictive value, or who may need medical treatment. In addition to failing an audiometric screening procedure, some other means is needed to identify children needing special otological and audiological attention. A history of earaches and ear discharge, especially when accompanied by otoscopic evidence of past or present infection, indicates a child · who needs special otological and audiological services. The frequency of occurrence of these conditions appears to be a measure of the urgency of this need.

In spite of all, however, screening audiometry does detect the children with moderate or severe impairment of hearing even if it will not detect those with mild impairments. It remains a primary method for the conservation of hearing in children.

Two general forms of screening audiometry were developed specifically for use in schools. One is *group speech audiometry,* developed by the Bell Telephone Laboratories. It screens a whole roomful of children at once. The youngsters write down on prepared blanks the numbers that they hear spoken at successively lower and lower levels. These test words are played from a phonographic disc. The other form is "sweep-frequency audiometry," carried out individually with a pure-tone air conduction audiometer. The very high and the very low frequencies may be omitted, and only one intensity or "screening level" is used. If these few test tones are heard, the child's hearing is considered to be within normal limits.

There is no great difference in the overall time per child between the two methods. Individual screening is likely to be further shortened by the omission of some of the test frequencies, but it is not yet clear just which frequencies must be retained.

The important point here is not the technique of screening or the criteria employed but *the concept of screening audiometry as part of an annual physical checkup.* This is the approach made by preventive medicine.

We note in passing that the emphasis that was placed for many years on hearing for the very high frequencies—8192, 11,584, and 16,000 Hz—has now evaporated. It was originally thought that these very high tones were particularly sensitive indicators of middle-ear disease or of beginning neural hearing loss. It now appears that, for purely physical and anatomical reasons, audiom-

etry above 6000 Hz is unreliable. No individual will give the same thresholds when tested on successive days. For one thing, small differences in the positioning of the earphone can cause large differences in standing wave patterns in the ear canal. Nor is the test valid. Even if high threshold levels for very high frequencies are confirmed on repeated tests, they do not now appear, as the result of the recent Pittsburgh study mentioned above, to give real and useful warning signs. For screening audiometry, 6000 Hz is high enough.

### Adults

Otitis media continues to be a threat but a diminishing threat to hearing throughout life. Adults are more aware than children of trouble with their ears or their hearing and are in a position to do something about it. Not so many adult ears suffer from sheer neglect. It is much easier to drain an effusion from the ear of an adult than from the ear of a child because the adult does not require a general anesthetic.

Otosclerosis strikes the ears of young adults but not children. As we noted in Chapter 4, there are no effective preventive measures against this disease. The problems of otosclerosis are the problems of surgery or of a hearing aid. Another danger to hearing confronts adults, namely, noise. Precautions can be taken against noise-induced hearing loss.

*Hazardous noise-exposure.* Noise hazards for hearing have for many years been associated with certain industries, notably boilermaking, drop forging, and weaving. The growth of heavy industry has increased the noise levels and also the number of workers exposed to them. The aircraft industry, particularly since the development of jet engines, has added new problems. Moreover, quite recently it has become clear that gunfire, including skeet shooting as well as artillery, machine guns, and small arms, and even the tractor on the farm are significant hazards to hearing. But noise-induced hearing loss develops slowly. Noises that are not painful or even really uncomfortable after the first week or two may gradually impair hearing if exposure to them is habitual.

For many years a sort of tacit conspiracy of silence kept the problem of noise-induced hearing loss from public view. Workers in very noisy places were pleased with their relatively high wages, and industry feared litigation, insurance problems, and compensation payments. (The problem of handicap and compensation is discussed in Chapter 9.) Now, however, "noise control" has become practical and popular, thanks to technical advances in acoustical engineering, to community concern about aircraft noise, and to a variety of military problems, including communication in noise. Court decisions in New York and Wisconsin first recognized noise-induced hearing loss as compensable under workmen's compensation laws, and similar recognition is being given in a rapidly increasing number of other states. Industry cooperated with the Research Center of the Subcommittee on Noise of the American Academy of Ophthalmology and Otolaryngology to gather more information, and it is now possible to state with considerable confidence just what is a hazardous noise-exposure to many common industrial noises.

Now that it is common knowledge that hazardous noise-exposures actually do exist, a major objective in the conservation of hearing of adults is to do something about the hazard, both in industry and in military situations. There are several approaches to the problem: to reduce the noise, either at the source or in the transmission; to remove all personnel from noise areas; to use protective devices such as earplugs or ear muffs; to identify noise-susceptible persons and remove them from noisy situations; and to institute "monitoring audiometry" to identify the persons who are actually beginning to develop a noise-induced hearing loss before they develop enough permanent threshold shift to constitute any practical handicap.

*Monitoring audiometry* was first formally defined and named in a symposium of what was then the Armed Forces–National Research Council Committee on Hearing and Bio-Acoustics on "Problems in Military Audiometry." The concept is very much the same as that of screening audiometry for children. We watch or "monitor" the hearing of all those who have a hazard of noise-exposure and find which ones require special attention. That attention may be ear muffs or it may be removal from the noise. Monitoring audiometry is regarded as part of a routine periodic health examination or physical checkup. The audiometry required is more elaborate than for screening schoolchildren but less elaborate than for diagnostic purposes.

## A GUIDE FOR CONSERVATION OF HEARING IN NOISE

The most complete and authoritative summary statement concerning hazardous exposure to noise and the application of a "damage-risk criterion" is a report prepared by a working group of the National Academy of Sciences—National Research Council Committee on Hearing, Bioacoustics and Biomechanics ("CHABA") at the request of the United States Army. The citation is given in the list of references at the end of this chapter.

A simpler, more elementary but very useful Guide for Conservation of Hearing in Noise, prepared for the benefit of industry, was issued in a revised edition in 1964 by the Subcommittee on Noise (in Industry). We reproduce in the following pages several sections from this Guide. The general principles are valid, and the sound levels and the durations stated in the Guide are certainly of the correct order of magnitude and can be accepted with fair confidence.

BASIC INFORMATION ABOUT HEARING LOSS AND NOISE-EXPOSURE [2]

Although there is still much to be learned about the relations of hearing loss to noise-exposure, we have accumulated enough information through experience and research to enable us to organize and conduct hearing conservation programs. This basic information is, in brief:

1. **Many noise-exposures can produce a permanent hearing loss that may affect communication by speech.**
2. Noise-induced hearing loss may be temporary, permanent or a combination of temporary and permanent.
3. Permanent noise-induced hearing loss is due to destruction of certain inner ear structures which cannot be replaced or repaired.
4. The amount of hearing loss produced by a given noise-exposure varies from person to person.
5. **Noise-induced hearing loss first affects man's hearing of sounds higher in frequency than those essential for communication by speech. Therefore, most early noise-induced hearing losses pass unnoticed unless they are detected by suitable hearing tests.**
6. **Four major factors characterize noise-exposure:**
   (a) **overall noise level**
   (b) **composition of the noise**
   (c) **duration and distribution of exposure during a typical work-day**
   (d) **total time of exposure during a work-life.**
7. Both hearing ability and noise-exposure can be measured reliably by competent, properly trained personnel. (The measurement and evaluation of impulsive noises, which are produced by explosions, drop hammers, riveting guns, etc., present special problems.)
8. **To be effective a hearing conservation program should include:**
   (a) **a noise-exposure analysis**
   (b) **provision for control of noise-exposure**
   (c) **measurements of hearing.**

INDICATIONS OF THE NEED FOR A HEARING CONSERVATION PROGRAM

**The initiation of a hearing conservation program should be considered whenever persons have**
1. **Difficulty communicating by speech while they are in the noise, or**
2. **Head noises or ringing in their ears after working in the noise for several hours, or**
3. **A temporary loss of hearing that has the effect of muffling speech and certain other sounds after several hours of exposure to the noise.**

\*     \*     \*     \*

Absence of pain when exposed to noise should not be construed to mean absence of hearing loss. Pain may be felt in the ear during exposure to noise levels of the order of 130 decibles: noise-induced hearing loss, however, may be produced at considerably lower noise levels. Pain and annoyance are not reliable indicators of a potential noise-induced hearing loss. The decision to initiate a hearing conservation program should not be influenced by the presence or absence of these symptoms.

Ultimately, the analysis of noise-exposure is the only completely satisfactory way of establishing the need for hearing conservation.

[2] These extracts from the "Guide for Conservation of Hearing in Noise" are reprinted by permission of the Subcommittee on Noise of the Committee on Conservation of Hearing, American Academy of Ophthalmology and Otolaryngology.

OUTLINE OF A HEARING CONSERVATION PROGRAM

A HEARING CONSERVATION PROGRAM CONSISTS OF THREE PARTS

## I. Analysis of Noise-Exposure

Noise-exposures are analyzed in terms of:
  (a) overall level
  (b) composition of the noise
  (c) duration and distribution of exposure during a typical work-day
  (d) total exposure time during a work-life.

Measurement of each of these four factors of noise-exposure is important for hearing conservation. Even though two different noises have the same overall level, their compositions may differ considerably (to such an extent, in fact, that one may produce a permanent hearing loss while the other may not). Also, the auditory effects of continuous noise-exposure are different from the effects of intermittent exposure to the same noise.

## II. Control of Noise-Exposure

Noise-exposure may be reduced by:
  (a) Environmental control
    (1) reducing the amount of noise produced by the source
    (2) reducing the amount of noise transmitted through air or building structures
    (3) revising operational procedures
  (b) Personal protection

The most satisfactory method of environmental control of noise-exposure is to control the noise at the source. Unfortunately, this is not always possible. When the amount of noise produced by the source cannot be sufficiently reduced, a combination of control methods may be required to conserve hearing.

## III. Measurement of Hearing

A hearing conservation program should include:
  (a) pre-employment and/or pre-placement hearing tests, and
  (b) routine periodic follow-up tests.

**These tests of hearing are the most important part of a hearing conservation program.** They provide a record of the initial status of an employee's hearing and make it possible to follow any subsequent changes in hearing ability. Pre-employment and follow-up tests help to identify persons who may be highly susceptible to noise-induced hearing loss. Test and retest results will show whether the conservation program is effective or not.

Even when noise-exposures are not severe enough to warrant a hearing conservation program, it is desirable to test hearing systematically as part of routine physical examinations. Hearing tests are as important and as necessary as tests of vision, or any of the tests which accompany a physical examination.

### RESPONSIBILITY FOR CONSERVATION OF HEARING

### Medical Responsibility

The conservation of any human function is primarily a medical responsibility. Hearing conservation is no exception. Prevention, diagnosis and treatment of hearing loss; validation and approval of audiometric records; and the final assessment of measurements of hearing are medical responsibilities. **Any hearing conservation program without medical supervision must be considered inadequate.**

Direct medical supervision of a hearing conservation program is highly desirable. A physician should be responsible for the organization and administration of the testing program as well as for checking and evaluating audiometric records. The physician himself does not perform all the operations necessary to the conduct of the program; he delegates responsibility for many of the technical activities to members of his staff, and sets up standards or limits within which they can operate semiautonomously. Whenever medical records show that control of noise-exposures may be inadequate, the physician in charge so reports. The responsibility for making necessary noise measurements and for effecting further environmental noise-exposure controls then devolves on the industrial hygienist, members of the engineering or safety departments or other persons assigned to the task. Although the actual operations of measurement and protection are performed by both medical and non-medical personnel, the physician ultimately is responsible for the health of the employee.

Medical supervision must be available if a hearing conservation program is to serve its dual purpose of preventing hearing loss and providing valid records for compensation claims. Many companies do not have a full time medical department and cannot provide direct medical supervision for a conservation program. These companies can, however, satisfy the general requirement of medical supervision by utilizing medical consultants.

## General Cooperation

The success of hearing conservation depends on the complete cooperation of employer, employee, and others concerned with the health and safety of employees. All groups stand to benefit equally from a hearing conservation program, and all groups should give the program their active support. Supervisory personnel should initiate noise measurements, make the environmental changes that are necessary for noise-exposure control, furnish any required ear protection and make it readily available to all employees, acquaint all employees with the benefits to be derived from hearing conservation, and, by example, promote attitudes that will benefit the program. Each employee should make proper use of the personal protection that is provided, obey environmental regulations, and participate willingly in the hearing testing program.

In the Guide there follows a section on technical information. Much of this material has been covered in Chapters 2, 3 and 4 of this book. Special problems, however, relate to the measurement of noise for purposes of hearing conservation, the assessment of noise-exposures to continuous or intermittent steady noises, and the establishment of criteria for noise control. Important developments have occurred since 1964 in these areas and at the present writing this section of the Guide is undergoing extensive revision. The following sections of this chapter draw extensively on a draft of the proposed new version.

## Methods of Measurement of Steady Noise

### A. *For Control of Noise*

Engineering control of noise at its source or by reducing its transmission requires measurement of both the over-all sound-pressure level of the noise and the distribution of energy across the frequency spectrum.

Over-all sound levels of steady noises may be measured with a sound-level meter (often designated SLM). The "C" or flat response scale of a sound-level meter measures the average over-all sound-pressure level in decibels relative to 0.0002 dyne per square centimeter. The meter indicator responds to irregular fluctuations present in steady noise and usually does not remain fixed in one position while a measurement is being made. Because of these fluctuations, the average of several readings taken at a measuring point is recorded as the over-all sound-pressure level of the noise at that location.

An octave-band analyzer (often designated OBA) consists of a series of electronic filters that select in turn for measurement each of several octave bands in the noise. Most standard analyzers are now designed to select eight octave-bands with center frequencies as follows: 63, 125, 250, 500, 1000, 2000, 4000 and 8000 Hz, as recommended by the United States of America Standards Institute (USAS S1.6–1060) and the International Organization for Standardization (ISO). Older instruments employed slightly different frequencies: the cut-off frequencies of each band were 37.5 to 75, 75 to 150, 150 to 300 Hz, and so on. Either set of filters is perfectly acceptable for engineering measurements related to noise-control. The differences in measurements of most noise spectra are small.

Some analyzers are designed to measure sound-pressure level in one-third octave bands or in narrow bands of constant width, for example, 5 cycles or 20 cycles. Such measurements are entirely acceptable, but are not necessary for determining the need for a hearing conservation program.

*The sound level meter and octave-band analyzer do not measure impulsive noise levels accurately.* If a noise-exposure includes impulsive noises, qualified acoustical engineers should make the noise measurements with special equipment.

### B. *For Assessment of Noise-Exposure*

"Sound level A" is the over-all sound-pressure level of a steady noise measured on the A scale of the sound-level meter. The electrical equivalent of the noise is passed through a broad-band filter that has a frequency characteristic very much like that of the human middle ear. The filter network and its scale were devised originally to assist in predicting the over-all loudness of relatively faint noises. The filter attenuates or excludes both high and low frequencies which may be physically present but to which the ear is relatively or completely insensitive. By coincidence the "weighting" it gives to the different parts of the spectrum corresponds very closely to the tendency of each part to produce a significant impairment of hearing. By "significant" we mean an impairment of hearing in the range of frequencies important for the understanding of speech. This correspondence is now widely recognized. The A scale has been incorporated in the method of assessing noise-exposure that is described below. A single reading on the A scale, in "dBA," is substituted for a series of octave-band measurements and the calculations necessary to reduce them to a single equivalent number.

Sound-level-A measurements should always be made at the approximate position of the employee's most exposed ear. To take account of the variations in noise level due to the schedule of operations, repeated measurements should be made during a single work day and also on different days of the week.

The use of a sound level meter with the A scale is simple and the use of a set of octave-band filters is not very difficult. Nevertheless there are technical pitfalls and these measurements should be undertaken only by skilled personnel who have had training and experience in making physical measurements with electronic equipment.

## Assessment of Noise-Exposure to Steady Noises

The reason for instituting a hearing conservation program is that habitual exposure to loud noise may, over a period of years, produce a permanent impairment of hearing. If the hearing of speech is impaired, the employee suffers a social handicap.

To decide whether to institute a hearing conservation program it is necessary to estimate the prospective noise-exposure of employees who work in noisy places and then to estimate the risk involved. *By risk we mean the percentage of persons who, because of noise-exposure, may be expected to develop a significant hearing handicap during their working life.*

This section deals with the estimation of the noise-exposure in a typical work day.

Noise-exposure implies a noise which has an intensity in dBA and also a duration of exposure in minutes or hours. Each of these factors enters into the risk of permanent injury to the ear. Fortunately we now know enough about the dependence of injury on each of these factors to be able to make several simplifications in our calculations.

One such simplification we have already mentioned, namely, to *measure the over-all intensity of the sound in dBA* instead of performing an octave-band analysis and a series of calculations.

The next simplification relates to changes of the intensity of the noise during a typical work day. If a steady noise is continuous at a given intensity over the entire work day we can say with considerable confidence what the workers' average hearing levels will be after a given number of years of such noise-exposure. Often, however, the noise is not continuous. It may change in intensity or perhaps cease entirely at certain phases of the operation, or the worker may not remain continuously in one place. The simplification that is made is to *calculate from the measured durations and intensities of noise-exposure the equivalent sound level A or $L_{eq}$ which carries the same risk of impairment of hearing as the actual exposure.* Such a single number is needed for the next step in the calculations.

The calculation of equivalent sound level A makes use of the "trading relation" that has been established between intensity (dBA) and exposure-time in minutes and hours. Laboratory studies of temporary threshold shift (TTS) have contributed greatly to establishing this trad-

TABLE 1A

PARTIAL NOISE-EXPOSURE INDICES CALCULATED ACCORDING TO THE 3-DB RULE

DURATIONS, 10 TO 120 MINUTES PER WEEK

| Minutes per Week | Sound Level A (class midpoint) (in dBA) | | | | | | |
|---|---|---|---|---|---|---|---|
| | 90 | 95 | 100 | 105 | 110 | 115 | 120 |
| 10 | | | 5 | 15 | 40 | 130 | 400 |
| 12 | | | 5 | 15 | 50 | 155 | 500 |
| 14 | | | 5 | 20 | 60 | 180 | 580 |
| 16 | | | 5 | 20 | 70 | 210 | 680 |
| 18 | | | 10 | 25 | 75 | 230 | 750 |
| 20 | | 5 | 10 | 25 | 80 | 260 | 840 |
| 25 | | 5 | 10 | 35 | 105 | 330 | 1040 |
| 30 | | 5 | 15 | 40 | 125 | 390 | 1250 |
| 40 | | 5 | 15 | 50 | 170 | 510 | 1660 |
| 50 | | 5 | 20 | 70 | 210 | 680 | 2070 |
| 60 | 5 | 10 | 25 | 80 | 250 | 780 | 2500 |
| 70 | 5 | 10 | 30 | 90 | 290 | 900 | 2910 |
| 80 | 5 | 10 | 35 | 105 | 340 | 1050 | 3320 |
| 90 | 5 | 10 | 40 | 120 | 380 | 1180 | 3750 |
| 100 | 5 | 15 | 45 | 130 | 425 | 1310 | 4150 |
| 120 | 5 | 15 | 50 | 160 | 500 | 1580 | 5000 |

The values in this table are calculated by means of the formula:

$$E_i = \frac{\Delta t_i}{40} \cdot 10^{0.1(L_i - 70)}, \text{ in which}$$

$E_i$ = partial noise-exposure index
$\Delta t_i$ = total duration in hours per week that the sound level in dBA is within a particular class
$L_i$ = midpoint in dBA of each class.

The 3-dB rule is incorporated in this formula.

TABLE 1B

PARTIAL NOISE-EXPOSURE INDICES CALCULATED ACCORDING TO THE 3-DB RULE

DURATIONS, 1 TO 40 HOURS PER WEEK

| Hours per Week | Sound Level A (class midpoint) (in dBA) | | | | | | | | |
|---|---|---|---|---|---|---|---|---|---|
| | 80 | 85 | 90 | 95 | 100 | 105 | 110 | 115 | 120 |
| 1 | | | 5 | 10 | 25 | 80 | 250 | 780 | 2500 |
| 1.5 | | | 5 | 10 | 40 | 120 | 380 | 1180 | 3750 |
| 2 | | | 5 | 15 | 50 | 160 | 500 | 1580 | 5000 |
| 2.5 | | | 5 | 20 | 60 | 200 | 610 | 1980 | 6250 |
| 3 | | 5 | 10 | 25 | 75 | 235 | 750 | 2380 | 7500 |
| 3.5 | | 5 | 10 | 30 | 90 | 275 | 880 | 2770 | 8750 |
| 4 | | 5 | 10 | 30 | 100 | 315 | 1000 | 3150 | 10000 |
| 5 | | 5 | 15 | 40 | 125 | 390 | 1250 | 3950 | 12500 |
| 6 | | 5 | 15 | 45 | 150 | 450 | 1500 | 4750 | 15000 |
| 7 | | 5 | 20 | 55 | 175 | 545 | 1750 | 5520 | 17500 |
| 8 | | 5 | 20 | 60 | 200 | 620 | 2000 | 6320 | 20000 |
| 9 | 5 | 5 | 25 | 70 | 230 | 700 | 2250 | 7120 | 22500 |
| 10 | 5 | 10 | 25 | 80 | 250 | 780 | 2500 | 7900 | 25000 |
| 12 | 5 | 10 | 30 | 95 | 300 | 945 | 3150 | 9450 | 30000 |
| 14 | 5 | 10 | 35 | 110 | 350 | 1100 | 3500 | 11100 | |
| 16 | 5 | 15 | 40 | 125 | 400 | 1260 | 4000 | 12600 | |
| 18 | 5 | 15 | 45 | 135 | 450 | 1420 | 4500 | 14200 | |
| 20 | 5 | 15 | 50 | 160 | 500 | 1580 | 5000 | 15800 | |
| 25 | 5 | 20 | 60 | 200 | 610 | 1980 | 6000 | 19800 | |
| 30 | 10 | 25 | 75 | 235 | 750 | 2360 | 7500 | 23600 | |
| 35 | 10 | 30 | 90 | 275 | 880 | 2750 | 8750 | 27500 | |
| 40 | 10 | 30 | 100 | 315 | 1000 | 3150 | 10000 | 31500 | |

See legend of Table 1A.

ing relation. The simplest rule that is approximately correct is that the risk of injury depends simply on the total sound energy of the noise-exposure, regardless of how the energy is distributed in time. *Thus for every halving of the duration of exposure, double the energy (i.e., an increase of 3 dBA) is permissible without increasing the risk.* This is the rule recommended by ISO/TC43/SC-1 (International Standards Organization, Technical Committee 43/Subcommittee 1) in 1969.

Some other organizations believe that the equal energy rule is too conservative when very short noise-exposures are concerned. Also it does not seem to allow adequately for the ability of the human ear to recover partially, during intervals of low levels of noise, from the effects of brief intense noise-exposures. For these reasons they recommend a 5-dB rule instead of the 3-dB rule, namely, *for every halving of the duration of a partial exposure the intensity of the exposure can be increased by 5 dBA without increasing the risk.* The 5-dB rule has been adopted by the Department of Labor in implementing the Walsh-Healy Act (see next section). The USA Standards Institute has not yet made its choice.

TABLE 2
RELATION BETWEEN COMPOSITE NOISE-EXPOSURE INDEX AND EQUIVALENT
CONTINUOUS SOUND LEVEL

| Composite Noise-Exposure Index | Equivalent Continuous Sound Level, dBA | Composite Noise-Exposure Index | Equivalent Continuous Sound Level, dBA |
|---|---|---|---|
| 10 | 80 | 1.250 | 101 |
| 15 | 82 | 1.600 | 102 |
| 20 | 83 | 2.000 | 103 |
| 25 | 84 | 2.500 | 104 |
| 30 | 85 | 3.150 | 105 |
| 40 | 86 | 4.000 | 106 |
| 50 | 87 | 5.000 | 107 |
| 60 | 88 | 6.300 | 108 |
| 80 | 89 | 8.000 | 109 |
| 100 | 90 | 10.000 | 110 |
| 125 | 91 | 12.500 | 111 |
| 160 | 92 | 16.000 | 112 |
| 200 | 93 | 20.000 | 113 |
| 250 | 94 | 25.000 | 114 |
| 315 | 95 | 31.500 | 115 |
| 400 | 96 | | |
| 500 | 97 | | |
| 630 | 98 | | |
| 800 | 99 | | |
| 1.000 | 100 | | |

The values for the equivalent continuous sound level ($L_{eq}$) in dBA are calculated by means of the following empirical formula: $L_{eq} = 70 + 10 \cdot \log_{10} \Sigma E_i$ where $\Sigma E_i$ is the composite noise-exposure index. The partial noise-exposure indices ($E_i$) are obtained from Table 1. The 3-dB rule is not involved in this formula or table.

The practical use of either of these two rules for assessing intermittent exposures to steady noise is greatly facilitated by tables, calculated in advance. Two different forms have been developed and an example of each is included below. One form is based on *partial noise-exposure indices* which correspond to different dBA levels and durations and which are summed to find the *composite noise-exposure index* (Table 1). The latter is related very simply to the equivalent continuous sound level in dBA (Table 2). This dBA value is then compared to whatever criterion value has been selected. (See next section.) Table 1 is based on the 3-dB rule, but a corresponding table could be prepared on the basis of the 5-dB rule.

The other form is illustrated by Table 3. In this form we find a series of columns of dBA levels, each headed by a *criterion level,* i.e., the level that is considered "permissible" or "acceptable" for continuous exposure to steady noise for 8 hours a day for a 40-hour work week. In the column below each criterion level are higher levels which are permissible for various shorter periods each day provided the dBA level during the remainder of the day is below the criterion level. If two or more different levels are above the criterion level, each with its own duration in hours per day, their indices may be combined according to the rule given in the legend of Table 3. The values given in Table 3 are calculated according to the 5-dB rule, but corresponding values could be calulated by the 3-dB rule if desired.

TABLE 3

EQUAL-RISK NOISE-EXPOSURES CALCULATED ACCORDING TO THE 5-DB RULE

| | Sound Levels in dBA | | | | | Corresponding Durations: Hours per Day |
|---|---|---|---|---|---|---|
| Criteria | 86 | 88 | 90 | 92 | 94 | 8 |
| Partial exposures | 88 | 90 | 92 | 94 | 96 | 6 |
| | 91 | 93 | 95 | 97 | 99 | 4 |
| | 93 | 95 | 97 | 99 | 101 | 3 |
| | 96 | 98 | 100 | 102 | 104 | 2 |
| | 98 | 100 | 102 | 104 | 106 | 1.5 |
| | 101 | 103 | 105 | 107 | 109 | 1 |
| | 106 | 108 | 110 | 112 | 114 | 0.5 |
| | 111 | 113 | 115 | 117 | 119 | 0.25 |

The figures in each column represent the intensity of noise in dBA for which the exposure shown at the right is equivalent to an eight-hour exposure to the "criterion value" at the top of the column. Thus 100 dBA for 2 hours daily is equivalent to 90 dBA for 8 hours, while for 1.5 hours it is equivalent to 88 dBA for 8 hours.

If during two or more periods per day the sound level (dBA) exceeds the criterion level, the combined effect is judged as follows:

The number of hours per day of actual exposure ($A_1, A_2 \ldots A_n$) at each sound level is compared with the total permissible time for such a sound level ($T_1, T_2 \ldots T_n$, from right-hand column) as if it were the only exposure above the criterion level. The series of fractions $\frac{A_1}{T_1}, \frac{A_2}{T_2} \cdots \frac{A_n}{T_n}$ is summed. If this sum exceeds unity, the risk from the combined exposure is greater than that of 8 hours continuous exposure at the criterion level. In this calculation the actual hours at the criterion level are included, but exposure time below the criterion level is disregarded.

The relations between duration of exposure and sound level given in this table are calculated according to the 5-dB rule.

## Life-Time Noise-Exposure, and Risk

The next step in estimating the risk of injury to hearing from noise-exposure is to estimate the years of habitual noise-exposure for the individuals who are at risk. With the help of Table 4 it can then be predicted *what percentage of each group of individuals may be expected to sustain a hearing impairment sufficient to constitute some handicap in everyday situations.* The relations given in Table 4 are based on 1) data from the Research Center of the Committee on Conservation of Hearing, 2) recommendations of the Committee on Conservation of Hearing for the evaluation of hearing handicap (Trans. of Amer. Acad. of Ophthal. and Otolaryng., March–April 1959), and 3) a study of the hearing of a considerable industrial population habitually exposed to noise. (W. L. Baughn, *International Audiology,* 1966, Vol. 5, pp. 331–338.)

Several simplifying assumptions have been made in preparing Table 4.

1. Hearing impairment (handicap) is defined as more than 26 dB (ISO) or 15 dB (ASA 1951) for the average of hearing levels at 500, 1000 and 2000 Hz.

2. Workers are assumed to enter the occupation in question at the age of 18 years.

3. The median hearing level of the workers at age 20 and with previous exposure levels of 80 dBA or less is assumed to be 10 dB (ISO) or 0 dB (ASA 1951).

TABLE 4
PERCENTAGE RISK OF DEVELOPING A HEARING HANDICAP

| Age<br>Exposure<br>(Age—20) | | | 20<br>0 | 25<br>5 | 30<br>10 | 35<br>15 | 40<br>20 | 45<br>25 | 50<br>30 | 55<br>35 | 60<br>40 | 65<br>45 | Years |
|---|---|---|---|---|---|---|---|---|---|---|---|---|---|
| | 80 | Total | 0.7 | 1.0 | 1.3 | 2.0 | 3.1 | 4.9 | 7.7 | 13.5 | 24.0 | 40.0 | |
| | | Due to Noise | NO INCREASE IN RISK AT THIS LEVEL OF EXPOSURE | | | | | | | | | | |
| | 85 | Total | 0.7 | 2.0 | 3.9 | 6.0 | 8.1 | 11.0 | 14.2 | 21.5 | 32.0 | 46.5 | |
| | | Due to Noise | 0.0 | 1.0 | 2.6 | 4.0 | 5.0 | 6.1 | 6.5 | 8.0 | 8.0 | 6.5 | |
| | 90 | Total | 0.7 | 4.0 | 7.9 | 12.0 | 15.0 | 18.3 | 23.3 | 31.0 | 42.0 | 54.5 | |
| | | Due to Noise | 0.0 | 3.0 | 6.6 | 10.0 | 11.9 | 13.4 | 15.6 | 17.5 | 18.0 | 14.5 | |
| | 95 | Total | 0.7 | 6.7 | 13.6 | 20.2 | 24.5 | 29.0 | 34.4 | 41.8 | 52.0 | 64.0 | |
| | | Due to Noise | 0.0 | 5.7 | 12.3 | 18.2 | 21.4 | 24.1 | 26.7 | 28.3 | 28.0 | 24.0 | |
| | 100 | Total | 0.7 | 10.0 | 22.0 | 32.0 | 39.0 | 43.0 | 48.5 | 55.0 | 64.0 | 75.0 | |
| | | Due to Noise | 0.0 | 9.0 | 20.7 | 30.0 | 35.9 | 38.1 | 40.8 | 41.5 | 40.0 | 35.0 | |
| | 105 | Total | 0.7 | 14.2 | 33.0 | 46.0 | 53.0 | 59.0 | 65.5 | 71.0 | 78.0 | 84.5 | |
| | | Due to Noise | 0.0 | 13.2 | 31.7 | 44.0 | 49.9 | 54.1 | 57.8 | 57.5 | 54.0 | 44.5 | |
| | 110 | Total | 0.7 | 20.0 | 47.5 | 63.0 | 71.5 | 78.0 | 81.5 | 85.0 | 88.0 | 91.5 | |
| | | Due to Noise | 0.0 | 19.0 | 46.2 | 61.0 | 68.4 | 73.1 | 73.8 | 71.5 | 64.0 | 51.5 | |
| | 115 | Total | 0.7 | 27.0 | 62.5 | 81.0 | 87.0 | 91.0 | 92.0 | 93.0 | 94.0 | 95.0 | |
| | | Due to Noise | 0.0 | 26.0 | 61.2 | 79.0 | 83.9 | 86.1 | 84.3 | 89.5 | 70.0 | 55.0 | |

EXPOSURE LEVEL IN DBA (left axis) · PERCENTAGES OF EXPOSED POPULATION (right axis)

The criterion for hearing handicap is an average hearing level at 500, 1000 and 2000 Hz of 26 dB (ISO) or more.

Noise exposure is assumed to be habitual from 20 years of age onward.

The percentage risk due to noise is the total percentage at each age and exposure level minus the corresponding percentage risk at 80 dBA or less (first line), which is due to causes other than noise.

The various simplifying assumptions employed in deriving Table 4 are listed in the text.

4. Each worker's equivalent sound level A of noise-exposure is assumed to be the same, year by year.

5. No significant sex differences are recognized in respect to presbycusis or to susceptibility to noise-induced hearing loss.

6. No hearing loss is induced by a life-time exposure to equivalent sound level A of 80 dBA or less. (This last assumption is very well founded on observations and measurements.)

It is common knowledge that hearing becomes worse with advancing age (presbycusis) and the data of the Research Center of the Committee on Conservation of Hearing show that *40 percent of the population who have not had habitual exposure to noise above 80 dBA nevertheless surpass the threshold of beginning handicap by the age of 63 years.* The expected percentage by age groups is given in Table 4 in the third line of every horizontal set of percentages. *It is obvious that even the most complete noise-control will not protect individuals from developing hearing impairments from causes other than noise.*

In Table 4 the term "percent due to noise" is used to express the *increased risk, due to noise-exposure,* of developing a significant impairment of hearing. These percentages are shown in boldface for each equivalent exposure-level-A from 80 to 115 dBA and for years of exposure from 0 to 45 years. The values were found by subtracting the percentages attributable to other causes from the total percentages actually observed in sample populations with habitual noise-exposure.

## Criteria for Noise-Control

The final step of deciding whether to institute a hearing conservation program and, if so, deciding what level of noise-exposure with its associated risk will be "acceptable," involves many social and economic considerations that must be taken into account by those who are responsible for such policy decisions. Many alternatives must be weighed, such as the relative merits and costs of noise control, of personal protection, of automation, of changes in operating procedures, and of careful monitoring of the hearing of noise-exposed employees and of changing the work assignments of those who begin to develop noise-induced hearing loss. There are imponderable humane and possibly political considerations, such as the certainty that those who have developed a noise-induced hearing handicap by the age of retirement at 65 years will inevitably develop more and more handicap with advancing years; a handicap more severe than it would have been without a large noise-induced component. The Walsh-Healy Act of 1969 [3] is an example of legislation which restricts noise-exposure in order to protect workers against this cumulative handicap in later years.

It should be obvious that there is no single criterion for the initiation of a hearing conservation program. It is clearly not feasible in many situations to try to eliminate all possibility of causing any noise-induced hearing loss in any individual. People vary too much in their susceptibility to noise and to other factors. Even at the 5 percent probability of producing a significant effect the statistical uncertainty is still rather large. On the other hand, a 50 percent chance of producing a significant hearing handicap after 45 years of exposure will probably be considered a rather high risk in most situations. It is certainly high from the medical point of view. But each organization must establish its own criterion in terms of acceptable percentage risk and the alternative means of protection to be provided.

In most discussions of proposed criteria it is generally agreed that 80 dBA is completely acceptable, with no clear risk at all, while 95 dBA is usually the highest that is considered as possibly acceptable. This equivalent sound level A approaches a 30 percent risk at 35 years. Actually *90 dBA has been the most frequent choice,* but usually with the recognition that personal protection and also careful monitoring of hearing for tell-tale losses of sensitivity beginning at 4000 Hz should also be employed.

## Use of the Methods of Calculation

The use the proposed method of calculation of equivalent sound level A and the importance of the choice of a criterion and also of the rule for dealing with intermittent noise-exposure will be illustrated by a specific example.

We will assume that the criterion level of 90 dBA has been adopted as a matter of policy and we wish to determine whether the noise-exposure of a particular employee is acceptable or whether some noise-control or modification of exposure time is required. Let us assume that

[3] Federal Register, Vol. 34, No. 96. Tuesday. May 20, 1969. Rules and Regulations 50–204. 10.

repeated measurements of sound level A at the position of this employee's ear is 96 dBA for 16 hours of a typical 40-hour work week. During the remaining 24 hours the level is 86 dBA. We will calculate first according to the "3-dB rule," using Tables 1 and 2.

Enter Table 1 at 16 hours in the first column headed "hours per week." In the column headed 95 dBA find 125 and in the column headed 100 find 400 as the corresponding partial noise-exposure indices. Our actual noise level of 96 dBA lies between 95 and 100 dBA and interpolation between 125 and 400 gives 180 as its partial index. Now reenter the table at 25 hours, the duration nearest to the actual duration of 24 hours. The index corresponding to 85 dBA is 20. A double interpolation, on the duration and also on the sound-level scale, gives an index of 27 for the combination of 24 hours exposure at 86 dBA. This is the second partial index. The sum of the two partial indices, 180 and 27, is 207. This is the composite noise-exposure index. Enter Table 2 with this value, which is just over 200. The corresponding equivalent continuous sound level is a little over 93 dBA. Our assumed criterion level is 90 dBA, and it is obvious that the equivalent sound level for this particular combination of noise levels and durations, calculated according to the 3-dB rule, exceeds the criterion.

The alternative calculation based on the 5-dB rule employs Table 3. Our criterion value is 90 dBA. Therefore select the column headed by 90 dBA. Our stronger noise-exposure level is 96 dBA. This obviously would not be permissible for 8 hours a day, five days a week, but it is permissible according to Table 3, for 3.5 hours per day. For a 5-day week this would be $5 \times 3.5 = 17.5$ hours. The ratio of the actual duration $(A_1)$ of 16 hours to the permitted duration $(T_1)$ of 17.5 hours is 0.91. The lesser exposure at 86 dBA is below the level which is permissible for 8 hours a day, and according to the method of calculation based on the 5-dB rule it may be disregarded. The combined quotient, $0.91 + 0.00$, is less than unity. Therefore the noise-exposure in question is permissible according to the 5-dB rule.

The result, in this particular example, depends on the choice of the rule and the corresponding calculation that is employed. The user of the method must decide which rule best fits his own context. We repeat that the USA Standards Institute has not yet issued a standard that deals with this question.

We believe that the over-all method presented above for assessment of noise-exposure is at least as accurate as, and is certainly simpler to employ than, previous methods, including the so-called Noise Rating Curves and the method described in the 1964 edition of the Guide. Table 4 gives numerical estimates of the risk of habitual noise-exposure. A trend toward general adoption of the 90 dBA criterion seems clear. The numbers in the various tables are, of course, subject to some future adjustments as our knowledge increases. *We can hope that in the future this method of assessment can be extended to include impulsive noises. At present it can be applied only to steady noises.*

The section of the Guide on ear protectors is also worth quoting:

## Use of Personal Protection

Ear protectors in effect reduce noise levels at the inner ear. Ear protection is particularly important when noise-exposures cannot be controlled adequately by environmental changes.

### Types of Ear Protectors

Ear protectors may be:
  (1) Ear plugs, or
  (2) Ear muffs.

*Ear plugs* are designed to occlude the ear canal. They may be made of rubber, neoprene or plastic. In general ear plugs should be made of non-porous pliable material; nothing made of hard material should be used. Contrary to popular opinion, dry cotton affords little or no protection. Material and shape have little to do with the effectiveness of commercially available plugs except as they affect acceptance by users.

*Ear muffs* are designed to cover the external ear. At frequencies above 1000 Hz, muffs provide about the same protection as plugs. At frequencies below 1000 Hz, certain correctly designed muffs provide more protection than plugs. (See Table 5 for some typical attenuation figures.)

TABLE 5
ATTENUATION IN DB FOR EIGHT DIFFERENT EAR PROTECTORS*

| Type | Frequency (Hz) | | | | | | | | |
|---|---|---|---|---|---|---|---|---|---|
| | 125 | 250 | 500 | 1000 | 2000 | 3000 | 4000 | 6000 | 8000 |
| Ear plugs | | | | | | | | | |
| A | | 21.9 | 25.0 | 25.9 | 33.4 | 38.0 | 41.2 | 33.0 | 37.5 |
| B | 15 | 15.9 | 16.2 | 21.3 | 28.8 | 33.7 | 33.7 | 32.9 | 39.1 |
| C | 8 | 16 | 16 | 19 | 23 | 29 | 27 | 34 | 40 |
| Ear muffs | | | | | | | | | |
| A | 8 | 23 | 30 | 32 | 33 | 40 | 39 | 39 | 28 |
| B | 19 | 30 | 38 | 38 | 42 | 44 | 45 | 40 | 35 |
| C | 7 | 13 | 23 | 31 | 34 | 34 | 42 | 40 | 35 |
| Cotton | 5 | 6 | 8 | 9 | 13 | 15 | 13 | 14 | 16 |

* Data derived from tests performed according to the American Standards Association method for the measurement of real-ear attenuation of ear protectors at threshold, Z24.22-1957.

The choice of plugs or muffs or both depends in part on the work situation. Will the employee's head be confined to a work space so small there is no room for muffs? Must he wear a hard hat in addition to ear protection? And so forth. There are advantages and disadvantages to the use of either plugs or muffs, and before a choice is made between the two, all the circumstances of a particular job should be considered.

### Fitting and Indoctrination

An employee's ears should be examined and his hearing tested at the time he is fitted with ear protectors. Plugs should be fitted individually for each ear: if the ear canals are not the same size or shape they may require plugs of different size. To promote the acceptance of ear plugs, an employee should be allowed to choose from two or three different makes at the time he is fitted.

As with other kinds of personal protection (hard hats, safety glasses, safety shoes or respirators) it may be difficult to convince employees that they should wear ear protectors. Successful personal protection programs are based on thorough indoctrination of personnel. An employee *must* be impressed with the importance of ear protection and the benefits to be gained from its consistent use. He should be told that:

(1) Good protection depends on a good seal between the surface of the skin and the surface of the ear protector. A very small leak can destroy the effectiveness of the protection. Protectors have a tendency to work loose as a result of talking, chewing, etc., and they must be reseated from time to time during the work-day.

(2) A good seal cannot be obtained without some initial discomfort.

(3) There will be no untoward reaction as a result of the use of ear protectors if they are reasonably clean. Ear plugs should be made of soft elastic material such as neoprene. Hard fixed material can injure the canal. (Skin irritations, injured ear drums, or other harmful reactions are exceedingly rare. A properly designed, well fitted and clean ear protector will cause no more difficulty than a pair of safety goggles.)

(4) The use of ear protection will not make it more difficult to understand speech or to hear warning signals when worn in a noisy environment.

Most of the available ear protectors, when correctly fitted, provide about the same amount of protection. The best ear protector, therefore, is the one that is accepted by the employee and worn properly. Properly fitted protectors can be worn continuously by most persons and will provide adequate protection against most industrial noise-exposure. The most effective way of evaluating the efficacy of an ear protection program is through follow-up hearing tests.

Ear plugs do not provide the same amount of attenuation in the field as in the laboratory, probably because of incorrect fitting and failure to maintain a good seal even with properly fitted plugs. Limited research data indicate that ear plugs provide on the average about 5 dB less attenuation under field conditions than in laboratory tests. A list of manufacturers of ear protectors is available on request.

## Auditory Analgesia: Loud Music

In the presence of very loud noise or music most subjects become less sensitive or insensitive to certain kinds of pain. Dental pain and obstetrical pain may be controlled in this way sufficiently to allow tooth extractions or childbirth without local or general anesthesia. Either music or white noise are given by earphones, and the patient has the volume under his own control, turning it up as necessary. Not all pain can be controlled in this way: for example, auditory pain in the ears at very high sound levels still persists. This form of analgesia has been given limited clinical trial, but concern about possible injury to hearing has discouraged its widespread use. Minimum standards to protect against this hazard were issued in 1961 by the American Dental Association.

The physiological and psychological mechanisms of auditory analgesia are not at all clear. We may think of a "saturation of the sensorium" and the principle of counterirritation, but these are little more than descriptions of the phenomenon. High sound levels of the order of 120 dB SPL are required. The experience is unusual and psychologically impressive, and it may explain in part the fascination of the very high noise levels in some modern dance halls. Playing in such orchestras night after night should be recognized as a hazardous noise-exposure.

## Conservation of Hearing in Elderly People

For elderly people the problem of hazardous noise-exposure becomes less and less important, and the maintenance of reasonable hygiene of the ear becomes more and more routine. There are fewer and fewer risks, as people grow older, from dirt and water or even from the common cold. The characteristic hearing loss of old age (presbycusis) is chiefly an inner-ear impairment, but we have no idea about how to protect against it. Neither can we protect against cerebral arteriosclerosis and the other conditions that we lump together as "senile changes." They are in the province of the new branch of medicine known as *geriatrics*.

Something can be done, however, to *protect communication by speech*. As hearing begins to deteriorate in elderly persons, they can begin to wear hearing aids and learn how to use them to their advantage. They can also take lessons in speechreading, and as their hearing losses become severe they can even learn how to keep their own voices pleasant and intelligible. These suggestions sound very simple and obvious, but the people who could benefit from them find them difficult to carry out, even if they can be persuaded to try. The problem is to *start soon enough* while the elderly man or woman is still adaptable, able to learn, and willing to make the necessary effort. As will be explained in other chapters, the person who becomes hard of hearing, particularly the elderly person, often does not recognize or admit his incapacity. He may blame others for not speaking up or for mumbling. By the time his hearing loss has become an obvious handicap it may be too late to "teach the old dog new tricks" and to alter his habits of a lifetime. To overcome such individual inertia and to create a healthy, constructive social point of view toward these and other problems of aging are the objectives of conservation of speech communication in elderly people.

## SUGGESTED READINGS AND REFERENCES

**Coles, R. R. A., G. R. Garinther, D. C. Hodge, and C. G. Rice.** "Hazardous Exposure to Impulse Noise," *J. Acoust. Soc. Amer.,* 43:336–343 (1968).
A technical report proposing damage-risk criteria.

**Cox, J. R., J.** "Industrial Noise and Conservation of Hearing," Vol. I, Chap. 18. *Industrial Hygiene and Toxicology,* F. Patty (ed.), 2nd ed. New York: Interscience Publishers, 1958.

**Davis, H., G. Hoople, and H. O. Parrack.** "The Medical Principles of Monitoring Audiometry," *A.M.A. Arch. Industr. Health,* 17:1–20 (1958).

**DeWeese, D. D., and W. H. Saunders.** *Textbook of Otolaryngology.* St. Louis: C. V. Mosby Company, 1964.

**Eagles, E. L., S. M. Wishik, L. G. Doerfler, W. Melinick, and H. S. Levine.** "Hearing Sensitivity and Related Factors in Children," Special monograph issue of *Laryngoscope,* 1963.
This is the "Pittsburgh Study" quoted in Chapter 5.

**Goodhill, V.** "Pathology, Diagnosis and Therapy of Deafness," Chap. 9. In *Handbook of Speech Pathology,* L. E. Travis (ed.). New York: Appleton-Century-Crofts, Inc., 1957.
A fairly detailed exposition of the medical and surgical aspects of deafness.

**Harris, C. M. (ed.).** *Handbook of Noise Control.* New York: McGraw-Hill Book Company, 1957.
Chapters 4 and 7 are particularly pertinent.

**Kryter, K. D., W. D. Ward, J. D. Miller, and D. H. Eldredge.** "Hazardous Exposure to Intermittent and Steady-state Noise," *J. Acoust. Soc. Amer.,* 39:451–464 (1968).
Prepared by NAS-NRC CHABA Working Group 46 to specify damage-risk criteria for exposure to sound.

**Kryter, K. D.** "Concepts of Perceived Noisiness, Their Implementation and Application," *J. Acoust. Soc. Amer.,* 43:344–361 (1968).
An excellent treatment of the problem of noisiness.

**Subcommittee on Noise** of the Committee on Conservation of Hearing (AAOO) and Research Center of the Subcommittee on Noise. "Guide for Conservation of Hearing in Noise," *Trans. Amer. Acad. Ophth. Otol.* (supplement, 1–40), 1964.
Available on request from Dr. A. Glorig, The Callier Hearing and Speech Center, 1966 Inwood Road, Dallas, Texas 75235.

**Ward, W. D. (ed.).** *Proposed Damage-Risk Criterion for Impulse Noise (Gunfire).* NAS-NRC Committee on Hearing, Bioacoustics, and Biomechanics, 1968. Office of Naval Research, Contract No. NONR 2300(05).
Report of "CHABA" Working Group 57.

**Williams, H. L.** *Ménière's Disease.* Springfield, Illinois: Charles C Thomas, 1952.
An exhaustive monograph by an eminent otologist.

# CHAPTER 6

## THE SURGICAL TREATMENT OF HEARING LOSS

### T. E. WALSH, M.R.C.S., L.R.C.P.

As described in previous chapters, the ability to hear requires an intact nerve of hearing to convey to the brain the nerve impulses set up by sound waves. For normal sensitivity of hearing there must also be an efficient apparatus to convey sounds from the outside world to the sense organ in the inner ear. This conduction apparatus consists of the external ear and canal for the collection of sound waves and the drum and ossicles of the middle ear. At the present time we are unable to restore any tissue that may have degenerated in the brain, the auditory nerve, or the inner ear. The surgical treatment of hearing loss is, therefore, aimed at correcting abnormalities of the conduction apparatus.

### SURGICAL TREATMENT OF THE MIDDLE EAR AND THE MASTOID

The function of the Eustachian tube in equalizing the pressure of air in the middle ear with that outside the eardrum has already been described. The tube normally opens only momentarily when we swallow or yawn. If any obstruction is present, so that the tube cannot open when it should, the air contained in the middle ear is partly absorbed, and the drumhead is pushed in by the air pressure outside. When the drum membrane is thus "retracted," its free motion is limited and its efficiency as a conducting mechanism is reduced. The result is a temporary, partial loss of hearing.

In addition to allowing the passage of air between the back of the nose and the middle ear, the Eustachian tube offers a pathway up which infections of the nose and throat can easily extend into the middle ear. Such infection is more likely to occur when the mouth of the Eustachian tube is surrounded by lymphoid tissue (adenoids), which easily becomes infected in colds or sinusitis.

The adenoids, tonsils, and sinuses are therefore doubly important as indirect causes of hearing loss. They may prevent ventilation of the middle ear, and they may favor infection. Enlarged tonsils and adenoids should therefore be removed surgically.

The spread of infection up the Eustachian tube is frequently helped by the improper forcible blowing of the nose, which is so commonly practiced. Children in particular should be instructed to blow the nose gently with both nostrils open so that the pressure does not force infected material from the nose up the Eustachian tube to the middle ear.

The condition of *serous* or *mucous otitis media* has been described in Chapters 4 and 5, and the necessity for removal of the fluid to restore hearing and to prevent the formation of adhesions has been pointed out. Often a simple incision of the drumhead or puncture by a needle with suction will clear up a serous effusion. Occasionally the condition can be relieved by inflating the middle ear by way of the Eustachian tube. Sometimes, however, adequate drainage cannot be obtained through the Eustachian tube, or perhaps the opening in the drumhead heals too quickly. In this situation the hole in the drumhead can often be kept open with a small piece of plastic tubing. In adults the puncture of the drumhead is usually done without anesthesia, but in children this procedure is not an easy one, especially if a plastic tube is to be inserted.

If the exudate in the middle ear is thick and the disease is of long standing, elimination of the large surface of the mastoid cells may be necessary. This requires the operation known as *mastoidectomy*, which will be described below.

Of course, if the accumulation of fluid is due to blockage at the nasopharyngeal end of the Eustachian tube, it may be relieved or recurrence prevented by removal of enlarged adenoids or by treatment of the overgrown lymphoid tissue by radiation. These measures are not likely to be effective, however, if the fluid is thick and mucoid.

The symptoms of inflammation of the middle ear, or *otitis media*, and its medical treatment by sulfonamides and penicillin were discussed in Chapter 5 as part of the medical treatment of the ear. If, however, the inflammation is not recognized early and is not promptly and efficiently treated, pus will form in the middle ear. This condition is technically known as *suppurative otitis media* and, popularly, as a "rising," a "bealing," or a "gathering" in the ear. If the drumhead is not incised promptly to relieve the pressure within, it may rupture spontaneously. Unless the infection is very mild, the drum should be opened *promptly*, if it has not done so of itself, and the pus within it allowed to drain out. Following a spontaneous rupture, the perforation does not always heal; but, if the drumhead is incised by the surgeon early in the course of the infection and the pus behind it is able to drain, the incision usually heals well with no residual loss of hearing. If, however, the infection is neglected, mastoiditis, with its attendant danger of further complications, may occur and the hearing be permanently impaired. *Prompt attention to infection of the middle ear will do much to prevent the loss of hearing that frequently accompanies perforation of the drumhead and chronic diseases of the middle ear.* Contrary to popular belief, the hearing loss which sometimes persists after mastoid surgery or incision of the drum membrane is due to the disease and not to the surgery.

A very mild infection or an infection treated by antibiotics may not develop into purulent or suppurative otitis media but may become instead a chronic mucous otitis media (see Chapter 5). The chief problem concerning mucous otitis media, particularly in children, is to recognize the condition. The treatment is to open the ear and remove the thick viscous fluid. Many such cases might be prevented by opening the ear earlier when the infectious process is a little more active and the secretion still thin and watery.

A more severe form of chronic otitis media, with continuing active infection, may follow acute otitis media if the acute otitis is not properly treated. The hearing becomes further impaired because, as a result of the infection, the ossicles become bound together with scar tissue or may actually be eaten away by the disease process. There is also the further danger that in certain cases the infection may spread into the skull and lead to meningitis and brain abscess. Operation for chronic otitis media is indicated to ensure the safety of the patient, to check the formation of scar tissue, and also to restore the hearing as far as it can be restored.

### Mastoidectomy

The operation of mastoidectomy for chronic otitis media has been considered a terrible and dangerous procedure by most laymen. It is usually, however, a lifesaving operation, and in the hands of a competent otologic surgeon it is not dangerous.

There are several kinds of mastoidectomy. The "simple" or "complete" mastoidectomy, performed for acute mastoiditis, aims to remove the diseased tissue in the mastoid bone and to establish free drainage of pus from the mastoid and the middle ear. "Radical" mastoidectomy is performed in chronic cases when the disease is not only in the air cells of the mastoid bone but in the middle ear as well. Its object is to remove all diseased tissues from both cavities and to create a single cavity that will eventually become lined with skin and cause no further trouble. "Simple" mastoidectomy, performed for acute infection of the mastoid air cells, causes no appreciable hearing loss if there are no other complications. The hearing may be expected to stay within normal limits. "Radical" mastoidectomy, on the other hand, performed most frequently for chronic running ears, usually leaves a hearing level for speech of about 45 dB because the middle ear is destroyed in the operation, even if it has not already been destroyed by the infection.

The final level actually represents an improvement of hearing in about one-third of all cases over the conductive loss which existed before operation while the middle ear was plugged with pus. For another one-third there is no significant over-all change in hearing, and for the remaining third the hearing is worse after the operation than it was before. Of course, if, as is frequently the case, there is also some sensory-neural hearing loss, the impairment due to it will remain and will be added to some 40 dB of conductive impairment produced by the operation. It should be clearly understood that *radical mastoidectomy is a lifesaving operation or is performed to prevent further deterioration of the inner ear and not for the sake of any possible improvement of hearing.*

## SURGICAL ALLEVIATION OF CONDUCTIVE HEARING LOSS

The two major diseases of the middle ear, otitis media and otosclerosis, have been discussed in some detail in previous chapters. The surgical treatment of acute otitis media is an important surgical procedure, but there are now also surgical operations that aim to combat a disease process as well as to improve the conduction of sound to the inner ear. One of these is *myringoplasty*, or repair of a persistent perforation of the drum membrane. Closely allied to this operation is the use of a "prosthesis," which is a mechanical substitute of some sort for a missing ossicle. The other two operations, aimed to relieve or circumvent the fixation of the stapes by otosclerosis, are *stapes mobilization* and *fenestration*.

We shall merely mention here in passing that surgery may be done to overcome congenital malformations of the external or the middle ear. If the external canal is closed (atresia), it may be opened by surgical procedures. Frequently, the benefit from such an operation is limited from the point of view of hearing because of malformations of the ossicles or other parts of the middle ear as well as of the external canal. Surgery is also often undertaken to improve the appearance of a malformed or missing external ear (pinna). This is usually done by a plastic surgeon rather than by an otologic surgeon.

### Tympanoplasty and Myringoplasty

There are many cases of chronic otitis media in which the disease is not sufficiently severe to warrant a radical mastoidectomy. However, the hearing in such cases is decreased because of the scarlike adhesions and perhaps because of other anatomical changes that have taken place in the middle ear, and perhaps also because of perforation of the tympanic membrane. For many years plastic operations have been performed in such cases either to re-form the middle ear or perhaps only to close the hole in the drum membrane. The more extensive operation was formerly known as "modified radical mastoidectomy," but it has recently been improved and popularized under the name "tympanoplasty." Here we should remember that "tympano-" refers to the entire middle ear, and not merely to the drum membrane. For the simpler operation, directed to closure of a hole in the membrane and nothing more, we use the term "myringoplasty."

The Committee on Conservation of Hearing of the American Academy of Ophthalmology and Otolaryngology approved, in 1964, the following statement and recommended set of definitions.

Until recently the modified radical and the radical mastoidectomy were the common operative procedures performed for chronic ear infection. These operations were designed primarily to eradicate this infection. More recently, the concept of surgery in chronic ear infection has changed to include both eradication of disease and reconstruction of the destroyed hearing mechanism. These more complex surgical procedures are being described by a multiplicity of terms. This multiplicity of terms to describe similar surgical procedures has caused considerable confusion. The common operations performed in surgery for chronic ear infection are listed below. It

is felt that, with rare exceptions, any operation for chronic ear disease could be classified as one of the following procedures. Technical surgical variations peculiar to one or another surgeon do not alter the fundamental classification:

1. Radical or Modified Radical Mastoidectomy

2. Mastoid Obliteration Operation

    An operation performed to eradicate infection when present, and to obliterate a mastoid or fenestration cavity.

3. Myringoplasty

    An operation in which the reconstructive procedure is limited to repair of a tympanic membrane perforation.

4. Tympanoplasty without Mastoidectomy

    An operation performed to eradicate disease in the middle ear and to reconstruct the hearing mechanism, without mastoid surgery, with or without tympanic membrane grafting.

5. Tympanoplasty with Mastoidectomy

    An operation performed to eradicate disease in the middle ear and mastoid, and to reconstruct the hearing mechanism, with or without tympanic membrane grafting.

*Myringoplasty.* In many cases the tympanic membrane has been perforated as the result of an old healed otitis media. The ear is perfectly dry. There is no discharge, but the patient's hearing is depressed because of the hole in the drumhead. Such holes can sometimes be closed by cauterizing, cutting, or scraping the edge of the perforation, and then providing some sort of scaffolding, such as cigarette paper or cotton, to assist the epithelium to grow across and thus heal the perforation. Some surgeons have had considerable success with these procedures, but others have not. A recent approach to the closure of perforations is to separate the epithelium from the fibrous portion of the drum membrane for a distance of about 2 or 3 mm from the edge of the perforation. A graft is prepared, usually from subcutaneous tissue (fascia) that covers the temporalis muscle, and is placed over the raw surface that has been exposed. It receives its blood supply from the raw surface. Often the fascial graft will "take" and close the perforation. Such operations may improve the hearing for speech from levels between 20 and 30 dB to a level of 15 dB or better, that is, within normal limits.

*Tympanoplasty.* When disease is still present in the upper part of the middle ear (the attic), a more extensive operation is required. The objectives are, first, to remove all diseased tissue from the middle ear, the attic, and the mastoid, and then to re-form a middle ear and ossicular chain. Defects in the drum membrane, or indeed a total loss of the membrane, can be repaired by the use of fascia from the temporalis muscle. When, as is most commonly the case, the incus is diseased and its long process (that part which is joined to the stapes) is missing, the remains of the incus, the body and short process, can be removed and a hollow drilled in the body. This hollow will then be placed on the head of the stapes and the short process under the handle of the malleus, so that the vibration from the drum membrane and malleus are conveyed to the movable stapes. In the event the crura of the stapes are destroyed by disease, the fascia graft forms a new drum membrane, and later fenestration of the horizontal canal can return hearing for speech to a level of between 20 and 25 dB.

Note that following this operation (without fenestration) the round window is walled off from the oval window by what remains of the drum membrane. The reduced middle ear cavity is still connected with the Eustachian tube (see Figure 6-2). The sound waves reach the oval window, exposed directly to the external canal and the round window, protected by the drum membrane, with somewhat different intensities and perhaps also with significant phase differences, and thus set up movement in the cochlear fluids.

### Stapes Surgery

The concept of forcibly breaking loose a fixed stapes and thus restoring its function is as old as it is simple. It was attempted many times during the last quarter of the nineteenth century and in the early nineteenth hundreds, but without much lasting success, and the operation was finally abandoned. Recently, the more complicated fenestration operation has been proved to be practical, lasting in its benefits, with high probability of success, but limited in the hearing-threshold level that it can yield.

A few years ago Dr. Samuel Rosen of New York revived the simple stapes mobilization. Although the immediate results are moderately successful, a rather high percentage of successfully mobilized stapes become immobile once more. In 1958, Dr. John Shea of Memphis suggested removal of all or part of the stapes. He used a piece of vein to close the oval window. He attached a small piece of plastic tubing to the incus, and the end of this tube rested on the vein. The sound vibrations were now carried from the ossicles to the fluids of the inner ear by this tubing. The hearing by this method was restored almost to normal in many cases. As time went on, other materials were tried for closure of the oval window and for the attachment to the incus. Gelfoam, fat, and vein were used, and also stainless steel wire. Teflon took the place of the plastic tube.

In stapes surgery the middle ear is approached by way of the external canal. The incision is made in the skin of the canal, and the skin is lifted off the bone and reflected forward, carrying the tympanic membrane with it. The head of the stapes is not readily visible from the ear canal but, by careful grinding with fine drills under a powerful microscope, enough bone is removed to obtain a good view.

With very fine knives, hooks, probes, and chisels, all specially made for this purpose, the head of the stapes is separated from the incus. The crura of the stapes are removed; the footplate is cracked across and removed in two pieces. The oval window is now open, and a piece of vein or other material is placed over it to close it and prevent the escape of perilymph. A plastic tube or wire is attached to the incus and rests on the material closing the oval window. The drum membrane and the skin of the canal wall are then replaced.

The advantges of stapes surgery are (1) it is, for the patient, a relatively minor operation requiring only a brief stay in the hospital, usually two nights and one day; (2) it is performed prudently, under local anesthesia; (3) it leaves a normal ear canal and drum membrane when healing is completed; (4) when successful the hearing level for speech is well within normal limits, often better than 10 dB.

Postoperatively there is very little discomfort. There is a slight earache which usually can be controlled by aspirin. There may be very slight dizziness, but much less than following the fenestration operation. Sometimes the sense of taste on the side of the tongue corresponding to the side of the operation may be modified so that food tastes unnatural and somewhat metallic. This effect, undoubtedly due to manipulation of the chorda tympani in the middle ear, is usually only temporary.

The percentage of immediately successful results is high. Most otologic surgeons achieve 85 to 90 percent—but no one can promise success with complete assurance in any particular case.

### Fenestration

The following historical account of the development of the fenestration operation, retained (with some small changes) from the first edition of our book, is of some interest in illustrating the step-by-step advance on an international basis.

Such a development is characteristic of most advances in medicine and surgery. As long ago as 1876, Kessel, in Germany, suggested removal of the immobile stapes. The removal, of course, left the oval window open. The opening was allowed to close with scar tissue, and Kessel hoped that the scar would be flexible enough to enable sound to enter the inner ear. His attempts were not successful because of the difficulty in removing the footplate of the stapes and because infection entered the inner ear from the middle-ear cavity.

In 1897, Passow, another German, tried a different approach. He made an opening into the basal turn of the cochlea and covered the opening with periosteum, the membrane which normally covers bone. Immediately after the operation his patient experienced a marked improvement in hearing, which, however, lasted only a few days. The danger of infection was a bugbear of this operation, and because of it and the consequent danger to life and the fleeting nature of the hearing improvement, the procedure was not generally adopted.

In 1910, Bárány, the great Swedish otolaryngologist (a native of Austria), suggested making an opening into the posterior vertical semicircular canal to reduce the danger of infection of the labyrinth. The surgical approach to the posterior vertical canal is made through the mastoid bone under aseptic conditions, and there is, therefore, little chance of infection. He performed this operation, and the immediate improvement in hearing was marked, but it lasted only two weeks.

In 1914, Jenkins, in England, opened the horizontal semicircular canal in two patients. In one case he covered the opening with a skin graft and in the other with a flap of skin taken from the posterior wall of the external auditory canal. The hearing improved markedly in both cases immediately following the operation, but it fell below the preoperative level in one case and was lost completely in the other shortly afterward.

Holmgren (1920), in Sweden, and Sourdille (1924), in France, continued working on this problem and gradually evolved improvements in approach and technique. It was Sourdille who evolved the flap of skin from the wall of the canal, which will be described in the next section, and left it attached to the drum. Some of his cases were successful, but in a large percentage of them the "fenestra" (from the Latin word meaning "window") closed, and the gain in hearing was lost.

Finally, since 1930, in America, Julius Lempert has further improved the technique of the operation. Whereas Sourdille performed his operation in two stages, Lempert devised a one-stage procedure. By attention to minute details of technique, Lempert improved his results. He, too, was disturbed, however, at the frequency with which the newly created fenestra closed and, in searching for a reason, argued that the window, made as it was in the limb of the horizontal canal, was so narrow that bone could easily bridge the gap. He therefore devised a new technique in which he placed the fenestra farther forward over

the wider, ampullated end of the horizontal canal and over the vestibule. He was now able to create a window a full millimeter in width. This added size alone made it less likely that the window would close, and now Lempert and his disciples seem to have finally solved the problem of how reliably to prevent the bone from healing over and closing the new fenestra. Close attention is given to removal of all bone dust and chips. The bone from the center of the opening is removed all in one piece. The edges of the fenestra are ground down thin and smooth, and the skin flap from the wall of the ear canal is pressed firmly down over the fenestra. The object is to bring the flap in contact with the membranous semicircular canal and with the edges of the cut endosteum that lines the bony canal on the inside. If the canal and the endosteum heal to the skin flap, the bone cannot grow over the opening. With present technique not more than about 1 percent of fenestras close again. Those that do close do so within the first year.

The principle of the operation, as developed by Sourdille, is illustrated in Figures 6-1 and 6-2. In Figure 6-1, which is a diagram of the correct anatomical re-

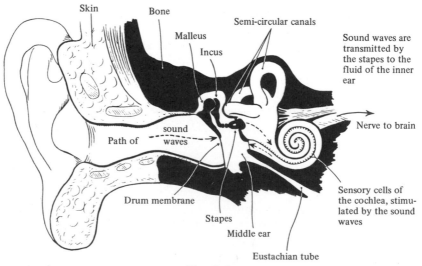

Fig. 6–1.

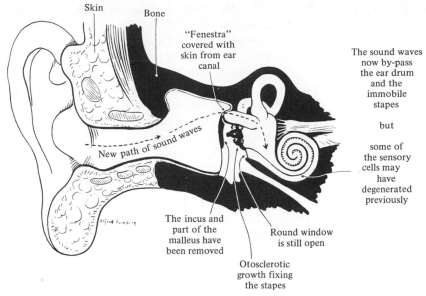

Skin     Bone

"Fenestra" covered with skin from ear canal

The sound waves now by-pass the ear drum and the immobile stapes

but

some of the sensory cells may have degenerated previously

New path of sound waves

The incus and part of the malleus have been removed

Round window is still open

Otosclerotic growth fixing the stapes

Fig. 6–2.

lationships as described in Chapter 3, the normal path of sound across the middle ear and into the inner ear by way of the stapes and oval window is indicated by arrows. Figure 6-2, another diagram, is intended to show (1) the fixation of the stapes by otosclerosis; (2) the degeneration of some of the sensory cells of the cochlea, which so frequently occurs in the later stages of otosclerosis; (3) the opening of a fenestra through the bony wall of the middle ear into the horizontal semicircular canal; (4) the skin flap from the ear canal covering the fenestra; and (5) the displacement of the eardrum and removal of the incus and most of the malleus. The new path of the sound waves is indicated, for simplicity, as entering the inner ear through the fenestra. Of course, both windows must be mobile, and both are affected by the sound pressure outside. The movement inside occurs because of the *difference* in pressure on the two windows at each instant. The pressure is probably greater on the average on the new fenestra than on the round window, which lies be-

hind what is left of the drum membrane. The pressure wave at the round window may also be a little earlier or a little later than at the fenestra ("out of phase," as we say), and this phase difference may increase the difference in instantaneous pressure. It does not matter much which way the fluid in the cochlea moves during the compression phase of a sound wave in the canal. What is important is *how much* it moves; and as a matter of experience the drum membrane over the round-window niche is an important factor in getting a good differential between the two windows.

*Description of the operation.* The present fenestration operation in the hands of a well-trained and competent otologic surgeon is not dangerous to life. The danger that is present, other than that of any operation in which an anesthetic is used, is that the hearing may be entirely lost in the operated ear. This can occur from difficulties at operation or may follow a postoperative inflammation of the delicate structures within the labyrinth. There have also been a few instances of facial-nerve paralysis. This condition, however, is only temporary, and recovery is spontaneous. In no case, in the care of a skilled surgeon, should there be danger of permanent injury to the facial nerve.

The operation may be performed under any type of anesthetic. A skin incision is made in the ear canal and the mastoid bone is exposed and entered. The spongy interior, composed of the partitions between the mastoid air cells, is removed sufficiently to allow approach to the enlarged ampullated end of the horizontal canal and to the middle ear. Great care is taken to control all bleeding, as the fenestra cannot be successfully made in the presence of any blood. The posterior superior bony wall of the external auditory canal is gradually removed until the joint between the malleus and the incus is exposed. This procedure is done with care so that the skin of the external auditory canal and the drum are not injured. Then the incus is removed, and the head and neck of the malleus are amputated. The skin of the external canal is now separated from the

bone of the posterior and superior walls, but its attachment to the drum is left intact. Thus, a flap of skin is formed which can be laid down over the fenestra. This flap of skin is carefully inspected for any particles of bone that might stick to it, and these are removed. All bleeding is again controlled. The fenestra is now made in the ampullated end of the horizontal canal by carefully burring through the bony capsule (Figure 6-3). The skin flap is then laid over the fenestra. The cavity is packed, and a dressing is applied over the ear.

*Course of events after the operation.* The average length of stay in the hospital is from five to seven days. Immediately after the operation, and even on the operating table if the operation is done under local anesthesia, hearing may return dramatically, and the patient, very hard of hearing before operation, may be able to hear the softest-spoken word. This degree of improvement may be diminished for the first few days after the operation because of some inflammatory change due to the surgery. It gradually improves after a period of two or three weeks.

After the operation the patient is somewhat dizzy for the first 24 hours. With the new techniques and the use of isotonic fluid for irrigation during the operation there is very little postoperative labyrinthitis, and most of the dizziness can be very easily controlled, so that the patient is expected to be out of bed the day after the operation, although he may be somewhat unsteady. Of course, certain movements of the head cause dizziness, and the patient must be careful to take things easy for a few days. It is unusual nowadays if the patient is not sitting up and eating full meals within 48 hours of the operation. The patient is urged to be up and walking about as soon as he is able after the operation, usually on the second or third day. On the fifth or sixth day the dressing is done, and all packing is removed from the

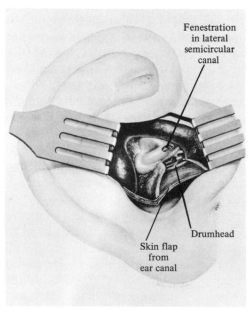

Fenestration in lateral semicircular canal

Drumhead

Skin flap from ear canal

Fig. 6-3.

ear. Only some sterile cotton is left to close the canal. The patient is allowed to go home the day that the dressing is done.

The first dressing is seldom uncomfortable and should never be painful. The ear must be treated at intervals until it is completely healed. These intervals are usually two to three weeks, depending on the techniques that the surgeon prefers. Healing is usually obtained in four to nine weeks.

When the patient leaves the hospital, there are precautions that must be taken for his safety. It must be remembered that the labyrinth has been disturbed and that sudden movements of the head may give rise to dizziness. Such sudden movements must therefore be avoided. For instance, when he is about to cross a street in traffic, the movement of looking each way should be a slow and deliberate one.

Because the horizontal semicircular canal has been exposed (except for its covering of skin) and is now quite accessible to the outside, it can easily be stimulated by changes in temperature. On cold days and when it is windy, cotton should be worn in the ear. The result of stimulation by the cold air is dizziness. It follows, of course, that swimming must be forbidden. It would be extremely dangerous to allow cold water to enter the ear canal following fenestration.

After complete healing has taken place, it is very important to have the cavity cleaned about every six months. Normally, the outer layers of skin all over the body shed dead cells. Elsewhere on the body surface these cells fall off unnoticed. In a cavity such as that left after fenestration, the dead cells may accumulate and must be removed.

Until healing is complete, superficial infections with parasitic fungi are rather common and may cause a delay in healing. It is important that the aftercare demanded by the surgeon be carefully followed.

The cosmetic effect of the operation is of minor importance, but it is well to know that in most cases no change in appearance from the normal can be noted when healing is complete.

### Evaluation

The fenestration operation and stapes surgery must be judged by the answers to four major questions:

For what kinds of deafness is it suitable?
What are the discomforts and dangers?
What are the chances of success?
How permanent are the benefits?

The first and second of these questions we have already answered. Both operations are theoretically suitable for conductive but not for sensory-neural hearing loss. Fenestration causes some temporary discomfort. Stapes surgery causes far less discomfort from vertigo, and the like, after the operation and does not require any periodic aftercare. The danger of losing the hearing of the operated ear entirely is about the same for the two operations. The danger to life is practically negligible for both of them.

The chances of success of both operations depend, of course, upon whether the operation is confined to suitable cases or whether it is tried on patients who have a good deal of neural loss in addition to their conductive loss. We must also set up some definition of "success."

*The objective of the fenestration operation and of stapes surgery is to restore the patient to a satisfactory hearing level for everyday speech.* By this is meant that he should, if the operation is successful, be able to hear ordinary conversation without a hearing aid. He should be able to hear adequately in most theaters, movies, and churches. A final hearing level for speech of 30 dB, which in the context of workmen's compensation laws corresponds to less than 25 percent handicap in the hearing of everyday speech (see Chapter 9), is generally accepted as the borderline of success, that is, a reasonably adequate level for practical everyday communication.

The fenestration operation is now so well standardized that if it is performed by an otologist who specializes in this operation, its outcome can be predicted within a very few decibels with considerable confidence. The reason for the consistency in the results is that the operation completely bypasses the fixed stapes and produces a new sound-conducting system. The new system, illustrated in Figure 6-2, is not as efficient as the normal ear with its complete drum membrane and its chain of ossicles, but it is simple and its performance is therefore predictable. It makes no difference how much conductive loss there was before the operation. After the operation the efficiency of transmission for speech is reduced by about 23 dB. For the "ideal" cases of purely conductive hearing loss it has been the uniform experience over a period of more than ten years for most of the leading otologic surgeons in this country that half of their patients show a final hearing level for speech of 23 dB or better. The variability from case to case is such that half of the cases fall in the range from 21 to 30 dB inclusive.

Of course, if the patient has any sensory-neural loss, the number of decibels estimated to be due to this cause must be added to the 23 dB that must be expected as the residual conductive impairment. The assessment of a small sensory-neural loss in the presence of a large conductive loss is not very easy because of the "Carhart notch" in the bone-conduction audiogram, as explained in Chapter 4.

The other sources of uncertainty about the result of the fenestration operation are the possibility of accidental injury to the inner ear during the operation (less than 1 in 100) and the possibility of closure of the fenestra (about 1 in 100). The closure occurs within one year if it occurs at all.

There are also a very few additional unexplained failures.

*In summary, then, in cases which show no evidence of sensory-neural loss, the over-all chance of a final hearing level for speech of 30 dB or better is about 80 out of 100. The chances are even for a final level of 23 dB or better. The chance of a final level of 20 dB or better is about 28 out of 100.*

The permanence of the result of the fenestration operation is now well established. If closure occurs at all, it occurs within one year. After the first few months the thresholds for speech become stable, and they have continued stable for periods up to 15 or 20 years without significant elevation beyond the normal elevation to be expected from advancing age. Fenestration does not prevent presbycusis, but neither does hearing loss increase faster than usual.

The permanence of stapes surgery is not yet clearly and fully established. The early operation of stapes mobilization was soon modified to stapes replacement because of the high incidence of closure or fixation within the first year or two. The late results with the various substitutes described above are much more encouraging, but there is some reason to think that the chances of permanent benefit will be influenced by the choice of materials. Only about five years have elapsed since the more successful combinations were standardized. It is too early to draw final conclusions as to permanence, but there is no doubt of the high percentage of initial success and excellence of the initial hearing levels in these cases.

## SURGICAL TREATMENT OF MENIÈRE'S DISEASE

Surgery can improve a sensory-neural hearing loss of one but only one variety. If the loss is due to pressure on the auditory nerve or the cochlear artery from a tumor of the auditory nerve, removal of the tumor may restore some or all of the lost hearing. Improvement is more likely if the hearing loss came on rather rapidly and the operation is performed promptly than it will be if the tumor grew slowly. In this case the nerve cells and hair cells are likely to be injured or starved beyond hope of recovery. The operation for removal of the tumor is not undertaken to restore hearing, however. It is undertaken to protect life, because further growth may cause pressure on vital centers in the lower brain stem.

Surgery may be employed in severe cases of Menière's disease, not to cure the disease but to give the patient relief from a disabling vertigo or an intolerable tinnitus. The "Day operation" or the "Cawthorne operation" is performed something like a fenestration operation, but the surgeon deliberately enters the inner ear and destroys the membranous labyrinth. The operations differ chiefly in surgical details of the means used to inactivate or destroy the labyrinth. Still another method (Arslan) employs high-intensity ultrasound, applied locally to the labyrinth, for this purpose. Such operations are justified because the brain compensates very well for the loss of the nonauditory labyrinth, although the vertigo from irritation and spontaneous discharge of this sense organ can be completely disabling. The only question is how long to wait for a spontaneous improvement or how severe must the symptoms be before operating.

At one time an effort was made to spare the hearing when the nonauditory labyrinth was destroyed. One method was to cut the vestibular nerve but spare the cochlear nerve. It soon appeared, however, that the hearing of the affected ear was so badly impaired by the same disease process, whatever it is, that speech could not be understood usefully, and there was often a very loud and annoying tinnitus. If there is reasonably good hearing in the remaining ear, the patient usually prefers unilateral deafness to the tinnitus and diplacusis; and he may get it whether he wants it or not as a result of the operation if the utricle, saccule, and semicircular canals are really thoroughly destroyed.

The Day, the Cawthorne, and the Arslan operations represent a type of operation that is now fairly common in neurosurgery. The neurosurgery does not restore a normal state, but distressing, undesirable symptoms are relieved by deliberate, well-placed, controlled destruction of a certain bit of tissue that is acting abnormally. A loss of function is often far preferable to faulty abnormal overactivity.

## HEARING LEVELS

It is important to note that all statements in this chapter concerning hearing level refer to the *hearing level for speech* actually measured by speech audiometry, using an instrument calibrated according to the American Standard for Speech Audiometers (1952) and the CID W2 spondiac word lists described in the Appendix. The calibration tone was adjusted to 22 dB re 0.0002 dyne per cm$^2$ (SPL). The hearing levels for speech were not inferred from pure-tone hearing levels, but they are actually quite closely comparable to ISO hearing levels for pure tones, as explained in Chapter 7.

## SUGGESTED READINGS AND REFERENCES

**Bilger, R. C., A. C. Goodman, and T. E. Walsh.** "The Fenestration Operation: A Perspective in Time," *Laryngoscope,* 69:141–163 (1959).

**Davis, H., and T. E. Walsh.** "The Limits of Improvement of Hearing Following the Fenestration Operation," *Laryngoscope,* 60:273–295 (1950).

**Goodhill, V.** "Pathology, Diagnosis and Therapy of Deafness," Chap. 9, in *Handbook of Speech Pathology,* L. E. Travis (ed.). New York: Applenton-Century-Crofts, Inc., 1957.
A fairly detailed exposition of the medical and surgical aspects of deafness.

**Schuknecht, H.** (ed.). *Otosclerosis.* Boston: Little, Brown and Co., 1962.
This symposium volume surveys authoritatively and exhaustively our present knowledge of otosclerosis and its surgical treatment.

**Shambaugh, G. E., Jr.** *Surgery of the Ear.* Philadelphia: W. B. Sanders Company, 1967.
A complete and authoritative treatise.

————. "Correlation of the Predicted with the Actual Result of Fenestration in 164 Consecutive Cases," *Laryngoscope,* 62:461–474 (1952).

# PART THREE

# AUDITORY TESTS AND HEARING AIDS

# CHAPTER 7

# AUDIOMETRY:
# PURE TONE AND
# SIMPLE SPEECH TESTS

## HALLOWELL DAVIS, M.D.

*Audiometry* means the measuring of hearing. There are many tests of hearing: some old and many new, some crude and some very refined and elaborate, some intended for screening and others designed for medical diagnosis. We shall make a rapid survey of these tests and name and classify or characterize most of those that are in current use in hearing clinics. We shall, however, be content to point out the principles that are involved and the kind of information that each test yields. We shall not discuss the details of technique and precautions. This is not a "cookbook of audiometry." Neither do we go far into controversial questions of theory or the "last word" from experimental psychophysics. Other authors and the current journals provide adequate treatment of these various topics. We are writing only a guide for the beginning student or the interested worker in a related field.

## OBJECTIVES OF AUDIOMETRY

There have always been two quite different reasons for measuring hearing. It is well to recognize these immediately because the choice of what aspect of hearing to test, the instruments and test materials or signals to be employed, and the whole conduct of the test depend on the objectives that are sought. A test or an instrument that is good for one purpose may be quite useless for another. Failure to understand the differences in objectives has led to considerable confusion and misunderstanding in the past.

One clear purpose of audiometry is to *assist in medical diagnosis*. The question to be answered is, *"What is wrong with the auditory system and where?"* The early simple tests, notably those that employed tuning forks, were clearly oriented to this purpose, and the first American standard for electric audiometers was specifically entitled "Audiometers for General Diagnostic Purposes."

Another purpose is *over-all assessment of hearing* to determine the fitness of the individual for certain tasks or duties, his need for special education or other assistance, his claim for compensation or in-

179

surance, and so on. The need for a hearing aid and the assessment of the benefit provided by a hearing aid fall in this general category. The central question usually is, *"How well can this person hear and understand everyday speech?"*

A third purpose is to identify quickly in a large population those with an impairment of hearing sufficient to require special attention. The final objective may be to cure or check the progress of the impairment or to provide special assistance to override it. This type of audiometry is called *screening audiometry*. The question is *"Who is in trouble but may not know it?"*

The fourth purpose is to detect any changes in hearing that may occur as a result of some recognized hazard to hearing. The typical hazard is habitual exposure to loud noise, usually in a military or industrial situation. This is called *monitoring audiometry*. Hearing is tested regularly, just as weight and blood pressure may be monitored by annual physical examinations. A record of the status of hearing, year by year, is kept. The question is, *"Has anyone's hearing changed enough so that his hazardous exposure should be reduced?"*

We shall consider below how audiometers, particularly electric audiometers, have been developed and tests with them specialized for each of these purposes. In general, diagnostic audiometry requires the greatest range of frequencies and the greatest dynamic range without sacrifice of accuracy. The assessment of hearing puts much more emphasis on speech audiometry, and screening and monitoring audiometry deal with large numbers of people; speed and simplicity of test are important.

### Organization of Chapters 7, 8, and 9

The following description of tests of hearing and their interpretation is divided broadly according to the main purposes of the tests as outlined above, but in part the organization is determined by the nature of the tests and the instruments employed.

In the present chapter, after a brief historical survey of simple tests of hearing, we give special attention to the electric audiometer as defined in the proposed United States of America Standard for Audiometers. We explain in some detail the standardization of audiometers and the audiogram, that is, pure-tone threshold audiometry as used for general diagnostic purposes. We include here the use of pure-tone threshold audiometry for monitoring and screening purposes. In the second part of the chapter we describe speech audiometry and the determination of the speech-reception threshold and discrimination scores. The discussion is organized around the standardized instrument and familiar materials.

In Chapter 8 we describe tests of hearing other than the determination of thresholds of hearing and simple articulation curves. The use of audiometry to assist in the selection of a hearing aid is included here. We consider many (but not all) of the audiometric tests that have been proposed for diagnostic purposes, particularly those oriented toward sensory-neural and central impairment. Here we also describe certain physiological tests of the ear, notably evoked-response audiometry and the measurement of acoustic impedance.

Chapter 9 is oriented to the problem of auditory handicap and to military and other standards of hearing. Special attention is given to the relation between audiometric measurements and workmen's compensation, and to the bearing on this general problem of the change from the ASA-1951 reference levels to the ISO values. The question of "normal hearing" in medicolegal context is also considered.

### NONELECTRICAL TESTS OF HEARING

In Chapter 2, "Acoustics and Psychoacoustics," it was pointed out that there are several different aspects of hearing. We may be interested in testing any or all of them, and different types of test are appropriate for each one. First and most obvious is *sensitivity*. How weak a sound can be heard? Then there is the *recognition of pitch*. Do pure tones sound pure and musical, and is the ear "in tune," so to speak? There is also auditory *discrimination*. How small a difference in pitch or in loudness can a person detect? Can he recognize difficult words? Can he pick out speech from a background of noise or of many voices as well as he should? And finally there is *tolerance*. At what intensity does a sound become uncomfortable or painful?

Originally the interest in audiometry lay almost entirely in sensitivity. From the medical point of view the object was to determine whether the fault lay in the sound-conducting mechanism of the middle ear or in the neural mechanism of the inner ear. More recently, however, the importance of tolerance, of correct recognition of pitch, and of auditory discrimination has been recognized, and tests for these other aspects of hearing have been developed. The otologist now wants to distinguish impairments of the sense organ from those of the auditory nerve or brain stem, and both such conditions from what we now call central dysacusis.

## Crude Tests of Sensitivity

To bring the study of hearing out of the realm of guesswork and to guide the medical treatment of its problems, we need tests and, above all, *measurements* of hearing. When someone is totally deaf in both ears, there is usually no doubt about it. However, to devise a simple and reliable test to determine whether a man's hearing is good enough for him to enter military service or bad enough to entitle him to compensation for injury is a very different matter. It is not easy or simple to measure the sensitivity of hearing accurately, partly because it requires complicated apparatus

to deliver sounds of known intensity to the ear and partly because physical sound has two major dimensions—frequency and intensity—and the loss of hearing for some frequencies may be much greater than for others. The difficulties are overcome by the electric audiometer; but the instrument is expensive, and the quiet surroundings required for accurate measurements of hearing may be expensive and difficult to provide. For rapid and approximate testing, therefore, the crude but time-honored methods—the *conversational voice,* the *whisper,* the *coin click,* and the *watch tick* —will still be used.

These four simple tests solve in different ways the problem of which frequencies to test. The voice and the whisper represent two kinds of sound that are most important for a man to hear, and if he can hear (and understand) the human voice, we do not much care whether or not he can hear the cricket's chirp. The frequencies most important for good understanding of speech extend from about 400 to 3000 Hz, and the voice test therefore gives some idea of the usefulness of hearing over this range. The watch tick and the click of coins, on the other hand, are high-frequency sounds, mostly above the range that is really needed to understand speech. They are useful because loss of hearing often begins with a loss of sensitivity for high frequencies, and the defect can be detected much earlier by the coin or the watch than by the voice or the whisper. In a very general way the hearing for speech is impaired most by conductive hearing losses, which affect all frequencies. Sensory-neural loss is most often a high-tone hearing loss, most severe above 2000 Hz. The spoken voice and the watch tick or coin click supplement one another in just this way, and *to the extent that they can be standardized* they are useful tools for rough-and-ready testing.

Two major difficulties with all simple tests, in addition to the necessity of providing a quiet room for testing with walls that do not reflect the test sounds, are standardizing the sounds and measuring their intensity. We have to assume that one man's voice is as easy to understand as another's, that watch ticks are alike, and that any two coins struck together in various ways will give off the same sound. Of course, many efforts to standardize these tests have been made. For example, certain key words, usually numbers such as "66" and "99," are regularly used in the voice test. Those who do much testing of this sort try to speak always with the same loudness and distinctness, and they do produce reasonably reproducible signals, but it is more difficult to match one voice with another.

The whisper test has the advantage over the conversational voice in that it is relatively easy to standardize the loudness of a whisper by whispering only at the end of an expiration. Incidentally, the whisper represents at fairly even intensity the range of frequencies needed for good understanding of speech. In an ordinary conversational voice the low frequencies are much more powerful than most of the high frequencies.

The intensity with which the sound of the voice, watch, or coin reaches the ear is varied by the tester coming closer and closer to the subject. This is theoretically a reasonable method because the intensity of sound varies inversely as the square of the distance it travels. (Twice as far away, one-fourth the intensity at the ear; three times as far, one-ninth; and so on.) In practice this rule almost always breaks down badly because of echoes from the walls of the room. Only in special sound-absorbent rooms does the rule mean much for distances of more than 6 ft or so.

When we test the sensitivity of the ear, we do not merely want to know that someone can hear our voice at 20 feet and our watch at 5, or that he can detect a tone of 1000 Hz at one ten-thousandth of a dyne per square centimeter. We want to know how the sensitivity of his ear compares with that of his fellow men. We

therefore establish the performance of a number of "otologically normal" men and women and express the performance of the man with poor hearing as a ratio with respect to the average expectation. "Otologically normal" means free of any obvious otological defect or impairment such as wax in the canal, a perforated drum membrane, or a history of earaches, discharge from the ear, or obvious difficulty in hearing. On the average, an "otologically normal" person just understands the standard whispered voice at 20 feet. If we must come closer to a man with poor hearing, say within 5 feet, before he can understand our whisper, we say that his hearing is 5/20 ("five over twenty" or simply "five-twenty"). Many standards of performance or hearing requirements, discussed in Chapter 9, are expressed in such ratios. The analogy to the Snellen chart test for visual acuity is obvious.

*Early tests of frequency range.* Among the first instruments employed for quantitative measurements of hearing were musical instruments (a small organ), the Galton whistle, and the Struycken monochord. The Galton whistle emits very high frequencies, like present-day ultrasonic dog-whistles, but the frequency is adjustable by a calibrated micrometer screw. The monochord is a taut metal wire activated by a bow like a violin or struck by a hammer like a piano. The intensity of neither instrument is closely controlled, but the threshold of hearing rises so sharply at the upper frequency limit that intensity is not very critical (see Figures 2-4 and 2-5).

The determination of the lower frequency limit of hearing was never satisfactory, but the broad distinction between high-frequency loss, as in presbycusis, and flat or low-frequency loss, as in otosclerosis, could be made. The whistle and the monochord are no longer used to any great extent.

*Tuning forks.* The most satisfactory and versatile simple instrument for testing hearing, which is still a very important part of an otologist's equipment, is a set of tuning forks. The octave frequencies of 64, 128, 256, 512 . . . Hz became established early as the standard frequencies. The forks emit a quite pure tone, and their damping is small so that the intensity decays slowly but regularly. With practice the fork can be activitated by striking it a standard blow. One quantitative measure is then the length of time that the patient can hear the tone when the vibrating tine is held close to his ear canal. More often, however, the otologist uses his own ear as a standard of reference. When the patient ceases to hear the tone, he quickly brings the fork to his own ear and hears for himself the loudness of a tone just below the patient's threshold. In this way a quick survey of the patient's sensitivity of hearing, octave by octave, can be obtained—at least by an otologist who himself has at least average hearing.

Tuning forks are particularly useful to the otologist because with them he can test hearing by bone conduction as well as by air conduction. If the rounded tip of the hilt (handle) of a vibrating tuning fork is pressed gently against a person's skull, either at the mastoid process, the forehead, the top of the head, or on a tooth, its sound is heard by bone conduction at pretty much the same loudness, for the average listener, as by air conduction. The following common diagnostic tests are based on this property.

The *Schwabach test* is a test of bone conduction. Instead of holding the vibrating fork close beside the entrance to the ear canal, the otologist places the tip of its hilt gently but firmly against the mastoid process of the skull behind and below the patient's ear. He then notes by how many seconds the hearing of the fork is shortened or prolonged relative to a normal ear, usually his own, in the same environment. "Schwabach-shortened" or "bone-conduction–decreased" means that the patient's

bone conduction is not as good as the average. This will be the situation if the patient has a sensory-neural hearing loss. If bone conduction is "lengthened" or "increased," a conductive hearing loss is suggested. The patient's hearing by bone conduction may actually be better than the examiner's because a conductive loss protects the bone-conducted tone against masking by air-conducted background noise, and it also prevents the radiation of acoustic energy out from the ear canal after it has reached the inner ear by bone conduction.

The *Rinne test* compares the patient's hearing by bone conduction with the patient's own hearing by air conduction. Like the Schwabach test, it is really a test of how much the ambient noise masks air-conducted as opposed to bone-conducted sound. The hilt of the tuning fork is applied to the mastoid as in the Schwabach test, but when the patient no longer hears the sound the fork is held close to the patient's ear instead of near the otologist's ear. If the patient again hears the tone he is said to have a "positive Rinne." It is normal to hear about twice as long by air- as by bone-conduction with the usual initial standard blow. If the patient does not hear the tone again by air, it is a "negative Rinne." The presumption in this case is a middle-ear conductive hearing loss in that ear.

The *Weber test* compares the hearing by bone conduction in the patient's two ears. This test also depends largely on differences in masking by the ambient room noise. The hilt of the vibrating fork is applied to the center of the patient's forehead and he is asked *where* he hears the tone. If both ears are normal, they will be equally stimulated and equally masked, and the sound will be heard as if it is in the center of the head. If there is conductive loss on one side, the sound is heard better by that ear (by bone conduction, of course). Thus the sound is heard in the abnormal ear, which is less masked. The Weber is said to be "lateralized" to the right or the left, as the case may be. If, however, one ear is normal and the other has a *neural* loss, the Weber is lateralized to the normal side. If the two ears are both abnormal but symmetrically so, the Weber will not be consistently lateralized to either side.

Still another tuning fork test, directed to detecting middle-ear conductive impairment, is the *Bing* or occlusion test. It depends on the increase in the loudness of bone-conducted sounds that occurs in the normal ear when the external auditory meatus is occluded. It will be recalled that one of the several pathways and mechanisms of bone conduction is a compression of the middle ear, with consequent movement of the tympanic membrane and ossicles, including the footplate of the stapes. This compression becomes much more effective when the meatus is closed. (Actually the placement of an air-conduction earphone with a flat cushion over the ear produces a significant occlusion effect.) Sounds below 2000 Hz are particularly enhanced. The effect does *not* depend simply on the exclusion of ambient masking noise from the occluded ear, although this may sometimes contribute to the effect.

The tuning fork, usually 512 Hz, is applied to the mastoid as usual. While the sound is still comfortably loud, the otologist applies the palm of his hand over the auricle, or presses the tragus enough to close the meatus, or inserts the tip of his finger or perhaps an ear plug into the meatus. The patient simply reports whether the sound remains the same (Bing-negative) or becomes louder (Bing-positive). (One precaution is to avoid trapping air under the finger or ear plug and thereby increasing the air pressure in the meatus and reducing the mobility of the tympanic membrane.)

In Europe many otologists routinely determine bone-conduction thresholds (with the electric audiometer) with the meatus open ("relative" bone-conduction threshold) and also with it occluded ("absolute" bone-conduction threshold). The comparison of absolute with relative bone-conduction thresholds is the equivalent of the Bing test.

Another old (1881) tuning-fork test is the *Gellé test*. This test is intended to detect fixation of the stapes, and depends on changing the air pressure in the external auditory meatus by means of an accessory nozzle, a tube, and a bulb. The sound from the hilt of the tuning fork is delivered through the nozzle or by bone conduction. Changes in pressure diminish the hearing, more for air conduction than for bone conduction and more for negative than for positive pressure in the meatus. Such changes constitute a "positive" result. If the stapes is fixed, there is no change in threshold with change in pressure: the test is "negative." With obstruction of the Eustachian tube, negative meatal pressure may *improve* hearing, particularly by air conduction. There is some disagreement whether hearing for low tones is more affected by changes of pressure than medium tones, and it is troublesome to standardize the equipment and procedure precisely, but when properly performed the test is valid and useful.

Many other tuning-fork tests have been suggested, but most of them are variations on these same themes. All of them, including those described, have their pitfalls and difficulties, but their value for initial orientation and for final confirmation, combined with their speed and simplicity, should not be overlooked by the electronically oriented audiologist. It should be noted also that all of these tuning-fork tests can be carried out with an electric audiometer. The advantage of the tuning fork lies in its speed and simplicity.

## THE ELECTRIC AUDIOMETER

### Definitions

There are several types and classes of electric audiometer. The following definitions are inspired by the latest draft of the proposed United States of America Standard for Audiometers which at present (1968) has been under discussion for several years in the United States of America Standards Institute (formerly the American Standards Association).[1] Our phrasing is different, but the substance is nearly the same.

Audiometric measurements can be made with pure tones or with spoken words or sentences. We therefore recognize two major classes of audiometer, namely the *pure-tone audiometer* and the *speech audiometer*. A single instrument may be designed to serve as both types.

Another distinction is *manual* versus *automatic*. This refers to the way in which the test tones or spoken material are selected and the results recorded.

*Pure-tone audiometers.* A pure-tone audiometer provides, as test material, pure tones of selected frequencies and of calibrated sound-pressure levels.

**Wide-range Audiometers** cover most of the human auditory range, both in frequency and in sound pressure level. They must have either one or preferably two air-conduction receivers, a bone-conduction vibrator, an on-off switch, and means for masking the opposite ear during tests by either air conduction or bone conduction.

**Limited-range Audiometers** have more restricted ranges of frequency or sound-pressure level, or both, but they must provide, at least, tones of 500, 1000, 2000, 3000, 4000, and 6000 Hz with a range of sound-pressure levels from 10 to 70 dB relative to the standard reference level. Facilities for bone-conduction tests and for masking are not required.

**Narrow-range Audiometers** are pure-tone audiometers with still more limited ranges of frequency and available sound-pressure levels. The frequencies and the

[1] This draft has now been approved and issued as USASI Specification S3.6–1969.

levels are usually those appropriate for particular screening tests.

*Speech audiometers.* A speech audiometer provides spoken syllables, words, or sentences at known sound-pressure levels. It comprises an acoustoelectric source, an amplifier, an adjustable calibrated attenuator, and one or preferably two earphones. The source may be a "live" voice with microphone or may be a disc, or magnetic or other record with an appropriate pickup. Means for masking the opposite ear are required.

**Limited-range Speech Audiometers** have restricted ranges of output sound-pressure level, and means for providing masking or background noise need not be provided. The ranges chosen are usually those appropriate for screening tests.

*Group audiometers.* Group audiometers present either pure tones or spoken material to a group of persons simultaneously. Means are provided for each individual to give reliable information as to which test tones are heard or which words or sentences are heard correctly.

*Threshold levels and sound-pressure levels.* The *hearing-threshold level* of an ear is the number of decibels by which its threshold of audibility exceeds a standard audiometric reference level.

The sound-pressure level of an audiometer is understood to refer to the sound-pressure level developed by the audiometer in a National Bureau of Standards 9-A coupler. Other couplers may be used only if suitable comparison data are available.

### Common Features of Pure-tone Audiometer

In a pure-tone audiometer an alternating current of the desired frequency is generated by an electronic oscillator circuit. Nearly all models now provide a series of fixed frequencies in octaves based on 1000

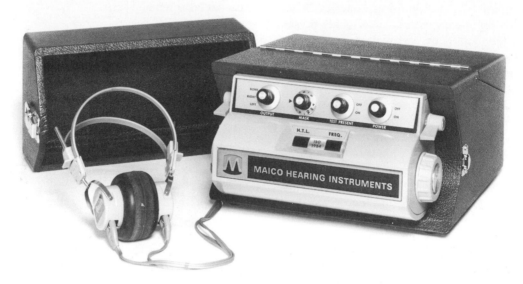

Fig. 7-1. A wide-range electric audiometer intended for general diagnostic purposes has air-conduction receivers, as shown in the figure, and also a bone-conduction vibrator (not shown). In the model shown the frequency is selected by turning the large knob at the right, the intensity (hearing level) by the large knob at the left. The interrupter controls are just above these knobs. Masking noise is provided. (*Maico Electronics, Inc.*)

Hz with some intermediate steps above 1000 Hz. The number and choice of frequencies depend on the particular use for which the instrument is designed. This is one basis of the definitions above. Formerly, instruments with continuous adjustment of frequency, such as the Peters, the Sonotone, and the Western Electric model 6B, were also popular, but the use of fixed frequencies has now become standard practice except for the patient-controlled recording type, described below.

The intensity of the sound output is regulated by means of a dial graduated, according to the U.S.A. Standard for Audiometers, in 5-dB steps. The electric current produces sound in a receiver or in an earphone that is held by a spring headband snugly against the subject's ear. Usually two receivers, carefully matched to one another, are provided, with a switch on the instrument so that the sound can be delivered to either ear at the choice of the operator. Sometimes one of the earphones

is a dummy, provided simply to exclude distracting sounds from the ear not under test. The receiver is provided with a rather firm sponge-rubber cushion that makes a good, but comfortable, acoustic seal against the side of the subject's head. The wide-range audiometer provides a range of intensities of as much as 110 or even 120 dB at some frequencies. An additional 10 dB of intensity is provided in some special instruments in use in schools for the deaf, but it is questionable whether the sense of hearing or the sense of feeling is being tested at these very high intensities. A remnant of hearing at such a high level is not very useful even with modern hearing aids. For ordinary testing the range of 110 or 120 dB is quite sufficient. Additional steps toward either very high or very low levels introduce considerable engineering difficulties.

The reference zero levels constitute a point of special interest and importance and will be discussed in some detail below.

The test tone is turned on and off by the operator. A special switching circuit is provided to cause the current to fade in and out gradually enough to avoid any audible click that might be produced by a sudden start or stop. On the other hand, the rise time is not more than one-tenth (formerly one-half) of a second so that it is quite practical for the operator to use very brief pulses of tone as test signals if he wishes. In the earliest models the test tone faded in and out very gradually and was normally on unless the operator interrupted it by means of the switch. Most modern audiometers can be operated with the tone either normally on or off. The thresholds obtained with the earlier models are practically identical with those obtained with more rapid interruptions or pulses, but the subject can usually make up his mind more rapidly and with less effort with the briefer signals. The net result of using rather brief pulses is a saving of time and fatigue on the over-all test.

Sometimes a signal circuit is provided whereby the subject holds down a pushbutton as long as he hears the tone and releases it when he ceases to hear. Most audiometrists, however, now prefer to have the subject raise his finger when he hears the tone rather than press a button. The speed and promptness with which the finger is raised give an observant operator much additional information as to the certainty with which the subject feels he hears the tone.

The heart of the audiometer, from the engineer's point of view, is not the generator that determines frequency or the "attenuator" that varies the intensity, since these are now routine in the electronic art; it is the receiver, which converts the electrical into acoustical energy. It is not easy to design and construct an earphone that is reasonably efficient for all of the frequencies we wish to test and that will maintain its original efficiency year after year. And the operator is at the mercy of the earphone. If the earphone is put out of adjustment by accidentally falling on the floor,

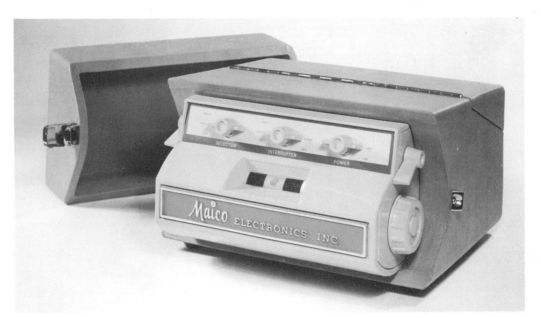

Fig. 7-2. A limited-range audiometer, suitable for monitoring or screening, does not have a bone-conduction vibrator or provide masking noise. Its range of intensities may be restricted and often the frequency range also. (*Maico Electronics, Inc.*)

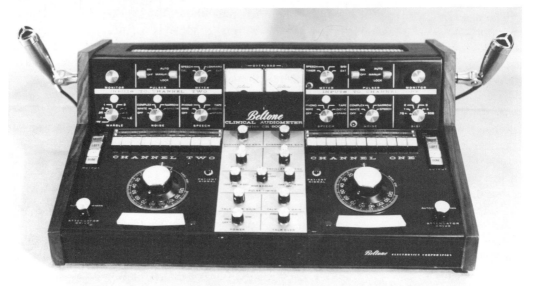

Fig. 7-3a. For certain tests, such as loudness balance, an audiometer requires two channels. In the model illustrated here each channel contains a microphone and a VU meter with which to monitor speech. Various other features may include automatic pulsing of the test tone and a "warble" (frequency modulation) of adjustable degree. (*Beltone Hearing Aid Company*)

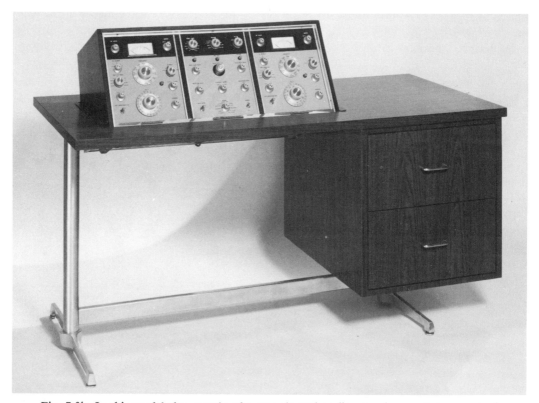

Fig. 7-3b. In this model the console of a two-channel audiometer is mounted as part of a desk-like unit.

its loss of efficiency in generating the sound will be interpreted as a lack of efficiency of the ear in detecting the sound. The scale on the instrument does not actually measure the sound but only the electric current that generates it. The careful operator therefore periodically tests his own ear, and if the instrument says that his ear is losing its sensitivity, he tests other presumably normal ears. If most of them show the loss of sensitivity, it is fairly certain that the "calibration" of the audiometer is no longer correct.

An important item for an audiometer intended for diagnostic purposes is a *bone-conduction vibrator* that delivers vibrations to the mastoid process of the temporal bone instead of generating sound waves in an earphone. The same electrical circuits are employed with no change except in the scale on which the hearing level is read. Still another accessory is a "masking circuit" that generates a masking noise to be delivered to the ear opposite to the one being tested. This may be necessary if the ear being tested is quite hard of hearing and the opposite ear hears well by bone conduction, and it is always required in tests of bone conduction. In older audiometers the masking sound was usually a buzz, produced by a sawtooth electrical signal. The types of masking sound recommended in the proposed USASI standard are either a narrow band of noise near the frequency of the test tone or a wide band of noise covering at least the range from 250 to 4000 Hz.

The more elaborate electric audiometers intended for diagnostic purposes may have still other features that allow the operator to perform tests such as loudness balancing or measurement of the difference limen for loudness in addition to determining hearing levels by air conduction and bone conduction (see Figure 7-3).

The specification of zero reference threshold levels presents special difficulties and will be considered further below.

## Standards for Audiometers

When electric audiometers were first introduced each company designed its own model with features that seemed best according to the judgment of its engineers and consultants. This situation led to some confusion and uncertainty, particularly with respect to just what values were taken as the reference levels on the intensity scale. There was also some concern that the purchasers of audiometers should have assurance of the accuracy of the frequency scale, stability of output with varying line voltages, and so on. To remedy this situation the Council on Physical Medicine of the American Medical Association, acting through its Consultants on Audiometers and Hearing Aids, set forth in 1945 certain minimal requirements and also certain additional recommendations for both audiometers and hearing aids, and for many years it maintained a program of so-called "acceptance" of instruments that met these requirements. Audiometers were accepted only after a sample of the model in question had been examined by an independent anonymous laboratory and certified as having met the published requirements. The AMA requirements were incorporated in a standard of the American Standards Association in 1951, but they were revised more frequently than the American Standards. By their recommendations the Consultants on Audiometers and Hearing Aids gave semiofficial guidance to the manufacturers concerning the needs and desires of medically oriented users of their instruments.

The program of acceptance of audiometers and hearing aids by the Council on Physical Medicine is no longer in force, but the Committee on Conservation of Hearing of the American Academy of Ophthalmology and Otolaryngology has established a Subcommittee on Audiometers. This committee announced in 1958 that it would "list" models of audiometers that were found, by tests made in independent but well-qualified laboratories, to meet the American Standards for Audiometers. This listing does not, of course, assure the purchaser that *every instrument* of that model necessarily meets all of the specifications quantitatively, but it assures him that the company in question has been able to produce such an instrument. The company at least has the necessary technical "know-how." This, after all, was the essence of acceptance by the Council on Physical Medicine. The listing by the Committee on Conservation of Hearing amounts substantially to a stamp of technical approval of the manufacturer. It gives useful backing to the voluntary cooperative effort represented by the USA Standards Institute.

The American Standards Association, renamed in 1966 the United States of America Standards Institute (USASI), is a voluntary association of manufacturers and consumers which has written standards for many branches of American industry. These standards are a convenience for all concerned and are regularly made the basis of specifications or procurement both by government and by industry. In the field of acoustics, for example, there is not only an American Standard Terminology, now known as the USA Standard Acoustical Terminology, but standard specifications for such items as the sound-level meter, octave-band filters, microphones, meters, and methods of sound measurement. The USA Standards are revised from time to time to keep pace with technical progress and the state of the art, and at the present writing (1968) the standards for all audiometers have been reviewed and will presumably soon be reissued in the form of a single new USA Standard for Audiometers.[2]

The National Bureau of Standards also cooperated in the development of the American Standards for Audiometers, and it preserves the instruments on which the

definition of the zero levels for audiometry rest. It serves as the final arbiter in any questions that may arise concerning the accuracy of calibration of new instruments in this country.

In addition to the various national standards organizations, like the USA Standards Institute and the British Standards Institution, there is an International Organization for Standardization (Organization Internationale de Normalisation). The name of this organization is abbreviated "ISO." It is composed of ISO "member bodies" in the various countries, and it develops and issues ISO recommendations for standards in various fields, including acoustics. Actually there is also another very similar affiliated organization, the International Electrotechnical Commission (Commission Électrotechnique Internationale), abbreviated IEC, which develops and issues recommendations for electrical instruments and equipment. Due to this division of interests at the international level one organization, ISO, deals with the reference zero levels for audiometers, because they are related to the sensitivity of human hearing, and its affiliate, IEC, deals with the audiometer as an electroacoustic instrument. The collaboration between ISO and IEC is so close that we may think of them as virtually a single organization.

Neither ISO nor IEC has any authority to enforce its recommendations. Like the United States of America Standards Institute, they are voluntary associations. They issue recommendations on the basis of a consensus which must represent close if not complete unanimity among the national member bodies, but for each country the only valid standard is the national standard of that country. In general, however, the ISO and IEC recommendations serve as models and are usually incorporated almost completely into the corresponding national standards. In some countries the member bodies are government

---

[2] Approved USASI Specification S3.6–1969.

bureaus, and their national standards have the force of government regulations. This is not the case in the United States.

The proposed USASI Standard for Audiometers mentioned in the previous section will replace three previous American Standards Association specifications: Audiometers for General Diagnostic Purposes (Z24.5–1951), Pure-Tone Audiometers for Screening Purposes (Z24.12–1952), and Speech Audiometers (Z24.13–1953). In these standards, both old and proposed, are many specifications concerning the accuracy of tone frequencies, the purity of the test tones, the accuracy of sound-pressure levels, the operation and the rise and fall times of the tone switch, the calibration of new varieties of earphone or bone-conduction vibrator, the headband, the ear cushions, unwanted sound, stability with respect to variations in temperature or in line voltage, shock hazard, and other items. Concerning all of these items agreement has been reached in the Committee on Bioacoustics of the USA Standards Institute. The issue of this standard has been delayed for several years, however, by failure of the Committee to arrive at the necessary "substantial consensus" concerning the standard reference threshold levels. To understand the situation some historical perspective is helpful.

### The Reference Zero Level for Audiometers: The Audiogram

When the famous Western Electric Co. 2A audiometer was designed in the Bell Telephone Laboratories in the early 1920s a basic decision was made concerning the reference zero level. An obvious choice from the engineering point of view would have been the dyne per square centimeter, the same for all frequencies. Then the sensitivity curve for hearing would have been plotted like the threshold curves in Figures 2-3, 2-4, and 2-5. This form of plotting facilitates comparison of human

hearing with other sounds, as in Figure 2-3, or specifically with the average intensity of speech, as in Figure 7-4. However the otological consultant to the project, Dr. Edmund P. Fowler, saw the new instrument as a *diagnostic tool* for the otologist, and wished to emphasize the *deviation from normal* of each subject. He believed, probably quite correctly, that this form of presentation of the results would promote the acceptance and general use of the electric audiometer by otologists. Dr. Fowler's counsel prevailed, and the intensity dial of the audiometer was labeled "hearing loss," meaning "decibels less sensitive than normal." The format of the audiogram (Figure 7-5) was devised with the reference zero level represented by a straight horizontal line near the top of the sheet and hearing loss (poorer hearing) plotted downward.

The next step was to determine experimentally for each frequency the voltage to be applied to the earphones that would produce a sound at the threshold of normal hearing. The particular earphone employed was the WE 705A, which was specially designed for stability of performance. Dr. Fowler selected a group of 85 young adults who worked in the offices or laboratories of the Bell Telephone Laboratories, people whom he found to have no signs or symptoms of disease of the ear. Such persons we now call "otologically normal subjects" (defined in the ISO Recommendation R389 as "a person in a normal state of health who is free from all signs or symptoms of ear disease and from wax in the ear canal, and has no history of undue exposure to noise"). The engineers at the Bell Telephone Laboratories then measured the thresholds of the 85 subjects with the laboratory model of the new audiometer. The actual readings were the voltages that had to be applied to produce a barely audible tone at each frequency. Each instrument was adjusted or "calibrated" so that when the intensity dial (later labeled "hearing

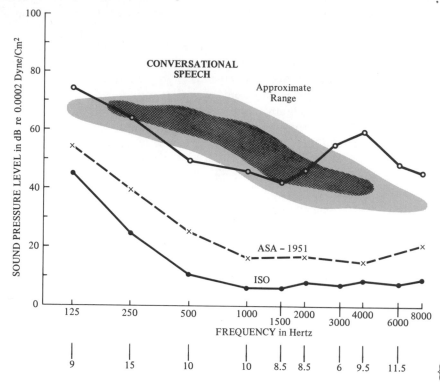

Fig. 7-4. The two lower curves show the ISO recommended reference zero levels (solid line and dots) and the ASA-1951 levels (dashed line and crosses). The numerical differences in decibels are given beneath the frequency scale. These *differences* are the same regardless of the type of earphone or coupler employed. The actual sound pressures plotted are for the WE 705-A earphone and NBS 9A coupler, and are the same as the data points shown by crosses (+) in Figure 2-5.

The upper curve (solid with open circles) is the hypothetical threshold curve of a man with impaired hearing, discussed in the text. The shaded area (slanting lines and stipple) shows the approximate range of the intensities and frequencies of the sounds of conversational speech at 1 meter. It is not strictly accurate to plot such *field* measurements of acoustic pressure on a graph of *coupler* pressures, for reasons explained in Chapter 2, but the orders of magnitude are correct nevertheless, and the comparison is valid for something as poorly defined as the area of conversational speech. The intensities measured from moment to moment would fall most often in the darkly shaded area, less frequently in the stippled area, and only rarely either above or below the stippled area.

loss") was set at zero decibels, the appropriate voltage was delivered to the earphone.

In the actual manufacture of audiometers, production control of earphones is maintained by measuring the acoustic pressure produced by each earphone in a small cavity known as a coupler or "artificial ear." The cavity is about the same size, 6 cu cm, as the human external canal and middle ear plus the space under the dia-

phragm of an earphone, but the walls are metal and the shape is simple. The pressures produced in this "coupler" are not quite the same as the pressures produced in the ear by the same earphone. The coupler pressures are, however, *reproducible* and serve to show that one earphone of a particular model is like another. A coupler was standardized by the National Bureau of Standards, and the present USA Standard for the zero hearing level is "stored" in the form of sets of acoustic pressures produced by certain models of earphone in an "NBS-9A coupler."

The actual set of threshold pressures, measured in the NBS-9A coupler, have turned out to be very close to later laboratory studies at the Bell Telephone Laboratories and elsewhere and also to the values finally recommended in 1964 by the International Organization for Standardization. The latter values are plotted as the lower curve in Figure 7-4. The pressures

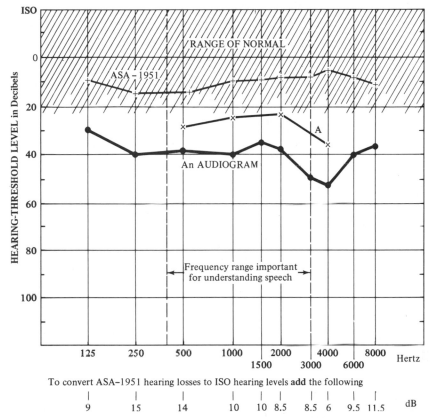

To convert ASA–1951 hearing losses to ISO hearing levels **add** the following

| | | | | | | | | | |
|---|---|---|---|---|---|---|---|---|---|
| 9 | 15 | 14 | 10 | 10 | 8.5 | 8.5 | 6 | 9.5 | 11.5 |

Fig. 7-5. On this ISO audiogram blank are shown (1) the reference zero level (horizontal at 0 dB), (2) the "range of normal," extending from the faintest tone provided by an audiometer to a transition zone between 15 and 22 dB hearing level, (3) the ASA-1951 reference zero level for pure-tone audiometers, (4) the U.S. Army "profile A," from AR 40–501 (see Chapter 9), (5) a hypothetical "flat" audiogram with a slight "4000 Hz notch," and (6) the range of frequencies important for understanding speech. The audiogram points do not fall exactly on the horizontal guide lines because the thresholds are supposed to have been measured on an audiometer calibrated to the ASA-1951 standard. The "hearing losses" were converted to ISO hearing threshold levels by adding, at each frequency, the number of decibels given below the frequency scale. For a discussion of the range of normal see Chapter 9. For otologically normal young adults the 95th percentile lies at about 12 dB HL (see Figure 2-5), but for older people it is lower, particularly at high frequencies.

In this figure the hearing threshold curve of 7-4 is plotted in the conventional format of the audiogram. The ISO reference levels are now the horizontal zero line. The position of the ASA-1951 zeros relative to ISO are also plotted.

The range of normal hearing is not precisely defined (see Chapter 9) but extends to 15 dB (ISO) and shades off gradually over the next 10 dB or thereabouts. This form of shading on an audiogram chart is a useful reminder.

differ slightly from one another for different frequencies from 500 Hz upward, and are significantly greater at 250 and 125 Hz than for higher frequencies.

In Figure 7-4 the upper solid curve shows an abnormal threshold curve such as might be obtained from a patient with a moderate conductive hearing loss. The approximate range of frequency and intensity of the sounds of conversational speech are also shown on the same diagram, and it is evident that he will not hear the higher speech frequencies, which are relatively weak, although the lower speech sounds lie mostly above his threshold. As pointed out in Chapter 2, this comparison of sound in an open acoustic field with sound pressures measured in a coupler is not exact, but as explained in Chapter 2 the error is only a very few decibels, and the diagram illustrates a principle.

In Figure 7-5 the same threshold curve is plotted as an audiogram. The horizontal zero line represents the ISO curve of Figure 7-4. The hearing-threshold levels are the differences between the ISO points and the actual threshold levels, plotted with increasing hearing-threshold levels (poorer hearing) downward. (These values are read directly from the dial of the audiometer.) In this diagram the emphasis is on the difference in sensitivity of the patient from "otologically normal subjects" of the 18- to 30-year group, and not on how well the patient hears ordinary speech.

In this way the reference zero hearing levels of the audiometer came to be associated with "normal hearing." We will consider in Chapter 9 the unfortunate and unforeseen difficulties that have arisen because of the various interpretations and connotations of the word "normal." Suffice it to say here that the word normal should be used only to refer to the subjects, not the hearing-threshold levels. We should say that *the reference zero hearing levels of the audiometer are the average (or mean or median) of the thresholds of otologically*

*normal persons between 18 and 30 years of age.*

In the 1930s each manufacturer determined experimentally his own set of reference zero levels, just as the Bell Telephone Laboratories had done for the Western Electric Co., and inevitably differences appeared among them. When the Council on Physical Therapy of the AMA prepared its first set of Minimal Requirements for Audiometers it adopted for the reference zero levels the values that had been determined in a field health survey that had been conducted by the United States Public Health Service in 1935–1936. The audiometric equipment, including the soundproof booths, was excellent. The survey was planned to obtain a cross section of the population of the United States, both rural and urban. Questionnaires and physical examinations made it possible to select from the data the threshold values for otologically normal subjects between 18 and 30 years of age. The modal values for each frequency were chosen, and later (1951) became the American Standard reference levels. These values, as coupler pressures, are plotted in Figure 7-4.

Those responsible for this choice were aware, of course, that the new reference levels were higher than the original Western Electric 2A values, but the difference was ascribed to the more representative selection of subjects in the USPHS survey, and they were accepted without question by otologists in the United States. The values seemed "realistic" in clinical practice.

Soon after World War II, however, when electric audiometers began to be used extensively in Europe and when various countries considered establishing national standards for audiometers, widespread dissatisfaction with the American Standard reference values appeared. The studies in England of the threshold of hearing, mentioned in Chapter 2, were carried out, and a British Standard, B.S. 2497 (1954), quite different from the American Standard, was based on it. Also independent studies were made in France, Germany, U.S.S.R., and by several investigators in the United States of America.

The problem of the "normal" threshold of hearing was taken up by the ISO in 1955, and a recommendation (R389) entitled "Standard Reference Zero for the Calibration of Pure-Tone Audiometers was issued in 1964. The values were based on 15 published studies (nearly half of them carried out in the U.S.A.) that seemed comparable in technique, precautions, and the selection of subjects. It is important to note that the subjects were not specially trained or experienced listeners, and the only "selection" was to reject those who were not "otologically normal."

The results of these 15 studies were in very good agreement. It was necessary to determine experimentally the relations between the coupler pressures produced by the different earphones in the different couplers used in France, Germany, the United Kingdom, the United States, and the U.S.S.R. In the ISO recommendation, values are given for five different combinations, but each one represents the same loudness produced in the human ear.

These ISO values have not yet (1968) been incorporated in a USASI standard for reasons that will be explained in Chapter 9, but they have been almost universally adopted by all European countries and by the otological and audiological professions and in many departments of the U.S.A. government, notably the Department of Defense and the Veterans Administration. As explained in an earlier chapter, the ISO reference levels are used exclusively in the present revision of this book.

Since the publication of the ISO values, the results of another United States Public Health Service survey have become available. The data were collected in 1960–1962. The population samples were chosen with great care, and the hearing levels have been analyzed with respect to age, sex, race,

region, and area of residence. The data that most closely correspond to the previous USPHS survey are those for the hearing in the better ear of men and women in the 18- to 24-year age group. These data are shown in Figure 4-6. From 1000 to 4000 Hz the average value is 3 dB (ISO). If the worse ears are included, the average hearing-threshold level is about 4 dB. (At 500 and 6000 Hz the divergences are greater, and no measurements were made in the survey at 125, 250, or 8000 Hz.)

The differences between the ASA-1951 levels and ISO average about 8 dB from 1000 through 4000 Hz. Thus the latest USPHS survey data fall between the ASA and the ISO reference levels but somewhat closer to ISO than to ASA-1951.

Another survey study, in Pittsburgh, was begun in 1958 and concluded in 1960. The subjects, over 4000 in all, were the children in four schools, selected to be representative of the entire school population of the city. The children ranged from 5 to 14 years of age. The study was conducted under the guidance of the Subcommittee on Hearing in Children, Committee on Conservation of Hearing of the American Academy of Ophthalmology and Otolaryngology. Special attention was given to otoscopic examination of the children and the relation of these findings to the audiograms. Suffice it to say here that the median audiogram (50th percentile) is at very nearly the same hearing level as that of the young men and women in the USPHS survey of 1960–1962.

Still another survey of children by the USPHS on a national basis has been completed, but the results are not yet available (1968).

The reasons for the difference between ASA-1951 and ISO have been debated at length, and the answers are not very clear. Evidently less than half of the difference can be attributed to the use of restricted populations (ISO) as opposed to a national survey with proper demographic sampling. Perhaps the audiometric technique and the time taken to determine each end point or perhaps the motivation of the subjects are the important differences. No one is sure (see also Chapter 9).

### Calibration for Bone Conduction

The bone-conduction vibrator is more difficult to standardize than the air-conduction receiver, and bone-conduction tests are more difficult to carry out properly. Skulls and skin differ to an annoying degree in their ability to conduct sound, and the force with which the bone-conduction receiver is applied to the mastoid is important. Some audiologists prefer to apply it to the forehead instead. The ear not under test must be "masked" by noise delivered through an air-conduction receiver. The ear under test must be open to the room. This makes it more vulnerable to masking by room noise than an ear that is snugly covered by an air-conduction receiver. No "artificial head bone" corresponding to the NBS-9A "artificial ear" has been standardized as yet, but rapid progress toward this end is being made in the International Electrotechnical Commission. This will be an important step.

In the meantime the calibration of the bone vibrator is left to each manufacturer. The standard practice for a good many

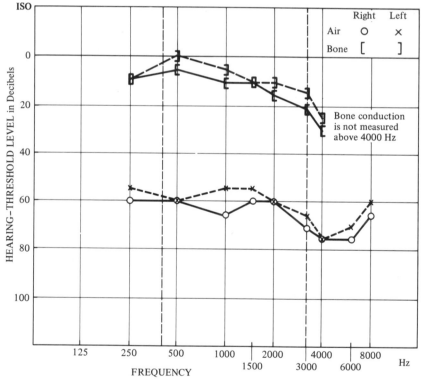

Fig. 7-6. These air-conduction and bone-conduction audiograms show the hearing-threshold levels in a hypothetical case of symmetrical middle-ear hearing loss with a slight additional inner-ear loss at the higher frequencies. Most of the bone-conduction thresholds are within normal limits. Note that each audiogram blank should carry the notation ISO (or ASA-1951) and also the code of symbols to be employed. The latter are not standardized. Often arrow heads (< and >) are used instead of brackets for bone conduction and often the convention for right and left is reversed. It is helpful to use color with red = right. This is a universal convention. Note also that it is difficult to make an audiometric chamber quiet enough to measure zero hearing-threshold levels by bone conduction at 250 Hz and particularly at 125 Hz.

years has been to label the scale for bone-conduction hearing levels in such a way that there will be no air-bone gap when air-conduction and bone conduction are determined on subjects with no conductive (middle-ear) impairment. The ears may be normal or may have pure sensory-neural impairment.

Like the air-conduction part of the equipment, the bone-vibrator portion should be tested periodically on presumably normal subjects. Calibrations are never permanent, and one of the great weaknesses of audiometry in the United States has been neglect of recalibration. *Annual recalibration by the manufacturer is strongly advised*, particularly if audiometric data are to be used in relation to insurance or other compensation.

## Automatic Audiometry

Probably the first automatic audiometer was the instrument developed by Békésy in 1947. This instrument introduced the novel feature of control of intensity by the subject, combined with graphic recording of his adjustments. The frequency of the test tone is automatically increased, slowly and steadily, as the audiogram chart advances under the recording pen. The patient presses a button when he hears the tone. The tone may be steady or else interrupted two or three times a second (see Chapter 8). The intensity of the signal is gradually reduced as long as the button is held down. When the subject no longer hears the tone, he releases the button. Now the signal becomes stronger and

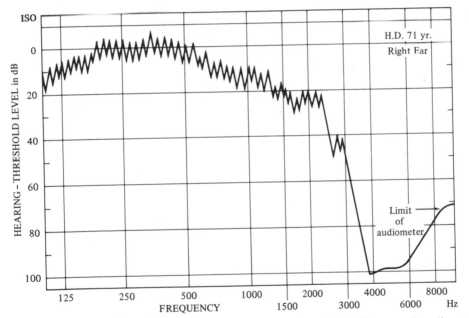

Fig. 7-7. Audiogram produced by an automatic patient-controlled (Békésy type) audiometer (*Grason Stadler Co.,* Type E-800). The chart moved steadily to the left as the frequency of the test tone changed continuously at the rate of 1 octave per min. The pen moved up or down at a rate of 2.5 dB per second. The direction of movement of the pen was upward (less intense) as long as the patient held his switch closed ("I hear the tone") but was downward (more intense) when the switch was open ("Don't hear the tone"). The subject for this test has an abrupt high-frequency sensory-neural hearing loss beginning just below 3000 Hz. He hears nothing above 3600 Hz in this ear. Part of the loss from 500 to 2300 Hz is due to presbycusis (71 years). The results of a monaural loudness balance test of this ear, 3000 vs. 2000 Hz, are shown in Figure 8-4. This ear does not show the narrowing of the trace that is very often associated with recruitment.

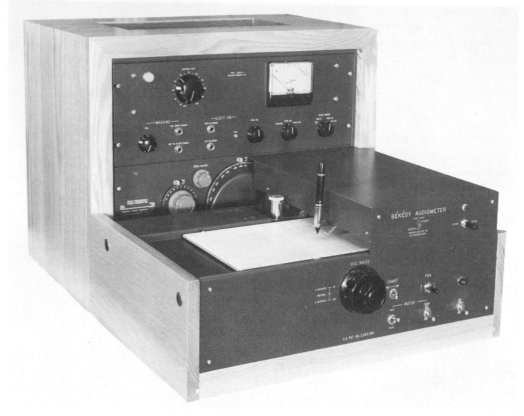

Fig. 7-8. This recording audiometer uses the patient-control principle. It may be operated either at a fixed frequency to study changes of threshold with time or with steadily changing frequency to trace an audiogram like that shown in Figure 7-7. It is usually known as a Békésy audiometer. (*Grason-Stadler Company*)

stronger until the subject presses the button again. Thus the pen zigzags up and down across the chart, reversing its direction each time the button is pressed or released. Usually there is an interval of 5 to 10 dB between the pressing (hears) and release (does not hear) of the button, as in Figure 7-7, but this range becomes very narrow in an ear that shows loudness recruitment.

The Békésy audiometer has been put to use in many research laboratories and hearing centers. It has yielded a vast amount of new experimental information on such topics as masking and auditory fatigue. Its accuracy is comparable with or better than clinical pure-tone audiometry. Automatic and semiautomatic audiometers will be

recognized in the next USA Standard for Audiometers, which is in preparation.

The military requirements for testing the hearing of many men, whether at induction or at discharge, or in monitoring programs for conservation of hearing, led to the development of the 1950s of several types of group audiometer and also of several automatic and semiautomatic audiometers, both group and individual.

Only one of these became popular, however, and the field of automatic audiometry at the present time (1968) is practically reduced to two representatives of the subject-controlled type, both for individual audiometry, known as the Békésy and the Rudmose, respectively. The Békésy pro-

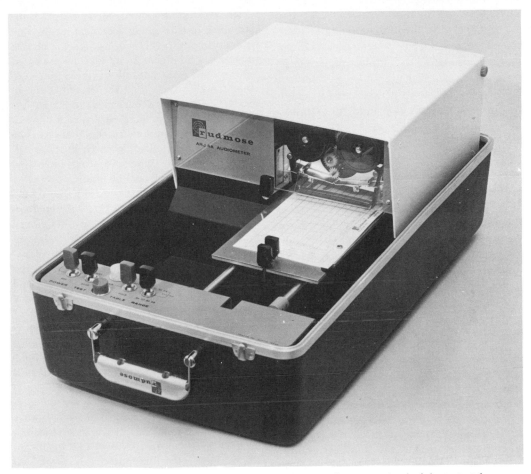

Fig. 7-9. This automatic recording audiometer uses the patient-control principle to test hearing at six frequencies in each ear. It does not require an operator except to start the machine. It is usually known as a Rudmose audiometer. (*Tracor Medical Instruments*)

vides either a continuously changing frequency ("sweep frequency") or a single selected frequency, and it yields a graph of the adjustments of intensity made by the subject. The Rudmose instrument tests each ear at six predetermined frequencies and records the thresholds on a card. With each type the operator only needs to start the machine. The Békésy instrument is versatile and well suited to diagnostic and research use, and the Rudmose instrument is particularly adapted to monitoring audiometry.

## Monitoring Audiometry and Identification Audiometry

The CHABA Council published, as part of the report of the meeting of 1955, a summary of the purposes and objectives of audiometry in the Armed Forces. The problems are the same as for audiometry in industry. In this summary "monitoring audiometry" was first formally defined. A later report (1967) of CHABA Working Group 43, concerned with intraservice standardization of audiometric tests, employs also the term "identification audiometry." The distinction between these two terms is stated in the following note: "Identification audiometry, or reference audiometry, deals with the initial preinduction tests that establish [a man's] reference hearing level. Recommendations for identification audiometry also hold for monitoring audiometry which deals with periodic check-ups."

The later (1967) report strongly recommends individual automatic audiometry of a type that makes unnecessary any intensity adjustment by the tester. A Békésy-type audiometer is mentioned as an instrument of this class. (The Rudmose modification is a member of this class also.) No mention is made of group audiometry.

We quote from the report of 1955.

### PURPOSES AND OBJECTIVES
### OF AUDIOMETRY

The purposes and objectives of audiometry in the Armed Forces, including their civilian employees, fall into five major categories:

1. to select or reject men as a part of the regular initial physical examination;
2. to provide information for the otologist concerning the extent and nature, the probable cause, and the progress of individual hearing losses in relation to the disease and to the effectiveness of treatment and preventive measures;
3. to establish the amount of hearing loss for compensation purposes, including the determination of the original state of hearing before any service-connected or employment-connected hearing loss has developed;
4. to enable personnel officers to determine whether certain individuals are qualified for certain military specialties that involve special kinds of hearing ability;
5. to obtain new information as to (a) the causes and the prevention of hearing loss; (b) criteria for hazards to hearing; and (c) the effectiveness of particular tests and instruments for accomplishing the above objectives.

A clear distinction must be made between: (1) the kind of hearing test; (2) the way in which the test is administered; and (3) the particular instrument or technical means that embodies both the chosen test and the chosen method of administration. Not all types of hearing test will suit all of these purposes equally well. There is at the present time no single "best" test of hearing, and much less is there any single "best" instrument for administering hearing tests in all situations. The kind of test best suited for each purpose will depend upon the kind of information that must be obtained from the test.

For example, the most generally useful kind of hearing test is pure-tone threshold audiometry by air conduction. This was developed originally for diagnostic medical purposes and is also well suited for screening at induction centers, for monitoring hearing conservation programs, for estimating disablement and appropriate compensation, and for many types of medical research. Another kind of hearing test is speech audiometry, including tests of ability to hear speech in noise. These special tests are appropriate for determining special hearing abilities needed in particular military specialties.

It is assumed that a pure-tone test of hearing is desired. There are a number of ways in which pure-tone tests can be administered, each with its advantages and disadvantages. Furthermore, the different choices are not all mutually exclusive, but can be combined in many ways, just as an aircraft can be designed for combat, transport or reconnaissance, may be large or small, may be piloted or a robot drone, and may be powered by reciprocating, jet or turbo-prop engines.

Among methods and types of pure-tone audiometry there are major choices that must be made between: (1) screening audiometry *vs.* monitoring audiometry *vs.* diagnostic audiometry, which implies a choice between a pass-fail test, a limited audiogram, or medically oriented audiometry including complete audiograms; (2) individual audiometry *vs.* group audiometry; and (3) manual *vs.* semiautomatic or fully automatic audiometry.

As to the means of embodying the chosen type and method in an actual instrument there are several choices at the engineering level, such as between electronic oscillators *vs.* tests recorded on discs or magnetic tape. The various choices listed above are more or less independent but, just as in the cases of aircraft, certain useful combinations are already well established. Audiometry was developed as a medical tool to assist in diagnosis and for this purpose the complete audiogram individually administered is universally employed. Furthermore, nearly all audiometers for diagnostic audiometry are manually operated and contain electronic oscillators. Semiautomatic recording audiometers for diagnostic purposes are under development, however, and may soon prove to be a useful supplementary tool in certain situations. The medical interest in diagnostic audiometry seems to lie in the development of new audiometric tests, rather than in new ways to facilitate the administration of pure-tone threshold audiometry.

For audiometry, as for aircraft, the choice of purpose is primary and the way of accomplishing the purpose depends on a balance of many factors, which include expense, personnel, and the availability of a particular instrument of established merit. The development of a means or instrument may make feasible a method that was previously not possible or practical. Such development is often an essential step, but a careful review of both old methods and new developments is mandatory before commitment is made on a large scale. There have been important recent developments in pure-tone audiometry for survey, monitoring, compensation and particularly for screening purposes. Such large-scale audiometry as is obviously required by the Armed Forces should be greatly facilitated by such new methods and instruments for group and individual pure-tone audiometry, both automatic and semiautomatic.

New methods and instruments alone will not insure good audiometry. Three other requirements are absolutely essential for *all* forms of audiometry. They are: (1) adequate acoustic environment, which means specially sound proofed, properly located booths and/or rooms to house the instruments and subjects; (2) trained personnel to administer the tests or to service any automatic devices that may replace the trained audiometrist; and (3) provision, both instrumentally and administratively, for periodic verification of the accuracy of audiometers in the field.

The uncertainties as to what are the best methods of audiometry for the Armed Forces appear to arise from the interplay of several factors. The most important factor is the recent laudable trend toward pure-tone audiometry as a required test of hearing to replace the out-moded voice and coin-click tests. The trend establishes a demand for audiometry on a large scale, but for audiometry that is quite different from the elaborate diagnostic audiometry that has for some time been employed as an adjunct to a medical specialty. Yet the concepts and the instruments for audiometry were developed for just these medical diagnostic purposes.

More recently screening audiometry, and group audiometry as a way of performing such screening, has been developed. Screening audiometry arose as a part of preventive medicine with particular orientation to the conservation of hearing in school children. The objective here was to identify rapidly those children who require closer examination and perhaps medical treatment. Such audiometry is roughly equivalent to the old voice tests and it has been rather taken for granted that it is the most appropriate type of audiometry for induction centers where a quick pass-or-fail test of hearing adequacy is the primary requirement. Screening audiometry, like diagnostic audiometry, is now a familiar and well-established concept.

An intermediate type of audiometry that we here term "monitoring audiometry" has more recently been developed in connection with conservation of hearing programs in industry. Its objectives are twofold. One is to establish the state of hearing of a relatively large number of individuals and to provide reference audiograms from which subsequent changes in their hearing are measured. The reference audiograms, particularly if they are pre-employment or so-called pre-placement audiograms, may be used to determine subsequent liability for later changes in hearing in connection with workmen's compensation. Its other objective is to detect changes in the hearing of individuals, relative to their reference audiograms, before the hearing losses become a practical handicap. Monitoring audiometry thus gives warning in time for instituting effective protective measures, such as the reduction of the noise itself, the reduction of the noise exposure of the individual or the use of individual protective measures.

Monitoring audiometry is more restricted than diagnostic audiometry. Only air-conduction tests are required for monitoring audiometry and a more restricted range of frequencies and intensities [is] sufficient. It differs from screening audiometry, however, in that it must measure auditory acuity and not merely give a pass-or-fail result. Usually, within the range that it covers, it must yield an audiogram comparable in accuracy with a diagnostic audiogram. The restricted range of a monitoring audiometer favors the development of group and of automatic or semiautomatic methods of administration. On the other hand, the necessity for accuracy and for an audiogram that is complete within the chosen range imposes serious difficulties both in the design of automatic instruments (particularly automatic group instruments) and in insuring their continued accuracy.

It seems clear that at present it is feasible to design and develop screening audiometers and monitoring audiometers that will expedite and make practical the screening and/or the monitoring of large numbers of individuals within reasonable limits of time, expense, space and trained personnel. It is not clear, however, that the same instrument should be expected to perform both functions. It is also possible that all monitoring audiometry need not be done in just the same way. In some situations an automatic individual audiometer, in other situations a manually operated group audiometer may have clear and overriding practical advantages. The general concepts of screening, monitoring, and diagnostic audiometry are well established, but there are several audiometric tests that fall in each class. There are various means or instruments for administering a given test and these differ in respect to expense, space, time and personnel required.

### Reduced Screening

Reduced screening employs 4000 Hz as a single monitor frequency to detect the beginning of hearing loss in situations that involve hazardous noise exposure. It is at this frequency that the first permanent threshold shift is noticed in exposure to most industrial or military noises. This shift produces the well-known "4000 Hz notch." *Single-frequency screening* at 4000 Hz may greatly simplify and expedite routine monitoring audiometry. It is very quick, and it has the great advantage of not requiring an acoustic environment any quieter than that of the average office. Some audiologists prefer to employ a second frequency, usually 2000 Hz, to back up the single-frequency test at 4000 Hz. Of course, all soldiers or workers whose hearing levels are found to lie above the screening limit, whatever limit may be chosen, must then be tested at all the regular monitor frequencies, and, if the loss is confirmed, should be given a full otological examination and diagnostic audiometry.

At the present writing opinion is divided as to whether *reduced screening* at two or perhaps three frequencies is sufficiently reliable to be used to expedite conservation of hearing programs for schoolchildren as well as for adults.

The Pittsburgh survey of hearing in children, mentioned earlier in this chapter, showed that even complete pure-tone audiograms were not as effective as had been hoped in identifying the ears with otological abnormalities that might be helped by proper treatment or preventive measures.

### Frequencies for Audiometers

When audiometry was new emphasis was placed on the measurement of hearing for very low tones, such as 64 Hz, and very high tones, such as 16,000 Hz. The trend over the years has been to concentrate attention on the range from 500 to 6000 Hz. It gradually became clear that measurements at the extreme frequencies are unreliable. At the high frequencies there are technical difficulties due to resonances in

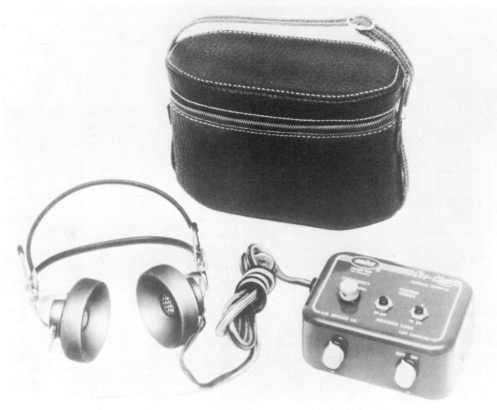

Fig. 7-10. A simple, two-tone (2000 and 4000 Hz) narrow-range audiometer with only two levels of output can be made very compact indeed. (*Ambco Electronics*)

ears and earphones, and at the low frequencies it is expensive to provide adequate exclusion of sound from audiometric booths at 250 Hz and below. Furthermore, the hearing levels for the whole lower half of the frequency range, from 1000 Hz down, can be very well predicted from the hearing level at either 500 or 1000 Hz. 4000 Hz is important as the most sensitive indicator of high-tone loss. The otologist may desire measurements at 250 Hz and perhaps at 8000 Hz, but for screening, monitoring, and identification these frequencies are quite unnecessary. More important are the intermediate frequencies of 1500 and particularly of 3000 and 6000 Hz.

The frequencies for audiometers required in the proposed USASI standard on audiometers and those generally used for certain particular purposes are given in the following table.

*Noise levels in audiometric booths.* In all audiometric work it is assumed that the tests are carried out in a room that is quiet enough so that the background noise does not interfere with the test. This is not a very difficult condition to meet if the patients are all very hard of hearing, as they are in a school for the deaf. If, however, we wish to measure normal or nearly normal hearing, special sound treatment for both the exclusion and the absorption of unwanted background noise is necessary. Prefabricated audiometric booths are available commercially, and, in general, have proved more satisfactory than reconstruction of a room in an existing building.

TABLE 1
REQUIRED FREQUENCIES (Hz)

| Class and Purpose | 250 | 500 | 1000 | 1500 | 2000 | 3000 | 4000 | 6000 | 8000 |
|---|---|---|---|---|---|---|---|---|---|
| **Wide range (USASI)** | | | | | | | | | |
| Diagnostic | | | | | | | | | |
| Air | 250 | 500 | 1000 | 1500 | 2000 | 3000 | 4000 | 6000 | 8000 |
| Bone | 250 | 500 | 1000 | 1500 | 2000 | 3000 | 4000 | | |
| **Limited range (USASI)** | | | | | | | | | |
| Monitoring and | | | | | | | | | |
| Identification | | 500 | 1000 | | 2000 | 3000 | 4000 | 6000 | |
| Air only | | | | | | | | | |
| **Narrow range (USASI)** | | No minimal requirements | | | | | | | |
| Screening | | | | | | | | | |
| Full | | 500 | 1000 | | 2000 | 3000 | 4000 | 6000 | |
| Two-tone | | | | | 2000 | | 4000 | | |
| Single | | | | | | | 4000 | | |
| **Military physical standards** | | 500 | 1000 | | 2000 | | 4000 | | |
| Calculation of hearing handicap | | | | | | | | | |
| AAOO guide | | 500 | 1000 | | 2000 | | | | |
| [California* | | 500 | 1000 | | 2000 | 3000] | | | |

* New York, Wisconsin, Missouri, and many other states follow the AAOO guide. Only California has a different specific requirement.

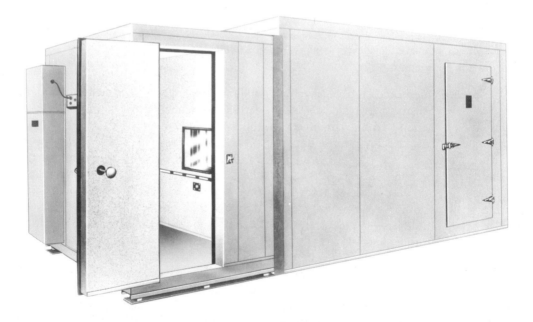

Fig. 7-11. Prefabricated sound-treated booths provide the quiet that is needed for accurate determination of auditory thresholds. The subject sits in a separate compartment from the tester. Both compartments are ventilated, but without raising the ambient noise level sufficiently to affect the desired threshold measurements. Specifications for such levels are given by the U.S.A. Standards Institute. (*Industrial Acoustics Company, Inc.*)

In a new building, however, acoustic engineers can design satisfactorily quiet rooms for audiometry at reasonable cost if they are consulted early enough in the planning. Sometimes the problem is very difficult for the acoustic engineer, as when the audiometric rooms must be located near washrooms, elevators, ventilating fans, or other machinery. The low frequencies are the most difficult and the most expensive to exclude.

The expense of a satisfactory booth will also depend critically on just what kind of audiometry is to be done in it. Are we content with measuring thresholds down to (but not below) 10 dB (ISO), that is, the American Standard zero? Such measurements are quite sufficient for monitoring audiometry in either military or industrial situations. Will an earphone always be over the ear under test or will we want to measure bone-conduction thresholds with an open ear canal? Do we want to measure thresholds at 125 and 250 Hz for diagnostic purposes, or will we be content to start at 500 Hz, as in monitoring audiometry.

Of course, the amount of sound treatment needed depends on the sound levels expected outside as well as on the permissible levels inside. The outside levels depend on local conditions, but for the guidance of acoustic engineers an American Standard tells what octave sound band levels are permissible in an audiometric booth if we are to measure zero hearing levels (American) using properly fitted earphones. (ASA S3.1–1960 "Background Noise in Audiometer Rooms.") This standard is now under revision. It is intended to provide two or three alternatives, one for measurements to 10 dB (ISO), another for 0 dB, and perhaps still another for −10 dB. The latter specification is difficult to meet unless the booth is located in a quiet area, but it is necessary if the threshold of hearing is to be measured in children. On the other hand, the requirements for

screening audiometry at perhaps 20 dB are relatively easy to meet.

A recent development that may assist materially in carrying out audiometric tests when the ambient noise is still a little above the desired standard levels is an earphone that provides *a circumaural noise-excluding shield in addition to the standard flat MX41/AR cushion that is applied against the auricle*. This device is known as an Otocup (Figure 7-12). The circumaural seal is made by means of a fluid-filled doughnut-shaped sac, something like a tiny partly-inflated inner tube, attached to the plastic shield. The advantage of the Otocup is that the earphone can be calibrated on the NBS 9A coupler. Loudness-balance transfer data for this combination should soon be available (1968). An alternative

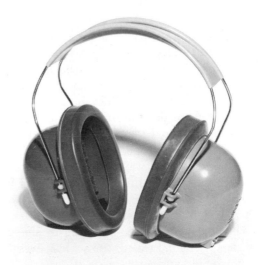

Fig. 7-12. The Rudmose RA-125 Otocups are earphone enclosures which allow the standard MX-41/AR audiometric cushions to rest against the pinna in normal fashion but provide noise attenuation by an outer plastic case with a conforming seal that fits around the edge of the case and makes circumaural contact with the side of the subject's head. Such devices supplement sound-treated booths in reducing background noise for audiometric tests. The illustration shows the outer cups only, without the earphones, as used for simple ear protection in noisy environments. (*Tracor Medical Instruments*)

uses only the circumaural seal. The volume of air enclosed is more than the standard 6 cc, and coupler calibration is difficult above 2000 Hz. This form is excellent for communication in noisy situations but is not suited to precise audiometry.

### Tests of Tolerance

A simple audiometric test that is very important in the selection of a hearing aid is the test of tolerance for loud sounds. It is usually performed with pure tones at 500, 1000, and 2000 Hz. One of the most important choices in the selection of a hearing aid relates to its maximum acoustic output, and this is determined by the subject's tolerance for loud sound (see Chapter 11). There are definite advantages in using a hearing aid that comes close to but never quite reaches the threshold of real discomfort.

The sensations of discomfort, of tickling in the ear, and of pain that are produced by very loud sounds have already been mentioned in Chapter 2 in the description of the auditory area. Here again, individuals differ as to the intensities of sound that merely cause discomfort, tickle, and pain. There seem to be tough ears and tender ears, or, rather, tough men and tender men. (Women, by the way, seem to be just as tough as men in this respect.) The man with one tough ear usually has another tough ear on the other side of his head. This toughness can be increased by simply listening to loud sounds for a while, even if the sounds are never made so loud as to tickle or become definitely uncomfortable. The increase in tolerance is likely to be greatest if the ear is unusually tender to begin with.

A test for tolerance is very simple in principle. It is like an audiometer or a speech test except that very loud sounds are used. Special apparatus may be required to make the sounds loud enough without distortion. The intensity is increased gradually until the listener indicates that he has had enough. Any such test, however, must be conducted with care, particularly on anyone with impaired hearing who has not yet become once more accustomed to hearing loud sounds. He may be startled, antagonized, or even frightened if the sound is made too loud too rapidly.

It was surprising to learn through a series of wartime experiments conducted at the Central Institute for the Deaf that the tolerance thresholds of the hard-of-hearing are on the average the same as those of normal ears. The hard-of-hearing may scatter a little more widely above and below the average, with some ears more tender and some tougher than the usual run of normal ears, but the differences are much smaller than had been expected.

### Speech Audiometry

Speech audiometry supplements pure-tone audiometry, although, as we shall see, it tests more than the ear. It's chief diagnostic use, as we shall see in Chapter 8, relates to impairments of the central nervous system. But if a *test of the over-all performance* of a subject in hearing, understanding, and responding to speech is desired, the directness and high face-validity of speech audiometry appeal to audiologists and to subjects alike. They all *like* speech tests. Also the tests for threshold, usually called the *speech-reception threshold* (SRT), have proved to be very reliable, and they have the advantage of giving the result as a single number.

Speech audiometry is particularly suitable for the general *assessment* of hearing and the estimation of the degree of practical handicap. Recall, for example, that in Chapter 6 all of the data concerning the improvement of hearing by surgery were based on speech audiometry. The speech-reception threshold has an advantage for *screening* audiometry also because a single pass-fail criterion can be established. Actually the screening by speech audiometry of the hearing of schoolchildren in 1927, using the Western Electric 4C audiometer, was the first use of speech audiometry and also of group audiometry. The success of this instrument and its method did much to promote the general acceptance of electric audiometers.

The principle of a *speech audiometer* is very simple. The test material is speech. Words or sentences may be spoken into a microphone ("live-voice testing") or, better, they may be recorded in advance in standard form and at known levels on either magnetic tape or a phonograph disc. In either case the speech signal becomes an alternating electric current. Its strength is varied by a calibrated attenuator. The listener may wear earphones, or sometimes listen with both ears to a loudspeaker. The listener determines, not when he can just hear the voice sounds, but when he can *identify* the words. He may repeat the test words aloud; check them on a multiple-choice list; or write them down; or, perhaps, if the speech material is a set of questions, he may answer the questions. Usually we take the "50-percent correct" level as the threshold. Or the subject may simply listen to the reading of some simple text and himself set the volume control so that he can just get the gist of what is being said. Of course, each form of test and each sample of speech material must be calibrated separately; that is, we must find the median (or modal) threshold for a reasonably large group of otologically normal listeners.

There are several *difficulties with speech audiometry*, some of which are quite apparent, although others are not. An obvious one is the problem of physical measurement of the intensity of the speech signal; others concern the choice of words or sentences; others, the voice of the talker; and others, the purpose of the test.

The problem of *physical measurement* has been adequately solved, even though measurement of speech is never as precise as measurement of pure tones because the intensity of the sound-pattern of speech is continually changing. The usual convention is to take a sort of running average of the largest of the excursions of the meter as it swings in response to the syllables of the words. A particular kind of meter, the VU ("vee-you") meter, or "volume indicator," is used for this purpose. The term "volume" in electrical engineering is used to mean exactly this kind of measurement of electrical speech signals, and the dial on a radio or a hearing aid that controls the intensity (loudness) of the output is therefore known as the "volume control." If the talker has the meter in sight himself, he can adjust, or *monitor*, his speech to a chosen standard level. A practiced talker can hold such a general level of conversation, or repeat a given word, within a couple of decibels, which is quite sufficient for our purpose.

More disturbing is the realization that all words, spoken naturally and in sequence, do not have the same physical power. Here we adopt the convention that all the words are to be spoken with the same *effort*, and the monitoring is done only on the strongest syllables. If single words are used, they are introduced by the same carrier phrase or word, such as, "Say the word _____" or "Would you write _____ now." The talker monitors on the carrier and lets the test word come naturally without any extra emphasis. The carrier also serves to warn the listener that the test word is coming so that he is at attention.

But now the *choice of material* becomes important because all words are not equally intelligible even when carefully monitored. Some can be understood even when barely audible, whereas others must be at a much higher level before even a practiced listener can identify them correctly. Familiar words are more intelligible than the unfamiliar; words of many syllables are easier than monosyllables; and words with weak vowels and high-pitched consonants, such as "thin" and "sift," are particularly difficult.

*Still other factors affect the intelligibility of speech.* Everyone knows that it is much easier to recognize a word in context in a sentence than when it is heard alone. Everyone knows also that it is easier to identify familiar words or names than those that are not familiar, and also that words are easiest to identify if they are spoken in a familiar dialect. It is obvious that nonsense syllables, which are used in research on the intelligibility of speech, are so difficult that they are not suitable for clinical use. What is not so generally recognized is the principle that *the size of the vocabulary that is used is important.* It is much easier to identify a digit—"one," "three," "eight," and so on—if we know that the test words are all numbers, than if the word may be any word in the English language. Context reduces greatly the number of probable alternatives among which the listener must choose. Certain combinations of words or phrases are probable; others are not.

*The development of speech audiometry.* The development of speech audiometry in the United States originated in the studies at the Bell Telephone Laboratories of the acoustic characteristics of speech, the psychoacoustics of human hearing, and the use there of samples of human speech to test the effectiveness of an electrical communication system, the telephone. We have already referred to the important part played by these laboratories in the early development of the pure-tone audiometer (the Western Electric 2A) and of the first screening speech audiometer (the Western Electric 4C). Another innovation was their use of speech material, ranging from nonsense syllables through single words to complete sentences, to test the effectiveness of a communication system.

This idea was exploited during World War II at the Psycho-Acoustic Laboratory at Harvard University. There the commu-

nication systems under test were at first military radio systems, used in the presence of loud noise or in other difficult acoustic conditions. Attention was later turned to hearing aids and the question of their best design. In each of these problems the intelligibility of standard lists of words or of sentences was the best if not the only basis on which to compare one radio system or one of its components with another, or one hearing aid with another.

In the tests of radio systems the listeners were average young men with average hearing. In the tests of hearing aids the listeners were hard-of-hearing men and women with different kinds and severity of hearing loss. It seemed a very simple and direct extension of speech testing to compare the hearing of people with impaired hearing (without hearing aids) with average hearing, using the same speech material and method of scoring that had been used to compare the radio systems or the hearing aids with one another. Those who took this step did not realize that two important hidden assumptions were involved. Unfortunately the assumptions were not justified, and speech audiometry has been overvalued for 20 years as a result!

This statement must be qualified immediately by recognizing that one type of measurement, a measurement of *sensitivity*, can indeed be made very successfully by speech audiometry. The speech-reception threshold, measured with suitable material such as digits, two-syllable (spondaic) words, simple sentences, or connected discourse, is as precise and reproducible as the pure-tone hearing-threshold levels of the audiometric frequencies of 500, 1000, and 2000, or 3000 Hz. In fact the correlation between these two measures of sensitivity, using easy speech material and pure tones respectively, is so good that the measure of the speech-reception threshold is redundant and therefore unnecessary in most cases. The more serious overvaluing has related to the measurement of the "speech-discrimination score" or the "discrimination loss."

The two major types of test for sensitivity and for discrimination, respectively, must be carefully distinguished. Very different types of material are (or should be) used, the administration of the tests is different, and the kind of information derived is very different also. The two types of speech test will be considered separately.

*Speech-reception threshold tests.* The speech-reception threshold is measured in decibels, like the hearing-threshold level for pure tones. The subject listens to simple, easy speech material. The level is sought at which the material is either "just intelligible" or perhaps "50 percent correct." His performance is compared with the average performance of a large number of otologically normal individuals of similar age, education, and linguistic background.

*The important requirements for the test material are familiarity of the test words and uniformity of presentation.* The vocabulary must be suited to the level of education of the subject, and the subject must be thoroughly familiar with the language (and dialect) in which the test is given. If it is a word test, such as Auditory Tests W-1 and W-2 (see Appendix), *the subject should be allowed to read a list, alphabetically arranged, of the words that he may hear.* This step in the procedure is very often neglected, but it is assumed if the standard calibration is to apply. Another general principle for threshold tests of speech is that *the listener must understand all of the items correctly at the highest intensity.* If he does not, the test material is not suitable for him, or else a threshold test is not the proper kind of test to apply for the disorder that he has. Most listeners hear correctly if the intensity is high enough, but as the intensity is reduced mistakes begin. The level at which half of the items are correctly understood is usu-

ally taken as the end point, or *threshold.* A rapid but reasonably accurate method is to adjust the volume of continuous speech, such as a simple text read from a book, until the listener can just easily follow the sense of what is being read. Such a continuous, even sample of simple, unemotional text is known in some laboratories as "cold running speech."

Probably the most popular recorded threshold tests for speech are the word tests known as W-1 and W-2, prepared by the Central Institute for the Deaf. They are direct developments from Auditory Test No. 9, standardized by the Psycho-Acoustic Laboratory of Harvard University for wartime use at the Army and Navy Aural Rehabilitation Centers. The words are all familiar words of two syllables with equal stress on each syllable (spondees) such as "railroad" (see Appendix). The very similar earlier list, used by the Western Electric Company in its 4C group audiometer, is a series of two-digit numbers, as, for example, "six four," "two three." Both sets of lists have been recorded on phonograph discs, with the words in groups, and each group weaker by a known number of decibels than the preceding group. Both sets have been carefully standardized, and the performance of listeners with otologically normal ears for each of them is known. With either list properly administered, the *hearing level for speech* may be measured with at least the same precision and reliability that we attain with the pure-tone test of a clinical audiometer. This accuracy is possible because, as their volume is reduced, the words pass quite abruptly from intelligible words to a mere trace of speech sound. The words were selected for uniform intelligibility by a laborious series of experiments. The use of several words in each group minimizes any errors introduced by a lucky guess or momentary inattention.

Slightly less, but still satisfactory, accuracy can be obtained by a trained talker reading the words into a microphone. Of course, he has his monitoring meter before him, and he adjusts the attenuator until the listener repeats half of the words correctly. Each talker must "calibrate" his own voice as well as the earphones (or loudspeaker and test room) by measuring the threshold of many otologically normal listeners of appropriate educational level. The calibration cancels out the effects of the talker's particular voice and tricks of pronunciation.

The Western Electric Company 4C group audiometer is now of only historic interest. A few of these instruments may still be in use for screening tests of schoolchildren, but they are no longer manufactured. The instruments had a magnetic pickup, no amplifier, and 20 or 40 pairs of earphones.

The American Standard "Specifications for Speech Audiometers" gives the important technical requirements of amplifier, earphones, and so on, and also the calibration. These specifications will be brought up to date in the forthcoming USA Standard for Audiometers.[3] For purposes of calibration it is recommended that a 1000 Hz calibration tone be recorded with the test material at the level determined as the running average of the largest excursions of the VU meter. The amplification is to be adjusted so that the coupler pressure produced by the earphone is 20 dB re 0.0002 dyne/per cm², for a TDH-39 earphone on a NBS 9A coupler. (This value is a slight readjustment of the former ASA-1953 value of 22 dB for a WE 705-A earphone.) This is to be the standard reference zero level for speech audiometry.

The above standard reference zero level is based on extensive studies of the speech-reception threshold, particularly at Northwestern University, using the W-1 and W-2 recordings prepared at Central Institute for the Deaf. However the speech-reception threshold is very nearly the same

³ Approved USASI Specification S3.6–1969.

for these recordings, for simple sentences or for simple continuous discourse.

*Uses of the speech-reception threshold.* The standard reference zero level for speech of 20 dB is, of course, higher than the ISO thresholds for the speech frequencies. The difference corresponds, obviously, to the difference between the threshold of *audibility* and the threshold of *intelligibility* of speech. Actually, as we have already noted, the speech-reception threshold level can be predicted very well from the average hearing-threshold level for 500, 1000, and 2000 Hz (or from the average of the two best of these three hearing-threshold levels). The greatest practical use of the speech reception threshold in a hearing clinic is as a confirmation of the results of pure-tone audiometry. If the two hearing-threshold levels, for pure tones and for speech, do *not* agree, it strongly suggests either a sense-organ disorder such as Menière's syndrome or a psychological or motivational situation such as simulated hearing loss (pseudohypoacusis), or an error of technique or failure of cooperation of the patient in one or both of the tests.

In this connection we should note that this agreement between the hearing level for speech determined directly and the hearing level for speech predicted from the average threshold level for pure tones did not exist when the ASA-1951 reference zero levels for pure tones and the ASA-1953 reference zero level (22 dB SPL) for

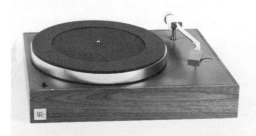

Fig. 7-13. A turntable is needed for recorded speech tests. (*Acoustic Research, Inc.*)

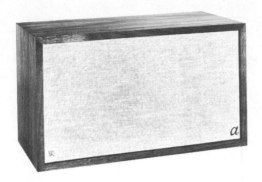

Fig. 7-14. A loudspeaker is used for free-field tests and for the assessment of hearing aids. (*Acoustic Research, Inc.*)

speech were used. The subjects apparently heard the pure tones better than the speech. Several clinics and the Veterans Administration adopted a higher reference level for speech (29 dB SPL) so that the direct and indirect measurements of the speech-reception threshold would coincide. It is now clear that the reference zero level for speech was almost exactly correct and that the ASA-1951 reference levels for pure tones were in error. The difference disappears when the ISO reference levels for pure-tone audiometers and the adjusted level for speech audiometers are employed.

The improvement in hearing that can be achieved by the use of a hearing aid (Chapter 11), or perhaps by surgery or other treatment (Chapter 6), can be very well described by the change in the speech-reception threshold.

*Speech discrimination tests and "articulation scores."* The second type of speech test aims to measure how well the listener hears words in general—all words. The test material is intended to be a sample of English speech as a whole, or at least that portion of English that is appropriate to the age, education, and linguistic background of the listener. The question is not at what level do easy words become intelligible but (1) how rapidly do words become intelligible as speech becomes louder,

(2) what is the maximum percentage of words (or nonsense syllables or sentences) that are intelligible at the most favorable intensity, and (3) how great is that intensity. Telephone and other communication systems, including hearing aids, are compared with one another on the basis of such information.

All the words in the English language are usually heard correctly by the average listener in ordinary face-to-face conversation; otherwise, the words would not have crept into the language in the first place. But some speech sounds, and therefore the words in which they are used, have a much wider margin of safety than others; that is, some of them can be understood at a much lower volume than others. (It will be recalled that by *volume* is meant the running average of the intensity of the strongest syllables in speech, and it is assumed that the weaker words and syllables are spoken with the same effort that is used in producing the stronger ones.) If we take a generous sample of familiar English words and speak them one at a time in a "carrier phrase" that offers no context to help the listener to identify the word, we find that some words, which we may call the "difficult" words, require a volume of 25 dB or more above the volume at which the first "easy" words are understood. By contrast, the lists of spondee words, matched experimentally to be equally intelligible, go from first-word–intelligible to all-words–intelligible in a range of about 6 dB (see Figure 7-15).

It is not always realized that the intelligibility of various word lists is a matter of the way the talker utters the words quite as much as it is of the "phonemic composition" of the words. Of course, some sounds—the weak fricatives, such as "th," "f," and "s," for example—depend for recognition on high frequencies in speech, and in speech the high frequencies generally carry less energy than do the low frequencies (see Figure 7-4). Actually the voice

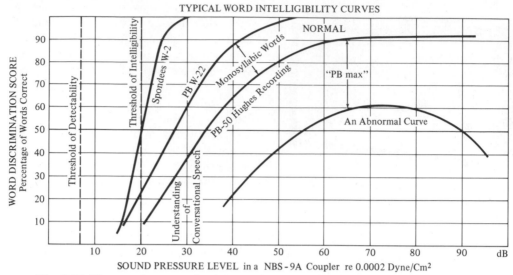

Fig. 7-15. The sound-pressure level for speech tests is defined relative to 0.0002 dyne per cm² for the calibration tone (1000 Hz) that is usually recorded on each disc. This meter reading for the calibration tone should match approximately the peaks reached by the VU meter during the carrier phrase.

The articulation curve for spondees rises more steeply than for monosyllables and is fairly constant from one talker or recording to another. The threshold of intelligibility for simple sentences and for connected discourse is practically the same as for spondees. This threshold is often called the speech-reception threshold. For monosyllables, however, the steepness and position of the curve vary from one talker or list of words to another. For some talkers, even normal listeners do not show perfect discrimination scores. For some abnormal ears the articulation curve goes through a maxmum and falls again at high speech levels. The plateau or maximum is called the "PB max."

and enunciation (or "articulation") of the talker are just as important. To be sure, an ear with severe high-tone hearing loss will not hear the high frequencies in speech; but the careless talker may fail to put them in in the first place.

Actually, in ordinary conversation we probably fail to hear correctly and completely many of the difficult words, but we do not realize that we have missed them because we hear part of the word, and the context gives us the rest. The context guides us in our choice among several possible words, any one of which we might have heard, just as it tells us which of several meanings of the same word, such as "run," "turn," "meat (meet)," or "so (sew)," is intended. Only when we come to unfamiliar proper names or something

out of context do we realize that the speech to which we are listening is something less than 100 percent intelligible.

We can describe someone's ability to hear speech *or* how well speech is transmitted by a communication system by means of an *articulation curve*. This tells us what percentage of a specified list of words the listener can identify as the words are spoken to him louder and louder. Of course, we should keep the talker constant from test to test, and the best way to do this practically is to use recorded word lists. The basic idea of describing speech reception by means of a curve instead of by a single index is no more complicated or subtle for the articulation curve than it is for the audiogram, although the quantities that are related to one another (that is, the percentage of words correctly understood and their intensity) are different from the intensity and frequency that enter into the audiogram. The articulation curve obtained for a group of listeners for one communication system is compared with the curve obtained for the same listeners with a standard comparison system. Or, in the context of a listening test, we can compare a man's articulation curve with an average or normal articulation curve for that particular recorded sample of speech.

The term "articulation" has been used to designate tests in which the listener tells what syllable, word, or sentence he has heard. This use of the term was introduced by communication engineers who were primarily interested in telephone or radio transmission between a talker and a listener. In a later chapter the term "articulation" will be used in its original sense (as it is employed in phonetics) to indicate how well a talker forms his words. In forming the consonants and fricatives, the tongue, lips, teeth, and other parts of our vocal apparatus fit together, or "articulate," with one another like the bones in our joints. The meaning has become extended, however, because the engineers speak of the "good articulation" of a telephone circuit when they mean that it effectively transmits to the listener the articulation of the talker. The tests by which engineers measured the articulation of telephones were called "articulation tests," and now, when the same kinds of tests are used to study the defects of someone's hearing, they are still called "articulation tests." The usage makes sense if we think of the word as meaning *the listener's ability to benefit by someone else's articulation* of the words to which he is listening.

Many *lists of sentences* as well as lists of words have been compiled for auditory tests of this sort. The most extensive and best known are the lists of the Bell Telephone Laboratories. They are framed as questions or as directions to tell or explain something, and the listener either answers the question or repeats the sense of it. Sample sentences include the following:

"What are some of the personal characteristics of the people of Japan?"

"Is the Hudson River salt or fresh water?"

"What punishment is inflicted upon a murderer in this state?"

"Explain how Jersey milk is obtained in Ohio."

More of the Bell Telephone Laboratories' sentences as well as sentences and words of the other tests that will be mentioned are given in the Appendix. Long lists are necessary because the same sentence cannot be used twice with one listener. His memory makes it much easier for him to recognize a sentence again even from a single key word. Sentence tests are therefore not so suitable for phonographic recording, but they have the advantage of being more interesting to the listener, and they have high face validity as samples of English speech.

The Bell Telephone Laboratories' sentences are too difficult in vocabulary and also require too much local knowledge of New York City to be satisfactory for general use elsewhere; and other lists based on more limited vocabularies and special interests—the military, for example—have been used to good advantage. Some sentences from a simplified Psycho-Acoustic Laboratory list (see the Appendix), designed as questions to be answered by a single word, are

"Which is larger, a man or a mouse?"

"Can you burn your mouth with ice cream?"

"Does a cow have kittens or horns?"

"What month comes after February?"

In an effort to obtain more accurate scoring, still another list was developed in which each sentence contains five key words. The subject repeats the entire sentence, but only errors in the key words are counted. This is a special sort of "word in context" intelligibility, useful for research work. A few samples, with key words italicized, are

> "*Clams* are *small, round, soft,* and *tasty.*"
> "*Sport* is *fun,* but *we need money.*"
> "The *boat tipped,* and the *fat lady screamed.*"
> "It is a *shameful act* to *wipe* your *mouth* on a *sleeve.*"
> "*Plug* the *leaky pipe* with a *wad* of *gum.*"

Another set of sentences was developed at Central Institute for the Deaf to provide a sample of "everyday speech." Special attention was given to the vocabulary, the length and form of sentences, and to idiom. The talkers, both male and female, were chosen as average with respect to "articulation." These sentences were intended for tests to determine the threshold of handicap (see Chapter 9), but they could also be used for easy material in an articulation test.

The best-known *lists of words used for articulation tests* are probably the *PB-50 Word Lists.* These are lists, 50 words each, of reasonably familiar monosyllables and were developed at the Psycho-Acoustic Laboratory at Harvard for wartime research on equipment for communication. Several complete lists are given in the Appendix. The abbreviation "PB" stands for "phonetically balanced." This means that nearly all the phonemes of the English language are represented in every list of 50 words. If only the initial consonants and the vowels are considered, the frequency of occurrence of the various sounds is fairly representative of English speech as a whole.

A rather similar set of 50-word lists, using a somewhat smaller and more fa-miliar vocabulary, was prepared at Central Institute for the Deaf. Two recordings of the CID lists have been made with different talkers. It so happened that one talker (Ira Hirsh) is highly intelligible, so intelligible in fact that the test has many of the properties of the spondee lists and does not reveal the limitations of hearing that we wish to measure. The other talker (Rush Hughes) clips his words so badly that some sounds are entirely missing by physical analysis, and even the best listener makes a perfect score only with the help of some fortunate guesswork. This recording is too "difficult" to constitute a good standard.

A list of words suitable for children was developed at the Clarke School for the Deaf, and other tests based on multiple choice rather than on simple repetition or writing down of the test word have been tried. Some of the most useful of these are given in the Appendix.

Actually a USA Standard for Mono-syllabic Word Intelligibility (S3.2–1960) has been issued. This standard specifies how word lists should be used to compare one communication system with another. The word lists contained in it are not quite identical with the PB lists used at the Psycho-Acoustic Laboratory or by the Central Institute for the Deaf, and represent an improvement with respect to familiarity of vocabulary. Still another set of lists prepared by Peterson and Lehiste is cited in the Appendix.

We are still without a proper standard articulation test for which normal values have been established. The administration of PB word lists by "live voice" is not satisfactory because talkers are not interchangeable. And even with the same talker the percentage of words correctly repeated by a given subject at a given intensity level may vary 5 or 10 percent from trial to trial even if the full 50-word lists are employed.

Nevertheless, certain generalizations can be made that are useful, assuming an "average talker." If a PB list (or any other list) is read too faintly, none of the words can be understood. As the voice becomes louder, more and more of the words are recognized, but even a normal listener does not make a score of 99 or 100 percent on a PB list until the intensity is at least 25 dB above the intensity at which he just recognizes one or two words. If lists are read at several different intensities, say 10 dB apart, the scores can be plotted, and an *articulation curve,* such as the one in Figure 7-15, can be drawn through the points. We know from thousands of experiments that the articulation curve is in general a smooth S-shaped curve that is steepest at or a little below its middle, and that at the upper end it levels off rather gradually to a plateau.

In Figure 7-15 it is evident that the articulation curve for the spondee words of tests W-1 and W-2 is much steeper than that for the PB-50 lists, and it lies farther to the left at lower sound-pressure levels. The steepness of the curve is due to the "homogeneity" of the list. The words were chosen and the level of each adjusted in the process of recording to bring about just this matching of intelligibility. As a result, the sound level corresponding to 50 percent correct can be determined very precisely. The less steep slope of the articulation curve for the PB words expresses the much greater spread in the "difficulty" of these words. The threshold for the PB words as recorded in test W-22 lies at a sound-pressure level about 7 dB higher than the threshold for the spondee words. This is chiefly because the monosyllabic PB words are more difficult as a group.

Another factor is the *larger vocabulary* employed. For the spondees the vocabulary is 36 words, and the subject reads the list before the test. For the PB test the vocabulary is very large. There are more than a thousand reasonably familiar monosyllables in the English language from which the listener makes his choice. If,

however, a list of only 25 monosyllables is used and the listener has read the list (alphabetically arranged) before the test, the monosyllabic threshold will lie appreciably closer to the spondaic threshold. Practically speaking, the effect of size of vocabulary becomes small for sets of more than 100 items.

If a few of the words are *unfamiliar,* it will have very little effect on the *threshold* (50 percent correct) *but will significantly reduce the level of the plateau* or "PB max."

In Figure 7-15 the difference between a "good" talker (W-22) and a "difficult" talker (Hughes) is well illustrated. The articulation curve for Hughes lies some 7 dB higher than for the W-22 recording, and its PB max is well below 100 percent.

For normal ears under good listening conditions, the plateau of the articulation curve is at 100 percent of words correctly understood; but if the words are heard through a communication system that does not transmit all the speech frequencies (or otherwise distorts the sounds), or the words are spoken against a background of noise, the curve may level off at some lower value such as 70 or 80 percent. This means that with an inferior communication system some words are never correctly understood, no matter how loud the speaker talks or how much amplification is introduced in the system. Just so, *a man with severe high-tone nerve deafness will always fail to hear certain sounds and will never make a perfect articulation score.* On the other hand, the same man may hear *some* words, the easy low-frequency words, as well as anyone else does. He may even have a normal speech-reception *threshold.*

It is a very convenient, although accidental, property of the PB and similar lists of familiar monosyllables that the volume at which 50 percent of the words are correctly understood when they are well spoken is about the level at which we can easily understand ordinary connected speech. It may seem remarkable that speech is readily understood when only about 50 percent of isolated monosyllables can be identified separately; but that is the experimental result both for normal and for hard-of-hearing listeners. In fact, if the connected speech is simple and deals with familiar material, it may be intelligible if the listener really pays attention at a level at which only about 25 percent of monosyllabic words can be correctly understood.

Practically, an important thing to know about someone's hearing is whether or not he can follow ordinary conversation. Is his hearing *socially adequate?* If not, the position of the 50 percent point on his PB articulation curve tells us how loud speech must be made (by a hearing aid) in order to make him socially adequate. Or we can measure his speech-reception threshold and add 8 or 10 dB to estimate the level for 100 percent correct on easy sentences or everyday speech.

We have described the articulation curve in general and the PB lists in particular because they show us the fundamental relationship between the *intensity* of speech and its *intelligibility*. The position of an articulation curve on the intensity scale is primarily a measure of *auditory sensitivity* (a threshold) and secondarily of the difficulty of the material for that listener. The height of the plateau that can be reached is a measure of *auditory discrimination,* that is, of how well difficult words are heard. For some abnormal ears the articulation curve not only reaches a plateau but actually goes through a maximum. Very loud speech is *less* intelligible than speech 10 or 15 dB less intense.

The important concept here is that there are two independent properties of speech and hearing. One is intensity. Usually this dominates the situation, and the intensity determines completely (for a given recorded test and a given listener) what the score will be, and if we know the threshold for speech we can predict the rest.

But this is not always true. Ears with the same threshold for speech may differ in the maximum percentage of test words they can hear correctly. To test this maximum, the words are given well above threshold. It is the maximum or the height of the plateau that is determined. This is sometimes called the *PB maximum.* A common cause for a PB maximum less than 95 percent is high-tone hearing loss. Another is poor enunciation by the talker. Another is distortion of the speech signal by a poor hearing aid.

## General Remarks on Speech Audiometry

Fifteen years ago the idea of the articulation curve as a measure of hearing was received with considerable enthusiasm by most audiologists and many otologists. It now appears that both the administration of the test and the interpretation of the results are more difficult than was then appreciated. We have pointed out in this chapter some of the sources of variability and uncertainty. For example, there is no accepted standard word list of monosyllables. Too much importance has been attached to phonetic balance of the word lists and not enough to the diction of the talkers, the familiarity of the words, the size of the vocabulary employed, and the test-retest variability of patients. The latter point is particularly troublesome because it obscures what we had hoped would be very useful information relating to the choice of hearing aids for particular patients. (We shall return to this question in Chapter 11.)

One reason for the present writer's early optimism in regard to the value of PB articulation scores and their possible use in diagnosis and assessment was an oversimplified concept of the phoneme as a unit of speech. He assumed that the difficulty in correctly hearing certain words depends primarily on the lack of intensity of certain elementary speech sounds (phonemes), notably the weak fricatives. These particular phonemes are rich in high frequencies, and therefore an ear with a high-frequency loss should be unable to hear them, and a poor ("low-fi") communication system would not transmit them adequately. The spectral composition of a phoneme was thought to be constant and to be a necessary and sufficient condition for its correct recognition. Words were thought of as mosaics of acoustically constant phonemes which are perceived and recognized independently. This is one reason why the phonetically balanced word lists were valued very highly.

The present writer is now told by his colleagues that a given phoneme does not always have the same sound spectrum, that the transitions from vowel to consonant and consonant to vowel are as characteristic and as important as the steady state (if any) of either the vowel or the consonant, and that the duration of a speech sound or the presence of a silent period may determine what it "sounds like" in a word. In short, speech is much more complicated than he once supposed.

Of course, the complexity of speech and the lability of the phoneme do not mean that the assumptions on which speech audiometry were founded are entirely wrong. It means that the assumptions were oversimplified. If high frequencies are not heard, as in the hypothetical case illustrated in Figure 7-4, the listener will certainly suffer some handicap in understanding speech. The extent of the handicap is hard to predict, however, because it will depend largely on how well the listener can employ other cues of timing, the modification of adjacent phonemes, emphasis, context, and so on, to offset his inability to hear the high-frequency components of some phonemes.

On the other hand, when large numbers of listeners and many trials are involved, articulation scores become quite stable and predictable. A very elaborate method of calculation of what is called the "articulation index" makes it possible to calculate from the spectrum and intensity level of a noise what the articulation scores (for monosyllabic word lists) will be for people listening in that noise, and a "speech-interference level" for that noise can be predicted. The method and concepts serve as useful guides in architectural planning and in noise-abatement programs.

We shall consider in Chapter 9 the "Social Adequacy Index of Hearing" that was proposed in 1948 for assessment of an individual's hearing. The difficulty in practice seemed to lie in the variability of the "PB max" scores of an individual and also in the dynamic aspects of speech. One factor that is clearly important and which has not been explicitly standardized is the speed of talking—both the length of time devoted to each word and phoneme and also the rate at which words or test items follow one another.

In summary, speech tests have several possible clinical uses, and different forms of test are required for each. One use is to measure the speech-reception threshold. For this the spondee word lists are very satisfactory, and easy sentences and connected discourse are acceptable. Speech-threshold audiometry has been standardized. Another use is medical diagnosis. Several special speech tests will be described in the following chapter, but the basic articulation curve gives only limited diagnostic information, such as a grossly reduced maximum articulation score. Another use is over-all assessment of hearing. The monosyllabic (PB) curves are descriptive and quantitative, but they test much more than the ear, and they are still inadequately standardized. A final use, the evaluation of hearing aids, would seem to be theoretically possible, but here articulation scores work poorly in practice. They are the right kind of a tool, but the tool is not sharp enough. Uncontrolled factors of various sorts make the test-retest reliability too low to assess the importance of actual differences among instruments except in extreme cases. In research, speech tests such as articulation scores are a very useful tool in areas such as hearing in noise and the advantages of binaural hearing, and also in the study of the relation of the physical characteristics of speech to speech perception and to linguistics. Here many special tests have been devised for special purposes.

## SUGGESTED READINGS AND REFERENCES

**Bunch, C. C.** *Clinical Audiometry.* St. Louis: The C. V. Mosby Company, 1943.
A monograph devoted to the development and use of the pure-tone audiometer.

**Davis, H.** "The Articulation Area and the Social Adequacy Index for Hearing," *Laryngoscope,* 58:761–778 (1948).
The articulation curves are based on the Rush Hughes recording and should be revised. The ideas may be of theoretical interest.

——, (assisted by the Subcommittee on Hearing in Adults for the Committee on Conservation of Hearing of the American Academy of Ophthalmology and Otolaryngology).
"Guide for the Classification and Evaluation of Hearing Handicap in Relation to the International Audiometric Zero," *Trans. Amer. Acad. Ophthal. Otolaryng.,* 69:740–751 (1965).

——, **G. D. Hoople,** and **H. O. Parrack.** "The Medical Principles of Monitoring Audiometry," *A.M.A. Arch. Industr. Health,* 17:1–20 (1958).
This paper is based on the report of a CHABA working group to the Air Force.

——, and **F. W. Kranz.** "The International Standard Reference Zero for Pure-tone Audiometers and Its Relation to the Evaluation of Impairment of Hearing," *J. Speech Hearing Res.,* 7:7–16 (1964). Also, *Trans. Amer. Acad. Ophthal. Otolaryng.,* 68:484–492 (1964).

**Eagles, E. L., S. M. Wishik, L. G. Doerfler, W. Melinick,** and **H. S. Levine.** "Hearing Sensitivity and Related Factors in Children," Special monograph issue of *Laryngoscope,* 1963.
This is the "Pittsburgh Study," also quoted in Chapter 5.

**Egan, J. R.** "Articulation Testing Methods," *Laryngoscope,* 58:955–991 (1948).
This is a condensation of the reports of the same title prepared at the Psycho-Acoustic Laboratory for the Office of Scientific Research and Development

(OSRD Report No. 3802). It contains a full description of the original phonetically balanced ("PB-50") word lists.

**Fletcher, H., and J. E. Steinberg.** "Articulation Testing Methods," *Bell Systems Technical Journal,* 8:806–854 (1929).
A classic article from the Bell Telephone Laboratories. It contains the complete list of BTL sentences.

**Glorig, A., ed.** *Audiometry: Principles and Practices.* Baltimore: The Williams & Wilkins Company, 1965.

**Hirsh, I. J.** *The Measurement of Hearing.* New York: McGraw-Hill Book Company, 1952.
An authoritative monograph that deals with psychoacoustic methods and principles.

————, **H. Davis, S. R. Silverman, E. G. Reynolds, E. Eldert, and R. W. Benson.** "Development of Materials for Speech Audiometry," *J. Speech Hearing Dis.* 17: 321–337 (1952).
This gives the background of the CID auditory tests.

**International Electrotechnical Commission.** "Pure-Tone Audiometers for General Diagnostic Purposes," IEC Publication 177. Genève, Suisse: Bureau Central de la Commission Electrotechnique Internationale, 1965.
Also available through the USA Standards Institute.

**ISO Recommendation R389.** "Standard Reference Zero for the Calibration of Pure-Tone Audiometers." Geneva, Switzerland: International Organization for Standardization (ISO), 1964.
Also available through the USA Standards Institute.

**Jerger, J., ed.** *Modern Developments in Audiology.* New York: Academic Press, Inc., 1963.
Chapter 1 ("The Measurement of Hearing by Bone Conduction," R. F. Naunton)
Chapter 2 ("Automatic Audiometry," W. Rudmose)
Chapter 3 ("Functional Hearing Loss," J. B. Chaiklin and I. M. Ventry)
Chapter 4 ("Measurement of Hearing in Children," D. R. Frisina)
Chapter 5 ("Electrophysiologic Audiometry," R. Goldstein)
Chapter 6 ("Middle-ear Muscle Reflexes in Man," O. Jepsen)
Chapter 7 ("Auditory Fatigue and Masking," W. D. Ward)
Chapter 8 ("Auditory Adaptation," A. M. Small, Jr.)
Chapter 9 ("Central Hearing Processes," E. Bocca and C. Calearo)
Chapter 10 ("The Theory of Signal Detectability and the Measurement of Hearing," F. R. Clarke and R. C. Bilger)
Chapter 11 ("Research Frontiers in Audiology," J. D. Harris)

**Kranz, F. W.** "Audiometer: Principles and History," *Sound,* 2:20–32 (1963).
Excellent historical review, including discussion of the reference level and the ISO standard.

**Newby, H. A.** *Audiology: Principles and Practice.* New York: Appleton-Century-Crofts, Inc., 1958.

**O'Neill, J. J., and H. J. Oyer.** *Applied Audiometry.* New York: Dodd, Mead and Company, Inc., 1966.
Recommended for the practical details of audiometric tests.

**Silverman, S. R., and I. J. Hirsh.** "Problems Related to the Use of Speech in Clinical Audiometry," *Ann. Otol.* 64:1234–1245 (1955).

**USA Standards Institute:** name changed (1969) to **American National Standards Institute.** 1430 Broadway, New York City 10018. *Standard Specifications for Audiometers,* S3.6–1969.
A recent revision of the three previous "American" Standards: *Audiometers for General Diagnostic Purposes,* Z24.5–1951; *Specification for Pure-Tone Audiometers for Screening Purposes,* Z24.12–1952; *Specification for Speech Audiometers,* Z24.13–1953.

——, *Background Noise in Audiometer Rooms,* S3.1–1960.

——, *Acoustical Terminology,* S1.1–1960.

**Watson, L. A. and T. Tolan.** *Hearing Tests and Hearing Instruments.* Baltimore: The Williams and Wilkins Company, 1949.
This monograph gives valuable details concerning electric audiometers and their use.

The citations in the literature for several additional word or sentence lists are given in the Appendix.

# CHAPTER 8

## AUDIOMETRY: OTHER AUDITORY TESTS

**H. DAVIS, M.D.**
**R. GOLDSTEIN, Ph.D.**

In the previous chapter we described the electric audiometer and also its use in determining pure-tone thresholds, the speech-reception threshold, the PB word-articulation curve, and the "PB max." This survey included most of the tests that are useful in the selection of hearing aids. We also described a number of simple diagnostic tests that can be performed with tuning forks or with a single-channel, pure-tone audiometer with a bone-conduction vibrator.

In the present chapter we consider a basic diagnostic strategy using simple tests and then describe several other diagnostic auditory tests that are suitable for cooperative adults and older children. Second, we consider the various tests for feigned impairment of hearing or pseudohypoacusis. In a third section we consider the auditory tests that are appropriate for young children, from neonates to the age of full understanding and cooperation. This includes reflex audiometry and electroencephalic audiometry: tests which are sometimes grouped together as *objective audiometry*. We include these tests of young

children here, although their purpose is more often assessment than diagnosis, because implicit in such testing is a search for conditions that can be treated medically or surgically. The final section of the chapter considers some of the tests used in otoneurology (or neuro-otology) to assess over-all auditory function and to assist in neurological diagnosis of disorders of the central nervous system.

We shall not describe the practical details of the various auditory tests. As in Chapter 7, we shall be concerned with the principles involved and with the logical relations among the tests. Full details of the instruments and tests, their historical development and their use, together with references to the publications in which they were originally described, are given in the books and review articles cited at the end of Chapters 7 and 8.

### DIAGNOSTIC TESTS FOR ADULTS AND OLDER CHILDREN

A primary reason for testing hearing is to assist in making a medical diagnosis. On the diagnosis rests the decision for treatment and also the forecast of the improvement or deterioration of hearing. Advice concerning use of a hearing aid, surgery for improvement of hearing, and so on, also depends in large part on a correct medical diagnosis. Furthermore, tests of hearing may be of real assistance to the neurologist and neurosurgeon in the diagnosis of disorders of the central nervous system, whether the basic trouble is auditory or not.

The otologist is always interested in the cause of the condition he finds. In order to treat it intelligently he should know not only *where* it is, but also *what* it is, and, whenever possible, *what causes* it. Of course, the anatomical and physiological distinctions establish certain classes of possible causes. Rarely, however, even for so simple a diagnosis as conductive hearing loss, does a physician base his opinion and course of action on a single symptom, a single sign, or the result of a single test. He always seeks confirmatory evidence, and he bases his final diagnosis on the balance of evidence in a total picture. Only the fully trained physician is competent to do this, although it is very tempting for an audiological specialist to begin to make diagnoses on the basis of the results of his hearing tests alone. An audiologist may be correct more often than not, but the experienced physician who considers audiometric findings as only one part of the total examination is in a better position to make a correct diagnosis. Above all, the physician will usually avoid the tragic mistakes that can so easily follow from oversimplification or from dependence on a single kind of information. For him the improbable but serious alternative, such as a brain tumor or a metabolic disturbance, is a very real alternative. He is better able to recognize these conditions that actually threaten life and to realize that the auditory symptoms that result from them are of only secondary importance for the welfare of the patient.

## Diagnostic Strategy

The diagnostic strategy of audiology is directed primarily toward identifying the anatomical location of impairments of hearing, whether in the middle ear, the inner ear, the auditory nerve, the central nervous system, or in some combination of two or more areas. This objective is desirable because it directs the otologist or neurosurgeon to the appropriate area and suggests the probable nature of the impairment. It is possible because the nature of the impairments that affect these areas cause characteristically different disturbances of function.

From the description of the anatomy and function of the different parts of the system given in Chapters 2, 3, and 4, it is evident that, broadly speaking, the impairments of the external and middle ear cause a conductive hearing loss, measurable in decibels, and that impairments of the central nervous system cause a quite different type of disorder, in general not describable in terms of hertz or decibels. The disorders of the inner ear cause impairments that may be partly conductive in nature, but which usually show other characteristic disturbances which may be identified with some degree of confidence by appropriate auditory tests. The major difficulties occur when two or more types of impairment occur in combination.

*The interview: informal spoken-voice testing.* An important first step toward a diagnosis can be made very simply in adults and older children on the basis of a direct interview with only the voice of the examiner as the test instrument. If the patient has difficulty in understanding the spoken voice at a conversational level but can hear and understand a loud voice, it is a strong indication that the difficulty is conductive and probably chiefly in the middle ear. In terms of audiometry, the thresholds for pure tones and for speech are elevated, but the articulation score at high intensity levels is high. Some otologists say, in this situation, that the patient's "cochlear reserve" is good. The prospects are good for alleviation of the impairment by aural surgery or for circumventing it by means of a hearing aid. Actually, if high-intensity speech is well understood, not only the cochlear reserve but the central functions of perception and understanding are good.

On the other hand, if the hearing and understanding of speech at high level are poor, or if the patient says that he hears but cannot understand the words, or complains of poor quality of musical tones or of interfering "head noises," or if he requires a very slow and deliberate presentation of words in order to repeat them correctly, then he probably has a more complicated disorder of inner ear, nerve, or central nervous system.

*Bone-conduction tests for middle-ear (conductive) impairment.* Let us suppose that by the simple spoken-voice test the patient's cochlear reserve appears good. The logical next step is to seek for evidence of middle-ear impairment. Most of the appropriate audiological tests relate to bone conduction and the presence or absence of an air-bone gap (see Chapters 3 and 4). Air conduction is impaired by middle-ear disease, but bone conduction is affected little or not at all. The simple tuning fork tests described in Chapter 7 give a quick approximate assessment of bone conduction. The Rinne test compares air and bone conduction, the Schwabach test compares the patient's bone conduction with that of a normal listener, and the Weber test compares the bone conduction of the patient's own two ears. The Bing test and the Gellé test are essentially quick tests for mobility of the stapes. These tests are not quantitative, however, and as performed in an otologist's office they may sometimes be confused by ambient noise.

The equivalent of the tuning fork tests can, of course, be performed with an elec-

tric audiometer if desired. The usual first step with this instrument, however, is the pure-tone audiogram, and then, unless the pure-tone audiogram is well within normal limits, a bone-conduction audiogram. As a first approximation the bone-conduction audiogram measures the inner-ear impairment, and the air-bone gap measures the middle-ear (conductive) impairment, including what may be due to fixation of the stapes. We repeat, however, that (1) the calibration of the bone-conduction vibrator is more difficult than that of the earphone, and the reference zero values are less clearly defined; (2) masking of the ear not under test is always necessary and may be disconcerting to the patient; and (3) very quiet surroundings are needed to avoid unwanted masking of the ear actually under test. Finally there are many anatomical pathways for bone conduction, some of which include the ossicles, and there is acoustic interaction between the inner and the middle ears. It is beyond the scope of this book to discuss the pitfalls and the limitations of bone-conduction tests. They are complex, particularly those related to masking a relatively good ear while testing the opposite (poorer) ear. In order to avoid some of the difficulties a modified bone-conduction test was proposed by Rainville in 1955.

*Rainville and sensory-neural acuity level (SAL) tests of bone conduction.* The new principle introduced by Rainville was to measure the masking effect on *air-conducted tones* produced by *bone-conducted noise*. The most familiar application (Jerger and Tillman, 1960) of the Rainville is the so-called sensory-neural acuity level or SAL test, but there are other modifications. The masking noise is applied to the mastoid (Rainville) or the forehead (SAL). A normal ear and an ear with only middle-ear impairment both have normal sensitivity for the bone-conducted masking noise. The difference in air-conducted sound level required to be heard in the presence of this bone-conducted masker, between a normal listener and the patient under test, measures the conductive loss (attenuation) of energy in the patient's middle ear. Of course the system must be calibrated on a group of otologically normal individuals, but it is not necessary to have the surroundings completely quiet, either for the calibration or for the actual test.

The SAL test is carried out by measuring two air-conduction thresholds: the threshold in quiet and the threshold in the presence of a fixed high-level bone-conducted noise. The difference in decibels between these two thresholds is then subtracted from the shift produced by the same noise in normal ears. The resulting number is the sensory-neural hearing level in decibels. This level is not quite the same as the conventional hearing level by bone conduction because it is determined with the ear partially occluded by the air-conduction receiver, although in the conventional method the ear is not occluded. The estimates of the air-bone gap, however, seem to be perfectly valid. The masking procedure is simpler than for the conventional bone-conduction measurements, but there still remains (1968) a technical difficulty in providing reliably a noise level by bone conduction as high as is desired for severe impairments.

*The acoustic impedance test.* If, from history, physical examination, and the foregoing audiometric tests it is concluded that there is a middle-ear impairment, there may still be doubt as to the cause and nature of the impairment. One distinction that may be difficult to make is between otosclerosis and a break in the ossicular chain. This question may be settled by measurement of the *acoustic impedance* of the ear. This is a purely physical measurement and requires no active participation by the subject. Clinical equipment for this test, known

as an impedance bridge, has been developed by Zwislocki (see Figure 8-1).

In principle a test tone is introduced into the external ear canal, and the sound that is reflected back by the tympanic membrane is measured. The amount reflected depends on the acoustic impedance of the ear. The impedance depends on the mass, the stiffness, and the acoustic resistance of the ear. Practically, a divided acoustic circuit (a "bridge") is used, and the acoustic properties of the ear are imitated by two adjustments of the counterpart of the ear. First the volume of the external ear canal is measured by filling it with alcohol, and a corresponding volume setting is made on the bridge. Then the remaining impedance of middle and inner ear is matched by a second adjustment. When the bridge is "balanced," the two reflected sounds cancel one another. The value of the impedance is read from a calibrated scale on the bridge. Measurements are made at several frequencies. The absolute values of impedance and their relation to frequency are characteristically different for (1) the normal ear; (2) a fixed stapes, as in otosclerosis; and (3) interruption of the ossicular chain.

We shall return to the measurement of impedance in another context, namely, the measurement of the threshold of the tympanic reflex.

*Simple speech audiometry in the diagnostic sequence.* Following the determination of pure-tone thresholds by air and by bone conduction the usual next step is to measure the speech-reception threshold and the maximum word-articulation score. These measures confirm and make quantitative the impressions gained in the initial interview. A numerical value can be assigned to the "cochlear reserve," namely, the percentage of monosyllables correctly repeated when heard at a comfortably loud level, at least 25 dB above the speech-reception threshold. At this level we sample

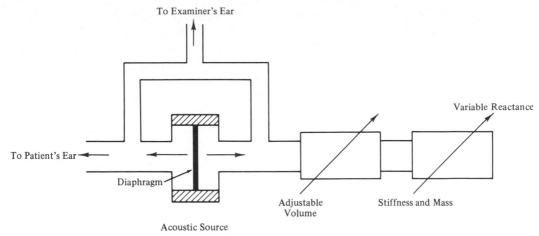

Fig. 8-1. Impedance bridge: schematic drawing, after Zwislocki (1961). The acoustic source is a symmetrical earphone which produces equal intensities of sound in the tubes that lead to the opposite faces of its diaphragm. The sound waves generated in the two tubes are in opposite phase and will cancel one another at the examiner's ear provided the sound reflected from the patient's ear at the left matches the sound reflected from the variable reactance at the right. An adjustable volume in series with the variable reactance is first set to match the volume of the patient's ear canal. Then the variable "reactance," which corresponds to a combination of stiffness and mass components, is varied until the bridge is balanced and the examiner hears no sound. (*Permission of Annals of Otology, Rhinology and Laryngology, 1961, 70:604*)

the plateau of the articulation curve, that is, the "PB maximum."

The speech-reception threshold itself usually gives little new information because it correlates so well with the average pure-tone hearing-threshold levels at 500, 1000, and 2000 Hz. A discrepancy is important however. It immediately points to something more than a conductive impairment. Of course a close agreement of speech and pure-tone hearing-threshold levels can be expected only if the patient has in the past had sufficient hearing to have learned speech and language in his mother tongue. Subjects who do not speak the language of the examiner present a special set of problems! Incidentally a discrepancy between pure-tone and speech thresholds, and particularly a discrepancy that varies from day to day, is a strong hint of pseudohypoacusis or feigning, although the combination may occur in sense-organ impairment also.

After the routine speech audiometry the audiologist must decide whether further tests are needed. Perhaps the diagnosis is clear at this point. Perhaps a final test would be the test of tolerance, to determine the power of a hearing aid that might be recommended.

The diagnostic analysis should continue, however, if the "cochlear reserve" (speech discrimination) is not good, or if the patient complains of the poor quality of the sounds he hears, or if there are any suggestions of a central neurological or a motivational problem.

*Inner ear (sensory-neural) impairment.* The impairments of the inner ear and auditory nerve comprise three major classes that can be distinguished fairly well by history, interview, and auditory tests, and which present very different problems of therapy and management. The first class includes noise-induced hearing loss, presbycusis, and most congenital defects of the inner ear. The second class is the type of sense-organ impairment that is encountered in Menière's syndrome. The third class is compression of the auditory nerve by a neurinoma. The classes may be combined, however, and the last two present rather difficult but important problems of differential diagnosis.

The common features of the first class, from the point of view of the results of simple auditory tests, are (1) elevated thresholds for pure tones by both air and bone conduction; (2) some elevation of speech-reception threshold and reduction of PB max, but no more than might be predicted from the pure-tone audiogram; and (3) no particular complaint about poor quality or "noisiness" of pure tones or speech. The absence of distortion of musical tones and speech makes the auditory impairment of this first class rather like a conductive impairment, and we have pointed out in Chapter 4 that inefficient mechanical (acoustic) action in the inner ear, particularly in the organ of Corti, may be one of the basic difficulties in many congenital defects and in presbycusis.

Clinically there is usually no difficulty in distinguishing among the three members of this first class. Presbycusis occurs in elderly people, congenital defects are nearly always noticed in childhood, and noise-induced hearing loss appears in late adolescence or adulthood with a clear history of habitual noise-exposure or an episode of acoustic trauma. We place here, with congenital defects, the abrupt high-tone hearing loss described in Chapter 4. This condition is identified by the air and bone audiograms. The chief diagnostic difficulty with this first class appears when presbycusis is superimposed on noise-induced loss or a congenital defect or when inner-ear impairments similar to those of congenital defects appear following or during an illness or suddenly with no apparent cause.

Noise-induced hearing loss represents an impairment of the organ of Corti. It is not certain to what extent sensory units (described in Chapters 3 and 4) are destroyed in whole or in part or else may simply have their thresholds permanently elevated. Whatever the pathology may be, one characteristic sign is the configuration of the audiogram with a high-frequency loss that is greatest at 4000 Hz (or sometimes 3000 or 6000 Hz). Even more characteristic is the presence of loudness recruitment accompanied by good discrimination for speech. Loudness recruitment is almost always associated with impairment of the sense organ; and so also quite frequently is dysacusis, manifested by poor quality of tones and poor articulation scores. We emphasize again, however, that recruitment and dysacusis do not always appear together, as illustrated in noise-induced hearing loss.

*Loudness recruitment.* Loudness recruitment is a very valuable sign because of its strong association with the sense organ. It is *not* produced by conductive impairment, either of the middle or of the inner ear; it is not encountered in central dysacusis; and it is relatively infrequent (not over 25 percent of cases) in acoustic neurinomas. We use the term in Fowler's original sense, referring to a more rapid than normal increase in loudness as the intensity of the test tone is increased (see Chapter 4). It is measured by the method of loudness balance. Unfortunately, as mentioned earlier, it is not always easy to test for it. In the alternate binaural loudness-balance test, when one ear is normal or nearly so, a series of comparisons are made, at one or two or even at three frequencies, of the hearing levels on the audiometer that sound equally loud to the two ears. Many audiometers designed for diagnostic purposes are equipped with two separate oscillators and attenuators to make loudness balancing easier. The results are usually plotted in either of the two forms illustrated in Figures 8-2, 8-3, and 8-4. In Figure 8-2, the key feature that shows re-

LOUDNESS BALANCES

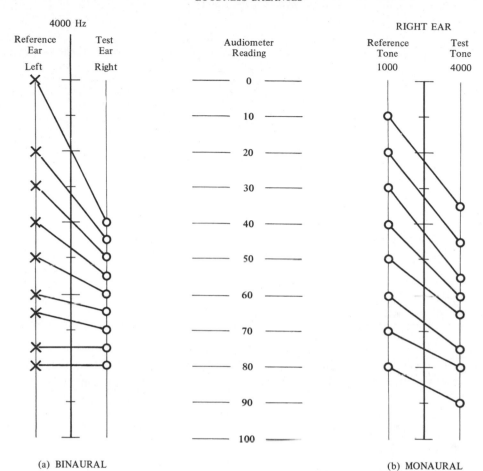

(a) BINAURAL    (b) MONAURAL

Fig. 8-2a. The results of binaural loudness balances at a given frequency are often plotted in this way (*Fowler*). One advantage of this form is that it can be superimposed on the regular audiogram. To do this, the values for the loudness balances are plotted about half an octave above and below the line corresponding to the frequency at which the balances are made and are joined by the straight lines. The conventional symbols for right and left are employed.

Fig. 8-2b. The results of monaural loudness balances at two different frequencies may be plotted as shown here or in the form of Figure 8-3. The hypothetical case illustrated shows "delayed" partial recruitment at 4000 Hz. The monaural balance must be used when the losses in the two ears are substantially symmetrical. The lower of the two frequencies, usually 500 to 1000 Hz, should show a better hearing-threshold level than the frequency to be tested.

cruitment is the change from the sloping lines near threshold (that connect equally loud settings) to horizontal lines at high intensities. In Figures 8-3 and 8-4 the corresponding feature is the approach of the observed points closer and closer to the diagonal line that is the locus of equal loudness in two normal ears.

A binaural loudness balance is more difficult for the subject than a simple threshold test, but with a little practice most subjects are able to do it quite well, even though they may protest that the job is difficult and that they have little confidence in their loudness matches. A monaural balance, in which a high tone is balanced

BINAURAL LOUDNESS BALANCE

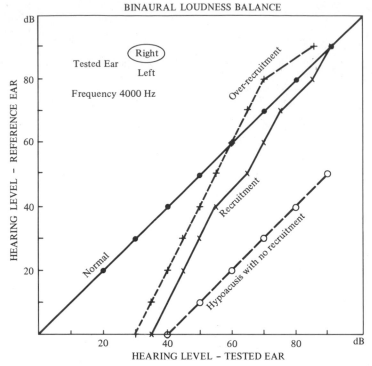

Fig. 8-3. The results of binaural loudness balances at a given frequency may be plotted in this way (Steinberg and Gardiner). If, as in the ideal normal case, the audiometer readings (hearing levels) are equal for every intensity setting, the points (solid circles) fall along the diagonal line labeled normal. A conductive hearing impairment shifts all the points to the right by an equal amount (open circles), and the line through them is parallel to the normal line. A hypothetical case of sensory-neural impairment with recruitment (x, solid line) is shown and also a hypothetical case with overrecruitment (+, broken line).

against a low tone, is more difficult, but it can be done by intelligent and cooperative patients.

Monaural loudness balance depends in principle on assuming that hearing is more abnormal at one frequency than at another. The "more abnormal" is identified by its higher hearing level and sometimes by its poor quality. A monaural loudness balance can show recruitment clearly only if there is a difference in threshold levels of 25 dB or so between the two frequencies that are compared. And sometimes there is recruitment even at the least abnormal frequency.

There is a strong tendency for binaural recruitment curves, when plotted in the form of Figures 8-3 and 8-4, to converge with the normal diagonal and with one another at the hearing level of 90 dB (Hood). The significance of this trend or of individual deviations from it is not clear however.

*Other tests for loudness recruitment.*

Some patients are not able to make reliable loudness balances, and sometimes there is no frequency at which hearing is within normal limits in either ear that can be used as the comparison tone. We must sometimes, therefore, infer the presence of loudness recruitment from tests other than loudness balance. These tests are useful qualitatively, but they are not quantitative.

The test of *tolerance for loud sound* may give a clear qualitative indication of recruitment if the threshold for a particular frequency is elevated, but its tolerance level is low. If the tolerance level is high, some recruitment may still be present, and at high sound levels the discomfort may arise in the middle ear and not simply because the sounds become uncomfortably loud.

An extension of the test of tolerance is to determine the *range of comfortable listening*. The patient judges or selects the level, at each frequency, at which he would be willing to listen to the radio for a long time. The range of acceptable values may

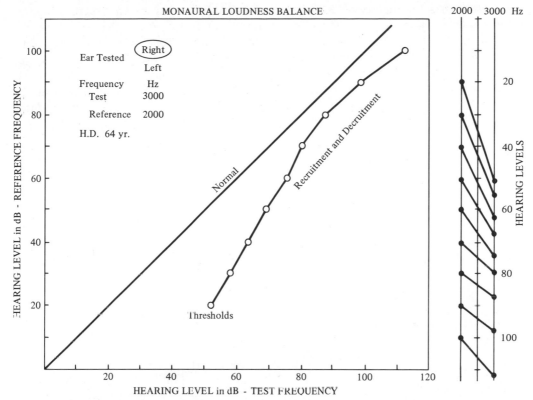

Fig. 8-4. The monaural loudness balances between 4000 Hz and 2000 Hz in curve A show partial recruitment followed, at high intensity, by "decruitment" or negative recruitment. The loudness that could be elicited by 4000 Hz in this ear seemed to approach a maximum at high intensity. These are actual data obtained from an ear with abrupt high-frequency hearing loss, illustrated in Figure 7-7. Curve B is hypothetical, to illustrate "overrecruitment" which is found occasionally.

The results of an actual monaural bifrequency loudness-balance test in a case of abrupt high-tone hearing loss are plotted in both the expanded and the compact form. There is recruitment at moderate intensities and "decruitment" at the highest levels. Note that the threshold for the reference tone (2000 Hz) is slightly elevated, at 20 dB (ISO), and some recruitment may be present at this frequency also. The test actually shows the difference in recruitment at the two frequencies. The complete audiogram for this ear is shown in Fig. 7-7.

be quite narrow in the presence of recruitment, and it may lie quite close to the threshold of discomfort. Determination of the range of comfortable listening is obviously important in assessing a patient for possible use of a hearing aid.

Another threshold that seems to be associated with the loudness of a sound is the *activation of the tympanic reflex,* that is, the contraction of one or both of the intra-aural muscles, the stapedius and the tensor tympani (see Chapter 3). The best way to detect the contraction of these muscles is by the resulting change in the *acoustic impedance.* The Zwislocki bridge can be used for this purpose, and other types of equipment have been developed and exploited by Metz, Møller, Klockhoff, Jepsen, and others. The numerical value of the normal threshold of activation of the reflex depends on the instrument used to detect the change of impedance and on the frequency of the test tone. It lies in general at about 70 to 90 dB hearing level.

The method has the theoretical advantage of not requiring the subject to make a loudness balance or other difficult judgment. It is not necessary to *measure* the acoustic impedance but only to balance the bridge and detect a *change* in impedance. The reflex is bilateral; the test tone may be applied in one ear and the reflex contraction detected in the other. The reflex is absent, however, if the nerves that innervate the muscles are injured from any cause. The clinical value of the method has not yet been fully evaluated.

The *Békésy audiogram* yields a simple sign that is often associated with loudness recruitment. The excursions of the tracing

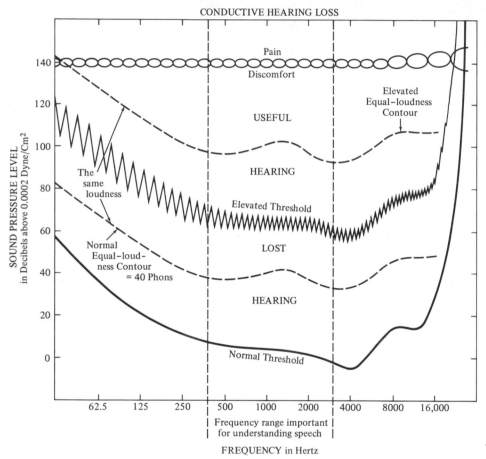

Fig. 8-5. Reduced auditory area in pure conductive hearing loss. The normal threshold zone and threshold for pain are shown as in Figure 2-4. The threshold for pain is uncertain above 4000 Hz. The elevated threshold represents a hearing loss of about 60 dB at all frequencies, a so-called "flat" loss, produced by a severe but purely conductive lesion such as otosclerosis. This is the greatest possible purely conductive loss. The case is theoretical, because a conductive hearing loss is rarely perfectly flat, and usually there is some high-tone sensory-neural loss associated with it. The equal-loudness contours are raised without distortion. Nothing sounds very loud. The high equal-loudness contours have been elevated above the threshold of pain. The threshold of pain is not elevated, although the zone of discomfort may rise somewhat. The elevated threshold is a monaural free-field threshold. It is represented as a zigzag line that can be interpreted as showing the individual variability in successive measurements or else as the tracing that might be shown on a recording patient-controlled (Békésy) audiometer as in Figure 7-7.

become shorter, meaning that the interval in decibels between "hear" and "don't hear" become smaller. In other words the crossing of the threshold becomes more abrupt. Some narrowing of the excursions at the higher frequencies is normal, as in Figure 8-5. Further narrowing, as in Figure 8-6 suggests that loudness recruitment is present and would be revealed by a direct loudness-balance test. This sign gives a partial indication of recruitment at thresh-

old, and does not test the upper part of the auditory area.

The *difference limen for intensity* is a test which theoretically should relate closely to loudness recruitment. It is the counterpart, at sound levels well above threshold, of the narrowed threshold trace of the Békésy audiogram. A pure tone at the desired level is presented to the subject, and small increases of intensity are introduced. The smallest increase that is detected with

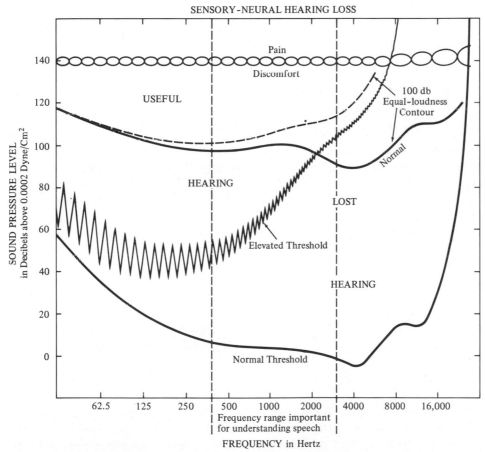

Fig. 8-6. Reduced auditory area in a hypothetical case of sensory-neural hearing loss. The normal free field, binaural threshold zone, and the threshold for pain are shown as in Figure 2-4. The threshold for pain is uncertain above 4000 Hz. The hearing loss is of the "gradual" high-tone type and is accompanied by strong "recruitment." The 100 dB equal-loudness contour is distorted but is only slightly displaced upward. High-level sounds are nearly as loud as for a normal ear. The threshold of discomfort is unchanged. The zigzag line, representing the elevated threshold as it might be shown by a patient-controlled (Békésy) type of automatic audiometer, covers a wide zone of uncertainty at low frequencies but a very narrow zone where the hearing levels are elevated and recruitment is present.

reasonable certainty is the subject's difference limen for intensity. A patient's difference limen is compared with values obtained with the particular instrument on a group of otologically normal subjects. The normal values vary as a function of both frequency and sensation level.

This type of test was introduced about 1950 by Lüscher and Zwislocki: it was modified by Denes and Naunton and later (1953) by Jerger. The best known modification is known as the *short increment sensitivity index (SISI test)*. The principle in all variations is the same: The ear with loudness recruitment can detect smaller changes in intensity than the normal ear, and this reduced difference limen is a sign of sensory-neural involvement. In the SISI test the patient listens to a tone 20 dB above his threshold for two minutes. An increment of 1 dB is introduced 20 times at approximately 5-second intervals. The increment lasts 200 msec and has rise and fall times of 50 msec. The patient signals whenever he detects an increase in loudness. The SISI score is given in terms of percentage of increments detected. Two or more frequencies may be tested. Patients with conductive or retrocochlear lesions make low scores; those with sense organ involvement tend to make high scores. This test has become fairly well established as a useful clinical test.

*Tests for pitch and tone quality.* Tests of *diplacusis* have been proposed, based on binaural pitch matching or on the difference limen for frequency. These are not so much tests for diplacusis as measures of the degree of diplacusis, and they are not widely used. The patient's description of the nature of his difficulty is usually sufficient, and it is not easy for him to match tones that are rough, complex, and noisy in one ear with pure tones presented to the other ear. The performance of the abnormal ear may fluctuate considerably. It is not the numerical values that are obtained

in such attempts that are important but the degree of difficulty that the patient has in the attempt to make matches or fine pitch discriminations. Much the same considerations apply to attempts to measure *tinitus*. Yet these disorders of discrimination are closely related to certain disorders of the sense organ and to impairment of discrimination for speech.

*Tests involving auditory fatigue or adaptation.* Gradually, since 1950, it has become evident that the threshold in some abnormal ears is not stable but rises more or less rapidly during auditory stimulation. The terms *auditory fatigue, fast adaptation,* and *tone decay* have all been used to describe this effect. The names of Dix, Hood, de Maré, Carhart, Miskolezy-Fodor, and Huizing are all associated with these early studies.

For some time there has been considerable confusion in the evaluation of various tests based on difference limens because the importance of adaptation was not recognized. Also validation was often in terms only of conductive versus normal versus sensory-neural, or else as a predictor of "recruitment." Now it appears that we may be able to make a very important generalization. *Fast adaptation is a strong indication of involvement of the auditory nerve, particularly by a rapidly growing acoustic neurinoma, but loudness recruitment, and also poor tone quality, and low speech discrimination strongly suggest impairment of the sense organ. None of these signs or symptoms is produced by conductive impairment.* Certain qualifications and limitations of these generalizations will be or have already been noted, but they are good guides and emphasize the importance of tests of adaptation in audiological diagnostic strategy.

*Tone-decay tests.* A simple test of fast adaptation at threshold is the threshold tone-decay test. A sustained tone is presented to the subject at his threshold level, and the subject keeps his finger raised as long as he hears the tone. If he continues to hear it for a minute, he has no significant adaptation.

A modification of this test is to present the tone 5 dB above the threshold level and then, when the tone is no longer heard, to raise the level 5 dB to make it audible again, and to continue making such increases until the tone is heard for some specified length of time, such as 30 seconds, or decays completely. A Békésy-type of audiometer with fixed frequencies is the most convenient instrument to use.

*Continuous tone versus pulsed-tone threshold audiometery.* Subject-controlled automatic (Békésy type) audiometry may be carried out either with a continuous tone of slowly increasing frequency or with an interrupted tone. The interruptions may be at the rate of 2 or 3 per second, and a duty cycle with 50 percent on-time is usually employed. The normal ear yields tracings that are completely (type I) or very nearly (type II) superimposable regardless of the interruptions. The Békésy type II audiogram shows a slightly better threshold for the interrupted tone, and both tracings may show the narrowing of the excursions mentioned as a "sign of recruitment." In the Békésy type III audiogram the continuous tone falls very rapidly below the tracing for the interrupted tone. In the Békésy type IV audiogram the continuous tone falls consistently below the interrupted tracing, usually without the narrowing of the excursions that is often present in type II. The amount of divergence depends somewhat on the rate of change of frequency in octaves per minute. The type III and type IV tracings are associated particularly with acoustic neuromas.

The gap between a continuous tone and the usual rate of interruption with intervals of about 200 msec can be explored by using shorter and shorter intervals. A *critical interval* appears for subjects with neural impairments at one or more frequencies. The threshold rises abruptly, as with a continuous tone, when the intervals are made too short. This test has not been formalized or widely exploited as yet (1968).

*Tests of vestibular function.* A final item in diagnostic strategy, when the issue is a decision concerning sense organ versus neural impairment, is a test of vestibular function. The test most widely employed is the caloric test. In a common version the external ear canal is irrigated with known quantities of water at two definite temperatures, one above and the other below body temperature. Such caloric stimulation induces rhythmic side-to-side movements of the eyes, known as *nystagmus*. The movements may be observed visually, or electric potentials related to the movements may be amplified and recorded on a moving tape. The duration in seconds of the nystagmus is observed for each ear and for each temperature.

From the durations of nystagmus and from its amplitude and speed a judgment can be made of normality or hyperactivity or hypoactivity of each labyrinth. We purposely omit all details concerning the technique of these (and other) tests of labyrinthine function as they are outside the scope of this book. Such tests are in the province of otology rather than audiology, and they figure prominently in the special area of otoneurology. They do assist in audiological diagnosis, however, because of the prominence of labyrinthine involvement in Menière's disease and the occasional encroachment of acoustic neuromas on the labyrinthine as well as on the cochlear portion of the eighth cranial nerve.

## Final Evaluation of Sensory-neural Impairment

We repeat a primary principle of audiological and, in fact, of all medical diagnosis: *a diagnosis is not based on any single sign, symptom, or test.* All of the available evidence, including the history and interview, are considered, and the diagnosis, therapy, management, and perhaps additional tests are determined accordingly.

Some differential diagnoses are more difficult and also more important than others, particularly those that involve possible acoustic neuromas. One reason for the difficulty is that the symptoms and the test results may be quite different for a very slowly growing tumor from those caused by more rapidly increasing pressure. The sensory units that are impaired but still active seem to be those that cause the tone decay, the poor speech discrimination, and so on. The same principles apply in Menière's disease. The picture is quite different during an acute episode as opposed to the quiet period between episodes. The nervous system seems to adapt to the complete and stable loss of some sensory units rather well. Particularly confusing is the simultaneous involvement of sense organ and nerve when the tumor compresses the cochlear artery as well as the nerve.

The general pattern or profile of audiometric test results in advancing nerve involvement is (1) absence of recruitment, (2) total tone decay, (3) type III or type IV Békésy tracings, (4) low SISI scores, (5) hearing-threshold levels only slightly elevated below 2000 Hz but more elevated for high tones, (6) speech-reception threshold in agreement with pure-tone levels, but (7) speech discrimination usually somewhat reduced, particularly at high intensities.

## FEIGNING: FUNCTIONAL OR NONORGANIC HEARING LOSS

In all of our discussions of tests of hearing, whether for pure-tone thresholds, speech thresholds, recruitment, or tone decay, we have assumed full cooperation by the patient. At worst, as in the case of babies or older autistic children, we assume indifference but not active deception. But when economic gain, "saving of face," or escape from danger is at stake, as in compensation for injury to hearing or discharge from military service, we may encounter a reversed motivation. The subject may not only make no real effort to hear; he may pretend not to hear at all or to hear much less than he really does. If the motivation to deceive for gain or safety is clear, this behavior is called *malingering*. If we are not sure of the motive, we call it *feigning*.

Two more general terms are also in widespread use: *functional* or *nonorganic* hearing loss. These terms describe hearing losses which cannot be ascribed to any "organic involvement." A more elaborate definition, given by Ventry and Chaiklin, is: "Functional hearing loss is the appropriate diagnosis when there are audiometric discrepancies and/or discrepancies between observed behavior and audiometric findings and when no apparent organic condition can be found to account for the discrepancies." The terms cover a wide range, from deliberate malingering to true psychogenic deafness. In Chapter 4 we gave our reasons for preferring the more neutral terms "feigning" and "pseudohypoacusis" to malingering.

We are particularly concerned here with tests or tricks to detect feigning and to determine the "true" threshold of hearing in spite of more or less conscious and deliberate efforts of the subject to deceive the tester. Many devices have been developed to catch off guard the man who is suspected of feigning. One consists of imparting to him in a rather low tone of voice some information that is interesting or important to him and observing whether he reacts to it. Typically the "test" is made outside of what appears to the subject to be the test situation. The giving of the information is made to appear unintentional. The basic principle for success of such tests is very simple: *The tester must be smarter than the subject, and a better actor.*

Not all audiologists are good actors, and more sophisticated tests take advantage of psychoacoustic principles which are probably unknown to the subject or which make it very difficult for him to control his behavior appropriately. Most of the formal tests to be described below are usually performed with a two-channel electric audiometer, but actually several of them are old tests that were originally carried out with tuning forks.

### Feigning of Monaural Impairment

*Stenger test.* The Stenger test depends on confusing the subject with respect to which ear is being stimulated. It is based on the fact that if two equally sensitive ears are stimulated simultaneously with an identical stimulus, the sound will be localized somewhere near the center of the head. If the stimulus is made more intense at one ear, then the listener will report that he hears sound only in that ear. He will not be aware of the weaker sound in the other ear. The threshold is determined on each ear for a tone of a particular frequency. The tone is then presented to the good ear alone at about 5 or 10 dB above its threshold. The patient will localize the sound to that ear. The tone is also presented to the supposedly bad ear the same number of decibels above its threshold. If the bad ear is as bad as the patient claims, he will probably localize the sound somewhere near the center of his head. If threshold is better in his bad ear than what he claims for it, the tone will sound louder in that ear and will be localized there. If the patient admits that he hears the sound in his bad ear, then this is a confession that he exaggerated the loss in that ear during the threshold measurement. Rather than admit that he hears in the bad ear he may claim that he hears

no sound. In this case the tester gradually lowers the intensity of the sound in the bad ear until it is less loud than the sound in the good ear, which has been constant all this time. If the patient now says that he hears the sound in his good ear, this is an admission that previously the sound in his bad ear had been strong enough to obscure the sound in the good ear. By this procedure a close estimate can be made of the actual threshold in the supposedly bad ear. The Stenger test can be modified for use with speech instead of with pure tones.

*Swinging voice test.* One's monitoring of which ear is being stimulated can also be disrupted by the swinging voice test (sometimes called the shifting voice test). If speech is fed alternately (for example, every half second) to one ear and then to the other, the speech will be very intelligible if both ears are stimulated at about the same sensation level. The listener is hardly aware that his ears are being stimulated alternately. If one ear is bad, however, the speech will lose much of its intelligibility. If a person claims a unilateral loss and still shows normal understanding of speech in this test, he can be suspected of feigning.

One modification of the swinging voice test is to present a prepared story to the listener, switching back and forth from the good ear, to both ears, to the poor ear. The story is presented at a level 20 to 30 dB above the threshold of the good ear and is written so that if the loss is unilateral, it still is perceived as a sensible story to the listener. The test is positive if the listener repeats the part of the story presented to the poor ear. If he does this, the threshold in his poor ear must be *better* than the level at which the story was presented. If he claims that he could not understand the story, even after several presentations, this should arouse the tester's suspicions. This test does not give a threshold measurement but simply an indication that the listener is not giving a true threshold.

### Binaural or Monaural Feigning

*Lombard test.* The Lombard test is based on the "voice reflex." In the presence of noise someone who is talking or reading aloud tends to raise his voice enough to hear himself speaking. We do this unconsciously when an automobile passes an open window or an airplane flies overhead. In the test, masking noise is introduced to both of the subject's ears while he is reading aloud. If he raises his voice when the noise is below his feigned threshold he gives himself away. The Lombard test can be used to detect feigned unilateral impairment by appropriately manipulating the noise levels at the two ears.

*Delayed side-tone test.* A different type of disruption of reading is used in the delayed side-tone test. The patient reads aloud into a microphone which delivers the speech to a tape recorder. The recorded speech is played back, with a delay of about 0.2 second, to earphones on the patient's ears. The delay corresponds to about one syllable. So long as the delayed sound is softer than the sound of the patient's speech within his own head, his reading will not be disturbed. As the delayed speech is made louder the patient will stutter or stumble, drag out his words, and usually raise his voice. With this test one can usually detect rather easily the feigning of a large hearing loss, but detection of small losses and the measurement of threshold are quite difficult.

*Doerfler-Stewart test.* One of the most extensively used quantitative tests for feigning has been the Doerfler-Stewart test and its modifications. This test depends on the interference by noise with the understanding of speech. The noise, however, must be at least as intense as the speech, and usually 10 to 15 dB greater, to make speech completely unintelligible. A person who is feigning may remember the loudness at which he pretends to begin understanding speech, but his monitor for loudness can be disrupted by the presence of noise. Both speech and noise, given to the same ear, are systematically varied in such a way that the person who is feigning cannot effectively retain the constant ratio of noise to speech expected from a cooperative patient and still remember at what level he is to stop "understanding." The details of the procedure are somewhat complicated, but a skilled examiner can manipulate the level of the test words, usually a spondee word list, and the masking noise in such a way as to arrive at a fairly accurate measurement of the "true" speech-reception threshold. The subject is concerned with the relation between the noise and the test words and pays little attention to the actual loudness of the words. He does not realize that a noise that just masks a test word sounds much louder than the test word.

*Békésy tracings in feigned hearing loss.* Sometimes the tracings obtained with a Békésy-type of recording audiometer reveal curious inconsistencies that assist in the identification of feigning or "functional hearing loss." Sometimes the thresholds are simply inconsistent with conventional pure-tone audiometry or with the speech-reception threshold. Particularly revealing, however, are Békésy tracings which regularly show better hearing for a continuous as opposed to an interrupted tone.

*Feigned total deafness.* On the whole, it is usually easy to catch the person who pretends to be totally deaf. Feigned deafness in one ear is fairly easy to detect and so is a pretended very large loss. The deception most difficult to detect is the addition of some 10 or 15 dB to a genuine hearing loss of between 15 and 30 dB. This, like a psychogenic overlay, can easily pass undetected and even unsuspected; yet it may make quite a difference in relation to military discharge or to the amount of workmen's compensation award.

*Signs and suggestions of feigning.* There are a number of signs or bits of behavior that should suggest the possibility of feigning to an alert audiologist. Prominent among these are (1) variations in thresholds on repeated trials, (2) incompatibility of different types of threshold, (3) bone conduction poorer than air conduction, (4) lack of agreement of speech or pure-tone hearing-threshold levels (or either of these) with history or clinical impression, (5) slow and deliberate responses, (6) partial (half-word) responses to spondee words, and (7) failure to respond to spondees at any level.

### Tests of Psychogenic Overlay

*Narcosynthesis, hypnosis, and suggestion.* At this point, for logical completeness, we refer to the method of narcoysnthesis, described in Chapter 4, and the related methods of hypnosis and suggestion. These are methods of treatment rather than diagnostic tests, but the diagnosis of psychogenic deafness or overlay, as distinct from deliberate feigning, can hardly be made except in retrospect following a cure by one of these psychiatric methods. As a matter of diagnostic strategy, feigning rather than psychogenic deafness should be assumed until the evidence to the contrary is overwhelming. As we noted in Chapter 4, psychogenic deafness is apparently very rare in the United States of America at the present time (1968). The diagnosis must be made by a psychiatrist.

*Physiological audiometry.* Physiological audiometry, to be described in the next section, particularly electroencephalic audiometry, may be very helpful in detecting and measuring the extent of a feigned or a psychogenic overlay, but it cannot distinguish between the two types. Very few cases

have been reported of electroencephalic testing in psychogenic deafness, but apparently the electrical responses of the brain are present with normal thresholds.

The principal methods of physiological audiometry depend on electrical responses from either the skin (electrodermal audiometry) or the brain (electroencephalic audiometry or "evoked-response" audiometry). In principle the physiological methods require only the passive cooperation of the patient, and they yield audiometric thresholds that are very close to the thresholds obtained by conventional clinical audiometry. The difficulties and limitations of the methods will be described in connection with their use in testing the hearing of children, but the Veterans Administration for a number of years has required an electrodermal test of threshold, at least at 1000 Hz in each ear, as part of the evaluation of claimants for compensation for service-connected hearing loss. If the threshold by either method of physiological audiometry is 10 dB or more better than his behavioral threshold, the subject is suspected of feigning an overlay during the behavioral tests.

The electrodermal response, as used by the Veterans Administration, is one component in the famous battery of the "lie detector" test. This fact is known rather widely, and this knowledge tends to discourage feigning in audiometric tests.

## TESTS OF HEARING
## FOR YOUNG CHILDREN

Most children who are 4 years old or older and some 3-year-olds can be tested by conventional behavioral audiometry. They can be instructed to raise a finger when they hear a tone and to lower it when they do not. The attention span is shorter in young children than in older children, but with encouragement and praise for correct responses 4-year-olds usually give quite reliable end points. Sometimes it requires two testing sessions to obtain complete pure-tone audiograms. The tester must be alert, however, for false positive responses by a child who is anxious to please, and therefore he must carefully avoid falling into a regular rhythm in the presentation of the test tones. It is usually easy to sense when the child understands what is expected of him and is cooperating well.

The real problems in testing the hearing of children arise when the child does not seem to understand or does not wish to cooperate. The children who require special testing methods are those (1) who are too young to understand, (2) who are mentally retarded, (3) who cannot make appropriate responses because of cerebral palsy even though they may hear something, (4) who are emotionally disturbed, (5) who respond only erratically or not at all to any stimuli (so-called "autism" or childhood schizophrenia), or (6) who may suffer from congenital or early acquired hearing loss so severe that they have failed to learn to pay any attention to such sounds as they may be able to hear. As we shall see, it appears to be quite important that children with early hearing impairment be given the benefit of amplified sound during their first two or three years of life in order to avoid this kind of "habitual disregard" of hearing.

The tests that are appropriate for young children may be divided into three classes. Some tests are effective for children of 2 to 4 years who are able and willing to respond. They are really devices to increase the child's motivation and keep him interested in the test. Tests of the second class depend on unconscious inborn reflex responses to sound. These reflex tests are particularly useful from birth to 2 years of age. The third class of test takes advantage of electrical reactions of the brain or the "electrodermal" response of the sweat glands. These are the physiological tests mentioned in the previous section in connection with feigned hearing loss or pseudohypoacusis.

## Methods Based on Increased Motivation

*Play audiometry.* Most children over 2½ years of age who are of normal mentality and without emotional disturbances can be taught to "play a game" with the tester. An auditory signal is used to tell the child that he may put a peg in a pegboard, turn over the leaf of a picture book, or do whatever is likely to interest a child of his age. Loud sounds are used at first until the child understands what he is expected to do; once this is accomplished, a pure-tone audiogram can be obtained. Perhaps the number of frequencies and intensities tested must be restricted or the testing spread over two or more sessions, but if the central processes of being able to attach meaning to a sound and of being able to keep attention concentrated are normal, it is just a matter of time to map out a peripheral hearing loss. The signals need not be pure tones. Valuable information can be obtained from a few clear responses to speech, to broad-band noise, or to the sounds of selected noisemakers. Unfortunately some children are very erratic on this and other tests, and some do not seem to be aware at any intensity of the auditory signals to which we wish them to respond. If the child is mentally retarded or shows negativistic "autistic" behavior, or has neurological difficulties, it may be very difficult to decide whether or not he also has impaired hearing. Such children simply do not learn to play this particular game.

*The peep show.* This test is basically a formalization and standardization of the informal "play-a-game" type of test just discussed. Both types, incidentally, can employ either earphones or an acoustic field. The older the child, the fewer objections to earphones, and with earphones the ears can be tested separately.

In one form of the peep show the child looks into an illuminated box at a picture. Then the light goes out. When a small signal light goes on the child can illuminate the box again and see a new picture by pushing a button, but he must wait until the signal light goes on. When he has mastered the idea, which most children over 3 years do quite easily, an auditory signal, usually a rather loud pure tone, is sounded along with the signal light. After several combined trials the signal light is omitted. If the child responds correctly by pushing the button when the tone is sounded alone, he obviously "hears" usefully, and his hearing can be mapped out in the same way that it is by the play-a-game method.

The numerical results and their significance are practically identical for these two methods. In each the consistency of response and the ability of the child to understand what he is expected to do are as important for interpretation as the hearing levels in decibels.

The peep-show type of test, and there are many variations, was obviously inspired by the concept of the conditioned reflex. The subject responds correctly to a stimulus and receives a reward, like a monkey or rat pressing a lever for food. It has been customary to speak of "conditioning" the child and to describe a failure of the test by saying that the child "failed to condition." The same vocabulary is often applied to play-a-game audiometry in order to preserve an objective attitude and not seem to draw inferences as to "understanding" or "insight."

The peep show has gradually declined in popularity during the last decade. Most clinics now rely chiefly on play audiometry and on the reflex, startle, and orienting responses described in the next section.

### Physiological Audiometry for Children

The following tests, including those using electrical responses, are sometimes called "objective" audiometry because they do not require a subjective judgment or decision by the child. We prefer the term "physiological audiometry."

The simplest variety of physiological test depends on simple inborn reflexes such as startle, waking from sleep, blinking (the auropalpebral reflex), or looking toward the source of sound (the orienting reflex). For these responses the child does not need to be "conditioned." The tests are appropriate for young babies, and they will be considered in the order of the age at which they are most effective.

Reflex tests are given in an open acoustic field, and only the orienting reflex makes any differentiation as to which ear may be most severely impaired. The reflex tests are relatively crude with respect to both frequency and intensity, but they are very useful indeed as screening methods to identify the babies who need follow-up tests and perhaps the immediate special management discussed in Chapter 16.

*Startle reactions.* The earliest startle response to a loud sudden sound is present at full-term birth and in many premature infants. At this stage it is known as the "Moro reflex," and consists of over-all movements of face, body, and limbs, and strong closing of the eyes. The full classical picture of the Moro reflex fades out during the first weeks of life, but clearly defined movements, blinking or grimacing, often with some turning toward the side from which the sound comes, persist and are the best reflex indicators of hearing up to the age of "play audiometry."

Considerable attention has been given to the best type of sounds with which to elicit startle reactions or orienting (turning) reactions. Sudden sounds are more effective than those with gradual onset. Any particular sound may elicit a clear startle response on the first one or two trials but then become ineffective. (The popular word here is "habituation.") Many audiologists believe that familiar sounds are more effective than unfamiliar sounds and that noises are more effective than pure tones. Much work has been devoted to selecting the best battery of noisemakers, such as "clackers," rustling paper, squeaking dolls, spoon-hitting-cup, and so on, and to standardize their intensity in order to gain the most information on the character and severity of the hearing impairment. We shall not attempt to summarize these efforts. Perhaps more attention should be given to narrow-band or "peaked-spectrum" noise. Noise seems to be clearly more effective than pure tones in eliciting reflex responses from infants or awakening them from sleep.

*Other reactions.* Many tests of hearing for neonates and young infants are essentially screening tests. In this context any movement of the body, or of a limb, or the face that seems clearly correlated with the stimulus may be used as an indicator. A change in the breathing rhythm or a momentary pause if the child is crying are among the many reactions to a sudden noise.

*Awakening from sleep.* Awakening from sleep is another well-defined response, particularly useful for neonates. Here there seems to be some preference for a high-frequency pure tone, usually 3000 Hz, or for white noise delivered from a small loudspeaker held by hand close to the child at one or two standard sound-pressure levels. The lower level is intended to be one which will awaken an infant with normal hearing within one minute. Failure to wake does not prove a hearing loss, but it does indicate the necessity for further trials or careful observation by parents in the home surroundings. It is sometimes difficult to control the depth of sleep of the infant under test.

An infant who awakens in response to a loud noise does not necessarily have normal hearing. Particularly deceptive in this respect are children who have fairly good hearing for very high tones or very low tones, or both, but poor hearing for the important speech frequencies. They may respond to many everyday noises and to voice sounds but not hear well enough to learn speech and language spontaneously. Reflex audiometry has many pitfalls.

*Orienting reaction.* More informative than simple awakening from sleep or a startle reaction to a sudden noise is the reflex turning of the head and perhaps the body also toward the side from which a new sound comes. This orienting response is usually well developed by six months when the child is able to sit on its mother's lap. It gradually becomes less clear after the first birthday and finally becomes submerged in general spontaneous movements and exploratory reactions. A skillful team can make a very good assessment of hearing on the basis of head-turning in response to noisemakers of various sorts, but great care must be taken to first attract the child's attention in the proper direction (forward), but not to attract it too much, and to avoid unwanted visual clues or air currents. Of course the simuli can be delivered by loudspeakers and can be standardized or calibrated in various ways. There are many variations on this theme and many different choices as to the best noisemakers, but the key to success is careful handling of the child and well-planned presentation of the stimuli, and above all careful observation. Habituation to sounds that were originally interesting presents one of the greatest difficulties.

Orienting reflexes are probably the best single method of reflex audiometry, and they have the advantage that they are at their best in the critical period from 6 to 12 months of age, when identification and approximate assessment of impaired hearing is so important.

A test based on conditioning a *visual* orienting response is closely related to the peep show (Suzuki and Ogiba). A strange visual stimulus, such as an illuminated doll, is presented to one side or the other of the child. The child looks toward the doll. This simple visual orienting response is now conditioned to a pure tone, as will be described below for the electrodermal response. As long as the tone is above threshold, the child turns his head *before* the doll is illuminated. This method is very simple and is one of the most reliable for children from 1 to 3 years old.

## Electrophysiological Tests of Hearing

Simple observation of children's behavior, supplemented by reflex audiometry, can be very effective in identifying for closer attention and study the young children with impaired hearing, but nevertheless it is common for the first recognition of impairment to be the failure of the child to learn to talk by the usual age of 18 to 24 months. In any case, and particularly if there are complicating circumstances such as possible mental retardation, cerebral palsy, emotional disturbance, and so on, there is need for a more definitive test of hearing suitable for children of all ages and particularly from 6 months to 3 years. The most successful definitive tests so far are three electrophysiological tests. All of them require fairly elaborate and rather expensive equipment, and they should be considered as final tests to be used in major hearing clinics—not as screening methods.

### Electrodermal Audiometry

The first electrophysiological method to be perfected is known as electrodermal audiometry (EDA). The response that is recorded is sometimes called the "skin galvanic response" or the "psychogalvanic skin response" (PGSR). The response is an activation of the sweat glands through the autonomic nervous system. It is detected by measuring the resulting change in electrical resistance (the Féré effect) or electrical potential (the Tarchanoff effect), or both, usually between the palm and the back of the hand. Usually it is the change of resistance that is detected. This requires the use of an external

source of current. Electrically the subject's hand constitutes part of one arm of a Wheatstone bridge. The bridge is balanced and then any change in the resistance of the subject is recorded by a pen on a moving strip of paper. Another pen indicates when electric shocks, sounds, or other stimuli are given.

The electrodermal response occurs normally in response to any painful stimulus, and it forms part of the pattern of many emotional reactions, and as such has been studied exhaustively both from the physiological and the psychological point of view. A very loud, unexpected sound may elicit the response, but a mild electric shock is a much more effective and reliable stimulus. The response does tend to habituate, however, meaning that repeated stimuli become less and less effective, and the response seems to represent an alerting or "orienting" reaction rather than a classical simple stable inborn visceral reflex.

The electrodermal response is made useful for audiometry by forming a conditioned reflex with sound (the audiometric test tone) as the conditioned stimulus. The conditioning shocks are applied through separate electrodes, either to the opposite forearm or to a leg. The first shocks are mild, but they are gradually strengthened until each shock elicits a clear electrodermal response. Sometimes the shocks must be made annoyingly uncomfortable and even painful. Tones are sounded from time to time, and shocks are given following some or all of them. The best interval between tone and shock is 0.6 sec. With some subjects it is sufficient merely to sound the tone without using any shock. Perhaps they already fear a shock, or perhaps they are sufficiently interested or startled by the sound to respond to it for its own sake. Usually, however, the acoustic signal must be combined with the shock in order to make it effective in bringing out an electrodermal response.

Some subjects respond very consistently

and clearly to the test tones, and by simply observing whether or not an electrodermal response appears at the proper interval after the beginning of the stimulus, that is, in about two seconds, we can, in principle, map out the audiogram of the subject. It helps if we reinforce the tones from time to time by giving the electric shock as well. In fact, one of the practical limitations of the test is the tendency of the response to "run down" (extinction). It gets smaller and occurs less frequently with repeated trials in spite of occasional reinforcement, and the strength of the shock usually has to be increased to keep a good conditioned response to the tones.

With sensitive subjects who respond consistently, the threshold of hearing can be mapped out with as great precision by electrodermal audiometry (EDA) as by the usual behavioral methods of clinical pure-tone audiometry, and the absolute thresholds by the two methods may be within a few decibels of each other. The theoretical advantage of this type of test is that it does not involve conscious response to the tones. The inference is that it should still be suitable for testing children (or adults) who cannot or will not respond voluntarily in conventional behavioral audiometry. No complicated process of concept formation, understanding what is wanted, or cooperating is involved. It is apparently a simple, straightforward conditioned-reflex test in the Pavlovian tradition.

The electrodermal response has been employed in several hearing clinics with rather considerable success. In favorable cases it gives quite definite and very useful information, and positive results obtained by this method are of great value. The difficulty comes in interpreting the failures of response. It is unfortunately true, although not generally known, that many normal individuals fail completely to establish the desired association between the auditory signal and the electrodermal response. In fact, some of them give very poor electro-dermal responses in the first place. Also, some individuals lose their conditioned associations very rapidly, and others may be quite erratic in their responses, sometimes responding and sometimes not to the same intensity of auditory signal. In others the base line is unsteady even without auditory stimulation, and it requires skill and experience as well as close attention to the proper latent period of response to identify the responses to the tone signals. And, most unfortunate of all, it appears that the very children who are uncertain and erratic in their responses to the peep-show or the "play-the-game" testing are the ones who are most likely to be erratic in their electrodermal responses.

In summary we repeat that EDA, as just described, is a very valuable method in expert hands, both as a test for children for educational assessment and as a test for possible feigning in adults, but it is neither infallible nor foolproof. A positive response means that the sound has stimulated the ear successfully, and the nerve impulses have reached at least the brain stem and have triggered off a response in the autonomic nervous system. Failure to respond, however, does not prove that there is a peripheral hearing loss.

The EDA test is objective in the sense that no voluntary conscious response is required from the subject. The tester, however, may find it difficult to decide whether a given deflection of the pen is actually an electrodermal response or not. It is possible to set up an elaborate system of labeling and coding the record of the resistance changes and judging them later as a group to be sure that the same criteria are used throughout the test and that the tester is not influenced by knowing whether the stimulus was weak or strong or whether the subject moved or cried in anticipation of a shock. Many testers prefer to make full use of all clues and behavior, as in the simple startle test, and try to decide whether the subject heard the tone, not whether his

EDR response was recognizable. This more liberal policy is good clinical practice.

Electrodermal audiometry enjoyed a period of considerable popularity, and a convenient instrument was developed and made available commercially; but now, because of its various difficulties, uncertainties, and limitations, it is falling into disfavor for use with children. It is not suitable for young children in any case because of the disturbing effect of the electric shocks. It cannot be applied during sleep, and drugs (even mild tranquilizers) seem to reduce the responses and interfere with the necessary conditioning.

## Electroencephalic Audiometry (EEA)

Another form of electrophysiological audiometry is *electroencephalic audiometry* (EEA). The brain is continually active, and in its activity it generates electric potentials like those in nerves and muscles. These potentials can be recorded by placing electrodes on a nerve or a muscle, or even in the general neighborhood of a nerve or muscle if the original signals are strong enough. The electrocardiogram is a familiar example of the distant recording of the electrical activity of a muscle, in this case the heart. The electroencephalogram (EEG) is to the brain what the electrocardiogram is to the heart. The electric potentials generated by the brain are strong enough to be detected by electrodes placed on the outside of the skull and even on the outside of the scalp. The potentials must be amplified, but the final patterns can be recorded by pens on a moving paper very much as the electrocardiogram or the electrodermogram is recorded.

The brain is continually active, and the pattern of electrical changes shows very well whether the subject is awake or asleep, and whether his eyes are opened or closed. Features of the pattern also depend on whether he is relaxed or very tense and anxious, whether he is a baby, a child, or an

adult, and a number of other factors. The record of an adult or of an older child is usually dominated by a surprisingly rhythmic series of waves at about ten a second, known as the Berger or alpha rhythm. These waves are strongest in the part of the brain (in the back of the head) that is associated with vision and are particularly sensitive to the degree of arousal, to whether the eyes are busy looking at something or whether they are closed, and to mild startle or other emotional reactions. The reduction or "blocking" of the alpha rhythm as a result of sound stimulation is called an electroencephalic response (EER). A number of efforts have been made to use EER in audiometry, either without conditioning or with conditioning by association with flashes of light or other independently effective stimuli.

It so happens that the change in the EEG pattern between waking and sleeping is a rather striking one and, furthermore, that a person who is lightly asleep shows rather dramatic transient changes in his EEG pattern (the "K-complex" and other changes) in response to sounds. The changes are in the direction of waking up, although the subject usually does not fully awaken but sinks back to the previous level of sleep. The K-complex and other electroencephalic responses do not have to be learned. They are inborn patterns just like the electrodermal response to electric shocks.

The recognition of EER to measured auditory stimuli in sleep seemed to be a very promising tool for physiological audiometry. It has been explored rather systematically. Many of the original hopes have been dissipated, but electroencephalic audiometry (EEA) has proved to be of considerable value nevertheless, especially when the patient is tested asleep. Actually, one of the limitations of EEA is the same as for EDA. The greatest difficulty is that people do not give a recognizable EER to *every* sound that reaches them while they are asleep, and the more frequently a given sound is repeated, the less likely is it to produce a reaction. Conditioning of EER to an annoying stimulus such as a shock is out of the question if the patient is to remain asleep. For another thing, the fluctuations of the EEG during sleep are many and complicated, so that it may be difficult to distinguish a response to a particular signal from a spontaneous change in the EEG pattern. Some subjects react very consistently, and their audiograms can be mapped either by blocking of the alpha rhythm while they are awake or by detecting K-complexes while they are asleep. Even so, the identification of K-complexes in a rapidly moving and changing record is a really difficult task for the tester. Objective procedures such as described for EDA, however, enable a person with no previous EEG experience to make a relatively accurate analysis of responses *after the test is completed* and if he has plenty of time to study each segment of the record.

There is a distinct advantage for EEA over EDA in that electroencephalic responsiveness is not limited by age. Consistent EDRs are difficult to elicit from very young children (three years and under) but EERs seem to occur as frequently in these young children as they do in older children or adults. A child is more easily controlled in EEA than in EDA. The entire EEA, from placement of electrodes and auditory stimulation to removal of electrodes, can be completed while a child is asleep. Mild sedation to induce sleep does not significantly reduce responsiveness. In EDA the child is conscious of the wires and phones and is disturbed by the annoying shock, and the resulting agitation frequently makes testing impossible. Sedation to calm the child unfortunately reduces electrodermal responses drastically.

### Electric Response Audiometry (ERA)

*Electric response audiometry* is a special form of electroencephalic audiometry.

The responses that are observed are electrical responses of the cerebral cortex which are imbedded in the electroencephalogram. Actually the K-complexes mentioned above that are seen in certain stages of sleep are electric responses, but in the waking state the responses are much smaller, and in order to make them visible, additional special equipment is necessary. On the other hand, except for children less than 18 months of age and a few older ones who are unruly, electric response audiometry does not require putting the child to sleep. With the child awake ERA is much simpler

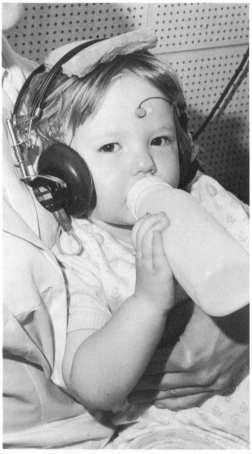

Fig. 8-7. Evoked response audiometry. The child, held by its mother, wears standard earphones. The electrode on the forehead is the ground lead. The "active" electrode is under the sponge rubber pad and the reference electrode is behind the right ear. (*Central Institute for the Deaf, photo by Harold Ferman*)

and quicker than conventional EEG audiometry. It is therefore described here as a third distinct variety of electrophysiological audiometry. It is often called *evoked-response audiometry,* but here the word evoked is redundant and electric is more informative.

The special equipment that is required for ERA is an *average-response computer* and the control circuits that are needed to synchronize the computer with the delivery of audiometric test tones. Some of the instruments that have been employed in the laboratory are fairly elaborate digital computers; others are somewhat simpler but still quite sophisticated analogue computers. All of them collect and combine in their memories the electrical activity following many similar stimuli. Some instruments do not *average* the responses in the strict sense of the word but simply *sum* them, exactly or approximately.

Averaging or summing is needed because the desired responses are almost always too small to be recognized in the raw electroencephalogram. They are obscured or masked by the spontaneous EEG activity. But this background activity is irregular and nearly random in its pattern, and if many samples are added together the negative waves tend to cancel the positive waves. Thus the average tends toward zero. On the other hand any time-locked pattern of activity that follows each stimulus will add up progressively. The result is an improvement of the signal-to-noise ratio, and a characteristic response pattern emerges clearly from the background of random activity.

Until very recently the rather slow response that is employed in ERA was interpreted as a diffuse response, generated over a large area of the frontal and parietal lobes and presumably activated by way of the reticular formation. Certainly the response in question is best detected by an electrode placed at the top of the head, that is, at the

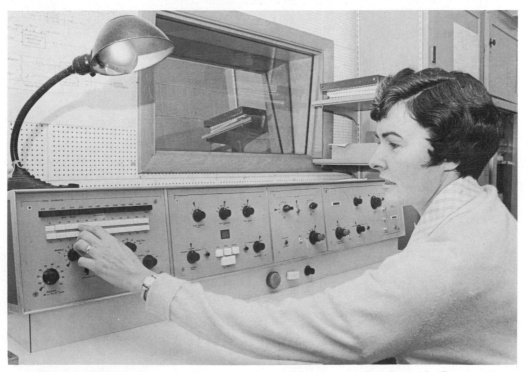

Fig. 8-8. Evoked response audiometer system (Princeton Applied Research Corp.). The operator is selecting the test tone. The records shown in Fig. 8-9 were obtained with this instrument at Central Institute for the Deaf. (*Photo courtesy St. Louis Post-Dispatch*)

"vertex," with reference electrodes on the ear lobes. For this reason it is often called the vertex potential or "V potential." Electrodes in this position record responses that are very similar for auditory and tactile stimuli and rather similar for visual stimulation.

The tactile and visual responses are most efficiently recorded if the "active" electrode is placed directly over the appropriate part of the primary somatosensory or visual projection area respectively. In these positions a series of early responses of the cortex, with latencies to peak of 50 msec or less, can also be observed. An electrode over the Sylvian fissure, where the auditory projection area is located, detects auditory responses very poorly, both the fast and the slow. The orientation of the auditory area, on the superior surface of the temporal lobe and perpendicular to the surface of the skull, is unfavorable for a recording electrode placed directly over it, but it favors the appearance of a potential difference between the top of the head (vertex) and the base of the skull (ear lobes,

mastoid or high postauricular area). Fortunately the electrode position that is most favorable for auditory responses also tends to minimize electrical artifacts due to eyeblinks or muscle potentials.

The pattern of the auditory V-potential response is a series of waves of progressively longer wavelength. The latency to peak of the first really clear (vertex-negative or $N_1$) wave is about 100 msec, the second peak (vertex-positive or $P_2$) is about 180 msec, and the third (vertexnegative or $N_2$) is about 300 to 400 msec (see Figure 8-9). (The tactile and particularly the visual latencies are a little longer.) The $N_1$-$P_2$ wave is the most stable and the easiest to recognize in most adults; the $P_2$-$N_2$ combination is sometimes more prominent, particularly in young children and in sleep. Actually the K-complex seems to be a member of the V-potential family with the $N_1$ and perhaps $P_2$ reduced and the later waves slowed and magnified by the sleep state.

The audiometric signals used in ERA are pulsed tones of perhaps 200 msec duration

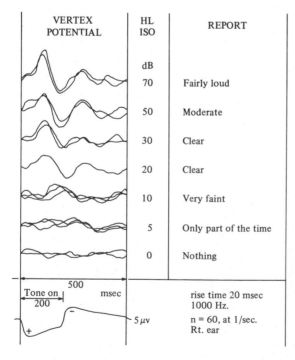

| VERTEX POTENTIAL | HL ISO | REPORT |
|---|---|---|
| | dB | |
| | 70 | Fairly loud |
| | 50 | Moderate |
| | 30 | Clear |
| | 20 | Clear |
| | 10 | Very faint |
| | 5 | Only part of the time |
| | 0 | Nothing |

Tone on | 500 msec
200

rise time 20 msec
1000 Hz.

5 μv

n = 60, at 1/sec.
Rt. ear

Fig. 8-9. The form, amplitude, and latency of the vertex (V) potential in response to 1000 Hz tone bursts at various hearing levels are shown in the tracings in the left column. The corresponding reports of the subjects are given on the right. The subject, an adult and a practiced listener with wellformed V potentials, was reading and paying no special attention to the audiometric signals except at the 5 and 0 dB hearing levels. For these she stopped reading and listened. Two or three trials were made at most of the hearing levels. Her reports were very consistent, and from them her behavioral audiometric threshold was estimated at 5 dB ISO.

Note the very slight reduction in amplitude of the V potential, its constant latency from 70 to 20 dB, and the rapid fall in amplitude and prolongation of latency from 20 to 5 dB. Duration of the tone bursts, time constants of the equipment, and so on, are shown by the calibration tracing at the bottom. (*Test conducted with a Princton Aplied Research evoked response audiometer, Model 140.*)

and 10 or 20 msec rise times. They are delivered either by earphones or, for infants, by loudspeaker. Actually the V potential is an "on" effect, and only the first 30 msec or so of each tone burst is really important. The pulses must not follow one another too rapidly. Intervals of 10 seconds or more are needed for maximum amplitude of response, and the responses become very small if the interval is less than half a second. The most efficient rates to get the largest summed response within a minute is one per second if the subject is awake, one every 2 seconds if he is asleep. Usually a total of from 50 to 70 responses are summed or averaged.

The equipment for electrical amplification of the ERA responses is exactly the same as for conventional EEG audiometry, and during the collection of the responses an EEG tape, moving slowly, provides a monitor to warn of excessive movement or other artifact. One commercially available ERA instrument writes out, through a second pen on the same tape, the cumulative total from the memory simultaneously with the addition of each new response. With the tape moving slowly only the amplitude of the response can be observed, but the tape is automatically speeded up just before the collection is complete. This gives a graphic record on an expanded time scale. Other methods of write-out are possible, but it is important both to see the average response immediately "on line," in order to decide what stimulus to use next, and also to have a permanent write-out. It is convenient to cut each sample, properly labeled, from the tape for later comparison with other responses. Small responses near threshold are identified by similarity of form and a slight prolongation of latency.

One difficulty with the method is that there are individual variations in the V potential, in voltage, latency, and wave form. Therefore a large clear "guide response" from a strong suprathreshold stimulus is very helpful if it can be obtained. A good

substitute is the response to a vibratory stimulus applied to the hand. The identification of responses near threshold is difficult if the subject has a low-voltage response with a poorly formed $N_1$ wave and at the same time a high-voltage background EEG.

A practical problem is to induce young children to hold still long enough for the collection of enough averaged responses. Adults or older children are allowed to read material of their choice. Younger children are amused by pictures, puppets, and a variety of toys appropriate to their age. An assistant skilled in the art of amusing children is an essential member of an ERA team. Very young children may be sedated with any of several drugs or tranquilizers and tested during sleep. Unfortunately, however, the responses are strong only in deep sleep and not in the drowsy or transition stage or in light sleep.

Experience is necessary, both for the administration of the test and for the identification of the responses, but with experience it is possible to detect children's electric responses at levels that correspond very well with those of behavioral finger or play-a-game audiometry. Part of the art here is to interpolate an estimated ER threshold between the level at which a clear response is obtained and one at which no response appears.

The over-all duration of the test is limited by the ability of the subject to sit reasonably still long enough. Even with one or two breaks for free movement, one hour under test or an hour and a half entrance-to-exit is the practical limit. This means that less than 30, and with young children less than 20, average responses can be obtained. It is advisable, therefore, to test the frequencies 250, 1000, and 3000 Hz in each ear first and then 500 Hz if time allows. The stimuli are presented first at what is expected to be a comfortably loud level, then increased or decreased in steps of 15 or 20 dB until the threshold has been bracketed.

The physiological significance of the evoked cortical V potentials is not known. The potentials do seem to be generated by the primary projection areas and perhaps also by the immediately adjacent areas, and their presence implies integrity of the entire pathway through the thalamus from sense organ to cortex. We may hope that, with further understanding, they may help us to evaluate brain injuries, congenital defects, and so forth, but as yet this is not possible.

Electric response audiometry is still (1968) in its infancy, but already it seems superior to both EDA and conventional EEA. It is unfortunate that the equipment is rather expensive, but it may be justified for major hospitals or hearing centers to provide a definitive test for difficult cases, notably for young children. It is also very helpful when feigning is suspected or to test hearing when mental retardation, autism, or multiple handicaps make other forms of audiometry uncertain or impossible.

## OTONEUROLOGY

In Chapters 3 and 4 we have discussed certain aspects of the functions of the central nervous system and its disorders, particularly as they relate to the auditory system. Here, under the title of otoneurology, we consider how certain tests that reveal abnormalities of auditory function may assist the neurologist or neurosurgeon toward a diagnosis or the localization of a lesion. The audiologist already renders this help to the otologist. We shall see, however, that his help to the neurologist and neurosurgeon is much more limited. The question for the audiologist or otologist is most often whether a demonstrated impairment of auditory function is adequately explained on the basis of sensory-neural impairment or whether a central impairment is indicated. On the other hand inter-

est in otoneurology is high, and in the future some audiological tests may be developed that have clearer diagnostic significance than those now available. Tests of labyrinthine function (caloric tests) through their relation to the ocular system (nystagmus) are much more advanced and useful in this respect than auditory tests.

### Aphasia

We shall not be concerned with the disturbances of the language function that are caused by certain lesions of the cerebral cortex. The impairment is a disturbance of the ability to communicate by speech, and it is related to injury of certain areas of the cerebral hemisphere that are "dominant" for speech, usually the left hemisphere (see Chapter 4). The impairment of function is obvious although its exact description may be difficult. The neurosurgeon tries to avoid as far as possible any injury to the "speech areas" in the dominant hemisphere. Our present point is that the audiologist has little to offer in the diagnosis or description of aphasia. The sensitivity for pure tones is normal or nearly so, not only in aphasia but in lesions of the cerebral cortex in general, as long as the patient can understand and respond adequately to the test.

We have discussed also in Chapter 4 the condition that has been called "congenital aphasia" and have pointed out that the condition is better described as a language disability or, better, a difficulty in learning language. We suggested the term "dysmathia" (difficulty in learning) or "dyslogomathia" (difficulty in learning language) as more appropriate terms. The reason for the difficulty in learning is not necessarily an organic brain lesion. The audiogram may be within normal limits, or it may show moderate or severe hearing loss. Such loss is due to peripheral organic impairment, usually in the inner ear, and not to any abnormality of the central nervous system. This situation reveals the complexity of problems of the central nervous system—to distinguish the organic from developmental, and from strictly functional or psychological difficulties, and to separate these from peripheral impairments that may also be present. The latter may seriously limit the input to the central nervous system and therefore its performance. In this situation it is probably best to think of a difficulty in *hearing,* which is an audiological problem, and a second difficulty in *understanding* or in *learning,* which is not.

### Tests for Brain-stem Lesions

Within the cranial cavity we shall subdivide the auditory system into only three parts: the auditory nerve, the brain stem, and the cerebral hemispheres or cortex. Some day we should be able to subdivide the brain stem into thalamic and infrathalamic levels, but we cannot do so usefully at present in terms of test results.

In general the disturbances of the brain stem rather resemble those of sense organ and nerve and may be explored by quite similar tests. For example a test of the change of threshold for a brief tone as a function of its duration has been proposed. We know that the normal ear becomes less sensitive by some 10 dB as the duration is reduced from 200 msec to 10 msec. Theoretically we believe that the "temporal integration" of loudness takes place in the brain stem, probably in or not far above the cochlear nucleus. So far clinical experience has not supported this prediction very well as the integration seems to be disturbed by Menière's disease but not by acoustic neuromas. This type of test may well be developed usefully in the future.

We must expect that the effects of brain-stem lesions will not be clearly predictable and will often be quite bizarre. This very feature may distinguish lesions of such a small, compact, but complicated piece of nervous tissue in which so many neurophysiological functions are carried out.

The first interaction between the inputs to right and left ears takes place low in the brain stem (see Figure 3-18). Such an interaction must be the basis for *lateralization* of the source of sound. Studies of the disturbance of this function have been carried out, but we shall not describe details or attempt to evaluate them.

Another binaural effect is the *masking level difference.* A pure tone between about 200 and 500 Hz or speech is presented to both ears simultaneously, mixed with masking noise. The masked threshold varies, depending on whether the tones in the two ears and also the noise in the two ears are in phase or out of phase with each other. With a certain combination of phases a masking level difference of as much as 15 dB can be produced by simply reversing the phase in one ear of the tone or of the masker. A test of brain-stem function based on this phenomenon has been tried, but the results reported so far with patients are difficult to interpret. Here, as with all other diagnostic tests, it is important to have trials on a large number of verified cases of relevant clinical conditions and a high correlation between the test results and the established diagnoses. A theoretical prediction that a particular result should be obtained is not enough.

### Tests for Auditory Cortical Function

In animal experiments the removal of the entire auditory cortex bilaterally causes two clear deficits. One is the inability to form a conditioned reflex (learn) to respond to a particular *sequence* of tones of different frequency. The deficit is in the temporal frame of reference and seems to involve short-term memory. The other defect is an inability to be guided by the *position* of a sound source. Here the animal does not move until the sound has ceased.

Short-term memory and perhaps the frame of reference of auditory space are apparently disturbed here also. These phenomena should suggest possible auditory tests of cortical function, but none such is now available.

By far the most revealing and successful tests of human cortical auditory function are based on modifications of speech audiometry. The recognition of speech, which is learned and not inborn, has a large cortical component. On the other hand good speech is quite redundant, and a word spoken poorly or heard incompletely may still be recognized quite effectively, particularly if the number of possible choices, that is, the vocabulary, is small.

The most sensitive tests for cortical impairment are not the monosyllabic words, although they too are useful, but garbled or *filtered speech* or *speech in noise*. The task which is difficult for the normal listener becomes extremely difficult or impossible for the impaired listener. A very effective way of modifying speech is to pass it through a low-pass filter with the cutoff at about 1200 Hz. Another is to mix it with either white noise or with a babble of other voices or with a competing message. All of these require a synthesis of a whole word or sentence from fragments. The task requires a good short-term memory and also nimbleness of wit.

Still another form of stress is to *speed up speech* by methods that systematically eliminate small bits from a recorded sample, not only shortening the pauses but the vowels and other sustained phonemes as well. This method preserves the original pitch of the sounds, and a doubling of the usual speed of talk does not usually reduce intelligibility.

It is no accident that the several types of stress that we have mentioned are exactly those that proverbially plague the elderly. Failure to discriminate speech in noise or in multiple conversation or to follow rapid speech are characteristic of the central-nervous-system component of presbycusis. When severe enough to affect word intelligibility in the quiet, it is "phonemic regression." But senile changes affect all parts of the brain, and no problem of localization is involved.

*Unilateral cortical lesions* that affect hearing do follow one important general rule. *The performance on any test by modified speech is worse when the material is presented to the ear opposite the affected hemisphere.* Of course it is assumed that the ears are normal or at least symmetrical by simple audiometric tests. Pure-tone thresholds and speech thresholds are *not* affected by the cortical lesion. The PB max *may* be relatively reduced for the contralateral ear, even without garbling or noise.

Note that in the above generalization the brain is symmetrical. There is no suggestion of a dominant left hemisphere. The task of simple *recognition* of words is evidently quite different from the *language* function that is impaired in aphasia. Also, even after hemispherectomy the contralateral ear does not become deaf. This is undoubtedly due to the rich crossing of auditory pathways in the brain stem.

Another interesting modification of speech is to give part of the input to one ear, part to the other. In this case the brain must integrate the inputs. Perhaps one ear receives high-pass the other low-pass filtered speech. Perhaps alternate samples of various duration (from a tenth of a second upward) are given first to the right and next to the left ear. Still another is to overlap spondee words in the two ears so that the first syllable to the right ear comes at the same time as the second syllable of the word to the left ear, or vice versa. This is called the *staggered spondaic word* (*SSW*) *test*.

All of these tests have shown promise, but none are fully standardized and validated. Validation will be slow because suitable cases for test with proved lesions that are both sufficiently extensive and sufficiently discrete are rather exceptional, and the number per year in any one clinic is small. We have, therefore, simply mentioned several types of test that seem to hold good promise for successful valida-tion. We must note, however, the credit due to two Italian otologists, E. Bocca and C. Calearo, who about 1955 pointed out clearly the possibilities of modified speech audiometry and stimulated much of the subsequent activity in this area.

## SUGGESTED READINGS AND REFERENCES

**Bocca, E., and C. Calearo.** "Central Hearing Processes," in *Modern Developments in Audiology* (J. Jerger, ed.). New York: Academic Press, Inc., 1963.
A useful review of speech tests in otoneurology from the point of view of the Italian innovators.

**Davis, H., S. K. Hirsh, J. Shelnutt, and C. Bowers.** "Further Validation of Evoked Response Audiometry (ERA)," *J. Speech Hearing Res.,* 10:717–732 (1967).

——— **(ed.).** "The Young Deaf Child: Identification and Management." *Acta Otolaryng. (Stockholm)*, Supplement 206 (1965).
Proceedings of a conference held in Toronto, Canada, on 8–9 October, 1964. (Organized by Percy E. Ireland.) Includes a survey and assessment of both screening and definitive tests of hearing in young children.

**Glorig, A. (ed.).** *Audiometry: Principles and Practices.* Baltimore: The Williams & Wilkins Company, 1965.
A useful volume but the multiple authorship reduces its effectiveness as a reference book for "how to do it."

**Jerger, J. (ed.).** *Modern Developments in Audiology.* New York: Academic Press, Inc., 1963.
The chapter titles and authors are:
1. "The Measurement of Hearing by Bone Conduction," R. F. Naunton
2. "Automatic Audiometry," W. Rudmose
3. "Functional Hearing Loss," J. B. Chaiklin and I. M. Ventry
4. "Measurement of Hearing in Children," D. R. Frisina
5. "Electrophysiologic Audiometry," R. Goldstein
6. "Middle-ear Muscle Reflexes in Man," O. Jepsen
7. "Auditory Fatigue and Masking," W. D. Ward
8. "Auditory Adaptation," A. M. Small, Jr.
9. "Central Hearing Processes," E. Bocca and C. Calearo
10. "The Theory of Signal Detectability and the Measurement of Hearing," F. R. Clarke and R. C. Bilger
11. "Research Frontiers in Audiology," J. D. Harris
Many of these chapters are excellent, and all are pertinent.

————, and T. Tillman. "A New Method for the Clinical Determination of Sensori-neural Acuity Level (SAL)," *Arch. Otolaryng. (Stockholm)*, 71:948 (1960).

Katz, J. "The SSW Test: An Interim Report," *J. Speech Hearing Dis.*, 33:132–146 (1968).
  Some details of experience with the staggered spondaic word test.

————, R. A. Basil, and J. M. Smith. "A Staggered Spondaic Word Test for Detecting Central Auditory Lesions," *Ann. Otol.*, 72:908–918 (1963).
  This is the original description of this test.

O'Neill, J. J., and H. J. Oyer. *Applied Audiometry.* New York: Dodd, Mead & Company, Inc., 1966.
  Up to date, well organized, well written and illustrated; probably the best available reference book for technical details of audiometric tests.

Ventry, I. M., and J. B. Chaiklin (eds.). "Multidiscipline Study of Functional Hearing Loss," *J. Aud. Res.*, 5:179–262 (1965).
  This will probably be the classic in its field for many years.

Zwislocki, J. "Acoustic Measurement of the Middle-ear Function," *Ann. Otol.*, 70: 599–606 (1961).
  The article is a clear statement of the principles involved in measurements based on acoustic impedance. Illustrative reactance curves are given for otosclerosis, for stapes mobilization, for interrupted ossicular chain, and so on.

# CHAPTER 9

## HEARING HANDICAP, STANDARDS FOR HEARING, AND MEDICOLEGAL RULES

### HALLOWELL DAVIS, M.D.

**AUDIOMETRIC EVALUATION**

Audiometry serves two major purposes that are quite different from one another. One of these is to assist in medical diagnosis. Here the pure-tone audiometer is the first instrument of choice. It is highly analytical, and the relations of hearing sensitivity to frequency that it reveals are often of considerable diagnostic significance. This has been discussed in Chapters 4 and 7, and various other diagnostic tests were reviewed in Chapter 8.

The other major purpose of audiometry is to assess the hearing of an individual in relation to the requirements of everyday life, of special tasks or occupations, or of his education. For such assessment it is very desirable to rate the individual in terms of a single number and to write various rules, standards, and requirements in such terms. Speech audiometry yields such a single number, namely, the speech reception threshold, which is very closely related to hearing handicap, and we shall see that most of the rules and standards

are in principle related to or derived from the threshold for speech. We shall also see that the difficulties of standardizing speech audiometry have led to the practice of estimating the threshold for speech by calculating the average pure-tone hearing-threshold level for what we shall call the "central speech frequencies," namely 500, 1000, and 2000 Hz. The assessment of handicap or of everyday hearing ability by rules based on this single measure is very satisfactory for individuals who have reasonably flat audiograms and no special problems of poor discrimination for speech. In short, it is very satisfactory for the majority of individuals, for statistical surveys, and for general standards and regulations. No single number or simple rule can suffice, however, for the exceptional cases of steep audiograms, or of sense organ or central dysacusis.

**MILITARY, ECONOMIC, AND SOCIAL COMPETENCE**

In 1949 a very broad scale of hearing was prepared by the Committee on Hearing of the National Research Council for possible incorporation in a set of physical standards appropriate to the peacetime needs of the Army and the Navy, to partial mobilization, or to total mobilization. The general principles of this broad original scale are reflected in the more recent and more detailed military standards.

In 1965 the Committee on Conservation of Hearing of the American Academy of Ophthalmology and Otolaryngology published a "Guide for the Classification and Evaluation of Hearing Handicap" which contains this scale in slightly modified form and expressed in terms of the ISO audiometric reference zero level. We quote the first two sections of that Guide, including the table that gives the classes of hearing handicap.

### INTRODUCTION
(References, at end of chapter, 2.1 through 2.6 and 3.1 through 3.5)

During the past several years the Committee on Conservation of Hearing has from time to time issued recommendations and approved for publication several articles dealing with the classification of hearing handicaps, the evaluation of hearing impairment, and the International Standard Audiometric Zero Level. These topics are interrelated and now, with the widespread adoption of the new International Reference Zero Level for Pure-Tone Audiometers, it becomes appropriate to restate and combine the recommendations and explanations with particular attention to the implications of the new audiometric scale.

### CLASSES OF HEARING HANDICAP
(2.3, 2.4)

Many persons, both children and adults, suffer from impaired hearing. The handicaps that arise from this are economic, educational and, above all,

social. These persons need help, both medical and educational.

In order to plan facilities for the medical treatment, for the rehabilitation and for the special education required by those with impaired hearing, we must know how many persons with hearing problems there are in various age groups and in various communities. In addition we must know the severity of their handicaps. Those who are profoundly deaf or have a severe handicap must be distinguished from those who are moderately hard of hearing, and these must all be distinguished from those who suffer only from the inconvenience of a minor handicap.

The first step in making such distinctions is to divide hearing impairment into categories of handicap. The Committee on Conservation of Hearing of the American Academy of Ophthalmology and Otolaryngology recommends the division of the handicap of hearing into classes or grades, according to the accompanying table. The over-all handicap of impaired hearing is best estimated in terms of ability to hear everyday speech well enough to understand it, but for statistical purposes the more precise measurements of pure-tone audiometry are preferable. This table defines each category in terms of pure-tone audiometric measurements such as are regularly made in surveys and tests of hearing, since it is possible to estimate a person's threshold of hearing for speech reasonably well from pure-tone measurements.

Specifically, each class in the table is defined in terms of the average hearing threshold level for three audiometric frequencies that are important for the understanding of speech. The numbers represent the simple average of the hearing threshold levels in decibels (dB) at the frequencies 500, 1000 and 2000 Hz,

## TABLE 1
### CLASSES OF HEARING HANDICAP

| Hearing Threshold Level dB (ISO) | Class | Degree of Handicap | Average Hearing Threshold Level for 500, 1000 and 2000 Hz in the Better Ear* | | Ability to Understand Speech |
|---|---|---|---|---|---|
| | | | More Than | Not More Than | |
| 25 | A | Not significant | | 25 dB (ISO) | No significant difficulty with faint speech |
| 40 | B | Slight handicap | 25 dB (ISO) | 40 dB | Difficulty only with faint speech |
| 55 | C | Mild handicap | 40 dB | 55 dB | Frequent difficulty with normal speech |
| 70 | D | Marked handicap | 55 dB | 70 dB | Frequent difficulty with loud speech |
| 90 | E | Severe handicap | 70 dB | 90 dB | Can understand only shouted or amplified speech |
| | F | Extreme handicap | 90 dB | | Usually cannot understand even amplified speech |

* Whenever the average for the poorer ear is 25 dB or more greater than that of the better ear in this frequency range, 5 dB are added to the average for the better ear. This adjusted average determines the degree and class of handicap. For example, if a person's average hearing-threshold level for 500, 1000, and 2000 Hz is 37 dB in one ear and 62 dB or more in the other his adjusted average hearing-threshold level is 42 dB and his handicap is Class C instead of Class B.

obtained with an audiometer that is calibrated according to the International Organization for Standardization's (ISO) Recommendation of 1964 (1.9).

The present classification is intended primarily for statistical purposes. It is not related to the problem of medical diagnosis. Deviations from audiometric zero within the limits of Class A (table I), or at frequencies above or below those that enter into the average, may be of medical significance for diagnosis or prognosis but they are not needed to estimate the hearing handicap as indicated in the table. Neither can the present table legitimately be used to classify individuals for educational purposes or for employment except as this classification is modified by the other considerations which are pertinent. These other considerations may sometimes completely supersede the present table. The classes of hearing handicap as defined here indicate, however, the usual handicap of the average individual under the varying circumstances of everyday life.

With a given audiometric hearing threshold level some persons will understand speech more easily and accurately, and others less easily and accurately, than is indicated in the table. Intelligence, quickness of perception, special training, general education, language background, motivation, ability to understand and time of onset all contribute to the degree of an actual handicap. Any impairment of the central nervous system may greatly complicate the situation. Any one of several of these various factors may be vital in determining a person's over-all economic or educational potentialities.

## Social Adequacy Index for Hearing

An attempt was made in 1948 to develop an index for the adequacy of a person's hearing on the basis of his threshold for speech (spondee words) and his discrimination for speech (phonetically balanced [PB] monosyllables). The central concept was that although everyday speech is a dynamic fluctuating affair and is heard at various sound-pressure levels and in various acoustic environments, there is, nevertheless, a broad statistical average of speech levels and conditions.

Otologists have been well aware of the concept of "social hearing." They know that a high-tone hearing loss at 4000 Hz and above does not really impair listening except for hi-fi music, and that there is so much noise in everyday living that a hearing level for speech of 30 dB is perfectly adequate and an excellent result for a fenestration operation. Even up to 40 dB hearing level for speech a person can "get by," most but not all the time, and only with some difficulty. Above the 40 dB hearing level for speech he definitely needs help, enough to have an operation or wear a hearing aid. On the average we hear speech at about 65 to 70 dB SPL (sound-pressure level) (see Figure 7-4). However, sometimes it is down to 45 dB and sometimes, as in a noisy subway or at a cocktail party, it is as high as 90 dB or more at ears. A man with a conductive hearing loss who has a hearing level for speech of 45 dB does beautifully at the cocktail party but may hear nothing at a lecture or in church.

With effort, he might be able to "get by" with everyday conversation about half of the time. If his hearing level is up to 55 dB, he probably will hear only in noisy places or when people really speak up for him, perhaps a third or a quarter of the time. People begin to leave him out of the conversation, or he must rely on speechreading. His hearing is now about at the threshold of social adequacy.

These relations are summarized in Table 1 in terms of hearing-threshold levels for speech. The social adequacy index provided a continuous scale of handicap and took into account the two dimensions of the hearing of speech, namely, sensitivity and discrimination. If a man's speech discrimination and his threshold for speech are normal, he will hear everyday speech, with its rich context, correctly nearly all the time. If his threshold for speech is elevated, he may be listening to speech somewhere on the rising slope of his *articulation* curve, as described in Chapter 7. He will have more or less difficulty with everyday speech. He will also have difficulty if his articulation curve reaches its maximum well below 100 percent, even if his threshold for speech is normal, because he will never hear certain words correctly.

The social adequacy index of hearing was conceived as the probability of hearing correctly a word of everyday speech, averaged across all words and all conditions. A table was constructed to express the trade-off between sensitivity and maximum discrimination score. The threshold of social adequacy of hearing was estimated to be at 55 dB (ISO) if discrimination was perfect and at a PB (Hughes) articulation score of 35 if the threshold level for spondees was 10 dB or better. We do not give the details because in practice the idea did not work out very well. One reason is that the PB recordings never have been standardized well enough to measure a man's discrimination with anything like the accuracy with which we measure his

TABLE 2

| Average Hearing Threshold Level for 500, 1000, and 2000 Hz in the Better Ear | | Presumed Ability to Understand Speech | Percentage |
|---|---|---|---|
| Total, above 40 dB (ISO) C + D + E + F | | | **2.7** |
| 41–55 dB | C | Frequent difficulty with normal speech | 1.6 |
| 56–79 dB | D | Frequent difficulty with loud speech | |
| 79–90 dB | E | Understands only shouted or amplified speech | **1.1** |
| over 90 dB | F | Usually cannot understand even amplified speech | |

threshold level. Also, we do not yet seem to know enough about the relation of the hearing and understanding of connected speech in words and sentences to its component frequencies, phonemes, and syllables.

Probably another dimension related to the speed of understanding should be added and perhaps still others. But the index was already as elaborate as it could well be for practical use. Our chief objective here has been to present the concept of a series of thresholds of various degrees of social adequacy of hearing. The various standards for hearing that will be presented below are based on such thresholds, but they are expressed simply in terms of threshold levels without regard for discrimination score.

**The Prevalence of Hearing Handicap**

Six categories of hearing handicap are defined in Table 1. In Table 2 is given the estimated percentage of the adult population of the United States that falls in the four most severe categories. The table is taken from "Characteristics of Persons with Impaired Hearing," based on data from the recent National Health Survey. The age range included is 18 to 79 years. Note that the hearing-threshold levels are measured, as in Table 1, as the average hearing-threshold level for 500, 1000, and 2000 Hz in the better ear. These are audiometric measurements of a demographic sample of the population of the United States.

In Table 3, from the same source, are

TABLE 3

PERCENTAGE OF PERSONS, 18 TO 79 YEARS OLD, WITH SPECIFIED SPEECH COMPREHENSION, BASED ON RESPONSE TO HEARING SCALE

| | Percentage |
|---|---|
| Total | 2.7 |
| Can hear and understand most spoken words. | 1.7 |
| Can hear and understand a few spoken words. Cannot hear and understand spoken words. | 1.0 |

given the percentages of responses to direct questions concerning the extent of hearing deficiency, addressed to all those persons reported as having some deficiency of hearing in the continuing nationwide household interview survey conducted by the Division of Health Interview Statistics of the National Center for Health Statistics. If a family reported that a member or members had "deafness or serious trouble hearing

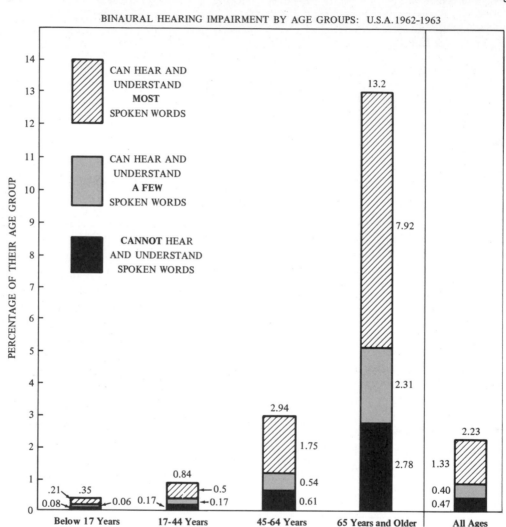

Fig. 9-1. Binaural hearing impairment by age groups, based on response to supplementary questionnaire of the Health Interview Survey (Public Health Service), United States of America, July 1962–June 1963. Ability is estimated *without the use of a hearing aid*. The percentages are shown separately for each of four age groups and for the entire population. The data for the age group below 17 years are based on the responses of parents. Those who were reported to have impaired hearing in the first interview, often by another member of the family, but who did not respond to the supplementary questionnaire, are excluded. If they are included, the percentage of binaural hearing for all ages becomes 2.7 percent, as in Table 1, instead of 2.23 percent. The percentage impaired is appreciably greater for males than for females in the two older age groups. (*National Center for Health Statistics, Series 10, Number 35*)

with one or both ears," a supplementary questionnaire concerning its extent and other details was mailed. About 90 percent of those addressed replied, or a parent or guardian replied for them.

Three questions asked in the follow-up correspond broadly to the degrees of impairment *assumed* to be associated with particular audiometric hearing-threshold levels in Table 2. The actual individuals questioned were not the same ones as those represented in Table 2, and the methods of collecting the data were quite different. Nevertheless the estimates of prevalence of hearing impairment are almost identical in Tables 2 and 3. The agreement gives added confidence to the estimate of 2.7 percent of adults who have "serious trouble with hearing" and also to the designation of classes of handicap in Table 2.

The data of Table 3 are broken down by age groups in Figure 9-1. The increase in incidence of hearing impairment with age is obvious. The same data are treated in Chapter 16 from another point of view (see Figure 16-1).

The agreement between the two surveys, audiometric and interview, is not so close when we try to estimate the total number of individuals in the United States who have a hearing handicap. The figure given in the 1960–1962 audiometric survey (National Center for Health Statistics, Series 11, number 11) for adults who have an average hearing level for 500, 1000, and 2000 Hz in the better ear of 26 dB (ISO) or worse is "about 8 percent or 9.2 million persons." The figure given for the interview survey, 1962–1963, is about 8 million persons reported to have impaired hearing in one or both ears, but of these only about 4 million were finally determined, by follow-up, to have impaired hearing in both ears. Obviously the criterion of impairment used by the respondents in the interview was more rigid than the one given in Table 1 for beginning handicap.

## Military Physical Standards for Hearing

Military service requires that a person be physically fit to perform certain required tasks and duties. Of course, there are some military duties that can be performed quite successfully by a man with a minor handicap, but a missing trigger finger, fallen arches, a leaky heart valve, a perforated eardrum, or dependence on a hearing aid quite properly disqualifies a man for unlimited service. For unlimited service a man must pass a whole series of screening tests. Failure on any one of these disqualifies him. The set of minimum requirements is known as the "physical standards." Hearing is one of the items in military physical standards.

Most of these physical standards could more aptly be called biological standards. They actually take their name from the doctor's "physical examination," in which he looks, feels, listens, and also measures with physical instruments such as scales, meter sticks, and blood-pressure apparatus. The audiometer is now one of these "physical" instruments.

Actually there is not just one set of physical standards but many. The military standards, however, are typical of the minimum requirements set up for their own purposes by various organizations—police and fire departments, commercial airlines, and many other groups.

There is a whole series of military physical standards. The primary set is for "unlimited" service. Then there are the more rigorous requirements for various special branches or activities such as aircraft pilot, submariner, or paratrooper. Sometimes a very specialized duty, such as sonar listening, may require the passing of special tests of hearing or other aptitude. More lenient standards are set for admission to limited duty. Still another set of standards concerns dismissal from duty entirely or from a special category. For obvious reasons a higher standard is required for admission to a particular duty status than is set for mandatory separation. Experience, the investment in special training, morale, natural deterioration to be expected from aging—all these enter the picture. The setting of initial physical standards is a difficult task of judgment, but separation involves many more conflicting interests and is even more difficult.

For many years the military physical standards for hearing were based entirely on the voice test, the whisper test, and sometimes the watch tick or the coin click (see Chapter 7). These old tests still survive in the regulations of many states and municipalities, but for military standards they now are used only as preliminary tests. The standards are based on pure-tone audiometry.

The hearing levels adopted by the Armed Forces represent what amount to *screening levels of hearing.* Different screening levels are needed for different purposes and situations. The sets of hearing levels or "profiles" given below are of general significance because they represent a large background of practical experience.

*Hearing profiles for service.* The Armed Forces are now (1968) making their transition from the ASA-1951 reference zero levels to the ISO reference levels. The latest available profiles, given below, are stated in terms of ASA-1951, with the instruction to translate any new ISO hearing levels to ASA by subtracting the appropriate number of decibels at each frequency (see Chapter 7). The recommendation has been made, however, and is presumably being implemented, that all of the profiles be reviewed and redefined in round numbers on the ISO scale in such a way as to keep the actual physical sound-pressure levels substantially the same as they have been on the ASA scale but to make minor readjustments to allow concise statement of the profiles in steps of 5 dB.

The profiles given below are adapted from Army Regulation AR 40–501.

Notice, in this table, that only four audiometric frequencies are considered, and that in many cases it is the average level for the three major frequencies most important for the understanding of speech that determines the adequacy of hearing. The levels given are ASA levels. The values will probably be 10 dB higher for the speech range and 5 dB higher at 4000 Hz when the rules are rewritten for the ISO scale. Notice also the differences in hearing levels that are related to the purpose of the screen, whether it is for capability for general unlimited military duty or merely for limited duty, and whether for enlistment in peacetime or for general mobilization. The standards for medical and dental registrants are included to illustrate the very different requirements set for a special highly trained group.

*The Medical Fitness Standard for Retention, Promotion, and Separation* deserves special attention as a standard appropriate to trained personnel at middle age or beyond. We quote from the pertinent section of AR 40–501.

Trained and experienced personnel will not be categorically disqualified if they are capable of effective performance of duty with a hearing aid. Ordinarily a hearing defect will not be considered sufficient reason for initiating disability separation or retirement processing. Most individuals having a hearing defect can be returned to duty with appropriate assignment limitations. The following is a guide in referring individuals with hearing defects for physical disability separation or retirement processing:

*a.* When a member is being evaluated for disability separation or retirement because of other impairments, the hearing defect will be carefully evaluated and considered in computing the total disability.

*b.* A member may be considered for physical disability separation or retirement if, at the time he is being considered for separation or retirement for some other ad-

TABLE 4
ACCEPTABLE AUDIOMETRIC HEARING LEVELS (ASA-1951 SCALE)

A. For Appointment, Enlistment, and Induction

|  | 500 | 1000 | 2000 | 4000 Hz |
|---|---|---|---|---|
| a) Both ears | Average of these three frequencies not over 20 dB with no one of them over 25 dB | | | 50 |
| or | | | | |
| b) Better ear | 15 | 15 | 15 | 30 |
| Worse ear | | No requirement | | |

B. Physical Profile Functional Capacity Guide (ASA–1951 scale)

| Profile Serial | | 500 | 1000 | 2000 | 4000 Hz |
|---|---|---|---|---|---|
| 1 | Each ear | Average not over 15 dB | | | Not over 40 |
| 2 | Both ears | Average not over 20 dB | | | Not over 50 |
|  | Better ear | Average not over 15 dB | | | Not over 30 |
| 3 | | May have hearing level at 20 dB with hearing aid by speech-reception score | | | |
| 4 | | Below retention standard (see text) | | | |

C. Medical Fitness Standard for Mobilization
   Hearing: Uncorrected hearing, average level (ASA–1951) at 500, 1000, and 2000 Hz, of 30 dB or more is unfitting for service.

D. Medicodental registrants
   Hearing: Hearing which cannot be improved in one ear with a hearing aid to an average hearing level of 20 dB (ASA) or less in the speech reception range is a cause of medical unfitness. Unilateral deafness is not disqualifying.

ministrative reason, the medical examination discloses a substantial hearing defect. This refers particularly to cases requiring hearing aids and those having hearing levels which may be rateable at 30 to 40 percent or more in accordance with the Veterans Administration Schedule for Rating Disabilities. It should be further noted that past performance of duty does not, per se, preclude separation or retirement because of physical disability caused by a hearing defect.

The guidance given in this excerpt is vague, presumably to allow the decision to be made by a medical officer on the basis of all aspects of each individual case.

### Civilian Standards

The foregoing military standards have been presented in some detail because they are probably the most realistic standards available. Many corresponding standards for civilian employment in state or municipal departments are still phrased in terms of voice tests, watch tick, and so on, and many of them are highly restrictive. We can hope that in the near future they will be restated in terms of ISO hearing-threshold levels, that the minimum hearing requirements bear a reasonable relation to the job requirements, and that the effective use of a hearing aid be specifically approved for all jobs or situations in which a hearing aid can reasonably be worn. One way to achieve this third goal would be to write the standard in terms of hearing level for speech, determined in an open acoustic field with or without the use of a hearing aid.

## THE PROBLEM
## OF MONITOR LIMITS

The object of monitoring audiometry (see Chapter 7) is to detect, by routine periodic tests of hearing, the individuals who show signs of incurring a significant noise-induced (or other) hearing loss. The specific rules and criteria for taking action must be evolved to fit the particular circumstances. "Monitor limits" appropriate in a military installation may be quite different from those suitable for a textile mill.

Of course, monitoring audiometry overlaps with screening audiometry and the problem of physical standards. Screening is oriented toward picking out those men whose hearing is so poor that they are not suited for or can no longer perform the duties to which they are assigned and toward detecting the men whose ears require medical attention. Inspection of the audiograms made in a monitoring program can serve this medical purpose. Monitoring audiometry does more than this, however. It singles out not only those who are already in difficulty, as shown by a hearing level that is beyond some arbitrary monitor limit, but also those who are *threatened* with handicap even though their hearing levels are still below the monitor limits. This is possible if *changes for the worse* are observed, judged by comparison of the most recent monitor audiogram with a reference audiogram previously established for that individual. The practical problem is to evolve a set of rules that is effective in picking up such changes for the worse but which eliminates spurious changes due to temporary threshold shift, transient middle-ear infections, and the like. The difficulty is to keep the rules simple and yet detect the significant changes, and to do this without overburdening the diagnostic center or the consulting otologist.

## MEDICAL RATING OF PHYSICAL IMPAIRMENT

We shall not attempt to write a history of the legal recognition of noise-induced hearing loss as an industrial disease that entitles a worker to compensation under workmen's compensation laws. The social wisdom of the laws and the legal justice of court decisions are irrelevant to the otologist and the audiologist in their professional capacities, but the otologist is called upon to assess or "rate" hearing for the purposes of payment of compensation. He is also asked to diagnose the type of hearing loss that a workman has so that a reasonable "causal relation" to noise-exposure can be affirmed or denied. His advice may also be asked as to the appropriate rules that should be followed by industrial commissions or even courts and legislatures in dealing with such cases, but more and more states are adopting explicit rules or codes.

Questions of the evaluation of permanent impairment, of causal relation, and the like, have been considered carefully and extensively by several groups and committees, however, and a consensus now seems to be emerging on most of the controversial points. Certain confusing terms, notably "disability" and "hearing loss," have been or are being redefined with more restricted meanings. This should greatly improve communication between the medical and legal professions. The issues, and also the responsibilities, involved in the evaluation or rating of impairment and of disability have been clearly stated.

We have already commented on the term "hearing loss" and the clarification that is made possible by adding the term "hearing level" to our vocabulary (Chapter 4). A term that has caused particular difficulty over the entire medicolegal field is "disability." The physician has used it as almost a synonym for impairment or handicap. But *to the lawyer the term "disability" means that a person's ability to engage in gainful activity has been reduced.* In other words, disability in the legal sense is not a purely medical condition. Physicians and their affiliates, such as audiologists, should carefully respect this legal usage of the term.

We now quote again from the "Guide for the Classification and Evaluation of Hearing Handicap."

### IMPAIRMENT, HANDICAP AND DISABILITY
#### (2.2, 2.3, 2.4, 2.7, 2.8, 2.9)

In various statements approved by the Committee on Conservation of Hearing, the terms *hearing handicap, hearing disability,* and *hearing impairment* have all been employed, usually with the intention of conveying substantially the same meaning, but some confusion exists because of connotations that are attached to each of the terms.

In the section on Classes of Hearing Handicap the meaning of *hearing handicap* has been stated once more. This definition of handicap is now almost identical with the definition of "impairment" that appears in the American Medical Association "Guides for the Evaluation of Permanent Impairment" (2.8), namely, "a medical condition that affects one's personal efficiency in the activities of daily living." It is further noted in the same guide that *disability,* as used in various workmen's compensation laws, involves nonmedical factors, such as may be related to actual or presumed reduction in ability to remain employed at full wages. "Permanent *impairment*" is therefore a contributing factor to, but not necessarily an indication of the extent of a patient's permanent *disability* within the meaning of the workmen's compensation laws. In other contexts, however, impairment does not imply a significant handicap but is used in a more general sense to denote any deviation from "normal." The impairment may be anatomical, or we may speak of an impaired function. The term is so useful in this very broad sense that *we are now departing from our previous usage and using "handicap" rather than "impairment" to make clear that we mean an impairment sufficient to "affect one's personal efficiency in the activities of daily living."* We shall thus speak of "percentage of hearing handicap" where formerly it was "percentage impairment of hearing," and at a still earlier date "percent hearing loss."

In summary, in this paper our definitions will be as follows:

*Disability:* actual or presumed inability to remain employed at full wages.

*Impairment:* a deviation or a change for the worse in either structure or function, usually outside of the range of normal.

*Handicap:* the disadvantage imposed by an impairment sufficient to affect one's personal efficiency in the activities of daily living.

### HEARING LEVEL VS. HEARING LOSS
#### (4.1, 3.2, 3.3, 3.4, 3.5)

The term *hearing-threshold level* is the complete and accurate designation for the measurement of an individual's hearing threshold by means of an audiometer. The shorter term *hearing level* may be used when we refer to the intensity of the sound produced by an audiometer at a particular setting of its intensity dial, just as in psychoacoustics we speak of *sensation level* when we mean a sound pressure level that is a given number of decibels above the threshold of a particular subject.

The term *hearing loss* should never be used when speaking of a particular number of decibels. It is properly used in referring to a general medical condition such as "conductive hearing loss" or "a noise-induced hearing loss." It emphasizes the impairment of function. It is illogical and very confusing, however, to speak of a hearing loss of 20 dB (ISO), for example, because this value lies well within the range of normal. It is very difficult to explain this fact to a layman. He automatically thinks of a hearing loss as an impairment and often as a handicap.

Throughout this document we have employed the term *hearing level* or *hearing-threshold level* to indicate the readings obtained on an audiometer. More precisely, hearing-threshold level means the number of decibels that the threshold of an individual's hearing lies above the reference zero level of the audiometer. Thus, hearing-threshold level may be measured according to either the ASA-1951 or the ISO-1964 scale. *In order to avoid confusion, for a period of several years it will be absolutely essential to designate explicitly which scale is being employed.* This is best done by means of the abbreviation *ISO* or *ASA-1951* placed in parentheses immediately after the abbreviation *dB*. Where tabular numerical recording is used, the *ISO* or *ASA-1951* may be placed opposite the date the audiogram was taken. It will be well to use *ASA-1951* rather than *ASA* alone because it is probable that a new American standard will some day be written that will incorporate the International Reference Zero Level.

## NORMAL HEARING AND THE THRESHOLD OF HANDICAP

Healthy young adults differ from one another with respect to the sensitivity of their hearing just as they differ with respect to height, weight, blood pressure, basal metabolism and many other anatomical and physiological characteristics. The sensitivity of hearing also changes systematically with age, slowly at first through adolescence and early adulthood, a little more rapidly through middle age, and much more rapidly beyond 60 years of age. This is part of the normal expectation of aging. *Normal sensitivity of hearing, even for young adults who have not yet suffered much decline, is a range and not a single hearing-threshold level.* This range is generally considered to extend from the least intensity available on an audiometer to about 23 dB (ISO), or 12 dB (ASA-1951). Hearing-threshold levels near either extreme may be considered unusual but not abnormal, although the occurrence of changes of sensitivity within the range of normal may have some diagnostic significance, particularly in children and adolescents.

The values chosen for the International Standard Reference Zero for Pure-Tone Audiometers were obtained by combining the hearing-threshold values measured on 15 different groups of young adults who had been screened to eliminate any who had visible signs or a history of otological disease. The average hearing thresholds are not a standard of normal hearing in a medical sense, but the values do represent the central tendency of the range of normal and are therefore the most logical selection for the reference zero. The ASA standard of 1951 was similarly based on the average values obtained from a population survey carried out in 1936. The probable reasons for the rather wide difference in values, about 10 dB, are discussed elsewhere (3.2).

The important point with respect to the evaluation of hearing handicap is that neither the ISO nor the ASA-1951 audiometric reference zero value corresponds to the threshold of handicap. Actually, *handicap is generally conceded to begin at about the upper edge of the range of normal, and more specifically at 27 dB (ISO) or 16 dB (ASA-1951).* We refer here to the average hearing-threshold level for the three frequencies

500, 1000 and 2000 Hz. *The percentage handicap is not proportional to the number of decibels that an individual's hearing threshold lies above the audiometric zero nor does it depend in any way on which audiometric zero is used to describe that threshold.* This is true because handicap depends upon the relation of an individual's threshold of hearing to the physical intensity of the everyday speech which he hears. There must be no confusion between the reference zero levels for audiometers and the hearing-threshold level at which hearing handicap begins.

### RULES FOR THE EVALUATION OF HEARING HANDICAP
#### (2.2, 2.6, 2.7, 2.9, 3.1, 4.2)

Ideally, hearing handicap should be evaluated in terms of ability to hear everyday speech under everyday conditions. The ability to hear sentences and repeat them correctly in a quiet environment is taken as satisfactory evidence of correct hearing for everyday speech. However, because of present limitations of speech audiometry, the preferred procedure is to *estimate the hearing-threshold level for speech from air-conduction measurements made with a pure-tone audiometer.* For this estimate the Committee on Conservation of Hearing recommends *the simple average of the hearing-threshold levels (in decibels) at the three frequencies 500, 1000, and 2000 Hz.*

In order to evaluate the hearing handicap it must be recognized that the range of partial hearing handicap, comprising classes B, C, D and E in the accompanying table, is not nearly as wide as the total dynamic range of human hearing. The audiometric reference zero level recommended by the International Standards Organization represents the average sensitivity of healthy young adults who have no indication of present or previous otologic disease. Thus, zero hearing-threshold level on the audiometer obviously represents very good hearing; it is not the point at which handicap begins. Actually, if the average hearing-threshold level at 500, 1000 and 2000 Hz is 26 dB (ISO) or less, usually no handicap exists in the ability to hear everyday speech under everyday conditions. At the other extreme, if the average hearing-threshold level at 500, 1000 and 2000 Hz is over 93 dB (ISO), the handicap for hearing everyday speech should be considered total. The possibility of utilizing any residual hearing beyond 93 dB (ISO) by means of a hearing aid is not taken into account in this evaluation. *For every decibel that the estimated hearing-threshold level for speech exceeds 26 dB (ISO), or 15 dB by the American Standard of 1951, allow one-and-one-half percent in handicap of hearing, up to the maximum of 100 percent.* This maximum is reached at 93 dB (ISO) or at 82 dB by the American Standard of 1951.

The Committee further recommends that any method for the evaluation of hearing handicap should include an appropriate formula for binaural hearing which will be based on the hearing-threshold levels in each ear tested separately. Specifically, the Committee recommends the following formula: The percentage of handicap of hearing in the better ear is multiplied by five (5). The resulting figure is added to the percentage of handicap of hearing in the poorer ear, and the sum is divided by six (6). The final percentage represents the binaural evaluation of hearing handicap.

The Committee also recommends that in the calculation of the percentage of handicap of hearing from the results of audiometric measurements no correction or allowance should be made for age.

### PROBLEMS OF CAUSAL RELATIONS
### (2.7, 3.1)

Often in evaluating a case of impaired hearing for purposes of compensation, an otologist will recognize two or more causes of the condition, perhaps acting simultaneously like aging and noise-exposure, or perhaps in sequence like chronic otitis media and an automobile accident. And sometimes, by virtue of pre-employment audiograms or periodic hearing tests for other purposes, the contribution from each cause may be estimated fairly accurately. If liability or compensation are involved, the question arises as to how to evaluate the various causal relations.

In some situations the various liabilities and the rules for calculating them are established by law or by administrative rules and interpretations. In other situations, and notably in circumstances where workmen's compensation laws and rules do not apply, the otologist must exercise his independent judgment. The proper division of liability in proportion to the contributions from two or more different causes is not easy, however. It is particularly difficult when discrimination loss or central dysacusis of any sort is combined with loss of auditory sensitivity. Even if the combined impairment is only a loss of sensitivity, the logic of the situation is complicated because, as noted in an earlier section, handicap does not begin at the zero of the audiometric scale. It is therefore necessary to *estimate first the extent of the total over-all hearing handicap and then, by an entirely independent calculation or estimate, apportion the liability according to the various contributing causes.*

An obvious simple example of diffi-culty in apportionment is the evaluation of binaural as opposed to monaural deafness. Monaural deafness is not half as handicapping as binaural, but it does involve half of the *peripheral* auditory apparatus. A less obvious example is the superposition of a mild otitis media on a hearing loss from industrial noise that was just below the level at which handicap and compensation begin. Neither condition alone is bad enough to cause a handicap but together they do. In some of these situations there are specific legal rules or precedents, but more often there are not.

### Stabilization of Hearing Thresholds

The guide from which we have quoted does not mention the necessity of assuring that the individual's hearing is stable before evaluating it for workmen's compensation or other monetary award. The usual practice is to make audiograms on three or more days, preferably spaced a week or so apart, to show that there is no progressive improvement of hearing, and to accept the best over-all audiograms as the basis for evaluation. Opinions and practice differ as to the minimum "waiting period" that should (or must by administrative rule) be allowed after the last hazardous noise-exposure or after an accident to allow full recovery from temporary threshold shifts. Two weeks is probably sufficient for industrial noise-induced hearing loss, but at least 6 months should be allowed after an accident or a sudden acoustic trauma. And of course whenever there may be a monetary award the audiologist must be alert for the possibility of feigning.

### PRINCIPLES OF EVALUATION OF IMPAIRMENT

The rules for calculating the percentage of handicap (or impairment) of hearing, as recommended by the American Academy of Ophthalmology and Otolaryngology and endorsed by the American Medical Association, have been stated in the foregoing section. Many of the principles on which these rules are based have been discussed in this or in previous chapters, but some of the rules are quite arbitrary. We summarize several of these principles as follows.

1. The threshold of handicap is related to the average intensity of everyday speech. It is in no way related to the range of normal hearing or to the reference zero levels of the audiometer (see Figure 7-4). The value of this threshold is at a speech reception threshold of about 25 dB (ISO). This value was based originally on the clinical experience of otologists, but it has been confirmed in the National Health Survey. The threshold of handicap lies about 10 dB above the most rigorous of the military standards for hearing.

2. In principle the evaluation of hearing handicap should be based on the speech reception threshold measured by direct speech audiometry, using samples of everyday speech. This is not feasible, however, because no suitable samples of everyday speech have been standardized. Such standardization is not likely because of difficulties related to vocabulary and to regional dialects and the specifications for an "average talker." The threshold for speech is therefore *estimated* by taking the average hearing-threshold level for the frequencies 500, 1000, and 2000 Hz. (In California the frequency 3000 is included also.)

3. The ceiling (100 percent) of hearing handicap is related to the power of the average human voice and to such social amenities as the distance from talker to listener and the acceptable loudness for group conversation. It is less clearly defined than the threshold of handicap,

and has been set, somewhat arbitrarily, at 93 dB hearing-threshold level. The exact value was chosen because it is reached by going up from the threshold according to the simple rule of 1.5 percent per decibel.

4. The simple linear relation stated above between percent handicap and decibels is arbitrary. It has the great advantage of extreme simplicity (see Figure 9-2).

5. The evaluation of percent hearing handicap can be made equally well on the ISO or the ASA-1951 scale of hearing level. Only the numerical values of the threshold and the ceiling are different.

6. The ratio of 5 to 1 in favor of the better ear in calculating the binaural handicap is arbitrary, but it is based on clinical observation and judgment.

7. No consideration is given to the possible benefits from a hearing aid or to known difficulty in obtaining such benefits. Thus many individuals whose handicap is rated as total (100 percent) for statistical purposes or for workmen's compensation are able to communicate quite effectively with the help of a hearing aid, but others can not.

8. No consideration is given to poor discrimination for speech, to tinnitus or other forms of dysacusis, or to any special importance of hearing to the individual because of his profession or employment. The rules as stated above were developed to meet the needs of workmen's compensation and of Veterans Administration rating of disabilities. Here the major types of hearing loss are conductive or noise-induced. For many other types of hearing loss the rules will considerably underestimate the actual degree of handicap.

9. No consideration is given to age and presbycusis. This is a rather arbitrary

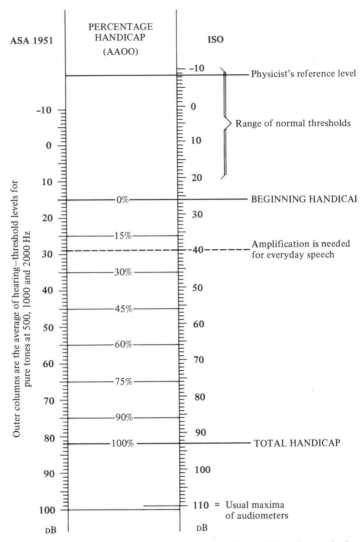

Fig. 9-2. The center column represents percentage handicap of hearing, calculated according to the rule originally formulated by the Subcommittee on Noise in 1958 and adopted by the AAOO in 1959 for use in cases involving compensation. "ISO" refers to the reference zero levels for pure-tone audiometers, recommended by the International Organization for Standardization. "ASA 1951" refers to the audiometric scale defined in the American Standard for Audiometers for General Diagnostic Purposes, Z24.5-1951 (*after Davis and Kranz*).

exclusion which will be discussed below.

### Previous Rules
### for Evaluation

Before the formulation of the AAOO rules for calculating percent handicap from pure-tone audiometric thresholds two other rules had been employed. The first of these, known as the "Fletcher point eight" rule, is almost as old as the electric audiometer itself, but it was never intended to be used as a measure of handicap! Harvey Fletcher, who was largely responsible for the early development of the audiometer at the Bell Telephone Laboratories, recognized early that an over-all evaluation of a hearing loss with a single number would be very desirable. For many purposes the audiogram is too analytical. He proposed the *percentage of normal hearing that had been lost*. He realized that the hearing of speech was the most important single function of hearing, and that the central frequencies, 512, 1024, and 2048 Hz, were the most important for this. He took the average hearing level, or hearing loss as it was then called, for these three frequencies. The dynamic range of the early audiometers at these frequencies was 120 dB. To convert the decibels of hearing loss to percentage of the total range he therefore multiplied the loss by five-sixths. This ratio was later approximated to 0.8 ("zero point eight"), which gave the name to the rule. The result was the percentage of originally available "auditory area" (in the speech range) that had been "lost," that is, the "percent hearing loss."

The rule is simple and easy to remember, and it effectively rank-orders hearing losses. Some otologists still use it. It is not satisfactory for calculating disability or insurance claims, however, because it disregards the concept of a threshold of handicap below which it is illogical to claim disability. It opened the door to many small claims, even on the basis of audiograms within the range of normal. On the other hand, it penalized those with severe hearing losses because 100 percent was not reached as long as any response to the audiometer was obtained in the speech range.

The second set of rules was issued by the American Medical Association's Council on Physical Medicine in 1947. It was prepared by Drs. E. P. Fowler and Paul E. Sabine. This method employed the four frequencies 512, 1024, 2048, and 4096 Hz but weighted them differently: 2048 = 40 percent, 1024 = 30 percent, and 512 and 4096 = 15 percent each. It made the important advance of introducing a thresh-

old and a ceiling. Both of these were near the present AAOO threshold and ceiling respectively. The increase in percent hearing loss was not linear as a function of decibels. The calculation of the over-all percentage required a chart that included a separate scale for each frequency. Probably it was because of the complexity that the method never became very popular. It was, however, the direct ancestor of the AAOO rules, which differ from it chiefly in their much greater simplicity and their total rejection of 4000 Hz from the calculation.

## THE PROBLEM OF NORMAL HEARING

We have discussed the question of the "normal" threshold of hearing in Chapters 2 and 7 in relation to the choice of the reference zero levels of pure-tone audiometers. "Normal" should not be interpreted as meaning "the very best," but rather as the median or mode of a distribution, because even ears that are entirely free of disease differ significantly in sensitivity. The standard deviations as well as the medians of thresholds of one group of healthy young men are shown in Figures 2-4 and 2-5. We repeat from Chapters 2 and 7 that there is not a *single* "normal" threshold but instead a *range of normal thresholds*. Even so, it is still necessary to specify the age and sex of the subject and the psychoacoustic procedure by which the threshold is determined if we are to judge whether a particular threshold is within its appropriate range of normal or not.

More serious confusion arises from the implication that normal means free of disease and that "abnormal" or "outside the range of normal" means disease or injury. The decision as to whether an ear is "abnormal" or not in this sense is a medical decision, involving much more than the determination of pure-tone thresholds.

The concept of a range of normal is very familiar to the physician, yet he always hesitates to draw a sharp line and say, "This is the limit. Anything beyond this limit abnormal," because to him and to most laymen "abnormal" implies disease or defect—something wrong. The 5 percent of subjects with the very best hearing lie outside the range of two standard deviations. Should we call their hearing "abnormally good?" On the other hand, the physician knows that as hearing gets poorer and poorer, the more likely is he to find *on closer examination* a disease or defect, such as otitis media or otosclerosis, that is responsible. But the significance of a hearing-threshold level of 30 dB, will depend on the age and the sex of the subject, among other things. And even if there is a considerable deviation, he is not likely to say "your hearing is abnormal." He will say "Your hearing is below average for your age. I shall try to find the cause (that is, make a diagnosis)."

The statistician, however, finds another way out. From the number and scatter of the original measurements he can calculate the limits within which any given percentage of new cases can be expected to fall. One common convention is arbitrarily to take two "standard deviations" as the range of normal, which practically means that we agree to call the most deviant 5 percent "abnormal" (without inquiring into cause) and to consider the other 95 percent as "within normal limits." This is illustrated in Figures 2-4 and 2-5. (For these data the distributions were symmetrical about the median. The situation is more complicated when, as in the National Health Survey, the deviations are greater in the direction of poorer hearing than of better hearing. Then the percentiles are a better way to express the deviations, as in Figure 9-3.)

Incidentally, it was in very nearly this way that the limits of normal for the 4C Group Hearing Test, described in Chapter 7, were established. A small but definite percentage of thresholds lay beyond the arbitrary cutoff point, and these were therefore automatically considered "abnormal." It later came as a shock to some people to learn that calculations from the results of the test, as applied to New York schoolchildren, showed that there must have been 3,000,000 hard-of-hearing children of school age in the United States. This result had been built into the test by statistical definition at the start.

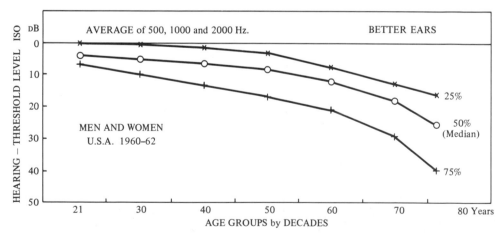

Fig. 9-3. Medians and quartiles of hearing-threshold levels by age groups for the better ears of men and women, average of values for 500, 1000, and 2000 Hz. (*Data from National Health Survey, United States 1960–1962, corrected to ISO reference level.*)

Above all *it must not be thought that the choice of a standard reference zero level for audiometry establishes a standard of normal in any legal sense*. It is true that the ISO levels do correspond closely to the mean or median threshold levels of otologically normal young adults. The ears tested had no detectable disease or history of it. Their hearing thresholds are convenient values for an arbitrary single reference level (ISO) at each frequency, but this does not mean that there is necessarily anything wrong with ears that are somewhat less sensitive. This should be obvious, but it is possible that some people who do not understand that the threshold of handicap is quite independent of the threshold of hearing may be misled by a careless statement that "the zero of the audiometer is the normal hearing threshold." They might think that therefore any poorer sensitivity, that is, a "hearing loss" in the old sense of the term, represents abnormality and injury and therefore automatically deserves compensation or payment for injury if any plausible causal relation can be established. This argument has actually been advanced in court in the past, particularly in connection with the "Fletcher point eight" rule, and it might be tried again in the future.

### "Actuarial" Hearing Thresholds

In 1966 the present writer introduced the term *actuarial hearing thresholds* to mean the average expectation of hearing according to age and sex. In a sense these are normal thresholds inasmuch as it is normal for the tissues of the body to change their characteristics with age (see Chapter 3) and for hearing to be very sensitive in childhood and less so in old age.

The National Health Survey of 1960–1962, to which we have referred repeatedly, has given us actuarial hearing thresholds for the United States for the age range 18 to 79, and soon the results of a similar survey of children's hearing will be available. The data have been analyzed and presented in many ways, according not only to age and sex, but with respect to race, region, area of residence, educational attainment, and many other factors, so that the average expectation (and for many items the interquartile range also) for almost any group can be stated with reasonable confidence. Figure 9-3 shows the over-all trend with age for men and women combined for the average of 500, 1000, and 2000 Hz (see also Figure 16-1).

### SUMMARY OF REFERENCE LEVELS, SCREENING LEVELS, AND STANDARDS

For convenience we assemble here, in ascending order of physical intensity, the various reference levels, screening levels, and physical standards that we have mentioned in this and other chapters. We shall refer to the average of values at 500, 1000, and 2000 Hz as the "central speech range." There are minor discrepancies between these numbers and certain graphs (for example, Figures 2-4 and 7-4) because ISO pressures are coupler pressures although some others are free field.

1. The physicist's reference level for sound pressure (SPL) 0.0002 $\mu$bar per cm$^2$ or $2 \times 10^{-5}$ newtons (N) per m$^2$, independent of frequency.
2. The ninetieth percentile of thresholds of hearing for young adults at the best frequencies. This corresponds quite closely to the physicist's reference level.
3. ISO reference zero levels for pure-tone audiometers. The median threshold of hearing for otologically normal young adults under laboratory conditions. A function of frequency. About 9.5 dB SPL (coupler pressure) across the central speech range (Figure 2-5).

4. US National Health Survey (1960–62) median for 18- to 24-year age group. Central speech range = 3.5 dB (ISO). (For other age groups see Figure 9-3.)

5. ASA-1951 reference zero levels for pure-tone audiometers, based on USPHS survey of 1936. A function of frequency. Central speech range = 11 dB (ISO) or about 20 dB SPL (coupler pressure). See also Figure 7-4.

6. Proposed USASI reference zero level for speech audiometers. Calibration tone 1000 Hz = 20 dB SPL (coupler pressure) or 11.5 dB (ISO).

7. Screening for schoolchildren. Central speech range = 25 dB (ISO).

8. The most rigorous US military physical standard (for appointment, enlistment, and induction). Better ear, central speech range = 26 dB (ISO) (Table 9-2).

9. Threshold of hearing handicap, AAOO rule. Central speech range = 27 dB (ISO).

10. More lenient US military standards such as profile 2. Central speech range = 31 dB (ISO) (Table 9-2).

11. Practical limit of hearing without amplification. Central speech range = 40 dB (ISO) (see Figure 9-3).

12. Usual level for recommendation of special management of children. Central speech range = 41 dB (ISO).

13. "Unfitting for military service" (mobilization) if uncorrected by hearing aid. Central speech range = 41 dB (ISO).

14. Beginning of marked handicap, AAOO classification. Central speech range = 55 dB (ISO).

15. Comfortable listening level. A range centering about 65 dB SPL (free field).

16. Beginning of hazard of habitual exposure to broad-band continuous noise, AAOO guide (see Chapter 5). Average octave band level, 300–2400 Hz, = 85 dB SPL (free field).

17. Total (100 percent) handicap, AAOO rule. Central speech range = 93 dB (ISO).

18. Threshold of discomfort. Almost independent of frequency. About 120 dB SPL or about 110 dB (ISO) (see Figure 2-5).

19. Threshold of tickle. Almost independent of frequency. About 130 dB SPL or about 120 dB (ISO).

20. Threshold of pain. Almost independent of frequency. About 140 dB SPL or about 130 dB (ISO).

## THE PROBLEM OF MULTIPLE CAUSES

Among the most difficult problems relating to handicap and insurance claims are those which concern "causal relation," particularly when two or more causes of the hearing impairment can be identified.

One classical case is that of *second injury,* in which a worker incurs some noise-induced hearing loss under one employer and then leaves to work for another employer. His hearing levels may be known when he terminates the first employment, and a preemployment audiogram may define them again a little later. Exposures in both employments contribute to the final impairment and handicap. Who should pay the workmen's compensation insurance claim, or in what proportion? In several states this situation is handled by special provisions in statutes or rules, and in some of them, for example in Missouri, a clear principle of *proportional liability* emerges. The situation is very unclear, however, when there is no record of the hearing of the employee at the start of his first employment. In any case it is difficult because handicap is proportional to decibels of hearing level *above a certain threshold,* 26 dB (ISO). The employee's original hearing was presumably better than this. He worked for some time in his first employment, losing hearing but without passing the threshold of handicap. To what extent, if any, should the first employer be liable for the subsequent handicap?

*Presbycusis combined with noise-induced hearing loss* is the other classical problem. Here the two causes, noise and aging, act simultaneously and in parallel. Perhaps neither one *alone* would have caused a handicap by the time a worker retired, but together they have done so, as illustrated in Table 4 in Chapter 5. What proportion of the liability does the employer bear? The AAOO rule says "all of it." Some states reduce the award by an arbitrary percentage related to age. Missouri requires a correction for age in terms of a certain number of decibels per year of age that are subtracted from the hearing levels before applying the AAOO rule. This procedure penalizes the worker very heavily. It seems to the present writer that the most equitable solution is found according to the principle of proportional liability, making use of the actuarial thresholds that are now available. In 1966 he (Davis) wrote as follows:

The actuarial threshold will become increasingly important if the principle of proportional liability is more generally utilized in medico-legal situations. Here is an example to illustrate the principle. An elderly patient who has been injured in an automobile accident complains of impaired hearing since that time. No previous audiograms are available. An otologist is called upon to decide what proportion of the impairment should be assumed due to natural causes, particularly his age. His present audiogram shows an average hearing level for 500, 1000 and 2000 Hz of 50 dB. The otologist may reason thus: "It is fair to assume that as a young man the subject had a hearing threshold level for the major speech frequencies at 500, 1000, 2000 Hz equal to the median value given for the 20-year age group in the statistical tables of the 1960–1962 National Health Survey. This value, his original actuarial threshold, is 3.5 dB. The subject is now 70 years of age. The actuarial hearing-threshold level for this age and for the same frequencies is 17.5 dB. The total shift of his speech threshold since he was 20 years old is from 3 to 50, or 47 dB. The shift that can be ascribed to aging alone, i.e., the difference in the actuarial thresholds is, from 3.5 to 17.5, or 14 dB. The amount to be attributed to the accident is therefore 47 − 14, or 33 dB. The proportion of the liability for the subject's hearing impairment that should be ascribed to the accident is 33/47 or 70 per cent."

*Notice that this calculation of proportional liability or "percentage responsibility" is completely independent of the threshold of handicap and of the calculation of the percentage handicap and the appropriate monetary award.* Those other calculations tell how big the pie is. The principle of proportional liability tells how the pie should be cut. Notice that a hearing impairment may be the sum of two or three separate impairments, each with a different cause. No one of the separate impairments need be severe enough to cause a hearing handicap alone, yet they may combine to give a very significant handicap. It does not seem fair or logical to place all of the responsibility on either one of the impairments, particularly when two impairments may develop slowly and concurrently, like aging and noise-induced hearing loss. It would seem fairer to assume, as the otologist did in the above example, that the responsibility should be divided according to the number of decibels threshold shift that can reasonably be ascribed to each cause. The actuarial thresholds provide a very reasonable basis for estimating the average effect of aging, including the everyday noise exposure of the general population. It also provides a starting point from which to reckon the threshold shifts in case no previous audiograms are available.

## PROBLEMS OF INDUSTRIAL AUDIOMETRY

In 1964, it was proposed in the United States of America Standards Institute to adopt the ISO reference zero levels for pure-tone audiometers in a revision of the old ASA standard of 1951. This proposal was opposed vigorously by many users of audiometers, notably organizations composed of industrial users engaged in hearing conservation in industry. Now (1968) nearly all of the original objections have been met by appropriate wording of the proposed standard, the inclusion of explanatory material, and the simultaneous rewriting of the USA standard for audiometric booths. The vote in favor of the ISO reference levels is not yet quite unanimous, but ultimate adoption seems inevitable.[1] It is worthwhile, however, to examine some of the more substantial objections raised during this debate.

The objections centered on the over-all average difference in level of about 10 dB between the ISO and the ASA-1951 contours (see Figure 7-4). The adjustment of the shape of the curve raised only temporary objection.

It was explained that the adoption of ISO values would not alter the actual sound pressures specified in existing rules and standards, although the numbers used to express them would differ. The objection was made that confusion and misinterpretation would still be possible, but this was tacitly withdrawn when various state and national bodies, notably several workmen's compensation boards or commissions, amended their rules to include explicitly the equivalent ISO values.

It was argued that it would be impossible to measure hearing-threshold levels at zero dB (ISO) in the noise backgrounds of existing booths. The counter argument is that it is not necessary to measure at zero dB (ISO) but only at 10 dB (ISO), which corresponds to the lowest level currently tested, that is, zero dB (ASA). The rebuttal was that a smart lawyer could confuse a jury or a referee by claiming that it should be possible to measure normal hearing, which is the meaning of zero dB. In fact *possible misinterpretation of the ISO zero*

reference level as a legal standard of normal hearing still remains a legitimate cause for concern. (This issue we have discussed above.)

A quite different argument was that the ASA-1951 standard actually expresses better than the ISO standard the average expected hearing of the young people who become industrial workers as opposed to college students or the usual laboratory subjects. No published data are available to support this claim, however, and the thresholds for all young adults found in the recent National Health Survey are closer to the ISO zero than to the ASA-1951 zero. Nevertheless the statement was repeated, probably quite correctly, "But that is what our figures show and that's what they found in the USPHS survey of 1935–36."

The probable basis for the difference between the ASA and the ISO standards was revealed in a report by Dr. Aram Glorig of two normal hearing studies conducted in successive years, 1954 and 1955, at the Wisconsin State Fair. Each year volunteer subjects were obtained, questioned, and examined otologically in the same way to obtain comparable groups of "otologically normal young adults." The audiometers and the audiometric environment were similar and fully adequate. In 1954 each subject was tested "only once, by the conventional manual procedure." The resulting average hearing thresholds at 500, 1000, and 2000 Hz corresponded almost exactly to those of the USPHS data, which are the basis of the ASA-1951 audiometric reference levels.

In 1955 the procedure was made more deliberate. At least three threshold crossings in each direction were made at each frequency. Also the audiometers had been provided with attenuators with 2.5 dB steps. The over-all test required 30 to 45 minutes. This was a laboratory atmosphere. The subjects became interested and tried hard. The data from this 1955 study agree very well with those of Dadson and King

---

[1] This draft has now been approved and issued as USASI Specification S3.6–1969.

in England (see Chapter 2) and are about 10 dB more sensitive than the 1954 Wisconsin State Fair thresholds. (Actually both the Dadson and King and the 1955 Wisconsin State Fair data are among the 15 studies on which the ISO reference levels are based.)

The factor which seems to differentiate the 1954 and the 1955 Wisconsin State Fair studies most clearly is the more deliberate pace and repeated trials in 1955 and the resulting improved understanding and motivation of the subjects. Glorig calls this factor the "test-subject relationship."

It seems reasonable to assume that patients who come to a clinic or doctor's office because of difficulty with hearing are well motivated, and a good audiometric technician does not rush the patient but establishes an atmosphere like that of the laboratory. The patients have come for help, and they try hard. It seems clear that the ISO standard is appropriate in this situation. On the other hand, in industrial audiometry the procedure may be more casual and geared to speed and efficiency rather than to deliberate study. In this situation the ASA-1951 standard has apparently given reasonable results in the sense that the subjects do not often show thresholds better than the ASA reference zero level, if, indeed, tests are ever made below this level. No wonder that industrial users are satisfied and wish to avoid the trouble, confusion, and expense attendant on changing to what, for their purposes, seems to be an unrealistically severe standard.

It is worth noting that in all of the studies on which the ISO standard is based, the pace was deliberate. In a discussion of the tests and calculations, P. Weissler writes as follows:

In most of the studies the age ranged from 18–25 years, although in one it was as low as 17 and another as high as 40. People tested were from five different countries. They were students, sophisticated laboratory personnel, naval recruits, volunteers at a State Fair, and inhabitants of a rural area. In a number of determinations, threshold was considered the lowest level for which two out of three signals were heard, while for two of the determinations, three out of three signals had to be heard. The means of ascending and descending thresholds were used in many studies, while in one, only the decreasing threshold was used. Testing time ranged from several different sittings for one subject to about 30 min per person. Although background noise was carefully measured in some cases, in others the test was reported to have been made in a "quiet" environment.

It is unfortunate if systematic differences in psychoacoustic method, notably the tempo of the test, and perhaps in the motivation of the subjects, have crept in and now separate industrial audiometry from medically oriented audiometry. The difference seems to be of the order of 10 dB for the expected initial threshold.

However, if the difference depends on a rapid as compared with a deliberate routine, the divergences in results should be less marked if the subject has suffered some noise-induced threshold shift. Then his thresholds become much sharper, due to recruitment. Also the end-point is now above the ASA-1951 zero, so that any bias of the operator in not expecting or seeking thresholds below zero is removed, and so is any possible effect of ambient noise in the booth. In any case the methods and the data of industrial audiometry are self-consistent and they serve a very useful purpose in the conservation of hearing.

## TRANSITION FROM ASA-1951 TO THE ISO SCALE

We are now (1968) in the period of transition from the ASA-1951 scale for pure-tone audiometers to the ISO scale, and this period will continue for several years until the ISO usage is universal. Even then there will be the problem of handling old audiometric data based on the ASA-1951 scale.

Recommendations to facilitate this transition in the Armed Forces were prepared (1967) by a Working Group of the NAS-NRC Committee on Hearing, Bioacoustics, and Biomechanics ("CHABA"). We quote those that still seem of general interest.

1. To translate "ASA-1951" audiometric data to ISO values
   a. The following *exact formula* may be employed for statistical, research, or special clinical purposes at the discretion of the individual user.

```
At ............. 250  500 1000 2000 3000 4000 6000 8000 Hz
Add to ASA-1951  15   14   10  8.5  8.5   6   9.5 11.5 dB
hearing levels
```

   b. Use the following *approximate formula* when translating individual audiograms from ASA-1951 in order to compare them with more recent ISO audiograms or to apply one of the regulations.

```
At ............. 250   500 1000  2000  3000 4000 6000  8000 Hz
Add to ASA-1951         15         10      5    10      dB
hearing levels
```

The average correction for 500, 1000, and 2000 Hz, sometimes called "the speech range," is 10 dB.

The exact translation formula represents the differences between the ASA-1951 values and the ISO values, rounded to the nearest half decibel. These exact differences are appropriate for certain statistical, research, and perhaps special clinical purposes. For translations for other purposes the approximate formula is a sufficiently close approximation and far simpler in application and results. The approximations are all exact multiples of 5, appropriate to the 5 dB steps in which pure-tone audiometers are calibrated. The greatest

deviation from the exact values is 1.5 dB, which is within the tolerances allowed in the ASA-1951 standard for audiometers. The average deviation for the three frequencies 500, 1000, and 2000 Hz is 10.8 dB, and for the four frequencies 500, 1000, 2000, and 3000 Hz it is 10.25 dB. The rounding errors are negligible for all practical purposes.

2. Prepare revisions of all regulations relating to hearing levels and the recording of audiometric data, including screening levels, physical standards, physical disability, and audiometric forms, using the approximate formula of paragraph 1. Consider minor modifications of the resulting requirements and criteria in order to simplify the resulting regulations. A blanket adjustment of 10 dB at all frequencies instead of application of the approximate translation formula will provide more uniform and more easily applied rules and regulations without changing the absolute sound pressure levels to a clinically significant degree. The blanket adjustment would not involve any substantive change of as much as 10 dB.

3. The present range of screening and monitoring audiometers, in terms of sound pressure levels, is satisfactory. These sound pressure levels will not be altered significantly by the recalibration, although the numbers that designate them will be different.

4. The requirements for sound-proof booths for screening and monitoring

audiometry will not be altered by the recalibration of audiometers to the ISO reference zero, because the regulations concerning screening levels, and so on, will be translated to ISO values and, therefore, the screening will be carried out at very nearly the same physical sound pressure levels as at present.

5. Inform all personnel who deal with audiometric data in any way clearly, immediately, and repeatedly about the nature and significance and also the importance of the change from the ASA-1951 reference to ISO-1964 reference zero. Label prominently, as by large rubber stamps, every audiogram or other record form made during the transition period and identify clearly in speech and in writing every hearing level as either ASA-1951 or ISO. A very important feature of this recommendation is the clear designation on each chart and record of the calibration of the instrument employed. *The data should be recorded as read from the instrument.* Any necessary translation to the other scale for particular purposes should be done by the subsequent user of the recorded information.

## SUGGESTED READINGS AND REFERENCES

**Army Regulations.** "AR 40-501, Medical Service—Standards of Medical Fitness." Washington: Headquarters, Department of the Army, December 1960.

**Davis, H.** (assisted by the Subcommittee on Hearing in Adults for the Committee on Conservation of Hearing of the American Academy of Ophthalmology and Otolaryngology). "Guide for the Classification and Evaluation of Hearing Handicap in Relation to the International Audiometric Zero," *Trans. Amer. Acad. Ophthal. Otolaryng.,* 69:740–751 (1965).

This is the article from which the extensive quotations in the text have been made. The following list of other guides, standards, and approved articles is taken from the same source, with additions.

1. *Standards*

   American Medical Association

   1.1 AMA Council on Physical Medicine. Minimum requirements for acceptable audiometers, JAMA, 127:520–521, 1945.

   1.2 AMA Council on Physical Medicine and Rehabilitation. Minimum requirements for acceptable pure tone audiometers for diagnostic purposes, JAMA, 146:255–257, 1951.

   1.3 AMA Council on Physical Medicine and Rehabilitation. Minimal requirements for acceptable pure tone audiometers for screening purposes, JAMA, 144:465, 1950.

   American Standards Association
   (USA Standards Institute: now American National Standards Institute)
   1430 Broadway, New York, 10018

   1.4 Audiometers for general diagnostic purposes. Z24.5–1951.

1.5 Specification for pure tone audiometers for screening purposes. Z24.12–1952.

1.6 Specification for speech audiometers. Z24.13–1953.

1.6a USASI Specification S3.6–1969

International Electrotechnical Commission

1.7 Publication 177, Pure tone audiometers for general diagnostic purposes.

1.8 Publication 178, Pure tone screening audiometers.

International Organization
for Standardization

1.9 ISO Recommendation R 389, Standard reference zero for the calibration of pure tone audiometers.
(1.7, 1.8 and 1.9 are available through the USA Standards Institute)

2. *Committee Reports and Guides*

2.1 AAOO Committee on Conservation of Hearing. The listing of audiometers, Trans. Amer. Acad. Ophthal. Otolaryng. 62:247–249, 1958.

2.2 AAOO Committee on Conservation of Hearing (Subcommittee on Noise in Industry). Guide for the evaluation of hearing impairment, Trans. Amer. Acad. Ophthal. Otolaryng., 63:236–238, 1959.

2.3 AAOO Committee on Conservation of Hearing. (Subcommittee on Noise.) Guide for the conservation of hearing in noise, revised 1969. Supplement to Trans. Amer. Acad. Ophthal. Otolaryng.

2.4 L. R. Boies et al. (AAOO Committee on Conservation of Hearing). Guide to the care of adults with hearing loss. 1966. AAOO, Rochester, Minn.

2.5 AAOO Committee on Conservation of Hearing (Subcommittee on Noise). The relation of presbycusis to hearing impairment induced by noise, Trans. Amer. Acad. Ophthal. Otolaryng., 68:695–696, 1964.

2.6 AMA Council on Physical Medicine and Rehabilitation. Principles for evaluating hearing loss, Trans. Amer. Acad. Ophthal. Otolaryng., 59:550–552, 1955.

2.7 AMA Committee on Medical Rating of Physical Impairment. Guides to the evaluation of permanent impairment, JAMA, 168:475, 1958.

2.8 AMA Committee on Medical Rating of Physical Impairment. Guide to the evaluation of permanent impairment; ear, nose, throat and related structures, JAMA, 177:489–501, 1961.

3. *Approved Articles*

3.1 Davis, H.: Missouri Senate Bill No. 167 concerning industrial hearing loss: an interpretation, Arch. Otolaryng., 72:87–95, 1960.

3.2 Davis, H., and Kranz, F. W.: The international standard reference zero for pure tone audiometers and its relation to the evaluation of impairment of hearing, J. Speech Hearing Res., 7:7–16, 1964.
Also Trans. Amer. Acad. Ophthal. Otolaryng., 68:484–492, 1964.

3.3 Davis, H., and Kranz, F. W.: The international audiometric zero, J. Acoust. Soc. Amer., 36:1450–1454, 1964.
Also Amer. Industr. Hyg. Ass. J., 25:354–358, 1964.
And Ann. Otol., 73:807–815, 1964.

3.4 Davis, H.: The ISO zero reference level for audiometers, Arch. Otolaryng., 81:145–149, 1965.

3.5 Davis, H.: International standard reference zero for pure tone audiometry, Trans. Amer. Acad. Ophthal. Otolaryng., 69:112–118, 1965.

**Davis, H.** "Reference Levels and Hearing Levels in Otology," *Ann. Otol.,* 75:808–818 (1966).
A review article, but introduces the "actuarial threshold."

————. "Application of the ISO Standard Reference Zero (Audiometric) (U)." NAS-NRC Committee on Hearing, Bioacoustics, and Biomechanics, Working

Group 51, September 1967. Office of Naval Research, Contract No. NONR 2300 (05).

————, **G. D. Hoople, and H. O. Parrack.** "Hearing Level, Hearing Loss and Threshold Shift," *J. Acoust. Soc. Amer., 30*:478 (Letter to the Editor).
This is the original proposal to distinguish hearing level from hearing loss.

**Glorig, A.** "A Report of Two Normal Hearing Studies," *Ann. Otol., 67*:93–112 (1958).

**Jerger, J. F., R. Carhart, T. W. Tillman, and J. L. Peterson.** "Some Relations between Normal Hearing for Pure Tones and Speech," *J. Speech Hearing Dis., 2*:126–140 (1959).

**National Center for Health Statistics**
Series 11, number 11: "Hearing Levels of Adults by Age and Sex: United States 1960–62," A. Glorig and J. Roberts (eds.).
Series 11, number 26: "Hearing Levels of Adults by Race, Region and Area of Residence: United States 1960–1962," J. Roberts and D. Bayliss (eds.).
Series 10, number 35: "Characteristics of Persons with Impaired Hearing: United States July 1962–June 1963," A. Gentile, J. D. Schein, and K. Haase (eds.).
The data are from the *National Health Survey,* Public Health Service, U.S. Department of Health, Education and Welfare.
These very informative pamphlets are for sale by the Superintendent of Documents, U.S. Government Printing Office, Washington, D.C. 20402. Price: Series 11—30¢ each. Series 10—45¢ each.

**Schmidt, P. H.** "Presbycusis: The Present Status," *Int. Audiol.,* Suppl. 1, 1967.
An excellent review.

**Tillman, T. W., and J. F. Jerger.** "Some Factors Affecting the Spondee Threshold in Normal-hearing Subjects," *J. Speech Hearing Dis., 2*:141–146 (1959).

**Weissler, P. G.** "International Standard Reference Zero for Audiometers," *J. Acoust. Soc. Amer., 44*:264–275 (1968).
This is a detailed report on the technical activities of ISO's Technical Committee on Acoustics No. 43, Working Group on Threshold of Hearing, which led to the ISO Recommendation R389, "Standard Reference Zero for the Calibration of Pure-Tone Audiometers," November 1964.

# CHAPTER 10

# HEARING AIDS

A. F. NIEMOELLER, D.Sc.
S. R. SILVERMAN, Ph.D.
HALLOWELL DAVIS, M.D.

A hearing aid is any instrument that brings sound more effectively to the listener's ear. It may simply collect more sound energy from the air, it may prevent the scattering of sound during transmission, or it may provide additional energy, usually from the battery of an electrical amplifier.

The first objective of a hearing aid is to make speech intelligible. The "quality" or naturalness of the speech may be sacrificed if necessary. Little thought was given to quality by those who used the old ear trumpets. They were well enough satisfied if only speech could be made loud enough to be intelligible. Even with early electrical instruments, the chief difficulty was still to deliver enough energy, and any necessary compromises were acceptable as long as speech could be understood. Now, however, the arts of electronic amplification and electroacoustic engineering have made it possible to deliver as much sound as the ear can tolerate. We can therefore raise our sights and say that a hearing aid should deliver sounds loudly enough to be heard easily, but without discomfort. The listener's hearing loss should be overcome and his auditory nerve stimulated in a pattern as nearly normal as possible. Of course, the instrument should not add new "internal" noises. Distortion of the original pattern of sound should be introduced only to the extent that it assists in bringing to the listener speech that is intelligible, comfortable, and of pleasing quality.

## MECHANICAL HEARING AIDS

The simplest hearing aid, used since man became civilized enough to grow old and become hard of hearing, is the hand cupped behind the ear. The hand intercepts more of the oncoming sound wave than does the ear alone and deflects more of its energy into the external canal. The larger the scoop, the more energy can be collected. The efficiency of the scoop can be improved if it is shaped to favor the delivery of the energy into the ear canal. The broad principle of the ear trumpet is illustrated in Figure 10-1.

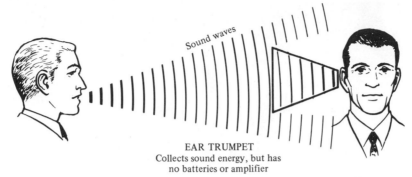

EAR TRUMPET
Collects sound energy, but has
no batteries or amplifier

Fig. 10-1. Ear trumpet. Collects sound energy, but has no batteries or amplifier.

The ear trumpet took many forms in efforts to compromise between effectiveness, convenience, and the user's vanity. Some of the varieties of shape and style are shown in Figures 10-2, 10-4, 10-5, and 10-6, photographs of the Goldstein collection of nonelectrical hearing aids at Central Institute for the Deaf. Some instruments were small and convenient, but not very effective. Others were built into cane heads, ear ornaments, or vases. Nearly all the instruments in the collection are black, probably to be as inconspicuous as possible, and all have in common a large surface or opening to catch the sound. Some also extend toward the speaker, where his voice is louder, and carry the sound to the ear in a tube without allowing it to scatter. When we recall that the intensity of sound in open air falls off rapidly with the dis-

tance the sound travels, we can see that much more energy can be collected if the ear trumpet reaches well out toward the speaker's mouth.

Most of the old-fashioned ear trumpets

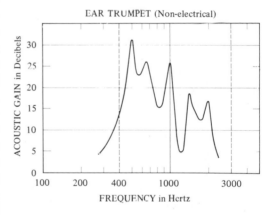

Fig. 10-3. This is the frequency characteristic of the ear trumpet shown in Figure 10-2. The acoustic gain is the difference between the sound pressure level measured in a 2-cc coupler attached to the ear trumpet and the corresponding level measured in a 6-cc coupler mounted in a plywood baffle cut to simulate the side of the head. The baffle and the microphone were placed normal to the incident sound at the position previously occupied by the mouth of the trumpet. Note the resonant peaks at 500 and 700 Hz and their multiples. Sharp resonant peaks of hearing receivers are exaggerated when an artificial ear (coupler) is substituted for an actual human ear. The gains for speech (spondees) of this ear trumpet for four hard-of-hearing listeners were 6, 11, 12, and 15 dB. (*Courtesy of J. R. Cox, Jr.*)

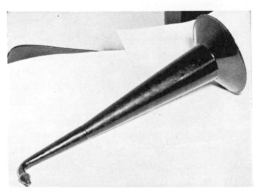

Fig. 10-2. An old ear trumpet.

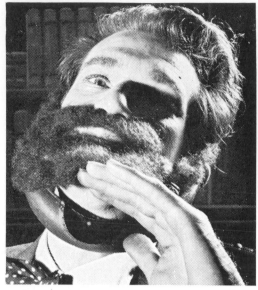

Fig. 10-4. Concealment by a beard of a large nonelectric hearing aid. (*From the Goldstein Collection, Central Institute for the Deaf. Photo, St. Louis Post-Dispatch.*)

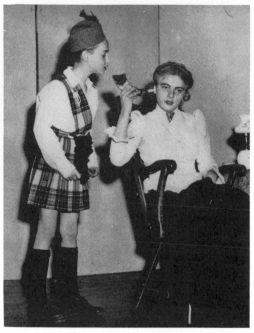

Fig. 10-6. Deaf children reenact the story of Alexander Graham Bell. (*From the Goldstein Collection, Central Institute for the Deaf.*)

were more than mere scoops to collect acoustic energy. They were also "resonators," tuned broadly to frequencies in the

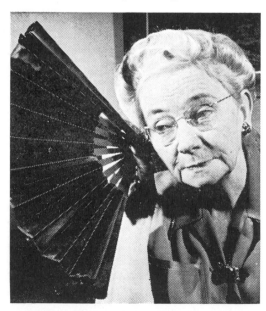

Fig. 10-5. An acoustic fan (*From the Goldstein Collection, Central Institute for the Deaf. Photo, St. Louis Post-Dispatch.*)

speech range. Sound pressures build up to higher levels at and near the resonant frequencies of the instrument, and at these frequencies the energy delivered to the ear may sometimes be increased in this way by as much as 10 to 20 dB. The external ear canal deals with sounds at frequencies near 4000 Hz in the same way. The tube of the trumpet is larger and longer than the ear canal and is thus "tuned" to a lower band of frequencies.

By empirically combining the principles of resonance and sound conduction, the ear trumpet or the speaking tube can be a fairly effective hearing aid. Those instruments are very simple and easy to use, and should not be forgotten in this electronic era. The gain for speech provided by an ear trumpet is likely to be about 10 to 15 dB. Even the cupped hand behind the ear gives us 6 or 8 dB. As we all know, this may make just the difference between understanding and not understanding a lecture or a sermon.

## "Louder, Please!"

The cupped hand at the ear also politely tells the speaker that the listener is having difficulty hearing him, and almost always, so universally is the sign understood, the speaker will raise his voice. An extra 10 dB of voice means only a little extra effort for most speakers. We instinctively and often unconsciously raise our voices this much in noisy surroundings when we begin to have a little difficulty hearing ourselves. The intensity of the voice is increased at the source, and the hard-of-hearing listener gets the benefit.

In the Psycho-Acoustic Laboratory the wartime project dealing with hearing aids was nicknamed "Louder, Please."

## Early Bone-Conduction Devices

Among the mechanical hearing aids of the last century it is interesting to find one, the acoustic fan, which took advantage of bone conduction. A sheet of metal or hard rubber, shaped and decorated like a fan, was held with one corner against the teeth. The vibrations of the metal were transmitted through the teeth to the bones of the skull and thus to the inner ear. More recently, men have used devices resembling pipes that employ the same principle. Bone conduction can, as we have seen, bypass a conductive deafness. The acoustic fan or pipe is unable, however, to collect enough energy from the air to be a very effective aid to hearing.

## Devices within the Ear

Formerly some otologists employed a "prosthesis," usually a bit of tissue paper to cover a perforation in the tympanic membrane or a wisp of cotton within the middle ear and touching the stapes, to improve the transmission of acoustic energy. Suitable cases were few, the improvements were only moderate at best, and the prosthesis had to be replaced frequently. The use of such devices in the middle ear has now been given up almost entirely in favor of the operations of myringoplasty or tympanoplasty, described in Chapter 6. The occasional temporary success of such simple prostheses nevertheless lent a glow of plausibility to a host of devices that were and probably still are advertised by unscrupulous individuals in uncritical newspapers and periodicals.

Complete restoration of hearing with a simple, inexpensive, but miraculous gadget that fits comfortably within the ear canal is the dream of everyone who is hard of hearing. Even the most sober and rational of us dream and wish. We are not very far removed from the days when the right ear of a lion was believed to be a cure for deafness or when we bought "snake oil" from the Indian medicine man. There are still enough wishful and gullible people to keep in business a few who are willing to promise enough at not *too* high a price. A thousand-to-one chance that the wonderful gadget may be a tenth as good as it is claimed to be seems to be worth a few dollars to many people. But actually there isn't such a chance. Claims of restoring hearing by "resonance" are a pseudoscientific smoke screen. Very rarely, it is true, something pushed blindly into the ear canal might open a passageway through or around a plug of wax. This might cause a real improvement; but, except for such cases, we may be quite sure that those who believed themselves benefited by mysterious nonelectrical within-the-ear gadgets were honestly self-deluded one way or another.

One of the most rigid laws of physics (although apparently not of human society) says, in effect, "You can't get something for nothing." What the hard-of-hearing man must get in order to hear is *more energy*. He may induce the speaker to provide it by saying, "Louder, please"; he may move closer to the speaker to intercept more of it; he may collect more energy in an ear trumpet or a speaking tube and bring it more efficiently to his ear; or he may provide it from the battery of an electric hearing aid.

Now, with the extreme miniaturization of modern hearing aids an electric hearing aid of moderate power can actually be worn within the ear, but it is not a simple or an inexpensive gadget.

## ELECTRIC HEARING AIDS

An electric hearing aid is a miniature telephone. It differs fundamentally from the mechanical aids we have just described in that *its batteries, and not the human voice, supply the energy of the sound that the listener finally hears*. The voice of the speaker merely serves to control the flow of electric current in the wires to the earpiece and gives it the pattern of the voice sounds. The receiver in the listener's ear, like the telephone receiver at the end of the line, converts the electric current back into sound. The point is that the sound generated in the earpiece, like the sound from a public-address system, may be made much louder than the sound that falls upon the microphone (transmitter) because its energy comes from the battery. A telephone is designed to produce at a distance a sound nearly as loud as the original voice. The energy from the battery of the telephone is required to overcome the losses in the long wires. A hearing aid is designed to produce a louder sound from a very small receiver at the end of a very short wire. Thus the energy of the battery serves to overcome the hearing loss of the listener.

### Types of Electric Hearing Aids

Electric hearing aids are of three general types: wearable, portable or desk types, and group.

Comfort, convenience, desire to conceal the instrument, and individual acoustic needs have all contributed to the development of a variety of types of wearable hear-

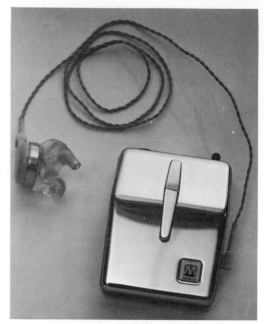

Fig. 10-7. A body-worn monaural hearing aid. (*Maico Hearing Instruments, Inc.*)

ing aids. Some types are more popular than others, depending on what the user considers most important to him. Later in this chapter we shall comment on the relative effectiveness of the different types in various listening situations.

Wearable instruments differ mainly in where they are worn on the body and in whether there is a receiver in one ear or in both ears. The following types are commercially available:

1. Conventional monaural: one instrument (microphone, amplifier, batteries) worn in the coat, shirt, or dress with receiver in one ear.
2. Monaural head-mounted: one instrument, housed in the temple of a pair of spectacles or in a case worn behind the ear or within the ear, with receiver in one ear.
3. Pseudobinaural or Y-cord: one instrument worn in coat, shirt, or dress with a receiver in each ear.
4. Binaural with conventional "packaging": two separate conventional instru-

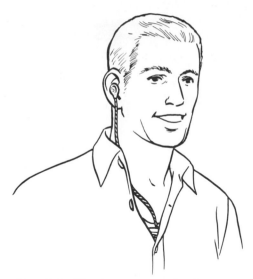

Fig. 10-8. Wearing a conventional monaural hearing aid. Men may wear the instrument in a pouch suspended from the neck under the shirt or they may clip it in a shirt, vest, or coat pocket. Women clip the instrument to a brassiere or slip or tuck it in a pouch and pin the pouch to a brassiere strap. (*Adapted from an illustration by Sonotone Corp.*)

ments worn on the chest, usually about eight inches apart, one for each ear.

5. Binaural spectacle: two instruments, "packaged" in the temples of spectacles, one for each ear.
6. Binaural head-mounted: two instruments on the head, usually mounted behind the ears, one for each ear.

These wearable types of earing aids are illustrated in Figures 10-7 to 10-15.

The portable or desk type of instrument can be used by a single hard-of-hearing listener who spends much of his time in one place. It may deliver more power with better quality than wearable instruments do, and it draws its power from a wall socket as a radio does. It does not require an insert receiver and frequently has two "over-the-ear" receivers. The portable hearing aid (Figure 10-16) may have multiple outlets, an advantageous feature for an itinerant teacher who wants to use the instrument with two or three children.

A group hearing (Figure 10-17) aid consists of one or more microphones, an amplifier, and as many as ten pairs of over-the-ear or insert receivers. Frequently a turntable is included for playing recorded speech, music, or sound effects. The effect of a group hearing aid may now be achieved with individual wearable instruments without connecting wires from the amplifier to the listeners. This is done by using electromagnetic transmission. One method uses an "induction loop," a loop of wire around the classroom that receives electric energy from the amplifier of the group aid. The magnetic field created by the loop current is sensed by a "telephone pickup," a small coil of wire in each of the conventional aids worn by the listeners. Movement of the listeners within the room is not limited by wires. For best signal-to-noise ratio, the speaker normally wears or carries a microphone held close to the lips.

Rooms equipped with induction loops

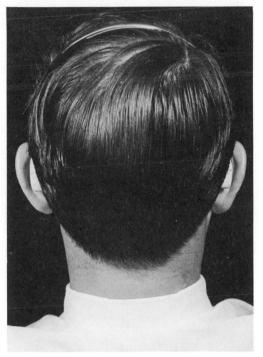

Fig. 10-9. A binaural "behind-the-ear" instrument. Clipped to a headband, it rests behind the ear. (*Maico Hearing Instruments*)

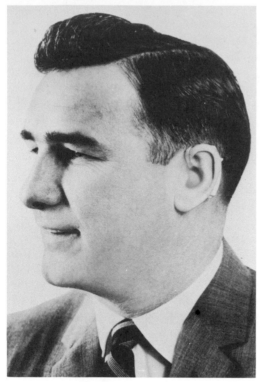

Fig. 10-10. Wearing a "behind-the-ear" instrufent. The instrument is held in place by the tube around the auricle. (*Maico Hearing Instruments*)

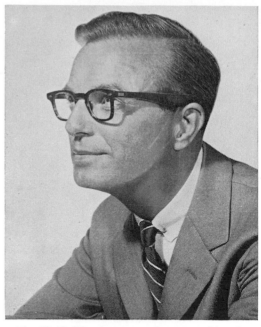

Fig. 10-12. Wearing an eyeglass type of hearing aid. (*Sonotone Corp.*)

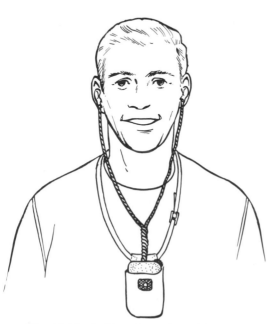

Fig. 10-11. A Y-cord hearing aid. Note the single instrument, with a receiver in each ear.

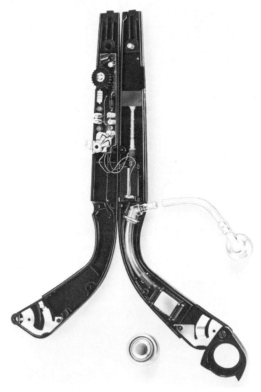

Fig. 10-13. Eyeglass hearing aid. (*Zenith Radio Corp.*)

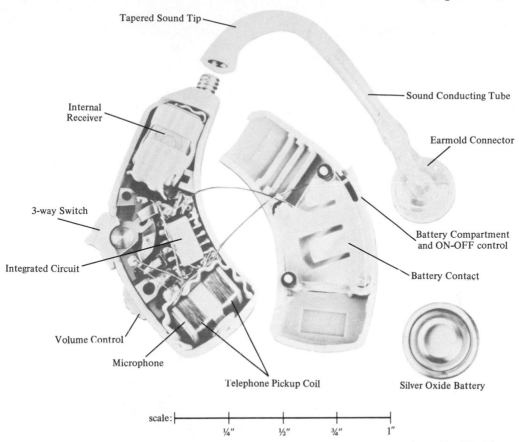

Tapered Sound Tip

Sound Conducting Tube

Internal Receiver

Earmold Connector

3-way Switch

Battery Compartment and ON-OFF control

Integrated Circuit

Battery Contact

Volume Control

Microphone

Telephone Pickup Coil

Silver Oxide Battery

scale: ¼" ½" ¾" 1"

Fig. 10-14. Cutaway view of components within a "behind-the-ear" hearing aid. (*Zenith Radio Corp.*)

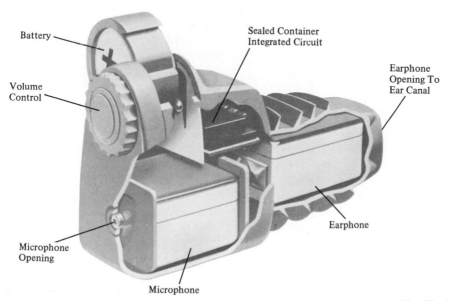

Battery

Sealed Container Integrated Circuit

Volume Control

Earphone Opening To Ear Canal

Microphone Opening

Earphone

Microphone

Fig. 10-15. Cutaway showing components within a "within-the-ear" hearing aid. (*Zenith Radio Corp.*)

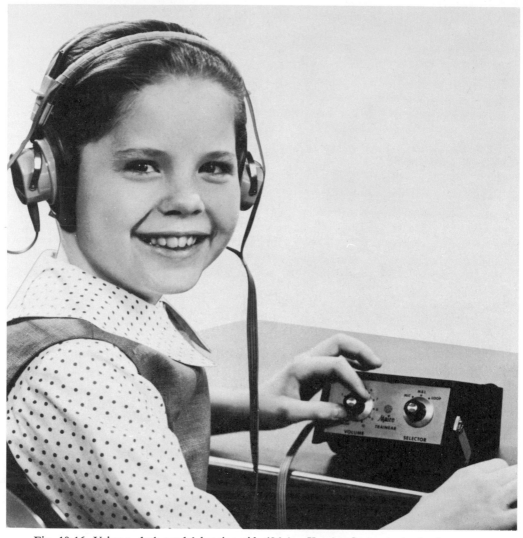

Fig. 10-16. Using a desk model hearing aid. (*Maico Hearing Instruments, Inc.*)

must be sufficiently far from each other to prevent excessive "crosstalk" from the loop of one aid to the listeners of another. Such crosstalk can be greatly reduced by using radio frequency (RF) transmission in which the speakers voice is used to modulate a "carrier" signal. The modulated carrier is "broadcast" through the loop to small radio receivers that are carried by each of the listeners and are tuned to the transmitted carrier signal. Adjacent rooms operate on different carrier frequencies, and receivers tuned to one carrier will reject all others. As with the conventional magnetic loop, two rooms with sufficient distance between them can operate on the same carrier frequency.

In some group hearing aids, it is desirable to free the speaker from microphone wires. This can be accomplished by using a "wireless microphone," actually a small portable RF transmitter, that transmits to a radio receiver whose output can be rebroadcast through either the conventional or RF loop systems or can be used to drive earphones directly. The radio receiver must be so-

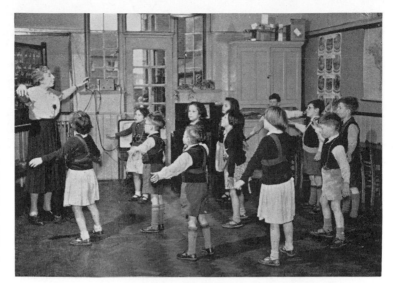

Fig. 10-17. An "inductance loop" group hearing aid. Note that the children's hearing aids are not wired to a fixed unit. The children may move about the room freely. (*Royal Residential Schools for the Deaf, Manchester, England*)

phisticated to have tracking capabilities to follow the frequency drift in the less stable "wireless microphone," and consequently, at present, it is rather expensive and too large to be carried on the person.

Group hearing aids are generally used in schols for the deaf and hard-of-hearing, in churches, in meeting halls, and in theaters. Binaural features are now being increasingly incorporated in these instruments.

### Basic Components of Electric Hearing Aids

The electric hearing aid is quite like a telephone or public address system. Each is an electronic system interposed between talker and listener to increase the acoustic signal at the listener to a level sufficiently above his "threshold" to make it intelligible. The threshold of the listener is controlled either by his aural sensitivity, by his noise environment, or perhaps by some combination of these. The basic components of each system are a microphone which transforms the acoustic signal from the talker into an equivalent electrical signal, an amplifier that increases the power level of that signal, and an output transducer that transforms the electrical signal back into the acoustical domain. Figure 10-18 illustrates these three basic components. The characteristics of

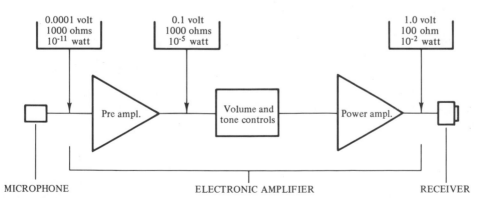

Fig. 10-18. Block diagram of an electronic hearing aid.

each, as they are related to the over-all performance of the hearing aid, will be examined.

### Microphones

The microphone is an electroacoustic transducer that transforms acoustic signals at its input into corresponding electric signals at its output. For microphones of high quality the transformation is linear with flat amplitude and phase response over the frequency range of interest. A typical hearing-aid microphone usually would not be considered "high quality" because some flatness of amplitude and phase response is normally sacrificed in order to make it sensitive, compact, rugged, and relatively inexpensive.

In recent years, three types of microphones, the crystal, the magnetic, and the ceramic have been used in hearing aids and each type has certain advantages and disadvantages. Since the "state of the art" of electronic circuitry and packaging is changing so rapidly and since microphones are described in detail in other texts, only an outline of the characteristics and principles of operation of each type that is used in hearing aids will be presented. Each microphone has a diaphragm that is set into motion under the influence of an acoustic pressure wave; the diaphragm is a mechano-acoustic transducer that transforms acoustic energy into mechanical energy. The diaphragm motion, in turn, is transformed into a voltage at the electrical terminals of the transducer. The method by which the mechanical energy is transformed into electrical energy is principally what distinguishes one type of microphone from another.

*The crystal microphone.* In a crystal microphone, the transduction element is usually a thin slab of Rochelle salt cut from a whole crystal. When properly cut, the crystal slabs are *piezoelectric* since a mechanical deformation of the crystal will produce an electric potential across its face. Moreover, the deformation and resultant potential are linearly related when the crystal is properly employed.

A typical crystal microphone is shown in schematic form in Figure 10-19. The crystal is rigidly mounted on three corners, and the fourth corner is mechanically connected through a stiff rod to a lightweight diaphragm. Acoustic pressure on one side causes motion of the diaphragm, and this motion is coupled through the driving rod to one corner of the crystal. The resultant deformation in turn induces a potential between the crystal faces which are coated with conducting foil or paint. Wires are then attached to the conducting surfaces to convey the potential to the amplifier.

Crystal microphones are adversely affected by excessive heat, moisture, dryness, or mechanical shock. Their electrical impedance is high, so that they provide reasonable transfer of power to the high input impedance of a vacuum-tube amplifier, but they are poorly suited for driving the lower input impedances of the solid-state amplifiers of most present hearing aids. For this reason crystal microphones are rarely used in modern hearing aids and are not likely to be used again because high-impedance ceramic microphones, which have certain advantages over their crystal counterparts, may be used.

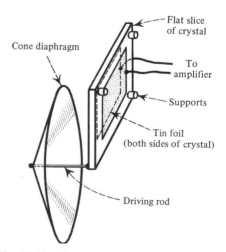

Fig. 10-19. Diagram of a crystal microphone.

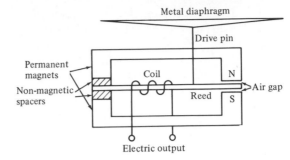

Fig. 10-20. Schematic drawing of a balanced-armature microphone.

*The magnetic microphone.* The magnetic microphone that is used in present hearing aids has a low electrical source impedance that matches the low impedance of most solid-state hearing-aid amplifiers.

The principal parts of a balanced-armature magnetic microphone that is widely used is shown in Figure 10-20.

Fluctuations of sound pressure cause corresponding motion of the diaphragm, which is coupled through the rigid drive pin to the reed or armature. The reed is a thin strip of soft magnetic metal and is positioned within a coil having turns of very fine wire. As the reed moves, the magnetic flux in the reed changes, and a voltage proportional to the rate of change of flux is induced in the coil.

The magnetic microphone is subject to damage when exposed to excessive mechanical shock but is relatively insensitive to normal changes of heat and humidity. Its inherent electrical noise is low because of its low electrical impedance.

*Ceramic microphones.* Ceramic and crystal microphones are physically and electrically quite alike except that the piezoelectric element of a ceramic microphone is ceramic, such as lead zirconate-titanate. Like crystals, ceramic elements have high electrical impedance and are best used with high-impedance amplifiers. Unlike crystals, ceramics are relatively insensitive to changes in temperature and humidity.

Although they have better low-frequency response than their magnetic counterparts, present use of ceramic microphones in hearing aids is quite limited because when they are matched to relatively high-impedance amplifiers the noise level out of the amplifier can be and often is relatively high.

### Electric Amplifiers

An electric amplifier is a system with electric signals at both input and output. If designed and used properly, the amplifier of a hearing aid will be relatively linear, and its self-noise will be low.

Although amplifiers all increase the power level of the signal, they are often designated as "voltage," "current," or "power" amplifiers according to whether their primary function is to increase the voltage, the current, or the power level of the signal.

A hearing-aid amplifier might appear schematically as in Figure 10-18. The *preamplifier* serves to increase the voltage level from approximately 0.0001 volts to 0.1 volts (60 dB voltage gain) without impedance change. This amplifier is therefore conventionally called a voltage amplifier even though there is considerable power gain (60 dB) as well. In contrast, the *power amplifier* serves principally to increase the power level of the signal from $10^{-5}$ watts to $10^{-2}$ watts (30 dB power gain) although there is also 20 dB of voltage gain. Note that through the entire amplifier the voltage gain is $10^4$ (80 dB) while the power gain is $10^9$ (90 dB). This means that the power into the receiver is a billion times as great as the power coming out of the microphone! The additional energy, of course, is supplied by the batteries that power the amplifier.

The art of packaging electronic circuitry is changing so rapidly as new electronic components are developed that detailed descriptions of electric amplifiers for hearing aids are inappropriate in this book. The reader is referred to the current engineering literature on linear electric amplifiers.

The history of electric amplifiers in hearing aids began in the early 1930s when a carbon amplifier was used to modulate battery power to a receiver. In the late 1930s the first vacuum tube aids were manufactured and used until the early 1950s when the first transistor aids appeared. By the early 1960s integrated-circuit amplifiers were being used, particularly in the "ear-level" and "in-the-ear" hearing aids where space is so important.

It has been possible, since the time of the vaccum tube aids to build amplifiers of high quality. However, the tradeoff between electronic excellence and cost, size, and ruggedness must be considered seriously by the manufacturer. Advances in the electronics and hearing-aid industries have lead to more efficient, rugged, and linear aids that are becoming smaller and smaller without significant increase in price. Several amplifiers from hearing aids of 1968 are shown in Figure 10-21.

### Receivers

A *receiver* provides the inverse function of a microphone; that is, it transforms an electric input from the hearing-aid amplifier to an acoustic output. The close relation between microphones and receivers goes beyond this, however. Most common microphones and receivers are *reciprocal;* that is, the microphones can act as receivers and conversely. As a result, for each type of microphone there is a corresponding type of receiver with the same basic principles of operation; only the configuration of the internal elements are different in order to enhance the quality of the device in that role for which it was designed. For example, there are both microphones and receivers of the moving iron, the crystal, and the moving coil types. The similarities of microphones and receivers of a particular type will be evident from the discussion that follows.

Receivers for hearing aids are of two general kinds: air conduction and bone conduction.

*Air-conduction receivers.* All air-conduction receivers for body-worn electric hearing aids are small enough to be worn in the ear. They are supported by an "insert" or "earpiece" of molded plastic. Even smaller than these are the type built into eyeglass hearing aids and the other tiny aids

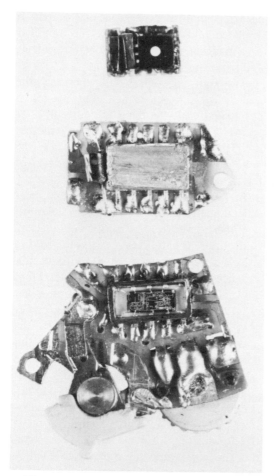

Fig. 10-21. Several types of hearing aid amplifiers: *A* and *B* employ integrated circuits. *C* is a miniaturized discrete component design. (*Zenith Radio Corp.*)

worn in or behind the ear. With the eyeglass and behind-the-ear types the sound from the self-contained receiver is carried into the ear canal through a transparent plastic tube which terminates in an individually molded ear tip. These tiny receivers represent one of the most difficult bits of electro-acoustic engineering in the hearing aid. These earphones must transform electric energy efficiently into sound, and at the same time they must avoid excessive mechanical resonance, which would emphasize some one frequency too much. All this is difficult to accomplish in such a small size. An ideal hearing aid would handle all the audible frequencies with equal efficiency. Such an instrument would preserve the natural quality of sounds and also avoid the discomfort from too great amplification of any one particular frequency. The ideal is being approached more and more closely, even in instruments that employ the small insert type of receiver, but we can hardly hope that it will ever be attained completely.

Receivers with the best acoustic characteristics, such as are used for audiometers and laboratory test instruments, are too large to be practical for wearable hearing aids. They are, however, included in many portable and group hearing aids.

The most common type of receiver used on larger, wearable hearing aids is the *moving-iron magnetic*. It operates on the same principle as the magnetic microphone but in reverse. A thin diaphragm of magnetic material is mounted close to a permanent magnet, as shown in Figure 10-22. The electric current from the amplifier passes through coils that are wound on cores of special magnetic material fastened to the permanent magnet. According to the strength and direction of the current through the coils, the magnet becomes stronger or weaker. The magnet thus pulls more or less strongly on the diaphragm. The diaphragm vibrates and sets up sound waves in the air.

The *balanced-armature magnetic* re-

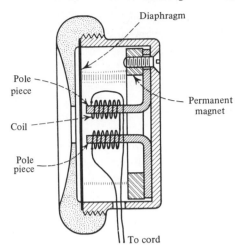

Fig. 10-22. A magnetic receiver.

ceiver that is used in many miniature headworn aids physically is quite like the balanced-armature magnetic microphone. Current through the coil causes the armature to move by changing the magnetic forces on it, and sound waves are produced by rigidly coupling the armature to a diaphragm.

The *crystal* earphone is very much like a miniature crystal microphone. The same kind of crystal is cut and mounted in the same way, and is connected mechanically to a thin metal diaphragm. The electric voltage from the output circuit of the amplifier is applied to opposite sides of the crystal, and the crystal bends in proportion to the voltage applied. The bending of the crystal moves the diaphragm and thus sets up sound waves in the air.

The *moving-coil magnetic* air-conduction receiver is known as the "dynamic" receiver. A light coil of fine wire is firmly attached to the center of a diaphragm, or cone. A strong permanent magnet is mounted so that the turns of the coil lie in its radial magnetic field. The varying electric current from the amplifier passes through the coil and causes it to move back and forth in the magnetic field in accordance with the variations in the current. The fundamental principle is used almost universally in radio and public-address loud-speakers. In the moving-iron and balanced armature receivers the coil is firmly attached to the magnet and varies the strength of the field that moves the diaphragm. In the moving-coil receiver, on the other hand, the coil is attached to and moves with the diaphragm.

*Bone-conduction receivers.* The moving-coil principle, in addition to being employed in most loudspeakers, is applied in some of the large high-quality earphones used for audiometers and other special purposes. New magnetic alloys, which make possible tiny yet permanent magnets, favor the development of this type of receiver, and a few hearing aids of the future may employ the moving-coil principle.

The most common type of *bone-conduction receiver* or *vibrator* is magnetic. It is designed to vibrate its case instead of setting up sound waves in the ear (Figure 10-23). Its diaphragm is attached rigidly to a plastic case shaped to fit comfortably against the mastoid bone behind the ear. The magnetic system is supported by the edge of the diaphragm. The pull of the magnet varies with the changes in the flow of electric current through the coil, and both magnet and case move in relation to one another. The inertia of the magnet is

considerable, however, and therefore the case, and with it the mastoid bone, vibrates appreciably. The case moves less than does the diaphragm of an air-conduction receiver, but it moves with considerable force and can therefore set up an adequate vibration in the skull. The vibrator is held in snug contact against the mastoid by means of a light spring headband, as shown in Figures 10-24 and 10-25.

Partly because of the way in which skin and bone transmit sound, it is difficult to design a bone-conduction vibrator that will deliver high frequencies to the inner ear as efficiently as it does some of the lower frequencies, but its range compares very favorably with the range of the usual air-conduction receiver.

*Comparison of bone conduction and air conduction.* In the chapter on the medical aspects of deafness, the principle of

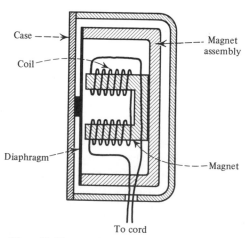

Fig. 10-23. A bone-conduction receiver or vibrator.

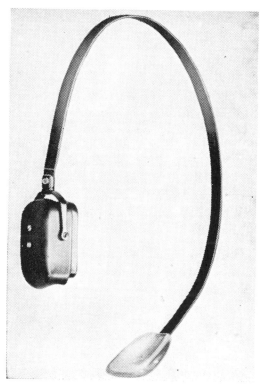

Fig. 10-24. A bone-conduction vibrator with its spring headband. (*Sonotone Corp.*)

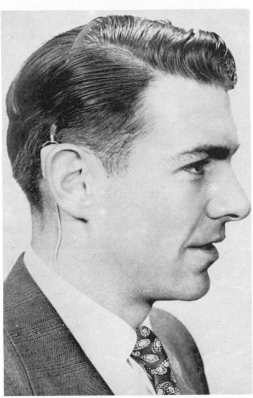

Fig. 10-25. A bone-conduction vibrator in place behind the ear. (*Sonotone Corp.*)

bone conduction was discussed. It will be recalled that bone conduction is definitely preferable to the insert type of receiver when, for any medical reason, the wearer cannot safely or comfortably use an insert earpiece. Bone conduction is most successful when the hearing loss is primarily conductive and the inner ear is still normal. We shall return to the problem of bone as compared with air in connection with the selection of a hearing aid; but it is worth noting that recent technical developments have favored air conduction somewhat more than bone conduction.

Thanks to the individually molded ear insert, a small in-the-ear air-conduction receiver can now deliver into the ear more sound of good quality than was formerly possible. A considerable fraction of the sound that reaches the inner ear from an air-conduction receiver may actually arrive

by way of the bone. The faithfulness of reproduction by a good air-conduction receiver is generally better, particularly for high frequencies, than by a bone-conduction vibrator. When the bone-conduction vibrator was first introduced, it was often preferred because it was less conspicuous and perhaps more comfortable than large, over-the-ear air-conduction receivers. Some wearers still prefer bone-conduction vibrators for the same reasons and find them perfectly adequate; but with the increased efficiency of small and less conspicuous air-conduction receivers that require no headband, the choice is based more and more often on the combination of greater convenience and simple effectiveness, and the majority of the hard-of-hearing prefer air conduction.

### The Volume Control

A volume control, or "gain control," makes it possible to adjust the over-all gain of a hearing aid to intermediate values. The volume control is usually a resistance that is provided with a sliding contact. It is usually located between stages of the electric amplifier. The full strength of the signal from the first stage is applied to the resistance, and the slider takes off and passes on to the next stage more or less of the signal according to its position.

### The Tone Control

The tone control is usually a complicated arrangement of condensers and resistances. It may be placed ahead of the first stage, or between stages; and the circuits actually employed in different instruments vary considerably from one another.

The tone control changes the relative strength of the high-frequency and the low-frequency tones in the signals that pass through it (see Figure 10-29). To obtain "high-tone emphasis," a combination of condensers and resistances is chosen that transmits high frequencies efficiently and low frequencies inefficiently. The low frequencies are reduced in strength, or "attenuated," more than the high, and thus a *relative high-tone emphasis* is obtained. High-tone emphasis may really be only *low-tone suppression;* but as long as plenty of gain is available, it makes no difference. The wearer simply pushes up the volume control, thereby increasing the strength of all frequencies equally, and the net result is an increase in the high frequencies with no loss in the middle or low range.

Low-tone emphasis is obtained by other combinations of condensers and/or resistors chosen to suppress the high frequencies.

Some makes of instrument do not have an adjustable tone control, but instead offer several models, each with its own particular emphasis of high tones, low tones, or middle tones. The purchaser then selects the model that best suits his particular needs. Other instruments have an internal adjustment for tone, which is set by the dealer when he sells the instrument; thus he "fits" the device to the purchaser's individual requirements. Still other instruments are "fitted" by selection of the appropriate receiver.

### The Cords and the Case

The cords of a hearing aid are obviously nothing more than light, flexible, insulated wires that carry the current from the amplifier to the receiver.

The problem with cords is to make them light and flexible and yet mechanically strong, durable, and electrically insulated. Furthermore, the covering must not generate static electricity or make a noise when it rubs on clothing, for noise carried mechanically by cords to the amplifier case and microphone can be a source of great annoyance. In addition, the covering of a cord must keep its insulating properties when moistened by perspiration.

The case deserves mention because it, too, must be strong, light, and durable. The shape of the case and its smoothness, as well as the material of which it is made, must be carefully planned and chosen to reduce as much as possible the noise made by the friction of clothing.

### The Molded Earpiece

An important accessory to all air-conduction hearing aids is the individually molded earpiece or insert (Figure 10-26). The earpiece is made of transparent or flesh-tinted plastic that is formed to fit snugly and comfortably into the wearer's ear. The receiver is made with a small tube-like projection or "nub" on its face that snaps into a recess in the earpiece and is held there by a spring, similar to that on a clothespin. The sound passes through this nub and through a hole drilled in the earpiece and is delivered well down in the external canal of the ear.

The first step in making an earpiece is to take an impression of the ear with a special elastic plastic. Dealers in hearing aids usually provide this service. They make the impressions and send them to a special laboratory, where the actual earpieces are made according to the patterns. The manufacturers of hearing aids have standardized the nubs on receivers so that an individual earpiece fits almost any make of receiver. Rarely is an adapter needed.

Occasionally acoustic leaks are deliberately introduced to "roll off" low frequencies. Usually, however, the earpiece is made to fit the ear snugly and prevent escape of sound around it. The close fit makes the action of the receiver more efficient, as no energy is then lost through leakage. If there is a leak, the sounds reaching the eardrum will be weakened, particularly in the low frequencies.

*Squeal.* If a loud sound is delivered within the ear, it is important that as little as possible should escape around the earpiece. If sound escapes, it may reach the microphone of the hearing aid and be picked up and amplified. The result will be a "squeal" resulting from what is known

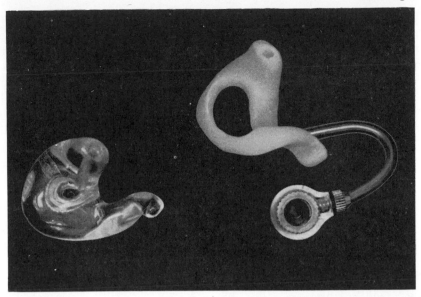

Fig. 10-26. Molded plastic eartips. On the left is a conventional eartip. In the "hideway" type on the right the receiver may be concealed and only the eartip is visible. The size and shape of the couplers that connect receivers to eartips are standardized for all hearing aids. (*Central Institute for the Deaf*)

as *acoustic feedback*. Not only is the "squeal" unpleasant; it may also drown out the sounds that the wearer wishes to hear. The development of the individually molded earpiece was an important advance. A hearing aid can deliver to the ear much louder sounds without squeal if the earpiece fits well than if it does not. Even so, even with a well-fitted earpiece, the gain of hearing aids worn at the ear is definitely limited by acoustic feedback.

The designer of a hearing aid must sacrifice some sensitivity if an instrument is to have a high acoustic output. He cannot rely on *all* the output staying within the ear. Even if the earpiece fits well, *some* sound inevitably escapes through the back of the receiver. A very sensitive, high-gain instrument with high maximum output goes into a squeal too easily to take advantage of its high gain.

Some ways of avoiding squeal are:

To improve the fit of the earpiece to the ear (and of the receiver to the earpiece)

To reduce the gain of the hearing aid

To move the microphone farther away from the receiver

To adjust the tone control for the best practical compromise.

### The Telephone Pickup

A telephone pickup is a feature of many of the more elaborate models of hearing aids. An inductive pickup coil is mounted within the case. A switch allows the user to substitute it for the microphone as the input to the hearing-aid amplifier. Thus when the telephone pickup is in use, there is no interference from the acoustic noise of the surroundings. The user simply throws the switch to the "telephone" position and holds the telephone receiver against the case of his instrument.

### Batteries

A battery is a reservoir of energy. The energy is stored in the chemical state and is transformed into electrical energy through electrochemical conversion when called upon. The *rate* at which energy is used by a hearing aid, that is its *power* consumption, is of the order of milliwatts and is determined by the amount of acoustic power that is required at the receivers and by the output and the efficiency of the microphone, electric amplifier, and receiver. One of the most significant improvements of the solid-state hearing aid over the vacuum-tube instrument is the increased efficiency of the amplifier and the resultant decrease in the cost and size of batteries.

The term "battery" is used to mean a group of electrical cells which are interconnected to provide electrical power, with the proper voltage and current, to the amplifier. Each cell has a voltage between its terminals of approximately 1.5 volts, the exact value being determined by the type of cell and the amount of energy that it has already given up. Cells can be rated according to their capacities for energy storage, measured in milliwatt-hours. However, since electrical power (milliwatts) is the product of voltage (volts) and current (milliamperes), the cell normally is rated in milliampere-hours which, given a constant output voltage, is also a measure of the stored energy. A 350 milliampere-hour, 1.5 volt cell, for example, could be expected to provide 5 milliamperes of current for 70 hours (525 milliwatt-hours). Two such cells when connected in series would give a 3 volt, 350 milliampere-hour (1050 milliwatt-hour) battery, and when connected in parallel would give a 1.5 volt, 700 milliampere-hour (1050 milliwatt-hour) battery.

### Carbon-zinc Cell

In a carbon-zinc or Leclanché cell a carbon rod is suspended within a zinc case and the space between these contains a black mix of manganese dioxide and an electrolyte paste of ammonium and zinc chlorides and water. The output voltage of this cell, with constant current drain, decreases rather uniformly with time, as

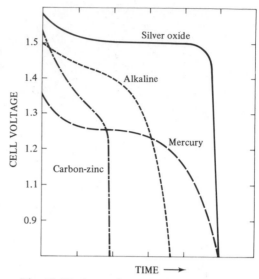

Fig. 10-27. Approximate voltage decay characteristics of several kinds of cells. The curves shown are drawn assuming constant current drain of cells of similar size. When the voltage falls below 0.9 volts, the cell is no longer useful.

shown in Figure 10-27. If the cell is drained with intermittent periods of rest, some of the voltage is regained after each rest period, and the battery life is prolonged. If the cell is drained beyond its normal limit, it may leak fluid and damage the hearing aid.

Other types of cells are not so susceptible to fluid leakage, have a relatively constant output voltage when drained over normal working periods, are not affected by adverse temperature and humidity, and store more energy per unit volume. For these reasons, carbon cells are not widely used in present (1968) hearing aids.

### Mercury Cells

The mercury cell operates on the same principle as the carbon cell, but typically one electrode is mercuric oxide, the other is a zinc-mercury amalgam, and the electrolyte is a solution of potassium hydroxide and zinc oxide. The cell container is a corrosion-proof, nickel-plated metal, so designed as to inhibit leakage. The energy density of these cells is quite high. They are not adversely affected by normal heat and humidity, and they maintain rather constant voltage (see Figure 10-27) over their useful life. Nominal voltage for these cells is 1.3 volts.

### Silver-oxide Cells

This type of cell has the greatest energy of those used in hearing aids. One electrode (anode) is zinc and the other (cathode) is silver oxide with an alkaline electrolyte of potassium hydroxide between them. The nominal voltage of 1.5 volts remains relatively constant over the life of the cell, as shown in Figure 10-28.

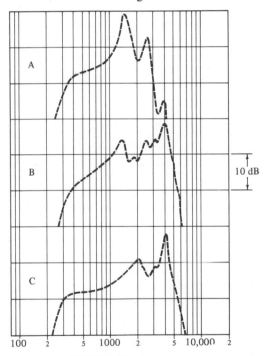

FREQUENCY in Hertz

Fig. 10-28. *Relative frequency responses of (A) the microphone, amplifier, and receiver; (B) the microphone and amplifier, and (C) the microphone of a hearing aid.* Curve (A) is the acoustic pressure in a 2-cc coupler. Curves (B) and (C) are voltage responses. All responses were made with the microphone, amplifier, and receiver "in situ" with constant sound pressure at the microphone. Thus, each curve reflects the combined responses of all stages preceding and the loading effects (if any) of all stages following the point of measurement.

### Zinc-manganese-dioxide (Alkaline) Cell

The alkaline cell has a zinc negative electrode (anode), a manganese-dioxide positive electrode (cathode), and a potassium hydroxide electrolyte. It is enclosed by a steel can which serves as a cathode current collector. The energy density of the alkaline cell is relatively high, and it can operate efficiently at high current drains. As the cell is discharged, the output voltage gradually drops but at a significantly slower rate than for the carbon cell. This is shown in Figure 10-27.

It is worth noting that in spite of the poor voltage-decay characteristic and relatively short life of the carbon-zinc cell, it is still the cheapest source of stored electrical energy per milliwatt-hour. The silver-oxide battery at present is gaining in popularity because its energy per unit volume is large (the battery does not have to be changed very often). Although its cost per milliwatt-hour is greater than that of carbon-zinc, it is less than the mercury cell, it is not sensitive to temperature and humidity, and it has a high output voltage and a relatively flat voltage-decay characteristic.

## ELECTROACOUSTIC CHARACTERISTICS OF A TYPICAL HEARING AID

In order to demonstrate more clearly the purpose, qualities, and limitations of the different basic components of hearing aids, we shall investigate in depth one hearing aid and try to point out those aspects of it that are perhaps not common to hearing aids in general. Clearly, hearing aids of different makes and models will have different electroacoustic characteristics. The aid that will be discussed is "typical" in its class, but it is not intended to represent an "average" hearing aid. This aid is a low-priced, "body-worn" hearing aid. It has a four-stage transistor amplifier with volume control and a two-position tone control.

### Frequency Response

The frequency response of the aid with 70 dB sound pressure level (SPL) at the input and 40 dB of acoustic gain at 1000 Hz is shown in curve *A* of Figure 10-28. The *response* in this case is the sound pressure that is produced by the receiver in a 2 cc coupler with constant sound pressure at the microphone.

To show how the signals are affected as they pass through the aid, the voltage-response curves at the microphone and amplifier output are also shown.

Other hearing aids with different components will have different response curves. In general, however, in present hearing aids the frequency response is limited at low frequencies by the magnetic microphone, and at high frequencies by the magnetic earphone. Sometimes frequency compensation is incorporated in the amplifier as a tone control (see Figure 10-29). Without compensation the amplifier normally has a very wide bandwidth. The frequency re-

sponse can also be changed by using different receivers as shown in Figure 10-30.

Behind-the-ear hearing aids and some body aids, in which the receiver is located behind the ear, use a small plastic tube to convey sound from the receiver to the ear. Often this tube contains acoustic damping in the form of sintered metal or lamb's wool. The length and diameter of the tube and the acoustic damping can each be varied to modify the response of the hearing aid. In general, the tube will introduce resonant peaks in the response curve, which result from standing waves in the tube, and a reduction in bandwidth. When the tube *length* is increased, the resonant peaks shift downward in frequency and the upper "cutoff" frequency is lowered. With an increase in tube *diameter,* high-frequency losses in the tube are reduced, and the response curve is raised for frequencies above about 1000 Hz. When an acoustical resistance is inserted in the tube, the resonant peaks in the response curve are damped.

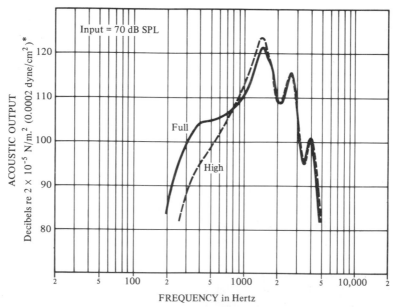

Fig. 10-29. Frequency response of a hearing aid for full-range and high-range tone control settings. Note: In this chapter the MKS system of units is used whenever appropriate. This system has been adopted in most modern engineering texts and standards. (The corresponding CGS units are given in parentheses.)

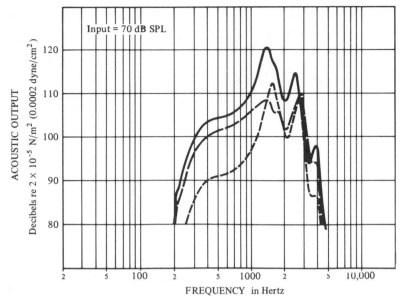

Fig. 10-30. Frequency response of a hearing aid with three different receivers.

The degree of damping is affected not only by the amount of resistance added but also by its location in the tube. Effects of the tube and damping are shown in Figure 10-31.

## THE OVER-ALL PERFORMANCE OF HEARING AIDS

The objective of hearing-aid design is to amplify speech without undue distortion but at the same time to protect the user against discomfort from too loud an output. The speech sounds are "packaged" for delivery to an elevated and more or less restricted auditory area (compare Figures 7-10 and 7-11). In addition the frequency bands above and below the important speech range are often deliberately suppressed so that noise in these bands will not annoy or distract the user.

The performance of a hearing aid is illustrated in Figures 10-32 and 10-34. Here the acoustic area of conversational speech extends from about 100 to about 8000 Hz, while the range important for good understanding of speech extends from about 400 to 3000 Hz. The sound pressure levels of conversational speech extend from a maximum of 66 dB in the lower frequencies to 30 dB or so in the high frequencies. The available auditory area of a user who has the common type of mixed hearing loss, that is, an over-all conductive loss plus some high-tone sensory-neural loss, lies largely above this area. His threshold of discomfort is assumed to lie at 120 dB, which is a likely level (Figure 10-32).

The frequency characteristic of a hearing aid is shown at the top of Figure 10-32. The flatness (or lack of flatness) of such a curve expresses the *fidelity* of the instrument. Its breadth measures the frequency range. The gain is negligible at very high and very low frequencies. The whole curve is moved up and down by changing the volume-control setting. The acoustic "gain" of a hearing aid is measured by comparing the sound pressure level developed in a 2 cc coupler with the sound pressure level (at 1000 Hz) measured in a free sound field before the hearing aid is introduced into it. The gain at 1000 Hz measured in

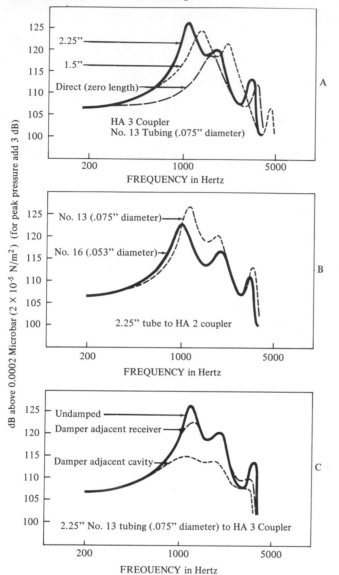

Fig. 10-31. Frequency response of a hearing aid receiver, showing (*A*) effects of tube length, (*B*) tube diameter, and (*C*) acoustical damping. (*Data from Knowles Technical Bulletin "Effects of Source Impedance and Acoustical Termination upon BK Receiver Response," Knowles Electronics, Inc.*)

this way may be 60 dB or more. (It is worth noting that the "gain for speech," measured as the difference in the threshold for speech of a hard-of-hearing listener with and without the hearing aid is often considerably less than the laboratory measurement of gain.)

There is, however, a maximum acoustic output beyond which the instrument cannot go, regardless of the setting of the volume control or the strength of the input signal. The frequency characteristic at maximum output (Figure 10-32) is flatter than it is in the normal operating range, but it has one or more maxima, because of the resonant peaks of the magnetic receiver. The position of this limiting maximum acoustic output curve describes the maximum "power" of the instrument.

In Figure 10-32 we see how the "area" of conversational speech is elevated and modified in shape by a hearing aid set to moderate gain and "low" tone control. Nearly all of the speech sounds now fall

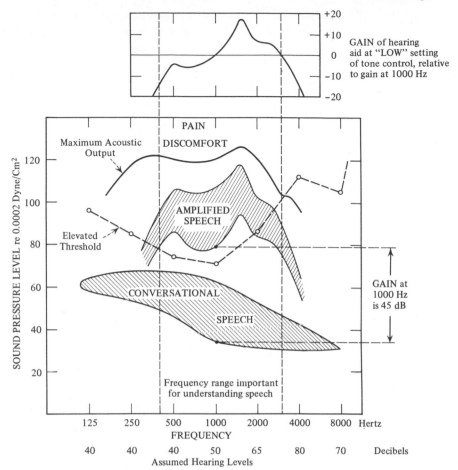

Fig. 10-32. Amplification of speech by a hearing aid without peak limiting. The area of conversational speech, as measured in a free acoustic field, is shown here with arbitrary sharp boundaries (see Figure 2-6). The upper boundary represents the level above which the peaks of speech, at that frequency, very seldom rise. The speech elements below the lower boundary contribute very little to intelligibility and can be disregarded. All of the measurements of output are made in a 2-cc coupler. The *gain of a hearing aid* at 1000 Hz is the difference between the sound-pressure level measured in the field before the hearing aid is introduced and the sound-pressure level measured in the 2-cc coupler. *The area of amplified speech* in this figure was found by moving the speech area upward by 45 dB at 1000 Hz and then modifying the shape of the area according to the over-all frequency characteristic of the hearing aid, as drawn above. This is the curve shown for the "low" setting of the tone control. The shape of the curve of *maximum acoustic output* is determined by the receiver. The level of maximum acoustic output is measured at 1000 Hz, and is here assumed to be 120 dB SPL, measured in a 2-cc coupler. This is close to the usual threshold of discomfort. Only occasional peaks of pressure at the frequencies near 1500 Hz reach this level. The limited auditory area for a hypothetical case of mixed hearing loss is shown. The amplified speech is delivered efficiently and with a minimum of distortion to this reduced "target area."

in the auditory area of the listener, but they do not encroach on his threshold of discomfort.

In Figure 10-34 we see how the distribution of the sounds of conversational speech would be modified by using a higher volume-control setting and at the same time altering the frequency characteristic to "high" by means of the tone control. The stronger low tones of speech are now deliberately amplified less than the weaker higher tones. The fidelity of the output is not as good as in the first example, but the speech may be easier for this particular listener to understand because another kind of acoustic distortion (which will be described below and which occurs when the maximum acoustic output is approached) is minimized.

In terms of these measures of performance—fidelity and frequency range, gain, and maximum power output—we can judge the performance of present-day hearing aids.

### Frequency Range

The frequency range of the hearing aid is determined mostly by the characteristics of the microphone and the earphone. The microphone becomes inefficient at the lower frequencies, and the earphone will not reproduce the higher frequencies. Both the microphone and the earphone have one or more resonant "humps" or "peaks." These are usually so located as to supplement one another and to give a relatively smooth and fairly flat frequency characteristic with quite acceptable fidelity over the middle range that is most important for speech. Modern hearing aids give ample practical coverage of the speech frequencies.

### Gain

An acoustic gain of at least 60 dB for the frequencies near the peak of the frequency characteristic is easily provided by a magnetic microphone, a transistor amplifier, and a magnetic receiver. The maximum *usable* gain is less likely to be limited by the electroacoustic apparatus than by an inadequate seal achieved at the ear. The individually fitted earmold has contributed greatly toward increasing the maximum usable gain of hearing aids. The volume control provides a variable gain in most

aids so that a range of gain of 30 to as much as 60 dB or more is available in many instruments. Sufficient gain is no longer a problem.

### Power

The maximum output of a hearing aid is inherently limited by the power of its battery and the power-handling capacities of its component parts. The acoustic distortion produced as maximum output is reached will be considered in more detail in a later section. Here compromises must be made, and both the designer of the hearing aid on the one hand and the user on the other are faced with a series of practical problems that involve the size and the expense as well as the performance of the instrument. Fortunately, for most users of hearing aids with moderate hearing losses, these problems are not often serious, as they rarely need to push their instruments to the limit of maximum acoustic output. On the whole, modern hearing aids are very well-designed and effective instruments, within the limits set by their objectives and by the engineering difficulties imposed by the desirability of making the instruments themselves as small and as comfortable to wear as possible.

## HEARING AIDS AND AUDITORY TRAINING FOR DEAF CHILDREN

Electric hearing aids for use with deaf children may be one of many varieties of three basic types: group, desk, or wearable. The advantages of a group hearing aid are its greater power output and a more desirable frequency response than the wearable aid and the possibility of minimizing acoustic feedback by keeping the microphone at a reasonable distance from the earphones. The improvements in wearable hearing aids, however, are reducing the importance of the differences.

Dr. E. Wedenberg of Sweden has suggested the principle of inserting appropriate filters "to compensate the lack of balance between the high and low portions of the speech frequency spectrum which accompanies auditory impairment. Thus the formant areas of higher frequencies valuable . . . to perceptibility may be 'raised' to a level at which they are audible along with the lower speech spectrum areas." This principle may be useful for children whom we can expect to achieve refined auditory discrimination. Whether this type of frequency response or the simple rising frequency characteristic suggested by the "Harvard Report" (of 1947), or other methods which have also been suggested, is best for hearing aids for deaf children is still under investigation.

The major advantage of a wearable hearing aid for the child is that he can have it with him at all times and benefit continuously from auditory stimulation. Frequently, children are first taught to appreciate sound over group instruments and then use their own wearable instrument outside the classroom.

There are a number of problems concerning features of group hearing aids for deaf children about which there is little experimental information. The desirability of compression amplification (described below) is generally recognized, but how restricted the dynamic intensity range of the compressed signal should be is another matter. For the deaf child who cannot make fine discriminations, the information contained in intensity changes in speech is important.

We also need more information about the value of binaural hearing aids for deaf children. The reference here is not to pseudobinaural hearing aids that use one microphone, one amplifier, and two earphones, which are little better than a monaural system, especially for localization of sound. A true binaural hearing aid is possible if each ear is aided by a system that is fed from a microphone mounted at that ear. Its advantage for a deaf child, in addition to his not too primary need for localization of sound sources, is now becoming apparent.

Other features of group hearing aids that are proving useful in practice are the insert type of earphones to increase comfort and to reduce acoustic feedback, ceiling-mounted microphones or inductance loops to increase freedom of action for the teacher and the pupils, acoustically treated rooms to reduce reverberation and distortion, visual aids to indicate intensity or pitch changes, and outlet boxes at blackboards.

## HEARING AIDS CANNOT DO EVERYTHING

*No hearing aid can ever compensate completely for a hearing loss.* Everyone who is thinking of getting a hearing aid should realize at the outset that there are limits to what *any* hearing aid can possibly do. Some limits are imposed by the ear and others by the nature of the sounds that we wish to hear. There are practical limits also, set by size, weight, and expense, to what can be built into a wearable hearing aid at the present time.

For example, an ear with sensory-neural deafness may be unable to hear high tones no matter how much they are amplified. If *all* the nerve fibers that are normally stimulated by tones above 3000 Hz have degenerated, then no conceivable hearing aid can ever make sounds above 3000 Hz audible again, except by transforming them to some lower frequency. This is the fundamental reason why hearing aids are usually of little or no assistance in the "abrupt" type of high-tone sensory-neural deafness.

Until about 1940 a practical limit of performance was set by the inability to provide enough amplification without undue distortion. Now, however, a powerful instrument can deliver a sound as loud as most wearers are willing to tolerate even after they have become accustomed to loud sounds. The limit of useful power is now set by the ear. A good hearing aid must, of course, bring sound above the threshold of audibility, but its output must never exceed the listener's threshold of discomfort.

In the hard-of-hearing ear the thresholds of discomfort and pain usually stay near the normal levels, so that *the range (in decibels) between the faintest audible tone and the loudest tolerable tone is diminished*. Now if we amplify all sounds equally, the strong sounds may become intolerable before the weak sounds are powerful enough to be heard. *Some suppression of the strong sounds may therefore be necessary if the weak ones are to be made audible.*

Speech is a mixture of sounds of different intensities, and the weakest sounds may be as much as 30 dB below the strongest (see Figure 10-32). If the range between audibility and discomfort is less (as it may be with a severe hearing loss), it may be possible to make speech audible and intelligible as well as tolerable, but only at the sacrifice of some "naturalness" or "quality." Fortunately, however, this compromise is necessary only when the hearing loss is very severe.

### Distortion in Hearing Aids

Whenever the output of a system is not some constant times its input, then the system is said to distort the signal. Since all physically realizable systems are power-limited and have finite bandwith, they are necessarily linear only for certain classes of signals. If the input signals are members of this class, the system is linear; if not, the system is nonlinear, and distortion results. Although this concept is simple, methods of accurately defining distortion are not. The reason is because, so far as a listener is concerned, some kinds of distortion are completely tolerable or even desirable, but other kinds will completely destroy his ability to receive information. For this reason there are many different measures of distortion, and it is up to the designer and user of the system (for example, a hearing aid) to decide which one best describes the nonlinearity of his system with respect to the expected signals in the system and the capabilities of the listener at its output. The relation between various measures of distortion in a hearing aid and the ability of an impaired listener to receive information is not fully understood. The problem is too complicated; there are too many kinds of signals of interest, too many kinds of nonlinearity, and too many kinds of hearing impairment. Nonetheless, there are some combinations of signals, nonlinearities, and listeners that are of special interest.

### "Limiting" of Output

The necessary protection against discomfort can be provided automatically. We have pointed out that an amplifier can deliver only just so much power from its last stage even when the "valve" is open wide. *One of the fundamental principles of selecting a hearing aid is to pick an instrument that has enough amplification but also has a maximum output that will be tolerable.*

When a hearing aid is used near its maximum output, as may be necessary if the hearing loss is severe, the strongest peaks of the electric waves will reach the maximum output of the instrument. We may think of the maximum output as a ceiling. The peaks of speech cannot surpass this limit, and the waves are therefore squared off, or "clipped," as shown in Figure 10-33. These clipped waves are tolerable, but obviously they are distorted in shape. That is why the quality of the sound suffers.

### Effects of Peak Clipping

Fortunately a considerable amount of simple peak clipping does not greatly reduce the intelligibility of speech even though it may make the voice sound

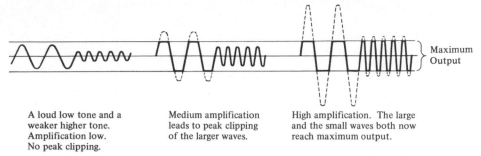

A loud low tone and a
weaker higher tone.
Amplification low.
No peak clipping.

Medium amplification
leads to peak clipping
of the larger waves.

High amplification. The large
and the small waves both now
reach maximum output.

Fig. 10-33. Diagram showing various degrees of "peak clipping" of speech waves.

harsh, rough, and unnatural. Ordinarily the low frequencies of vowel sounds, which are the most powerful of the speech sounds, as indicated in Figures 10-32 and 10-34, reach the limiting maximum acoustic output first and consequently suffer from peak clipping. The change of quality in the speech is most noticeable in these vowel sounds. It is actually rather surprising, however, to see on an oscilloscope how severely the speech waves may be squared off and distorted by simple peak clipping before the speech becomes really difficult to understand.

In order to reduce or avoid the distortion and loss of quality introduced by peak clipping it is desirable to amplify the higher frequencies of speech more than the lower frequencies, so that both the high frequencies and the low frequencies reach the limit of maximum acoustic output together. Such "high-tone emphasis" is introduced by reducing the amplification of low tones, as shown in Figure 10-29. This moderate high-tone emphasis allows for the use of the greatest gain before the clipping level is reached. It uses most efficiently the restricted auditory area of most hard-of-hearing listeners, as illustrated in Figure 10-34.

One reason that the intelligibility of speech suffers so much more from peak clipping of the low tones than from corresponding clipping of the high tones is that some of the harmonics that are introduced by the peak clipping of low frequencies are clearly audible, and for high frequencies most of the harmonics lie above the range of speech frequencies and are very inefficiently transmitted by the receiver of the hearing aid. If the listener has a high-tone hearing loss, these high-frequency distortion products are doubly excluded and of no consequence.

With the proper combination of high-tone pre-emphasis and appropriate limiting of the output by peak clipping, plenty of amplification can be used in a hearing aid to make faint sounds audible while at the same time the ear is protected against discomfort. Intelligibility is well, although not completely, preserved. There is some deterioration of quality when the peak clipping becomes severe. We must pay for the protection, so to speak, but the price in quality need not be very high. The high-tone emphasis must be introduced *before* the peaks are clipped, as was pointed out in the Harvard Report. That is why we speak of high-tone *pre*-emphasis. No additional high-tone or low-tone emphasis should be put in by the receiver *after* the clipping.

In order to get the best combination of protection and intelligibility, a receiver with good acoustic characteristics must be used. Some hearing aid receivers are too "resonant," meaning that they respond too well to one particular band of frequencies. After the amplifier has clipped the peaks

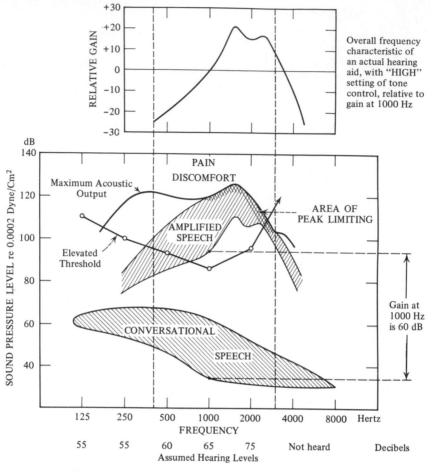

Fig. 10-34. Amplified speech with peak limiting. The hearing aid is now set for maximum volume, assumed to be 60 dB gain at 1000 Hz, and for *high* tone control. The hypothetical hearing levels, shown below, leave only a small target area below the threshold of discomfort. The maximum acoustic output is 120 dB at 1000 Hz. The amplified speech (shaded area) is delivered efficiently to the target area. Peak limiting occurs at frequencies above 1000 Hz, but not below. This holds distortion to a minimum. This result is achieved by the sharply rising frequency characteristic of the microphone-amplifier combination. The input is assumed to be ordinary conversational speech. Of course, with loud speech there would be more peak limiting.

of the waves electrically, the receiver should deliver all parts of the speech spectrum to the ear at about the same maximum level, a little below the threshold of tolerance.

A receiver that has a resonant peak will amplify not only that frequency of the input but also the second, the third, or even the fourth harmonics that are introduced by the peak clipping of lower frequencies.

Not only may the resulting high peak pressures reach the threshold of discomfort; they also cause a further deterioration of the intelligibility of certain vowel sounds, to say nothing of the unpleasant ringing quality that it introduces. For example, a receiver with a resonant peak at 1500 Hz gives a strong response at this frequency to inputs in the neighborhood of 750, of 500, and of 375 Hz when these are strong

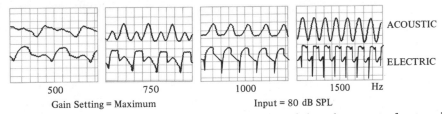

ACOUSTIC

ELECTRIC

500      750      1000      1500      Hz

Gain Setting = Maximum                    Input = 80 dB SPL

Fig. 10-35. For this figure the electrical waves were recorded at the output of a transistor hearing aid across the terminals of the receiver. The peak clipping in this instrument is unsymmetrical, and a sharp transient peak is introduced by the output transformer. The receiver has a resonant peak at 1500 Hz. It smooths out the sharp irregularities of the electrical waves, but it accentuates the first two or three harmonics of frequencies that are an octave or more below its resonant peak. For these oscillograms the input was 80 dB SPL, the gain setting was maximum, and the tone control at "low." (*Courtesy of J. B. Cox, Jr.*)

enough to reach the clipping level. The output wave forms are shown in Figure 10-35.

### Compression Amplification

Another way of limiting the output of a hearing aid is by *compression amplification*. Compression amplification is equivalent to a rapidly acting automatic volume control. The strong sound waves themselves reduce the gain of the amplifier. The output of the instrument is limited to a definite maximum, and the method has the advantage that the wave form is less distorted than it is by simple peak clipping. Automatic gain control is now incorporated in some hearing aids.

### Harmonic Distortion

If a pure tone of frequency $f_o$ is applied to a linear hearing aid, the only signal that will appear at its output will be a pure tone of frequency $f_o$. At most, the amplitude and phase at the output will be different from those at the input. If the hearing aid is nonlinear, harmonics of the input frequency $f_o$, namely $2f_o$, $3f_o$, . . . , will appear in the output. The ratio of the power in the harmonics to the power in the fundamental frequency $f_o$ gives a measure of "harmonic distortion." The harmonics, either singly or in combination, are easily measured and for this reason harmonic distortion is often used to specify distortion in a hearing aid. The amount of harmonic distortion in a system varies with the fundamental frequency; low frequencies will have many harmonics that fall within the system pass-band and higher frequencies will have fewer. This is shown in Figure 10-36.

### Intermodulation Distortion

Most input signals to hearing aids, even relatively "steady" signals, are not pure tones; they contain many frequencies. Therefore, it can justifiably be argued that

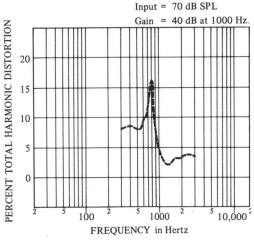

Input = 70 dB SPL
Gain = 40 dB at 1000 Hz.

Fig. 10-36. Total harmonic distortion in a body-worn hearing aid. (See Figures 10-28, 10-29, and 10-30 for response curves relevant to this aid.)

perhaps a more valid measure of system distortion in *intermodulation distortion*. A linear system with input frequencies $f_1$ and $f_2$ will have only those two frequencies in its output. A nonlinear system will have the two input frequencies plus their harmonics, plus the sums and differences of the input frequencies and their harmonics. The measure of intermodulation distortion of the system is the ratio of the power of the output signal at frequencies other than the applied frequencies relative to the output-signal power at the applied frequencies. There are several methods for measuring harmonic distortion. They differ in the kinds of input signals that are used and the kinds of output signals that are measured. All methods attempt to give an estimate of power at distortion frequencies relative to the power at applied frequencies, and in practice none is easily implemented.

### Ringing

Speech is inherently a transient kind of signal; bursts of energy are often followed by periods of relative silence. If speech is applied to any band-pass system and to hearing aids in particular, we notice that the response of the system lags behind the excitation. In particular, the output

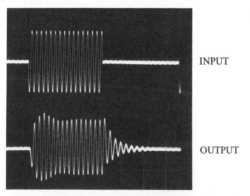

INPUT

OUTPUT

Fig. 10-37. Response of a hearing-aid receiver to a 2000-Hz tone burst. The output builds up gradually and does not terminate immediately or abruptly.

will continue for a short time after the input has been abruptly turned off, much as a bell will continue to ring after being struck. This kind of distortion is called "ringing." The measure of ringing that is often used is the time required for decay at the output when a pure-tone input has been abruptly squelched. Like other forms of distortion, ringing is frequency-dependent. Unlike other forms, ringing occurs in *linear* as well as in nonlinear systems. Ringing in the receiver of a modern hearing aid is shown in Figure 10-37.

### Use of Hearing Aids in Noisy Environments

The use of hearing aids in noisy environments is perhaps best understood by considering an example. Suppose two people are trying to communicate in a noisy environment. One has impaired hearing and uses a hearing aid. In many situations, both indoors and out, ambient noise levels are relatively constant over a region in which two people are talking. This is assumed for the example.

In relatively echo-free spaces the noise and speech levels at the microphone of the hearing aid might appear as shown in the lower two curves of Figure 10-38 when plotted as a function of distance to the talker. Notice that the signal-to-noise ratio, the difference in decibels between speech and noise levels, decreases as the distance from talker to listener increases. Six inches from the talker's lips the S/N ratio is large (24 dB), and eight feet away the signal and noise levels are equal. *Speech intelligibility will decrease as the S/N ratio decreases* independent of whether or not the listener uses a hearing aid. Therefore, for good communication the talker and listener should be close together. In this respect the person with a hearing aid even has an advantage over the person with normal hearing, since it is sometimes possible to put the hearing-aid microphone

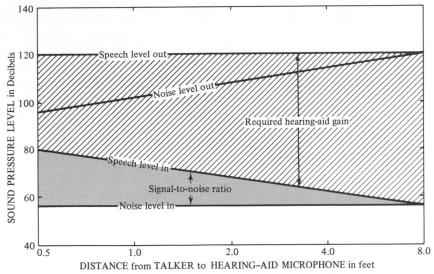

Fig. 10-38. Effects of distance between talker and hearing-aid microphone on the signal-to-noise ratio and required hearing-aid gain.

quite close to the talker's lips. There is on the present market (1968) at least one body-worn hearing aid that has a removable microphone for just this purpose.

In regions that are more reverberant, where the speech levels do not decrease as shown in Figure 10-38, the case for making small the distance between talker and listener can still be made. As the distance between talker and listener increases in a reverberant space, the ratio of *direct* to *reverberant* speech levels will decrease even though the *total* speech level does not decrease appreciably. For a given total speech level, intelligibility decreases as the ratio of direct to reverberant energy decreases.

If the listener adjusts his hearing aid so that at any distance the speech level of the output remains the same (see Figure 10-38), then the required acoustic gain must increase as the speech level input decreases. That is, the hearing-aid user would increase the gain as he backs away from the talker. With respect to the hearing aid, high gain is undesirable because the self-noise, which arises within the hearing aid itself, generally will be higher for higher gains. In addition, and perhaps more important, when the high gain is accompanied by poor signal-to-noise ratio at the input, the *total* power that must be supplied by the aid must be greater in order to achieve a given output speech level because the aid must supply power for both the amplified speech *and* the amplified noise. If the noise is comparable in level to the speech, a considerable portion of the available power from the aid must then be used to amplify the noise.

A final argument can be advanced in favor of low gain and high speech-input level by observing that the impaired listener will hear his own voice through his hearing aid at a comfortable level only if his voice level and the speech level from the person with whom he is communicating are equivalent at the hearing-aid microphone. If the aid is worn on the head or body, this means that the two people must be close together so that the speech levels from both persons will be high compared to the noise, and the hearing-aid gain can be low.

## BASIC PRINCIPLES FOR THE SELECTION OF HEARING AIDS

Of course, a hearing aid should be as small, light, durable, and inexpensive as possible, and it should amplify sound without unnecessary impairment of quality. But when we use the terms "as possible" and "unnecessary," we admit that we are prepared to compromise. If he cannot have both, the user will sacrifice quality in order to obtain intelligibility. We have pointed out some of the features that make a hearing aid "good" in general, but exactly the same instrument may not be the best for everyone. People differ too much in their hearing losses and in the loudness of the sounds that they will tolerate, not to mention in the size of their pocketbooks! Different features will be more important for one man than for another. Let us illustrate with a few examples.

Miss Brown has a moderate conductive hearing loss with hearing-threshold levels at about 55 dB (ISO) in the "Speech range." The maximum intensity of average speech is about 65 dB (SPL). Faint speech becomes just intelligible to a person with 0 dB hearing-threshold levels at approximately 20 dB (SPL), but speech must be at about 75 dB for Miss Brown to understand it. Miss Brown may catch a word or two of average speech now and then but no more. But a hearing aid that provides 30 dB of amplification will raise all but the faintest sounds of average speech above her threshold. Since her loss is conductive in nature, and therefore without recruitment, the amplified speech will not sound particularly loud to her, but it should be fully intelligible. She will do well in ordinary social situations when there is not a confusion of many voices or other noise. This 30 dB of assistance is Miss Brown's first requirement.

Miss Brown's second requirement is that the amplified sound must not cause discomfort. Most persons, whether their hear-

ing is normal or hypoacousic, do not feel discomfort until the peaks of speech reach at least 115 dB (SPL). If Miss Brown's threshold of discomfort is at about 115 dB, she should select a hearing aid that has a maximum output just under 115 dB. There is no conflict between her two requirements. The 30 dB of amplification raises average speech peaks from about 65 dB to only 95 dB. There is still a margin of 20 dB before the hearing aid's maximum output of 115 dB is reached. This margin will allow Miss Brown to hear loud speech naturally and without noticeable peak clipping. The distortion of peak clipping will seldom occur, and Miss Brown is therefore not much concerned about how the instrument sounds when it is "overloaded." The limiting feature is for her merely an emergency protection that guards her against great discomfort from sudden unexpected noises. She should easily find an instrument that gives her practically perfect intelligibility whether the speaker talks loudly or softly.

Miss Brown will probably find, if she shops around, that several different makes of instrument are about equally effective, clear-toned, and attractive. Certain models may not sound as pleasant as others, but two models or combinations of the same brand may very well differ more in "how they sound" than two similar models made by different companies.

Suppose that Miss Brown goes to a laboratory and is tested with different hearing aids by elaborate and time-consuming articulation tests. She would probably make a nearly perfect score with each of several instruments. Then even the expert who tested her would be unable to say with certainty that *one* instrument is better for her than any other. Miss Brown is easy to "fit."

But consider Mr. Jones, who has a really severe hearing loss. He has not been able to find an instrument that can "get through" to him without hurting his ears.

His audiogram shows about 90 dB hearing level for low and middle frequencies, and he cannot hear 4000 Hz at all. He obviously needs a great deal of amplification. The critical point for him is to find an instrument which will provide this high gain, and yet not be uncomfortably loud even when it is driven to its maximum output. The 65 dB or so of amplification that Mr. Jones requires, added to the original 65 dB of average speech, makes a total of 130 dB (SPL). This total is at least 10 dB more than the usual threshold of discomfort. The fact that Mr. Jones is hard of hearing does not mean that his ear is any "tougher" than normal. We will assume that his threshold of discomfort is 120 dB. For comfort, therefore, Mr. Jones must be satisfied with less than the full amplification that he apparently needs. He must find a hearing aid with just the right maximum output. The instrument must "package" speech accurately by clipping its peaks or by compression, and must deliver it into the very restricted range between Mr. Jones's threshold of hearing and his threshold of discomfort. Success or failure may depend on whether the receiver is "flat" instead of "resonant" and on whether the tone control suppresses the low frequencies enough to keep speech intelligible when it is distorted by peak clipping. Mr. Jones is difficult to "fit."

If Mr. Jones has not used a powerful hearing aid before, he is likely to profit considerably by auditory training. Listening systematically to sound that is loud but not quite uncomfortable may increase his tolerance so that he can use an instrument with greater maximum output. Such an instrument will have more "elbow room" and will not clip the peaks of speech so heavily. Speech will then sound more natural and probably be more intelligible; but Mr. Jones's high-tone loss is severe, and he must not expect any instrument to give him a perfect articulation score.

Mrs. Smith is quite hard of hearing, but she is not so badly off as Mr. Jones. She has hearing-threshold levels of 70 dB at 500 and 1000 Hz, increasing to 110 dB at 4000 Hz. Figure 10-32 shows this kind of a sensitivity curve and how a fairly powerful hearing aid should make speech loud enough for her. She can probably find several instruments that (1) are tolerable, even for loud speech when the gain control is well up; (2) make faint or distant conversation intelligible; (3) make nearly all words intelligible under good listening conditions; and (4) have a "quality" that is acceptable to her.

In making comparisons of instruments, Mrs. Smith should listen at both low and high levels. Two hearing aids may sound very much alike at low levels; and yet one may be obviously superior to the other when loud sounds drive them to the limit of their output and force them to clip and distort some of the sound waves. On the whole, Mrs. Smith will probably do best with an instrument that has a definite high-tone emphasis, but she may prefer the quality of an instrument without the high-tone emphasis. This compromise is probably best settled by Mrs. Smith herself, but her decision is easier if she can choose an instrument that has an adjustable tone control. Then she can increase or decrease its high-tone emphasis according to the situation.

We will not discuss the special problems of old Grandpa Tompkins or little Mary Johnson, but the same general principles of compromise apply to all of them. Additional practical hints regarding the selection and use of hearing aids are given in the next chapter.

### Selective Amplification and Individual Fitting

We have deliberately spoken of "selecting" rather than "fitting" a hearing aid. "Fitting" suggests too strongly the fitting of a pair of eyeglasses or a suit of clothes. The differences among hearing aids are not as large and as obvious as they are among eyeglass lenses and suits of clothes, and it is difficult to judge with sufficient precision the success of the "fitting" of a hearing aid.

*Selecting a suitable hearing aid is, first, a series of tests of adequacy in fundamentals, and then a series of judgments of intangibles or a series of compromises.* There is usually no one best fit that is demonstrably best under all circumstances.

The idea of precise individual fitting is a survival from the days of feeble amplifiers and sharply resonant receivers and microphones. Perhaps we should explain in more detail that a mechanical vibrating system like the diaphragm of a telephone receiver operates most efficiently near its "natural period," but may be much less efficient for frequencies that are an octave or two higher or lower. Resonance may be made less sharp by "damping" the diaphragm, but the maximum efficiency is reduced at the same time. When amplifiers were weak, the necessary efficiency was obtained by deliberately making the receiver and the microphone quite sharply resonant without much damping. The same compromise was made in the early telephones. The quality was poor, as those of us who remember the telephones of 50 years ago can testify, but the sound was loud enough to be heard, and most words could be understood. A reasonable compromise was achieved by making the microphone and the receiver resonant for different frequencies so that a wider band of frequencies was transmitted with fair but adequate efficiency. For the early electrical hearing aids an assortment of receivers and microphones, resonant at different frequencies, was provided, and the wearer determined by trial which combination gave *him* the best quality and intelligibility with adequate loudness. There was actually considerable variation

among receivers of the same model, more variation than there is in modern instruments; and "fitting" was a three-way trial-and-error effort to get the best combination of microphone, amplifier, and receiver for the particular listener. The intelligibility was sometimes so poor that small differences in instruments might be quite important. Speech might be usefully intelligible with one combination and nearly unintelligible with another.

The idea of "fitting" a hearing aid was supported by the very plausible argument that a hearing aid should compensate for each person's particular hearing loss by amplifying some frequencies more than others. The audiogram was taken as the guide to show which frequencies needed "selective amplification." This principle seems obvious, but for several reasons it does not work out in practice.

For one thing, if we should compensate fully for the abnormality of the audiogram, we would usually compensate too much. It was pointed out in Chapter 4 that *the hearing for loud tones is usually more normal than the hearing at threshold,* particularly with sensory-neural hearing loss. If we correct strictly according to the audiogram, we are therefore likely to get a caricature of the proper correction.

Really accurate compensation for the audiogram has never been tried. Most audiograms are irregular, and the frequency characteristics of a hearing aid are nearly always irregular also. Only by chance can an exact compensation at all frequencies ever be achieved.

Finally, the principle of selective amplification overlooks the effects on the intelligibility of speech when the hearing aid is operated at high gain, and peak clipping occurs.

In a series of wartime studies at the Psycho-Acoustic Laboratory, at Harvard University, it was found that *an instrument with good over-all characteristics and true square-top peak clipping that amplified a wide range of frequencies about evenly or with moderate emphasis of the high tones gave the best results.* Hard-of-hearing listeners made as good (or better) articulation scores with it and had more "elbow room" than they had with any other combination that was tried. This was true for all of the common types of hearing loss. Other "compensations" that were tried (but with no better results) included several that more nearly followed the principle of selective amplification. The details of these experiments are available in book form for the technical reader (see Suggested Readings at the end of this chapter).

In general, similar results were obtained by British investigators (1947) and were made the basis of the design of the Medresco (Medical Research Council) hearing aid that is manufactured for, and distributed by, the British government.

### The Audiogram as an Aid to Selection

What remains of the principle of selective amplification and of fitting according to the audiogram boils down to something like this: It doesn't work out well to give a real low-tone boost. The choice for the best understanding of speech lies between undistorted reproduction and a moderate low-tone suppression (or high-tone emphasis). Hard-of-hearing listeners are likely to prefer natural reproduction as the best for quality, but with a high-tone hearing loss, speech is often better understood if moderate high-tone emphasis is given. If the hearing loss is severe, regardless of whether it is "flat" or "high-tone," a high-tone emphasis (introduced by the microphone or the amplifier) is very desirable because it preserves the intelligibility of speech when the hearing aid is pushed to its maximum output. In the selection of a hearing aid the audiogram is most useful as a guide to *how powerful*

an instrument will probably be needed— not as a guide to the best frequency characteristics. The audiogram also reveals the subjects with abrupt high-tone nerve deafness that cannot be helped much by any hearing aid because their ability to hear high tones has been lost completely.

### Other Tests for the Selection of Hearing Aids

Other tests were developed during the 1940s that employed measurements of the threshold and discrimination for speech described in Chapter 7. We shall mention one fallacy that is common to several tests, so that the hard-of-hearing and their advisers alike may be warned.

It was suggested, for example, that if, with instrument A, a listener can *understand fainter speech* than with instrument B, then instrument A is the better instrument for him. *The weakness of this type of test lies in the problem of how to set the gain control of the hearing aids.* The listener is usually instructed to set it himself so that average speech comes to him at "the most comfortable loudness." Unfortunately, many subjects on repeated trials do not duplicate their own settings for most comfortable loudness. "Most comfortable" seems to cover a range of a good many decibels. Of course, if instrument A happens to have its gain control set higher than B, it has just this much advantage when the final test is made. It will be able to pick up fainter speech than can instrument B. Tests of this sort are likely to be tests of how the listener happens to set the gain control, not of how well the instrument "fits" or how "efficient" it is. All that we can usefully find out with faint speech is whether an instrument has *some* gain setting that will allow the wearer to pick up speech that is as faint as he is likely to encounter in everyday life. Most present-day hearing aids can do this. Of course there will always be the unusual case with unusual requirements. Our comments apply, however, to the majority of people with impaired hearing.

Another frequent misunderstanding concerns the "noisiness" of a hearing aid. Of course, any crackling or hissing generated in the instrument is undesirable, but sometimes instruments with high amplification are wrongly rejected as "noisy." The trouble may be that the wearer has happened to set the gain control higher than he needs to, and all the background noises therefore sound unpleasantly loud. Perhaps a different setting of the tone control may make the noise less annoying. It is not the fault of the instrument that it amplifies all the sounds that reach it and that it cannot pick out the voice and reject the noise when they happen to be sounds of the same frequencies.

Among other limitations on the "fitting" of hearing aids are the rather poor reliability (reproducibility of results) of discrimination tests, the mental "set" of Mr. Jones when he takes the test, and the influence of the order in which various hearing aids are tested.

The audiologist helps make the crucial decision on whether a hearing aid is indicated. He makes his decision on the basis of a careful case history, an interview, and certain tests. The more conventional tests are pure-tone and speech audiometry described in Chapter 7. Sometimes the tests will be made in controlled noise. Despite their limitations, these tests, when they are properly interpreted, along with the counseling discussed in Chapter 11, are helpful to Mr. Jones in guiding him in the selection of a hearing aid.

Audiologists are now using to a greater and greater extent tests of the performance of hearing aids under conditions of stress. One such condition is the controlled noise mentioned in the previous paragraph. Others include a reverberant room, competing voices, and a variation of the direction of the source of the sound.

## SUGGESTED READINGS AND REFERENCES

**Briskey, R. J., W. H. Greenbaum, and J. C. Sinclair.** "Pitfalls in Hearing Aid Response Curves," *J. Audio. Eng. Soc.,* 14: 317–323 (1966).
Discusses the ambiguities of interpreting hearing-aid measurements in the form of frequency response curves in a 2-cc coupler with respect to the subjective measurements of loudness in an actual ear.

**Davis, H. et al.** *Hearing Aids: An Experimental Study of Design Objectives.* Cambridge, Mass.: Harvard University Press, 1947.
This is a technical report of experiments conducted at the Psycho-Acoustic Laboratory under contract with the Office of Scientific Research and Development, frequently referred to as the "Harvard Report."

————. "The Selection of Hearing Aids," *Laryngoscope,* 56:85–115, 135–163 (1946).
A reprinting in full of report "PNR-7" issued December 31, 1945, by the Psycho-Acoustic Laboratory, Harvard University, Cambridge, Mass. It in-

cludes a theoretical analysis of the general problem of "fitting" a hearing aid and a critique of several "fitting" procedures.

**Greenbaum, W. H.** "Miniature Audio Amplifiers," *J. Audio. Eng. Soc.,* 15:438–444 (1967).
Miniaturized discrete components and integrated circuits as used in hearing-aid amplifiers are discussed.

**Committee on Electro-Acoustics.** "Hearing Aids and Audiometers." Medical Research Council, Special Report Series No. 261, London: His Majesty's Stationery Office, 1947.
This is a technical report of experiments in Great Britain to specify the design of hearing aids and audiometers.

**Hirsh, I. J.** "Use of Amplification in Educating Deaf Children," *Amer. Ann. Deaf* (in press for November, 1968).
Various kinds of wired and wireless group hearing aids are discussed along with their advantages and disadvantages.

**Anon.** "Effects of Source Impedance and Acoustical Termination on BK Receiver Response," *Knowles Technical Bulletin,* Knowles Electronics, Inc., 3100 N. Mannhein Rd., Franklin Park, Ill.
Discusses the effects of the impedance of the electrical source and of the acoustical load on the response of receivers used in miniature hearing aids.

**Lybarger, S. F.** "A discussion of hearing aid trends." *Int. Audiol.,* 5:376–383 (1966).
A discussion from the point of view of a manufacturer of hearing aids.

**Silverman, S. R.** "Tolerance for Pure Tones and Speech in Normal and Defective Hearing," *Ann. Otol.* 56:658–678 (1947).
A summary of investigations at Central Institute for the Deaf under contract with the Office of Scientific Research and Development. They dealt with the mapping of thresholds of discomfort and pain in listening to loud sounds.

**USASI,** Standard Method of Expressing Hearing Aid Performance. United States of America Standards Institute (now American National Standards Institute, 1430 Broadway, New York, 10018); USAS: S3.8 (1967).

**Victoreen, J. A.** *Hearing Enhancement.* Springfield, Ill.: Charles C Thomas, 1960.
A good popular presentation of principles and background of hearing aids.

# CHAPTER 11

## COUNSELING
## ABOUT
## HEARING AIDS

### S. R. SILVERMAN, Ph.D.
### HALLOWELL DAVIS, M.D.

Two major responsibilities of the audiologist who is considering a hearing aid for his client are to perform the kinds of tests cited in Chapter 10 on which to base his recommendations and to give advice about selection of and adjustment to instruments. This chapter deals with the questions about hearing aids that are likely to occur to a prospective user, particularly to a first-time user. In a sense, the suggested "friend" referred to in the chapter may well be the audiologist counseling his client. This is the point of view of the chapter.

A hearing aid may be ridiculed as a "tin ear." It may be thought to detract from a person's appearance or suggest premature old age. But the man or woman whose hearing is failing should want so earnestly to hear that he will not worry about such real or imaginary trifles. His friends will welcome his use of a hearing aid because it spares them the painful necessity of having to shout and repeat for him. In fact, *it shows lack of consideration for his family and friends when the* *hard-of-hearing person does not wear a hearing aid if he can possibly do so and benefit by it.* Moreover, his hearing aid opens to him a broad vista of enriched social experiences which every person, hard-of-hearing or otherwise, needs for a happy adjustment to our complex world. Let it not be said of the hard-of-hearing, "Vanity, vanity, all is vanity."

## TO WEAR OR NOT TO WEAR
## A HEARING AID

According to Table 1, taken from the National Health Survey, approximately 1,214,000 persons had ever used a hearing aid. The survey also indicated that 882,000 were using them in the period July 1962 to June 1963. From the point of view of this chapter it is interesting to note, from Table 1, the basis for selection of an aid, with dealer advice predominating. From Table 2 we find that the degree of satisfaction from the use of a hearing aid varies, with more than half of the users either very satisfied or fairly satisfied.

It is interesting to estimate the propor-

318

TABLE 1

NUMBER AND PERCENT DISTRIBUTION OF PERSONS WITH A BINAURAL HEARING IMPAIRMENT WHO HAVE EVER USED A HEARING AID, BY BASIS FOR SELECTING AID AND ACCORDING TO SPEECH COMPREHENSION GROUP: UNITED STATES, JULY 1962–JUNE 1963

| Basis for Selecting Aid | Total[1,2] | Persons Who Have Ever Used an Aid | | |
|---|---|---|---|---|
| | | Cannot Hear and Understand Spoken Words | Can Hear and Understand a Few Spoken Words | Can Hear and Understand Most Spoken Words |
| | Number of Persons in Thousands | | | |
| All persons.................. | 1214 | 468 | 294 | 444 |
| | Percent Distribution | | | |
| All bases.................... | 100.0 | 100.0 | 100.0 | 100.0 |
| Prescribed by doctor................ | 12.9 | 16.7 | *10.5 | *11.0 |
| Prescribed by clinic............... .. | 18.1 | 15.8 | 21.4 | 18.2 |
| Advised by dealer.................. | 33.7 | 29.9 | 35.7 | 36.5 |
| Saw it advertised.................. | 7.8 | *7.1 | *7.1 | *9.2 |
| Recommended by friend or relative.... | 11.9 | 13.0 | *10.5 | 11.5 |
| Other and unknown................ | 15.7 | 17.5 | *14.3 | 13.5 |

* This figure is approximate.
[1] Includes persons whose functional degree of hearing impairment was unknown.
[2] Without the use of a hearing aid.
(*Data from Table 11. "Characteristics of Persons with Impaired Hearing." U.S. Department of Health, Education, and Welfare, Public Health Service Publication No. 1000—Series 10–No. 35, April, 1967.*)

tion of users as related to age. In Figure 11-1 we present our rough guess of this relationship. As our criterion of those who can be "helped" by a hearing aid, we have chosen a hearing-threshold level of 40 dB or more at one end of the scale and the ability to receive communication satisfactorily (socially) at the other end. We note that the greatest percentage of people who need help fall between the ages of 20 and 60. Statistics from the National Health survey bear this out. In the top portion of the figure we have attempted to indicate when certain conditions related to hearing impairment manifest themselves. This information essentially leads us to the rationale of the graph.

We do not mean to imply that all individuals with such conditions as noise-induced hearing loss and presbycusis can be helped substantially by hearing aids, but we believe that it is important to keep in mind the prevalence of these circumstances in arriving at estimates of the distribution of potential users.

Whoever has difficulty with his hearing in everyday conversations should think seriously of getting a hearing aid. The difficulty may vary with different situations, depending on the distance from the source of sound, the surrounding noises, the clarity of the speech or music; the lighting, which may help or interfere with speechreading; and many other factors. For example, someone with a moderate hearing loss may not need amplification

TABLE 2

NUMBER AND PERCENT DISTRIBUTION OF PERSONS WITH A BINAURAL HEARING
IMPAIRMENT WHO HAVE EVER USED A HEARING AID, BY DEGREE OF SATISFACTION
WITH THE AID AND ACCORDING TO SEX AND SPEECH COMPREHENSION GROUP:[3]
UNITED STATES, JULY 1962–JUNE 1963

| Sex and Degree of Satisfaction with Hearing Aid | Persons Who Have Ever Used an Aid | | | |
|---|---|---|---|---|
| | Total[1,2] | Cannot Hear and Understand Spoken Words | Can Hear and Understand a Few Spoken Words | Can Hear and Understand Most Spoken Words |
| | Number of Persons in Thousands | | | |
| Both sexes................... | 1214 | 468 | 294 | 444 |
| Male........................... | 625 | 210 | 134 | 274 |
| Female......................... | 590 | 258 | 160 | 170 |
| | Percent Distribution | | | |
| All degrees.................. | 100.0 | 100.0 | 100.0 | 100.0 |
| Very satisfied..................... | 32.5 | 37.6 | 28.6 | 30.0 |
| Fairly satisfied.................... | 29.0 | 30.3 | 32.3 | 25.7 |
| Not satisfied...................... | 9.1 | *8.3 | *9.9 | *9.7 |
| Not currently using aid.............. | 27.4 | 21.8 | 28.2 | 32.4 |
| Unknown......................... | *2.1 | *1.7 | *1.4 | *2.3 |

* This figure is approximate.
[1] Includes persons whose functional degree of hearing impairment was unknown.
[2] Without the use of a hearing aid.
[3] Data are based on household interviews and a follow-up mail supplement and refer to the living, civilian, noninstitutional population.
(*Data from Table 13 "Characteristics of Persons with Impaired Hearing," U.S. Department of Health, Education, and Welfare, Public Health Service Publication No. 1000—Series 10–No. 35, April, 1967.*)

for ordinary conversation but may need it for lectures, sound movies, and church, and in social gatherings where there is likely to be a background of many voices. Also, obviously, the accurate understanding of speech is more important for some than for others. The businessman who must know exactly what goes on in conferences needs it more than the elderly person who merely wishes to hear the radio, the television, or casual conversation more easily. In the long run, each man and woman must decide for himself whether his hearing loss makes him socially (or economically) inadequate.

If a man is in doubt as to his need for a hearing aid, the audiogram is a very helpful guide. Generally, *if the hearing level for speech in the better ear is worse than 40 dB, a hearing aid is needed*. But the prospective user must realize that, in spite of optimistic advertisements, a hearing aid is not a perfect instrument. It does not provide complete compensation for hearing impairment. It will benefit the wearer only in proportion to his willingness to accept it, short of unattainable perfection, and to his patience and effort in learning to make the most of it.

Some types of hearing loss are less apt than others to benefit from a hearing aid. For example, a man's audiogram may

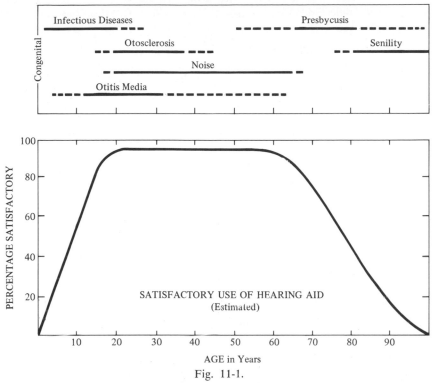

INCIDENCE of HEARING LOSS by AGE and CAUSE

Fig. 11-1.

show a slight impairment (20 to 30 dB) in the low frequencies and a precipitate drop beginning at 1000 Hz. He will probably complain, "I hear, but I can't make out what you are saying." This is understandable, since the frequencies above 1000 Hz convey sounds which are very important for the intelligibility of speech. For example, "fin" may sound the same as "thin" or "sin." Ordinarily, a hearing aid alone is of little value in overcoming this difficulty. However, even in such a case a proper hearing aid, *supplemented by a program of intensive auditory training* in discrimination of the sounds which make up speech, can be of great assistance. This is true even if the auditory training and instruction in specch turn out to be more helpful than the hearing aid! It is well, however, to repeat that in addition to whatever reduction in dynamic range and frequency response the user must learn to tolerate, he must also accept

the fact that he will suffer many extra listening failures, brought on by reduced signal-to-noise ratios, in work-a-day situations *even after full auditory training and full acclimatization to his instrument*. Acceptance of these limitations in hearing-aid use can lead to greater satisfaction in the benefits which it does bring.

### Hearing Aids for the Aged

The use of hearing aids by elderly people is likely to present another special problem. Their deafness is usually of the sensory-neural type, technically known as *presbycusis*. Their ability to hear high frequencies decreases with advancing age. As we have just pointed out, such a pattern of hearing loss often results in imperfect discrimination. In younger people, intensive auditory training and constant use of an instrument help the listener learn to make use of all auditory clues.

When the other problems of advancing

age are added to deafness, the situation becomes still more difficult. We must frequently reckon with poor health and gradual failure of other faculties, particularly of vision, which is so helpful as a supplement to hearing. Not only do old people often become very dependent on others; they may also find themselves unable to "keep up with the times." In addition, many of them live alone or with children who "have their own lives to lead." All these factors may lead to tensions, fears, and general nervousness, which are hardly conducive to the concentration essential for effective and comfortable use of a hearing aid. Nevertheless, we should be encouraged by the favorable reports of the Veterans Administration of its experience with elderly users of hearing aids (see Chapter 19).

Each elderly person should be evaluated in terms of his particular temperament and way of living. When there appears to be any possibility of benefit, we strongly suggest a trial period with a hearing aid during which the person is encouraged but not forced to use the instrument. If he himself then expresses a desire to have the hearing aid, it should be purchased.

### Hearing Aids for Children

There is a great difference of opinion, again without much supporting evidence, on when a child is ready to wear a hearing aid. One point of view holds that the early years are the years in which the child learns the meaning of sounds, particularly speech, and hence he should wear a hearing aid at all times from the moment it is discovered that he is deaf. This appears to be the predominant point of view. On the other hand, some workers believe that the child must first be trained to some degree of awareness and discrimination of sound, since failure to benefit from the instrument will discourage its use.

Furthermore, some young children may be frightened by the loud sound of an instrument and become conditioned against it. Some audiologists fear possible damage to an ear exposed to the high sound-pressure levels generated by a hearing aid. This is a rather remote possibility, but, as we have seen in previous chapters, the cause of lack of response to sound may be elsewhere than in the periphery, and it would be unfortunate to damage an intact end organ.

### Will a Hearing Aid Endanger Hearing?

The prospective user of a hearing aid often asks, "Will the use of a hearing aid destroy the remainder of my hearing by overloading it?" We want to emphasize that *a hearing aid neither injures nor cures an abnormal ear,* nor does it alter the status of impaired hearing (see also Chapter 4). It merely enables the user to make better use of the hearing that he possesses and keeps his hearing in practice. He remains attentive to sound. If, however, the new hearing aid makes the wearer "nervous," he should break it in by using it for short periods daily, gradually increasing the length of each period of use. We have to repeat that we must be cautious when we are not sure of our assessment of hearing in a very young child.

### Hearing Aids and Speechreading

There is no truth in the rather prevalent notion that the use of a hearing aid will diminish one's skill in speechreading. On the contrary, the hearing of speech is likely to reinforce speechreading because auditory clues assist in the discrimination of words that look alike on the lips. For example, in the sentence, "The package is heavy," the word "baggage" might be substituted for "package." The context, which the speechreader ordinarily uses to distinguish words that look alike on the lips, is no help here, since both words fit the context. But a hearing aid might enable the speechreader to discriminate between the initial "p" and "b" and between the "ck" and "g" in the two words. Of course we have chosen an extreme example, but long-time users of hearing aids generally report that *the continuous association of hearing and seeing speech is mutually advantageous.* Even in cases of extreme hearing loss, in which complete understanding of speech is not attainable, a hearing aid may furnish enough auditory clues, such as stress and intonational patterns, to supplement speechreading quite effectively.

### Ear-level or Body-worn?

We have seen in Chapter 10 that hearing aids can be worn on the body or at ear level, either behind the ear or mounted in an eyeglass frame. Most users prefer an ear-level instrument because it is convenient, inconspicuous, and free of clothing noise. Furthermore, it enables the listener to turn his microphone easily to the source of sound. However, users with hearing-threshold levels over 50 dB(ISO) require so much power that it may result in squealing in an ear-level hearing aid even with a perfectly fitting earmold. In cases of such severe loss, trials under a variety of conditions should precede the final decision.

### Air Conduction and Bone Conduction Compared

Air- and bone-conduction hearing aids differ in the construction of their receivers and in the pathways over which the amplified sound is delivered to the inner ear. The buttonlike air-conduction receiver, coupled to the external auditory canal by a fitted plastic earmold, delivers sound through the normal pathway. The rectangular bone-conduction vibrator, on the other hand, makes contact with the mastoid bone behind the ear, and its vibrations are transmitted by the bone directly to the inner ear (see also Chapter 10).

We might suppose that a bone-conduction instrument is indicated whenever the deafness is of the conductive middle-ear type. The obstruction that interferes with the passage of sound presumably can be bypassed by bone conduction, and the intact nerve endings can pick up the sound waves as they come, relatively unimpeded, directly through the bones of the skull. However, physical difficulties limit the performance of bone-conduction units. Bones and the skin that covers them vary in density and elasticity and, therefore, in their ability to transmit sound. It is more difficult to get efficient delivery of speech sounds by bone conduction than by air conduction. Full bone-conduction efficiency is difficult to achieve with ear-level aids. The bone system has been incorporated in some eyeglass type of units, but the bone vibrator is then hard to isolate from other parts of the hearing aid, inducing feedback; and sufficient pressure against the skull is hard to maintain. Moreover, many good prospects for bone units (persons with conductive loss) are good candidates for middle-ear surgery for restoration of their hearing. As a consequence, clinicians generally report that not more than 1 percent of their subjects can use bone conduction more satisfactorily than air conduction. This rather small percentage suggests that, if the prospective user of a hearing aid is still in doubt after listening by both air and bone conduction, unless he has competent advice to the contrary, he should choose air conduction.

Bone conduction is definitely preferable, however, when the user suffers from chronically discharging ears. Also, a few users who can hear over the telephone without a hearing aid, but who cannot quite follow face-to-face or group conversation, find it a great convenience to have the ear free for direct contact with the telephone receiver. However, a telephone pickup, described in Chapter 10, makes an air-conduction instrument also very convenient for telephone conversations.

### Individually Molded Earpiece

Anyone who expects to use an air-conduction hearing aid should have an earmold that has been fitted to the contours of his own external ear; an earpiece that is not properly fitted may irritate the ear canal and may also interfere with the efficient transmission of sound. As was pointed out in the preceding chapter, a well-fitting individual earmold not only is more comfortable and more secure; it allows the hearing aid to deliver sounds as it is designed to deliver them, that is, with the greatest efficiency and fidelity. Even for the person who had not yet made his final selection of a hearing aid, be it body-worn or ear-level, a molded earpiece is a good investment because it will fit almost any make of air-conduction receiver to which it is attached. For adults the fit is permanent, but growing children obviously require a periodic change of earmolds. It takes considerable instruction and practice to get the earmold in and out properly, and some modification for comfort may be critical for acceptance in the early days.

### Monaural or Binaural?

Of great interest to hearing-aid users is the advent of the binaural hearing aid. We need to remind ourselves of the illustrations in Chapter 10 which distinguish between the Y-cord and binaural instruments. The Y-cord hearing aid consists of one microphone and amplifier with a receiver going to each ear. A binaural aid is made up of two complete instruments, one for each ear. Since the microphone is the new ear for the user, the binaural aid at-

tempts to duplicate nature by providing two "ears." The conventional means of "packaging" the binaural aid is to house an instrument in each temple of a pair of spectacles as shown in Figures 10-12 and 10-13. Of course, individual aids of the type shown in Figures 10-9 and 10-10 can be worn behind the ears.

Research on binaural hearing aids has now progressed to the point where some conclusions can be drawn with high confidence. The first conclusion is that the major handicap imposed by using only one hearing aid (assuming an ear-level instrument) is that about half of the time this aid is on the wrong side of the head and is hence shadowed from the primary message. In such an event, a second hearing aid with its microphone on the favored side will yield much more efficient reception for the moment.

The second conclusion is that *binaural* help does occur. It gives secondary but real advantage to the aforementioned monaural reception. This advantage is equivalent to improving the speech-to-noise ratio about 3 dB. Such a modest benefit, however, is frequently obliterated, during which time binaural reception will be no better than monaural reception. Thus, it is unrealistic to expect a new dimension of intelligibility in everyday listening because of binaural interactions. Instead one should expect the second aid to be helpful because it combines a little binaural facilitation with more continuous favorable monaural reception (see Chapter 2).

The third conclusion is that the modest binaural facilitation of intelligibility is essentially independent of the binaural benefit to localization. When two hearing aids can recreate an auditory sense of space, the user achieves a sense of orientation which may make him much more comfortable. For some people, this comfort is a reason in its own right for wearing a second instrument. However, the sense of comfort does not mean that intelligibility against competing sounds is improved more than the 3 dB mentioned above.

### Right Ear or Left?

The audiogram is a useful guide to the choice of the ear on which to wear the hearing aid. If both ears show hearing levels for speech between 40 and 75 dB, the hearing aid should be worn on the *worse* ear. The better ear is left free, and it is still good enough to be of some use without a hearing aid. If, however, one ear or both ears have a hearing level worse (numerically greater) than 75 dB, the *better* ear should be fitted. If the level is worse than 75 dB, it is difficult enough to get good hearing with the better ear. There is usually a good deal of sensory-neural hearing loss in such a case, and intelligibility may be poor even with a powerful instrument. Furthermore, the margin between the threshold of hearing and the threshold of discomfort begins to get rather narrow when the hearing level is worse than 75 dB. Of course, there are exceptions to these rules, but experience has shown this rule to be a good guide in a majority of cases. If an audiogram is not available, the user should wear the aid on the worse ear if his hearing loss is only mild, but on the better ear if he is severely handicapped without any aid at all.

### Hearing Aids for Unilateral Hearing Loss

A person with unilateral hearing loss may have difficulty in three ways: in hearing a person who addresses him from the side of his poor ear, in determining the location of the source of sound, and in hearing in the presence of a background noise. To deal with these difficulties Harford and his co-workers have suggested and demonstrated the value of Contralateral Routing of Signals (CROS) for certain cases of unilateral deafness.

Harford describes CROS as follows:

A behind-the-ear air-conduction hearing aid is mounted in a headband with a wire extending from the amplifier, across the headband, to a hearing-aid earphone mounted on the other end of the band. With this arrangement, signals originating on the side of the impaired ear are picked up by the hearing-aid microphone mounted near that ear, amplified slightly, and routed *electrically* across the head to the earphone mounted near the good ear. A plastic tube carries the acoustic signals from the earphone into the otherwise open canal of the good ear.

CROS can also be adapted to a standard eyeglass hearing-aid frame.

CROS offers the unilateral case (with normal hearing in one ear) escape from adverse head shadowing in noisy surroundings when the wanted sound is on his "bad" side. Furthermore, he is actually helped in this case by the imperfections of reproduction inherent in the contemporary ear-level hearing aid, since these imperfections introduce a difference in the quality of the redirected signal. This quality difference helps him recognize the side from which the wanted sound is coming.

The use of CROS in cases of high-frequency loss is simply a way of restoring high-frequency components with a relatively sharp filtering out of the low frequencies. The advantage CROS offers here is to reduce the feedback problem. The most important thing is that the sound from the hearing aid is being fed into the ear via an open earmold, so that unaided sound can be received directly at the same time. This is a neat way to achieve selective amplification without plugging the ear.

## HOW TO CHOOSE A HEARING AID

The medical aspects of deafness have been discussed in Chapter 5. In summarizing these rules for the choice of hearing aids we assume that the prospective user has consulted his family physican or, better, an otologist, and that the medical profession has done all that it can do. The otologist will presumably take an audiogram for his records and to assist him in his diagnosis, and he will give reliable advice as to whether a hearing aid is indicated.

We believe that a qualified audiologist should be consulted in all decisions about hearing aids for children. As mentioned in Chapter 10, there are now many clinics that offer unbiased advice on the selection of hearing aids, whether for children or for adults. These problems are complicated, and it is difficult for even an expert audiologist to pick out objectively and scientifically the hearing aids which best "fit" each individual. Furthermore, many persons are forced to rely on themselves, their friends, and the distributors of hearing aids in making their selection (see Table 1). Otologists will continue to give assistance.

The hearing aid dealer is obviously not a disinterested party except for assistance in the selection of the most suitable model from his own particular offerings. Most purchasers must rely very largely on their own judgment and be prepared to discount some of the claims for special methods of "fitting" put forward by competing manufacturers. For this reason auditory tests and the basic principles of selection were described at length in the preceding chapters. Now let us consider how a person who wants to buy a hearing aid may, without the benefit of expert advice or special apparatus, make a reasonably satisfactory selection from the makes and models of instruments that may be available in his community. Fortunately, the selection among the better instruments is no longer as critical as it once was or as is suggested by some advertisements. *Any one of several choices is likely to be a good one,* thanks to the great advances in recent years by the hearing aid industry and its distributors.

## Available Dealers

It is generally not wise to buy a hearing aid by mail if there is any practical alternative. Direct personal contact with the dealer is most desirable. The prospective user should find out first, therefore, which hearing aid companies have local representatives in his district His choice is practically restricted to the makes of instrument which are available to him for inspection and trial. Nearness to a dealer is also a great advantage for subsequent repair and replacement service.

## Services, Batteries, and Earmolds

Specific inquiry should be made about the availability, quality, and cost of service, including the replacement of batteries. Hearing aids, like automobiles, must sometimes be repaired. If repair service is not immediately available, the user may be deprived of his instrument for long periods of time. Some dealers replace the entire hearing aid, others lend an instrument while an aid is at the factory for service, and others may be able to replace immediately such major parts as amplifier, microphone, or receiver. Unnecessary repairs at exorbitant prices are to be avoided, and the user is cautioned against being "high-pressured" into buying a new model of an instrument to substitute for an older model that happens to get out of order. It is wise to look into the company's policy regarding trade-in value of old instruments in the event that new models appear on the market.

Some spare cords should be purchased, particularly if the dealer is not easily reached. As a matter of fact, *we suggest a complete spare hearing aid if the cost is not prohibitive.*

Dealers in hearing aids arrange for the manufacture of the individually molded earpiece. The contract of purchase should clearly indicate whether the cost of the earpiece is included in the final price of the instrument.

## Size, Cost, and Convenience

Even when expert advice is available, the decision on size, weight, cost, style, color, and convenience of the instrument is the user's own. Only he can strike the balance of his preferences. He must, however, weigh these items against the performance of the various instruments in overcoming his own particular hearing loss. There are three major items of expense in a hearing aid: the initial cost, repairs and replacements, and batteries. Low cost of one of these items does not necessarily mean low cost of the others.

Issues related to pricing, distribution, and servicing of hearing aids by the industry are discussed in a report of hearings before the Subcommittee on Antitrust and Monopoly of the Committee on the Judiciary, United States Senate, Eighty-Seventh Congress (1962).

## Simple Tests of the Performance of a Hearing Aid

In general the prospective user may rely on the dealer to recommend the particular combinations of amplifier, earphone, and tone-control setting that are most likely to be suitable for him. An audiogram will usually help the dealer arrive at his conclusions, and some dealers make their own audiometric tests. Each company that relies on the audiogram or other tests usually has a system or formula to show which of its several instruments or combinations is most likely to give satisfaction. The systems have been worked out with care, partly on theory and partly from the experience of actual users, and the choices based on them are usually rather good. It is advisable to try the first two or three combinations suggested by a dealer, but it is rarely necessary to try more.

No simple set of rules for self-selection

will do for everyone, because some people are much more seriously handicapped than others. The following method should work well, however, for someone who is just becoming really hard of hearing but can still "get by" if people will only speak up loudly enough. The principles have been explained in the previous chapter; if the rules obviously do not fit your case, you can probably judge readily enough what feature of a hearing aid is most important for you and how to test for it. The general principle is this: Test for the essentials; follow your preferences thereafter.

The features of performance that should be tested when a hearing aid is chosen are:

Tolerability
Intelligibility of ordinary speech
Intelligibility of faint speech
Intelligibility of difficult words
Freedom from internal noise
Aesthetic "quality"
Intelligibility under difficult conditions

It is not possible to test these items *accurately* without elaborate apparatus; but with the help of a friend it is not difficult to come to a useful opinion on most of them. The assistance of a friend is essential, however, because *the tests should all be made under similar conditions and with the same voice and the same set of words and sentences.*

The ideal arrangement is a loan or trial period with each of several instruments, so that they may all be tested at leisure at home under the same conditions and in the same place, and the more promising ones tried in actual everyday situations. Trial periods are not generally encouraged by dealers because some unscrupulous "prospects" have no intention of purchasing the instrument and because others will not take responsibility for damage. A compromise can be worked out in most instances. Perhaps it may be possible to rent an instrument or to make a deposit for the trial period that will be applied to payment for the hearing aid if it is purchased, but otherwise the deposit will be sacrificed by the user.

If arrangements cannot be made for home testing, the prospective user should ask a friend to go with him to the various agencies and try to carry out the same trials and tests in each case under as nearly the same conditions as possible. The friend must have a good, normal voice and be willing to practice the trick of speaking test words and reading some selected passage from a book or magazine over and over in just the same tone and *with the same loudness*. If he can standardize three different voices—average, faint, and loud—so much the better. During the trials he must keep his distance with care. A distance of 5 feet, which is an average conversation distance, is good; but 3 feet is better if the room is small or if there is some unavoidable noise. For most of the tests a quiet room is very important.

The desirability of obtaining an individually molded earpiece has been mentioned. For the very first trials one of the "universal" earmolds provided by the various companies will have to do. With them, however, it may not be possible to test the instruments at full gain, because, as has been explained, a hearing aid is more likely to "squeal" if the earpiece does not fit snugly.

Each of the instruments should be worn as they are meant to be worn. They should not merely be held in the hand. The body reflects, absorbs, and distorts sound waves and is part of the acoustic system of the hearing aid when the instrument is actually in use. During the actual tests the friend should be faced, but the eyes should be closed to avoid unconscious speech-reading.

### Tolerability

*Tolerability* is very important but is very difficult to test unless you are already an experienced user of a hearing aid. Sounds that are uncomfortably loud at first become tolerable with a little practice. The unfamiliar experience of hearing a really loud noise may be terrifying to someone who has been hard of hearing for a long time. Therefore, feel your way with a little care. Unless your hearing loss is quite severe, an instrument of only medium or low power may be better at first. However, with your friend, you should cautiously *try the maximum output of the instrument before the final choice is made*. But remember: *An otherwise satisfactory instrument should not be rejected simply because it is very loud, but only if it is really intolerable*. Unless your hearing loss is severe and you must use nearly full gain, you will rarely hear the loudest output except by accident, as when a door slams, and then only for a very short time.

### Intelligibility

*Intelligibility* of speech can be tested in three ways. First, your friend reads a selected passage from a book or newspaper in an ordinary but even voice. The same passage of connected speech should never be listened to more than once for purposes of judging intelligibility. Experiment with the volume control and the tone control *to be sure that you can find a combination that makes it easy to understand what he is reading*.

If more than one instrument makes ordinary speech easily intelligible to you, the test can be made more difficult. Let your friend read in a *very quiet voice*. This is, of course, equivalent to "hearing at a distance." It is important to vary the position or orientation of the hearing aid to the sound source. Most users can benefit from ear-level instruments. Care should be taken that the instrument is worn firmly and placed for best reception of sound with the proper length of tubing and at the right angle. A higher setting of the volume control may be necessary, but be sure that you can find *some* setting that will do the job. Some instruments may fail on this test. Eliminate them from the competition, and center your attention on those that pass.

Now comes the test with difficult words. You should have prepared in advance a set of word lists with each word written on a separate card. These can be prepared from the lists in the Appendix. Shuffle the cards each time they have been read. Prepare a number of such little packs with the words in each pack alike except for one sound. A series of words to test the vowels is *bat, bite, boot, beat, boat, bout, bit, bait, but, bet, bought*. For consonants, the following words can be used: *vie, by, high, thy, shy, why, thigh, die, lie, tie, rye, pie, fie, my, sigh, guy, nigh*. If you know that you have difficulty with certain kinds of sounds, it is easy enough to make up a list that is heavily loaded with just the words that you find most confusing.

Your friend should read the words in an ordinary voice and all at the same volume. It may help him to say "now" before each word to get his voice going smoothly. You should set the volume control so that the words come to you quite loudly, but not uncomfortably so. This is not a test of sensitivity of the instrument but a test of how well it enables you to discriminate among and to recognize correctly the sounds that ordinarily are difficult for you. Loud sounds are easier to discriminate than faint ones, so the instrument is "given a break" by being set so that words will not be missed simply because they are too faint.

It is a good plan to put some words two or three times over on the same list. The important points to keep in mind are these:

Use the same list, reshuffled each time, for all instruments.

Your friend must keep his voice, his distance, and all other conditions as nearly the same as possible.

Avoid speechreading.

Keep score systematically.

This test is about as elaborate and rigorous as is practicable without special apparatus. The remaining "tests" depend much more on your opinions and preferences, but your friend can be very helpful by making sure that all points are considered systematically and by noting your comments. Let him be scorekeeper. Without some sort of scorecard, it is very difficult to compare the performance of one instrument heard in one shop with another heard somewhere else and perhaps on another day. Remember, however, as we have said in Chapter 10, that hearing aids cannot do everything.

### Internal Noise

By the time you have finished the test of intelligibility, you have probably formed some opinion of the "quality" of the instrument, that is, whether or not you "like its sound." If the instrument has any great internal noise, either electrical or from friction against your clothing, you will certainly have noticed it by this time and will have scored a black mark against that instrument.

### Quality

As to "quality," it is well known that men and women who have heard high tones poorly for some time, as well as many with normal hearing, prefer the quality of a hearing aid (or radio) that does not emphasize—and may even suppress—high tones. They describe its sound as "smoother, more mellow, more comfortable, more pleasing." When the high tones are emphasized, or even merely restored to their normal strength, such listeners say the voice or music is harsh and unpleasant, even though words may be crisper and easier to understand. Remember, therefore, that if your hearing has been subnormal for some time, you are likely to prefer the instrument with the "full, smooth tone," even though the word test may show that you understand difficult words better with an instrument that emphasizes the high tones a bit. Your friend will probably remind you of the importance of understanding correctly. He represents your "talking public." Other people, too, are interested in having you understand them readily, and to them *your ability to understand is more important than how mellow their voices sound.* If the word tests do not show any great difference, then pick the instrument that "sounds best" by all means, but remember that *the quality preferences of those who have heard poorly for some time are notoriously misleading.* You may have forgotten how speech *should* sound.

As a final word of advice, when you are scoring an instrument on quality, lean toward the crisp rather than the mellow. You are likely to get the best results with it in the long run, even though some practice will probably be necessary before you realize the full benefits.

### Difficult Conditions

But it is not enough to judge the quality of an instrument under good conditions only. An instrument may work very well when its volume control is set low or when your friend talks in an ordinary voice; but it may lose its clarity when the control is set high or when your friend suddenly raises his voice. The reasons for this were explained in the preceding chapter. The point to remember is this: Compare instruments for *loud* as well as for average voices *without moving the volume control from the position that makes the average voice easy to understand.* This test gives some idea of the leeway the instrument has before it either loses quality from "overloading" or else becomes intolerably loud. Plenty of leeway, techni-

cally called a "good operating range," is important for those whose auditory area has been much restricted by a severe hearing loss. But, in this test your friend should raise his voice by degrees. Don't invite someone with a distorted sense of humor to help on this one! It is particularly helpful to listen under different conditions of instrument orientation and noise to more than one person talking at the same time. This is known as a "competing message" test.

There is no very good way to find out without actual trial periods how different hearing aids sound in noisy places. Your friend may have a fairly standard voice, but he cannot carry a kit of sound effects with him. We have mentioned the desirability of a trial period if the dealer will consent. It is not necessary to make such trial of *every* available instrument. The tests that you and a friend can do on the spot should be enough to narrow the field down to two or three leading instruments.

It is an open question whether anyone who has not already had experience in wearing a hearing aid is really qualified to judge the performance of an instrument in noise. The novice is likely at first to suppress the high frequencies with the tone control, then turn down the gain control, and end by "throwing out the baby with the bath." If there is much noise around you, you must listen to noise if you are to hear voices also. Normal listeners must put up with the noise and often must struggle to understand. The tone control of a hearing aid may take some of the sting out of the noise, but no instrument can magically sort out speech from noise or one voice from another when both sounds occupy the same part of the frequency spectrum and come from the same direction. Here is where two hearing aids may be much better than one.

A trial period gives a better idea of the strong and the weak points of an instrument; but *play fair with the first instrument you try. Give it another trial after you have tried other instruments.* You are likely to do better in everyday situations with the second or third instrument and also to like them better because you are learning how to wear and use them. After you have gained this experience, a second trial of the first instrument may show that it is better than you thought.

Families and associates of hearing-aid users *should not shout* into the microphones. It is better to speak naturally but distinctly and to face the listener so that he can take full advantage of speechreading. Slamming of doors and pounding, which are nerve-racking to most wearers of hearing aids, should be avoided.

If a hearing-aid user has difficulty hearing the radio or television clearly enough for his enjoyment, he should consider having his set equipped with a socket into which he can plug an earphone. High-grade telephone receivers are now available, and they may reproduce music and voice more faithfully than can a hearing aid. It may be very helpful to avoid the unnecessary transformations, first into sound by the radio and then back into electrical signals by the hearing aid. All noises in the room are thus excluded. The arrangement should offer no difficulty for a good radio or television serviceman.

Some persons with a long-standing hearing loss may not like a hearing aid simply because it sounds "strange." They have often forgotten what it means to hear well, and therefore their judgment of how things should sound is not very reliable. They must be as patient with a hearing aid as they are with a new pair of shoes, and their families must be equally patient with them.

No one but an expert should ever open the case of a hearing-aid amplifier. Even opening and closing it may cause trouble, and to poke around inside may cause severe damage that will be expensive to repair. If you must satisfy your curiosity and see the inside, your dealer will be glad to show it to you. Remember, if you do damage through opening up the case (and don't think your dealer will fail to detect it), it is liable to void your service guarantee! As explained in the previous chapter, the miniaturized transistor amplifiers of many modern hearing aids cannot be repaired, even by an expert, but must be replaced as a unit in case of failure.

## SUGGESTED READINGS AND REFERENCES

**ASHA Reports, Number 2.** "A Conference on Hearing Aid Evaluation Procedures." American Speech and Hearing Association, Washington, D.C., 1967.
Very useful discussions of the problem.

**Carhart, R.** "The Usefulness of the Binaural Hearing Aid." *Trans. Amer. Acad. Ophthal. Otolaryng.,* 62:120–128 (1958).

**Committee on the Judiciary, United States Senate.** *Hearings before the Subcommittee on Antitrust and Monopoly.* "Prices of Hearing Aids." Eighty-Seventh Congress, U.S. Government Printing Office, Washington, D.C. (1962).
Contains testimony from the hearing-aid industry, economists, audiologists, and others about issues related to the distribution of hearing aids.

**Harford, E., and E. Dodds.** "The Clinical Application of CROS: A Hearing Aid for Unilateral Deafness," *Arch. Otolaryng.* (Chicago), 83:455–464 (1966).

**Hirsh, I. J.** "Binaural Hearing Aids: A Review of Some Experiments," *J. Speech Hearing Dis.,* 15:114–123 (1950).

**Jerger, J., C. Speaks, and C. Malmquist.** "Hearing Aid Performance and Hearing Aid Selection," *J. Speech Hearing Res.,* 9:136–149 (1966).

**National Center for Health Statistics.** Series 10, Number 35. "Characteristics of Persons with Impaired Hearing: United States, July 1962–June 1963." (A. Gentile, J. D. Schein, and K. Haase, eds.)
Data from the *National Health Survey,* Public Health Service, U.S. Department of Health, Education and Welfare. (For sale by Superintendent of Documents, U.S. Government Printing Office, Washington, D.C. 20402. Price 45 cents.)

**O'Neill, J. J., and H. J. Oyer.** *Applied Audiometry.* New York: Dodd, Mead & Company, 1966.
Chapter 11 is an excellent discussion of hearing-aid evaluation, with historical perspective.

**Prosthetic and Sensory Aid Service.** The following articles appear together in *Bulletin of Prosthetics Research,* 10–7, 5–92 (1967): published by Department of Medicine and Surgery, Veterans Administration (252 Seventh Ave., New York 10001).
E. F. Murphy. "Hearing and Hearing Aids—A Layman's Notions."
W. O. Olsen and R. Carhart. "Development of Test Procedures for Evaluation of Binaural Hearing Aids."
R. N. Kasten and S. H. Lotterman. "Azimuth Effects with Ear-level Hearing Aids."
J. Jerger. "Behavioral Correlates of Hearing-Aid Performance."
E. D. Burnett. "A New Method for the Measurement of Nonlinear Distortion Using a Random Noise Test Signal."

**Round Table on Hearing Aids,** *International Audiology,* 5:373–393 (1966).
This is a round-table discussion held at the VIII International Congress of Audiology in Mexico City in 1966. The contributors and titles are:
Davis, H. "Hearing Aids: Introduction to the Round Table."
Lybarger, S. F. "Discussion of Hearing Aid Trends."
Ewertsen, H. W. "The Fitting of Hearing Aids in the Danish Hearing Rehabilitation Centres."
Decroix, G. "Stéréoaudiométrie et Appareillages Stéréophoniques."
Hirsh, I. J. "Recent Development in Hearing-Aid Use."

**Shore, I., R. C. Bilger, and I. J. Hirsh.** "Hearing Aid Evaluation: Reliability of Repeated Measurements," *J. Speech Hearing Dis.,* 25:152–170 (1960).

**Shore, I. and J. C. Kramer.** "A Comparison of Two Procedures for Hearing Aid Evaluation," *J. Speech Hearing Dis.,* 28:159–170 (1963).

# PART FOUR
# REHABILITATION FOR HEARING LOSS

# CHAPTER 12

## SPEECHREADING

### MIRIAM PAULS HARDY, Ph.D.

Speechreading, or lipreading, is an integral part of communication. We have unconsciously learned that if we watch the speaker, we do not have to listen as intently. We get more information more readily when we can see and hear the speaker. Most of us prefer to turn on the television set, rather than the radio, to hear the President's address to the nation. We crane our necks in order to peer around the woman with the large hat or an elaborate coiffure sitting in front of us at a lecture. In a critical verbal exchange, we watch intently, not only to enhance the verbal message, but to take in the facial expression, the gestures, the subtle postural changes, as well as the situational cues that can convey so much information. In noisy situations such as are found at large social gatherings, riding on the subway, or in industrial plants, we become even more dependent on visual cues if we are to communicate effectively.

There are wide variations in ability to speechread. Some are "born lipreaders"; the majority have reasonable facility in utilizing visual cues, but some find it most difficult. The factors that make good speechreading have been explored in various studies that will be discussed below. There is reason to suspect that there may be biologic factors that underlie the process that are not fully understood. Speechreading skills can be sharpened with training, determination, and practice, but individual differences seem to persist despite training—at least with the kind of training we have commonly employed to date.

People with normal hearing utilize visual cues subconsciously. Since they are seldom in a situation in which they are dependent on them, they are usually amazed, then intrigued, when it is demonstrated that they can and do speechread. On the other hand, the hearing-impaired individual is forced by the very nature of his handicap to utilize speechreading as a major support for diminished auditory information that may also be distorted. It behooves him to become as expert as possible.

## LANGUAGE AND SPEECHREADING

Language is man's most unique characteristic. It can be defined as the mind's use of a common symbol code. It is the core of all aspects of human communication, whether it be the comprehension of oral language through hearing or through seeing (speechreading), the comprehension of written language (reading), or the formulation and expression of language, speaking, and writing.

We learned language and to talk because and as we heard. Because we talked, we learned through auditory, visual, and kinesthetic feedback to refine gradually what we heard and what we said. It is a closely interlocked system, each input and output modality enhancing the others. As Lashley said in 1951, "The processes of comprehension and production of speech have too much in common to depend on wholly different mechanisms."

Language comprehension demands being able to process rapidly incoming bits of acoustic and visual information in temporal sequence and patterns in milliseconds of time and to derive language meanings almost simultaneously. It requires good short-term memory and also ready storage and retrieval, both into and out of the long-term language memory bank.

Speechreading is a process similar to reading. Both employ the visual modality. Like learning to read, learning to speechread has two steps. First, one must learn how to decode (identify and discriminate) and hold in immediate memory a sequence of visual patterns; and, second, how to comprehend the message that is conveyed by the language code. One must have an adequate command of language in order to read, or to speechread, for comprehension. The adult who had language firmly established before acquiring a hearing loss has a problem very different from that of the child who has never heard or

who has never heard well, and who must slowly and painfully acquire his language in spite of a defective auditory system. One cannot readily understand vocabulary or language forms that one does not know, either from the lips or from the printed page.

Decoding spoken language (speechreading) is a more difficult process than reading the printed page. In both processes one is identifying and discriminating fleeting visual events that must be held in short-term memory as the language message unfolds. For the speechreader, however, these patterns are never fixed, as they are on the printed page, and he cannot review unless the speaker repeats. To further complicate the process there are wide variations in the visibility of the phonemes that make up spoken words, phrases, and sentences. Likewise, there are variations in the visual patterns that are presented by different speakers even when saying the same material. All this is further affected by lighting, distance from the speaker, the angle at which the speaker must be read, and the like. Although speechreading involves the same processes as scanning the printed page, it demands more of the speechreader in terms of visual perception, visual memory, and visual "fill-ins."

## FACTORS IN SPEECHREADING

The factors that contribute to speechreading ability have been suggested by experienced teachers, by investigators, and by speechreaders themselves. Jeffers, in a thoughtful overview (1967), has organized the factors and analyzed the research relating to them. She emphasized three primary factors. One is *perceptual efficiency,* which includes the ability to identify speech sounds or elements and to perceive them rapidly, and also the ability to gain information from the face when the focus is on the mouth. Associated with these processes are visual acuity and attention and speed of focusing and peripheral vision. The second factor is *synthetic ability,* which includes the ability to identify parts and patterns (words and phrases) and the gist of a message. The third primary factor is *flexibility,* which fosters the ability to revise tentative identification of a message. Among major secondary factors are the amount and kind of training, language proficiency, motivation, and reaction to frustration and failure.

Associated with language proficiency is intelligence and also the extent and pattern of the subject's impairment of hearing, its duration, and his age at its onset. In general, investigations confirm the importance of visual perception, the ability to fill in missing words, and training. Language proficiency, as might be expected, is important for the speechreading skill of deaf children, but it seems not to be important for the adult population who already possessed language when their hearing failed. Duration of hearing impairment seems to be important, but the influence of hearing level is not clearly established.

*One is on safe ground in stating that speechreading is a composite skill consisting of subskills that might be teased out and measured.* It should be possible to develop a test battery that describes a person's capabilities and limitations prior to training and, on the basis of these findings, to devise an instructional program that best meets his needs. Although we may find that there are biologic differences that are not overcome by training, we may also be able to delineate the factors that can be improved with a specific kind of training.

O'Neill (1967) advocates that visual communication be studied apart from its therapeutic implications. When we understand better what is involved in visual communication, we will then be in a position to devise better techniques for working with the individual who is in trouble.

## THE TASK OF THE SPEECHREADER

### Visibility of Spoken Language

Speechreading, or lipreading, can be defined as the skill that enables a person, regardless of whether his hearing is normal or impaired, to understand language by attentively observing the speaker. It is appropriate to analyze all that is implied by the words "attentively observing."

Spoken language is a rapid succession of utterances that are composed of some forty-odd meaningful sounds of varying degrees of visibility. These sounds have been divided into two major categories: vowels and consonants. The speechreader must be able to recognize all the visible movements, and he must fill in those that are invisible. Fortunately, sounds like 'f,' 's,' 'th,' and 'ch' that are relatively difficult to hear are easy to see on the lips. Likewise, the sounds that are more difficult to see (like the short vowels) are easier to hear because they have more energy in the low and midfrequency range where the majority of hard-of-hearing people have useful residual hearing. The forty-odd sounds are produced by changing the shape of the mouth and the relative position of the tongue, teeth, lips, and jaw. It is these rapidly changing movements that the speechreader must observe and interpret. To help him fill in the gaps in what he hears and sees for only about one-third of speech sounds are clearly visible), the speechreader can learn to use the sensations that he imagines or actually feels in his own speech muscles as he watches the speaker. Note what even an expert speechreader does when puzzled. He silently imitates the movements he sees. This imitation helps him translate a visual image into a motor speech image, and usually gives him a valuable clue. This use of the muscle-feeling sense is a valuable training device.

It may seem impossible to speechread

when only one-third of the sounds are clearly visible, but we are all accustomed to the same sort of confusion, albeit to a lesser degree. Two or more words like "ice" and "eyes," or "up" and "cup," or "come" and "gum" may look alike on the lips, and the speechreader must derive from context which one is said. This is not different from what all of us must do with words that sound alike, such as "their" and "there," and "sow" and "so," and "sew," or the words that have different meanings depending upon how they are used in a syntactical array. The speechreader simply has many more choices to make as well as blanks to fill in. He must learn to hold in mind the visual pattern as it unfolds on the lips and automatically translate it into meaningful language. He must maintain an anticipatory set, yet remain flexible so he can shift as he gets more information.

Lashley, in his discussion of the problem of serial order in behavior, cleverly builds up to a superb illustration of this kind of mental gymnastics. "Rapid righting with his uninjured hand saved from loss the contents of the capsized canoe." Note that the associations that give meaning to "righting" as against "writing" are not activated for at least 3 to 5 seconds after hearing (or speechreading!) the word. However in reading one is on the right track by the second word in the sentence.

In vocal utterance, there are no pauses between words as there are on the printed page. For example, the phrase "plenty of potatoes" has the same number of syllables as "plenipotentiary." Both are said within the same time span with no division between syllables. The division into words is an interpretive process that takes place in the mind. It is never seen on the lips or, for that matter, heard by the ear.

The speechreader must be cognizant, too, of the rhythm and flow of the sentences; each language has a characteristic rhythm determined by its syntactical structure, as well as by the pronunciation of specific words. An appreciation of this basic rhythm and syntactical order helps him to fill in the many gaps in what he actually sees and hears. In addition, there are the less regular rhythms of phrasing and emphasis. Stress patterns markedly affect what the speechreader sees. By noting the prolongation of certain syllables and the pauses between syllables, he gets additional information. The same group of words said with different emphasis and phrasing has its meaning changed completely. Read aloud the following sentences, stressing the italicized word, and note the results. Then watch to see the differences in timing when someone else says them, and you will have a better appreciation of this point.

"*Good!* By God, we're going to Kansas."
"Goodbye, *God.* We're going to Kansas."
"Goodbye! *God,* we're going to *Kansas.*"

### Looking and Listening

In addition to these factors, the cues provided by the general situation are very helpful. Facial expression, gesture, and postural changes are frequently as revealing as the words uttered. Often an object handled, or pointed to, gives a valuable cue, and the place and the particular speaker shed light on the topic under discussion. For example, we can easily anticipate what the clerk behind the counter at the grocery store will say, or the remarks of the airplane hostess, or the comments of the motorcycle cop who has signaled us over to the side of the road for running a red light.

The deaf and hard-of-hearing must learn to recognize and employ the details of every speech situation. The more limited his hearing, the greater the strain on the speechreader, for his attention is concentrated on this rapid succession of ever-changing movements that vary with each

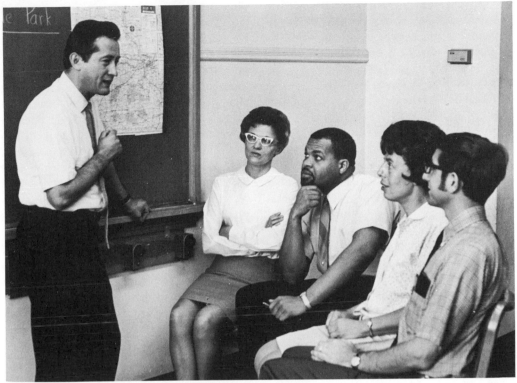

Fig. 12-1. Instruction in speechreading. (*Central Institute for the Deaf, photo by Harold Ferman*)

speaker. This rapid flow of speech must be grasped in a fleeting instant, for there is no opportunity for review. Interpretation must be almost instantaneous. Attentive observation of all these factors demands such alertness that tension and fatigue are produced in a relatively short time. Then, too, poor lighting, distance, noise, confusion, and distracting movements can defeat even the most experienced speechreader. Many a hard-of-hearing person, depending on speechreading alone, is so fatigued by the demands of his daily job that a social evening hardly seems worthwhile.

For most hearing-impaired individuals, these difficulties can best be helped by use of an appropriate hearing aid or hearing aids. Most people with a moderate to severe hearing loss can be brought within the range of good function with carefully selected amplification appropriate to the nature and degree of loss. Therefore, they can rely on hearing as the primary modality and use speechreading as the supportive skill.

Unfortunately, there are those who, by the very nature of their auditory problem, cannot use amplification or can only profit from it to a limited degree. For the profoundly deaf, its value may be limited to auditory support from stress and rhythm patterns, and serve as an alerting device. One of the major benefits may be to help him monitor his own voice. There are others with more complex auditory problems, whose ability to discriminate speech is seriously affected and for whom amplification only adds additional loudness without additional clarity. For others increased loudness is intolerable.

We communicate best with a combination of looking and listening. The use of a hearing aid does not eliminate the need to speechread. The two processes are complementary and should be so employed by the hearing-impaired individual.

## METHODS OF TEACHING SPEECHREADING

### Conventional Approaches

Prior to 1940, when help for the hearing-impaired was limited chiefly to a course of 30 or more lessons, a number of methods were developed. The originators, as well as the teachers who adopted and adapted a particular method, were usually hard-of-hearing individuals, who, after they learned to lipread, became interested in helping others. Consequently several schools of lipreading (speechreading) developed, each with its firm advocates. There were few college courses in speechreading prior to World War II, so the courses for instructors tended to emphasize known approaches and were not concerned with underlying theory. A very interesting and rewarding historical overview, as well as a succinct evaluative description of the various methodologies, is found in Deland's *The Story of Lipreading* (1968). Fortunately, this book is once more available after being out of print for nearly a quarter of a century.

It is eminently worthwhile for anyone interested in the field to read the textbooks that were written by the pioneers, especially Bruhn, Nitchie, Kinzie, Bunger, and Ewing. Although they tend to be overly structured, outlining materials and procedures in detail, they do contain the distillation of years of experience and hard-earned wisdom that is not available elsewhere. Many people have learned to speechread by each of these methods. There is no evidence to date that one approach is more effective than another.

A prospective teacher of speechreading should be thoroughly familiar with at least one and comfortable with all, so as to be able to develop an eclectic approach that is suitable to a particular student or group. Careful review of the different methods suggests that they have much in common. All stress the need for synthesis, rather than analysis, for successful speechreading; also, in varying degrees, they stress the value of auditory and kinesthetic cues in enhancing visual cues. The major differences lie in the way the speech positions and movements are presented to the student so that he learns to recognize and discriminate among them on the lips. All systematically employ syllable drills using the movement or position of the lesson, and then provide practice using it in words, sentences, and stories. All but the Jena method proceed from the visible to the less visible and from the simple to the complex as the lessons are developed in a course.

The Jena method is unique in its presentation of an over-all introduction to phonetics in the first few lessons, then relying on rhythmic syllable drills and talking-together exercises to enhance automatic recognition. Its proponents hold that this makes for interlocking speechreading with auditory training and speech production, and has the additional advantage of permitting more freedom in the construction of the lessons themselves by not restricting the students to a particular sound per lesson. Instead, each lesson is centered around a topic, such as dining out, shopping, travel, and the like. Interest is sustained by the unity of the topic, and valuable experience in anticipating the turn of the conversation can be set up, as a wealth of materials can be employed around the central theme.

### Group and Individual Instruction

Cogent arguments can be made for both group and individual instruction. Group teaching is more efficient when professional services are limited, as well as being less expensive for the student. However, the students must all have about the same aptitude for the task so that the material can be challenging, but not over-whelming, for each member of the group.

Screening tests administered prior to instruction usually demonstrate that prospective students fall into three groups in facility for speechreading: excellent, average, and poor. Tests administered to these same individuals after a period of instruction show that, although each student demonstrates improvement, he tends to remain within the same relative groupings. This suggests that these differences are significant and should be respected.

Individual instruction has the advantage of being flexible to the immediate needs of each student. It is essential for those who have had their hearing suddenly wiped out by illness or trauma and are plunged into a silent world. This is a catastrophic experience that requires immediate expert management on a highly individualized basis.

The effectiveness of group instruction was demonstrated in the Army and Navy Hearing Rehabilitation programs during World War II, where it was necessary, because of the pressure of numbers, to plan the most efficient and effective program for a large turnover of hospitalized patients with a limited staff. It required adapting old techniques and creating new ones. However, the advantages of well-planned group instruction were retained on their own merits. Results can often be obtained with a group that are difficult to achieve with individual instruction. The association with others, similarly handicapped, continually reminds the student that his case is not unique. He is less inclined to self-pity, and he profits by the successes, the observations, and even the errors of his classmates. The element of competition enters, and the interplay of personalities as well as the spontaneous comments of the group produce the easy natural atmosphere favorable for learning. These same com-

ments develop the student's ability to anticipate, as well as the mental flexibility to deal with abrupt changes of subject. It provides a rich experience with the speech patterns of the varied personalities within the group.

## SPEECHREADING IN THE TOTAL PROCESS OF HEARING REHABILITATION

As we see throughout this book, advances in the medicine and the surgery of the ear and the emergence of clinical audiology as a professional field have done much to improve our understanding and management of auditory disorders. With the perfecting of the modern wearable aid, speechreading is no longer considered the only help. Nevertheless, it holds its own as an integral part of a total hearing-rehabilitation program.

A careful diagnostic evaluation is the first step in any hearing-rehabilitation program. For certain individuals, a complete physical examination, with various specialists contributing to the total picture, may be required. Any indicated medical or surgical treatment should be carried out, not only for improving hearing but for general health. The audiologic evaluation should not only measure the nature and degree of the hearing impairment, but, what is even more important, it should assess the total communicative function of the individual and the communicative demands of his particular "world" and how he can be better prepared to meet them.

A detailed communicative evaluation as well as a psychological appraisal are indicated for children. The psychological evaluation should be a sophisticated one that does not penalize the child for his language retardation and the effects of sensory deprivation, yet establishes a reasonable estimate of his intellectual potential and points up factors that interfere with learning. The objective is to describe as fully as possible the child's capabilities and limitations, so that an effective program can be initiated. It must be recognized that a significant number of children with hearing impairment have multiple problems. In addition to the hearing loss, there may be a language disorder, other specific learning disabilities, attentional peculiarities, limited intelligence, or emotional problems to complicate the learning process. These must be identified, if the child is to have an appropriate program to help him learn through and around his difficulties (see Chapter 16).

If otologic and audiologic findings indicate a hearing aid, its selection should be guided by the audiologist, and he should help the subject learn to use it as effectively as possible over a period of time (see Chapters 10, 11, and 13). With this kind of management, it is possible to plan a training program that is hand-tailored to the needs of that individual. There are rarely two similar, much less identical, problems; one is dealing with people, not "ears."

The experience gained in the military rehabilitation programs during World War II laid the groundwork for current concepts of hearing rehabilitation. In a military organization one has complete control over the patient and his time. Thus it was possible to have concentrated daily instruction for 4- to 8-week periods. Such a program is not practical for the average adult engaged in earning a living or managing a busy household. Thus most programs must be worked out in terms of feasibility as well as need. Such a concentrated program might profitably be considered, however, for hard-of-hearing children for whom little or no special help is available in their local community. With an intensive short-term program, even in a residential facility, many children who are now floundering could better maintain themselves in the regular educational stream (see Chapter 17). We need imaginative approaches, for

the hard-of-hearing child is far too often a neglected youngster in our schools.

The major role of the itinerant speech and hearing therapist in the public schools is not just giving the child speechreading lessons or auditory training, or struggling to correct an off-pressure 's', but to ensure that the child's vocabulary and language are expanding as rapidly as possible. Most hard-of-hearing children have mild-to-severe language handicaps which contribute the major obstacle to their progress in the regular classroom. Curricular tutoring as indicated, as well as other kinds of imaginative supportive help, should make it possible for most hard-of-hearing children to keep up with their peer group.

Two basic approaches are required: First, the individual must understand the nature of his hearing impairment and face objectively the problems it poses, and he must be helped to assume responsibility for meeting them. It is profitable to instruct the members of the family so that they better understand the problem and learn how they can and must help. With schoolchildren, this information needs to be given to the classroom teacher as well as to the parents. Second, the three aspects of the communicative process, speechreading, auditory training, and speech correction, must be developed in a close-knit fashion with emphasis on which aspect is most pertinent for the individual. There can be no "cookbook" approach.

Just as important as the initial otologic and audiologic evaluation is regular reassessment over the years by the otologist, the audiologist, and other specialists who may be needed. The physical status may change, the hearing loss may vary, and hearing aids may wear out. The nature of the problems that arise, particularly for children, shifts in the process of growth and maturation. The problems are not static, and there can be no single diagnosis that provides "the truth" for all time.

## PRACTICAL ADVICE
## FOR THE SPEECHREADER

Speechreading is seldom easy, because so many critical factors cannot be controlled. A poorly lighted room that throws deep shadows on the speaker's face or a seating arrangement that forces the speechreader to look into a bright light are deleterious. The friend who attempts to help by buttonholing the speechreader merely presents an additional problem. At close range the speechreader cannot readily follow the speech, nor can he observe any situational cues. Approximately 6 feet has been found to be the most comfortable distance. Furthermore, it is well worth the speechreader's efforts to seek a position from which he can observe most comfortably all members of the group without facing the light. Confusing and disturbing movements and noises only serve to divert his attention and increase his fatigue.

As we have pointed out, the very character of speech itself presents a major problem. Ideas must be grasped in a fleeting instant, for speech is never static. Much of it is invisible, and every new combination of syllables produces minor changes in the individual sounds. No two mouths are alike; no two individual's speech patterns are identical. Poor speakers impose a burden, for their articulation is careless and indistinct and therefore hard to see. *The greatest help is good quiet speech.* The well-intentioned person who shouts or exaggerates his speech pattern only increases the difficulties. One who covers his mouth or turns while talking, or has annoying mannerisms, presents similar problems. Likewise, it is well-nigh impossible to follow the speech of a man who has his teeth clamped on a pipe or has a cigarette dangling from his lips. An impassive, expressionless face is more difficult than a mobile one. The considerate speaker, however, can materially reduce all these problems.

The sociable person, keenly interested in people and events, usually makes rapid progress in speechreading, while the shy, reserved individual and the unimaginative, phlegmatic type are at a disadvantage. The secret of successful speechreading lies in the ability to grasp an idea intuitively and develop its meaning without attempting to follow every word. A too literal person, or one who clings tenaciously to a preconceived idea about where the conversation is headed, always has serious difficulties. An illuminating answer was given the author by a relatively uneducated pupil. Pressed for an explanation of his unusual skill in speechreading, he replied "Well, Missy, I figures out where you're going and I beats you there!"

Essential as it is to be on the alert to catch significant trends and changes in a conversation, it is also true that undue tension and fatigue may cause a mental "block." Therefore the speechreader must strive to maintain a happy balance.

From the outset, a speechreader needs a sense of humor to help him surmount many failures. Speechreading can best be improved by constant practice in everyday living rather than by repeated returns to the classroom. The student's progress depends largely upon himself, for the teacher can only chart the way. The student's intelligence, application, and determination are vital factors in achieving success. It cannot be too strongly emphasized that a person with a hearing loss should frankly face this fact. The natural tendency is to ignore the hearing impairment or to attempt to conceal it. These efforts, even though partly successful for a time, lead to an increasing strain. Eventually both social and business life will be affected.

A handicap in hearing can be successfully overcome only by the efforts of the individual himself. Instruction and guidance will provide the groundwork. Continual practice of speechreading in daily contacts will usually develop the skill to carry on a normal life comfortably.

### Aids to Communication

Anyone with a hearing loss may profitably consider the following suggestions for ease of communication.

1. Remember that hearing is the natural and normal way to understand speech. Therefore, be fitted with, and get instruction in the use of, the best possible hearing aid for *your* particular impairment.
2. Be determined to develop good speech-reading skills. Don't forget that it can help you in every conversation.
3. Do not strain either to hear or to see speech. A combination of looking and listening enables you to understand most speakers readily. Actually, how you get it doesn't matter, just as long as you understand.
4. Keep relaxed, but remain alert and tuned in. Anticipate what may be said, but be ready to shift as the ideas develop.
5. Do not expect to get every word. Follow along with the speaker, and as you become familiar with the rhythm of his speech, key words will emerge to enable you to put two and two together.
6. Try to stage-manage the situation to your advantage. Since lighting is important, avoid facing a bright light, and try not to allow the speaker's face to be shadowed. Keep about 6 feet between you and the speaker, so that you can more readily observe the entire situation.
7. Try to determine the topic under discussion. Friends can be coached to give an unobtrusive lead, such as "We are discussing the housing problem." This is particularly helpful in large conversational groups.
8. Maintain an active interest in people and events. Being abreast of national and world affairs, as well as of those of your community and intimate social circle, enables you to follow any discussions more readily.
9. Remember that conversation is a two-way affair. Do not monopolize it in an attempt to direct and control it.
10. Pay particular attention to your speech. A long-term hearing loss or a sudden profound loss may cause a marked deterioration of voice and articulation. This requires professional help, for a pleasant, well-modulated voice and intelligible speech are a great asset.
11. Cultivate those subtle traits of personality that do so much to win friends and influence people. A sincere, ready smile, an even disposition, and a genuine sympathetic interest in other people can do much to smooth your path.
12. Remember that the education of *your* public is your responsibility. Many people are embarrassed because they have no idea of how to talk with the wearer of a hearing aid or with a speechreader. Put them at ease, and assure them that quiet, natural speech is their greatest favor to you.

## SUGGESTED READINGS AND REFERENCES

Black, J. W., P. P. O'Reilly, and L. Peck. "Self-administered Training in Lipreading," *J. Speech Hearing Dis.*, 28:183–186 (1963).

**Bruhn, M. A.** *The Muller-Walle Method of Lip-Reading.* Lynn, Mass.: The Nichols Press, 1929.

**Bunger, A. M.** *Speech Reading—Jena Method.* Danville, Ill.: The Interstate Press, 1954.

**Deland, F.** *The Story of Lipreading,* Washington, D.C.: Volta Bureau, 1968.

**Ewing, I. R.** *Lipreading and Hearing Aids.* Manchester, England: Manchester University Press, 1944.

**Frisina, D. R.** *"Speechreading," Report of the Proceedings of the International Congress on Education of the Deaf and the Forty-First Meeting of the Convention of American Instructors of the Deaf, U.S. Document No. 106,* U.S. Government Printing Office, Washington, D.C., 191–207 (1964).

**Haspiel, G. S.** *A Synthetic Approach to Lip Reading.* Magnolia, Mass.: Expression Company, 1964.

**Jeffers, J.** "The Process of Speechreading Viewed with Respect to a Theoretical Construct," in *Proceedings of International Conference on Oral Education of the Deaf,* Washington, D.C.: Alexander Graham Bell Association for the Deaf, 1530–1561 (1967).

**Kinzie, C. E., and R. Kinzie.** *Lip-Reading for the Deafened Adult.* Philadelphia: The John C. Winston Company, 1931.

**Lashley, K. S.** "The Problem of Serial Order in Behavior," in *Cerebral Mechanisms in Behavior, The Hixon Symposium*, L. A. Jeffress (ed.), New York: Hafner Publishing Company, 112–135 (1967).

**Nitchie, E. B.** *New Lessons in Lip Reading,* Philadelphia: J. B. Lippincott Company, 1950.

**O'Neill, J. J.** "Frontiers of Research in Visual Communication," in *Proceedings of International Conference on Oral Education of the Deaf,* Washington, D.C., Alexander Graham Bell Association for the Deaf, 1562–1571 (1967).

**O'Neill, J. J., and H. J. Oyer.** *Visual Communication for the Hard of Hearing, History, Research, and Methods.* Englewood Cliffs, N.J.: Prentice-Hall, Inc., 1961.

# CHAPTER 13

## AUDITORY TRAINING

### IRA J. HIRSH, Ph.D.

Babies with normal hearing accompanied by good intelligence *learn* to respond to, and to distinguish among, an enormous variety of sounds. They seem to differentiate the sounds of different persons approaching, to recognize speechlike sound from adults and from other children, and eventually to control through hearing their own production of speech (see Chapter 14). Furthermore, through their auditory reception of speech around them, they appear to acquire the rules for making words and sentences in their own language.

There are two special cases in which these normal steps of auditory learning are not taken at all or are not sustained over long periods of time. The first is the child or adult who once had normal hearing, who learned to speak and to use language properly, but who subsequently lost some of his hearing through disease or accident. The second is the child who was born with impaired hearing and whose original learning and experience therefore did not have the usual auditory components. In both cases the normal course of learning and the

normal use of auditory cues must somehow be compensated by special additional auditory learning or training. The principles underlying this special training are the subject of this chapter.

## HEARING AND AUDITORY PERCEPTION

When we speak of *hearing* we refer to any of the various ways in which human beings react to sound waves. When the clinician makes an audiogram, he is reporting on only one facet of auditory response, namely, the sensitivity to very weak tones at different frequencies. In the course of testing the hearing further, to know something about the nature of the hearing impairment, he may test still other functions, like sensitivity to differences between intensities, between frequencies or between durations, or between judgments of the loudness of different sounds or sounds heard at one or the other ear. In addition, when the clinician uses speech audiometry, he may be interested in the weakest levels of speech that a patient requires for a certain degree of intelligibility, or he may be interested in the percentage of speech items in a list that the patient can repeat correctly, sometimes in the quiet and sometimes when the speech is presented against a background of noise. These clinical tests of hearing represent only a small sample of the auditory functions that might be tested, and they do not very often exhaust those that the listener actually uses in everyday life.

One of the most common uses of hearing is in communication by speech. In such a situation we know that the talker and listener must be able to discriminate sound from nonsound, speech sounds from nonspeech sounds, and particular speech sounds from other speech sounds. In addition to these purely auditory discriminations the listener must have sufficient memory to hold a short string of received sounds in storage long enough to fit them into the pattern of a sentence, and he must have learned something about the rules of his language in order to use this auditory memory span appropriately. In the sections that follow we shall try to analyze these global descriptions of hearing into what appear to be the most important parts and then to discuss which of these parts are impaired by the loss or absence of hearing.

### Sensitivity to Sound

Even the apparently simple response of raising a hand or finger whenever a tone appears is a complicated interplay between response systems and the several subsystems of hearing. A young child being tested for the first time will not automatically respond to levels of sound that are as low as those to which he will respond after some experience and training. In short, even the simple audiogram can be "improved" with training. This claim has suggested to some that training affects the auditory sense organ or perhaps the auditory nerve, whereas it is much more likely

that the principal effect of the training is to increase the likelihood of response.

Teachers of young deaf children emphasize that the first step in an auditory-training program is to develop an "awareness of sound." This expression probably refers to the fact that these children have had no experience in making responses to sound, particularly responses that have been rewarded; that is, they are insensitive to certain sounds around them. But they can become sensitized to them through training. It should be obvious that the original lack of sensitivity does not show what sound levels will eventually define a child's audiogram. In short, as many clinicians recommend, *a child's hearing cannot be evaluated reliably until after several testing sessions which have been separated by periods of training*.

### Sound Discrimination

Even if a person can respond to any of a large variety of sounds, by raising his hand or otherwise, he does not "hear very well" unless he can also distinguish the sounds one from another. Some persons are called "tone deaf," which would imply that to them all of the notes of the musical scale sound the same. This extreme condition probably does not exist, but people do differ greatly in their ability to remember musical pitches and intervals. In any case the utility of auditory perception is based upon the ability to respond differently to different sound patterns. The listener can know that the talker was happy or sad only if he can distinguish one melody pattern from another in the voice. The pedestrian is safer if he can distinguish sound coming from the left from that coming from the right. Listeners to speech must be able to distinguish different frequency patterns in order to distinguish among the vowels and among certain consonants in speech. This list could of course become very long, but the basic notion is that auditory perception is based upon many sub-abilities to discriminate between pairs of sounds, sounds which differ acoustically according to one or another feature or cue.

### Pattern Perception and Recognition

Although we might devise tests for sound discrimination with a variety of sound pairs, it is clear that such sounds do not often come in pairs, nor does one deal with only one feature or cue at a time in everyday listening. A listener can easily distinguish the words "father" and "petroleum." In fact, we could hardly list all of the cues that allow a listener to discriminate those two words (number of syllables, beginning consonants, vowels, and so on), but such a distinction does call our attention to the fact that packages of features arrive in patterned ways to be processed by listeners. Although "pattern recognition" is a term most often used in the psychology of vision, it is quite clear that similar processes of recognition take place in auditory perception. A difference is that usually the auditory patterns are spread out in time, and visual patterns appear to be spread out in space. The main reason for drawing a distinction between sound discrimination and pattern perception is that the former is defined in terms of acoustic features taken one at a time, whereas pattern perception emphasizes the ability of listeners to *derive information from sequences of acoustic events over rather long periods of time* (like those of words, sentences, melodic phrases, or even whole symphonies) in arriving at categories or "pigeon holes" of perceived patterns that can then be dealt with relatively quickly. Here again we must note that *the ability to recognize patterns depends upon learning.*

### Perception of Speech

In our very verbal society where, according to one pundit, "speech appears to be for some the easiest form of breathing," the commonest use of our hearing is in understanding the speech of others and in monitoring our own speech. The auditory abilities required correspond to the three levels discussed above, namely, sensitivity to sound, discrimination of sounds, and recognition of patterns. In addition they are conjoined with those parts of our experience and memory that contain the vocabulary, the phonemic rules, and the structural aspects of our language.

For a listener to understand the speech of a talker, the sounds emitted by the talker must of course be audible to him; that is they must lie above his threshold. None of these speech sounds is like the pure tone of an audiometer, but instead each one of them contains many frequencies simultaneously. How the energy is distributed among the different regions of frequency varies from speech sound to speech sound and is in fact one of the most important cues for recognizing the individual speech sounds. For example, when the mouth is shaped to produce the vowel /u/ (oo), the principal resonances of the vocal tract lie in the low frequencies, namely around 300 to 400 Hz, higher or lower depending upon the age and sex of the talker. On the other hand, when the mouth is formed to say the vowel /a/ (ah), the principal resonances lie in a slightly higher frequency region, namely 600 to 800 Hz. If a listener is to distinguish between these two vowels or to recognize one or the other, he must be able to detect or recognize in which part of the frequency range these principal energy peaks or *formants* lie. Similarly, in order to distinguish a consonant like /s/ from /sh/, he must be able to discriminate between a peaking of energy around 7 kHz, which characterizes the former, and a peaking around 5 kHz, more typical of the latter.

The features illustrated by these two examples are *spectral features,* meaning that the principal cue to determining which speech sound has been spoken is the form of the spectrum and the region of frequency in which the peak or peaks are most pronounced. But there are other features as well. The consonant sounds may be divided into two broad classes: voiced and unvoiced. Since all consonant sounds involve a constriction or interruption of the breath stream, as we see in Chapter 14, all are characterized by some kind of noise. In addition, however, the voiced consonants contain both this noise and that due to the simultaneous vibration of the vocal bands. Therefore the distinction between a voiced and an unvoiced consonant like /s/ and /z/ is based upon the presence of noise alone or the presence of noise plus the complex tone of the vocal bands.

Aside from the spectrum and the presence of tonal or line components, there is another rather large category of *temporal features* in which speech sounds are identified by the way in which the evolve in time. For example, the unvoiced plosives /t/, /p/, and /k/ are characterized by the relatively abrupt starts preceded by a brief period of silence, and they last only a short time. Unvoiced fricative consonants, on the other hand, like /f/, /s/, and /th/ have gradual onsets and last for relatively longer times. The spectra of /s/ and /t/ may be very similar, but their temporal forms are quite different and are presumed to be the features by which the listener distinguishes them.

The cues that we have discussed so far have to do with the identification of individual speech sounds or phonemes. The understanding of speech requires, in addition, the temporal cues that talkers use to segment their speech into syllables and words. There are also melodic features that permit the listener to identify intonation patterns of the fundamental frequency of the voice. Such intonation patterns supply a context of meaning on which phoneme identification is then imposed, and they are probably recognized very early by young children, even before they begin to differentiate the speech sounds themselves.

## AUDITORY TRAINING IN REHABILITATION

In focusing on *rehabilitation*, we mean to imply that our aim is to restore, as far as possible, functions that have previously been normal. The concept applies to children or adults who, as a result of sickness or accident, lose some of their ability to hear. The various kinds of hearing losses have been reviewed in Chapters 4 and 5, but we will recount some of the auditory symptoms that accompany such hearing loss, particularly those that affect the perception of speech.

### Nature of the Problem

Consider a young adult who has sufficient intelligence, hearing, and other human abilities to have completed high school or perhaps college and to have taken up gainful employment. He has learned his language well, can communicate easily with others in a variety of acoustic environments, enjoys listening to music, attends plays or movies, and enjoys a variety of programs on radio and television. He may attend church and meetings of the PTA or political groups and can hear the speakers in such circumstances without difficulty. His first symptoms will be a noticeable increase in the effort with which he must attend and concentrate in order to understand the minister or lecturer, and his family members may begin to notice that he prefers to have the radio or the television sound at a higher level than is desired by other members of the family. Usually, except in cases of accident or in certain types of disease, the hearing loss will gradually increase over a period of months or years. Only rarely do the auditory symptoms appear suddenly.

The particular problem will of course depend upon the type of hearing loss. In otosclerosis, for example, the impairment is almost purely conductive and the primary problem is one of sensitivity, which deteriorates gradually over a period of years. Such a patient notices that he does not have great difficulty when people are talking loudly enough, in a noisy automobile, in a television program in which he can turn up the volume, or in a noisy office or factory environment where everyone hears badly because of the noisy background. If his loss in sensitivity cannot be alleviated through surgery, this kind of patient can be greatly helped by amplification. In stating that the essential problem is a loss of sensitivity, we mean to imply that if the sensitivity is restored surgically or is compensated for by amplification, then the other aspects of auditory perception, which are not affected by the disease, are still available for his use.

He will still have difficulty, however, because the surgical or prosthetic remedies were not called into play immediately. Several aspects of auditory perception involving discrimination, pattern recognition, and language usage, which had been less used, must now be relearned. This important point means that even though the loss of sensitivity is the principal problem in a conductive impairment, the clinician cannot assume that everything else will fall into place as soon as the sensitivity is restored. Depending upon the severity of the loss, *rehabilitative procedures that focus on auditory training, speechreading, and improved monitoring and production of one's own speech must often accompany surgery or a hearing aid.*

Problems associated with sensory-neural hearing loss are somewhat more complicated. There is the problem of sensitivity, defined by the audiogram. Very often, but not always, there is a greater loss of sensitivity in the high frequencies than in the low frequencies. Amplification through a hearing aid is not so easily accepted since sensitivity may be normal in the low fre-

quencies. Even so-called "selective amplification," which provides more gain for the high frequencies than for the low, may not restore adequate hearing, as we have seen in Chapter 11. In addition, sensory-neural hearing loss often affects other auditory functions besides sensitivity. Patients tested above the threshold may not show normal responses. Abilities to discriminate changes in frequency or intensity are often abnormal, and the ability to discriminate or recognize short words in the discrimination test of speech audiometry (see Chapter 7) is often impaired. Here, not only have auditory functions fallen into disuse because of the change in sensitivity, but also the ability to handle even the audible sounds is reduced. These patients must use a new acoustic code which changes slightly as the hearing changes over time.

In summary the role of auditory training for the patient with a progressive conductive impairment, with or without surgery or a hearing aid, is to make explicit for him those listening rules, cues, and strategies that he used when his hearing was normal. The more complicated varieties of sensory-neural hearing loss, unequal at the different frequencies, require rehabilitative procedures that not only reteach what was once known but also attempt to substitute other ways of listening. This includes supplementing of listening with looking to substitute new cues for those that are no longer available, even with a hearing aid.

### Difficulties in Speech Perception

We can apply some of these general notions about the problems of hearing loss to more specific considerations in connection with speech perception. Consider again the patient with a purely conductive loss and hearing threshold levels at approximately 50 dB at all frequencies. Figure 13-1, which is an elaboration of Figure 9-1, illustrates the difficulty that this patient has with conversational speech from a talker who is about 1 meter away. Note

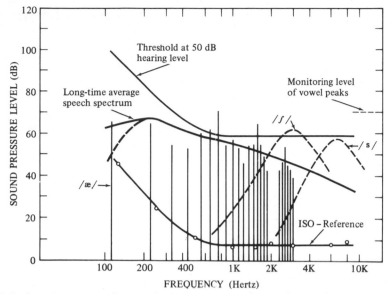

Fig. 13-1. Sound spectra of several phonemes, showing their relation to the long-time average speech spectrum and to the 50 dB hearing threshold level.

that the patient's threshold of audibility is shown here as sound pressure level at different frequencies, and it is located 50 dB above the average threshold of audibility (see Chapters 2 and 9). Now we have superimposed on his threshold curve an averaged speech spectrum that is characteristic of a talker about 1 meter away. Note that on the average such speech is completely inaudible to this listener. By "on the average" we mean the averaged energy *between* those bursts of loud sound in speech, the weaker speech sounds, and those periods of silence that mark the borders of syllables, words, and sentences. We have also put on this figure three individual speech sounds: the vowel /æ/, and the consonants /s/ and /sh/. The vowel is shown as a series of harmonic lines peaking in those regions of frequency that are called "formants." It is those peaks that presumably allow the identification of this vowel in contrast to other vowels. These formant peaks are audible to this patient when they are present. The spectra for the sounds /s/ and /sh/ are continuous, like noises, and only /sh/ peaks just above the

patient's threshold curve. Of course, whether or not these sounds are audible depends upon their intensity, and they have been plotted in this figure as closely as possible to their individual intensities, as related to the 70-dB, long-time average speech spectrum.

Figure 13-1 should make at least one feature of the difficulty in speech perception clear, namely, that if the energy in particular speech sounds is less than that required for audibility, then obviously no further processing can take place. In short, we must change the relation between the energy in these speech sounds and the patient's threshold to make enough of them audible. This relation can be improved either by moving down the patient's threshold curve (as by successful surgery) or by moving up those lines that represent the spectra of speech sounds (as by a hearing aid).

It has already been noted in Chapter 7 that there are some cases in which compensation for lack of sensitivity is insufficient, because as the intensity of speech is increased, as with a speech audiometer, the intelligibility of monosyllabic words reaches a maximum score of perhaps 60 percent and never goes any higher. These low discrimination scores, which cannot be improved by increased intensity, mean that there are certain aspects or cues to speech perception that are not available. Investigators are only now, in the late 1960's, beginning to apply new techniques of testing and of analysis to ascertain which classes of phonemic cues are most often associated with different kinds of hearing loss. Summarizing the case material in the literature, we can state that the very high-frequency sounds give frequent trouble, such as distinctions between /s/ and /sh/, between /i/ and /u/, between or among the unvoiced plosives, and so on. We do not really know whether initial consonants give more trouble than final consonants in single syllables, how important vowel confusions are, nor whether patients with such difficulties in speech discrimination profit more than—or as much as—persons with normal hearing when intelligibility is aided by the addition of context.

### Auditory Training Program

Although it is not our intent to produce here a manual on auditory training, the rationale for the basic steps can be summarized.

It is not likely that the hard-of-hearing adult or older child needs to be taught again to be aware of sound. On the other hand, gradual loss of hearing will be accompanied by a failure to attend to those aspects of sound that become more difficult to hear. Such patients, newly equipped with hearing aids, must not be sent out to unscramble for themselves the new buzzing confusion that is now upon them. Attention to weak, not recently heard sounds must be focused, and gross discriminations must be carefully retrained. With higher frequencies again available, the telephone bell and the doorbell can be distinguished, but such discriminations may not be im-

mediately obvious and therefore must be made part of a training program.

With respect to speech perception, several goals must be kept in view. Through audiometric testing, the clinician knows something of the character of a loss. This information plus the results of ingenious analysis by master teachers will show which auditory cues are available to the listener, which can be made available through training, and which are not likely to be available at all. The emphasis here, of course, is on the individualization of the program.

Drills and exercises are particularly useful for adults, especially when the items contain contrasting elements based on cues that the patient is to learn. Recognition based on such cases must be carefully trained through several stages. At first the cue may be used in isolation and slowly enough that the listener can succeed. Then speed becomes important, especially as the cue is introduced into syllable and word contexts, such as *b*ed and *r*ed. Finally, the availability of the cue must be demonstrated and trained as it occurs in the rapid exchanges of conversation. Teachers in many fields find that proceeding from easy, rewarded steps to the finer, more difficult ones will produce better learning with less frustration than when the most difficult and challenging aspects of auditory perception are introduced early.

## AUDITORY EDUCATION OF THE DEAF CHILD

As indicated earlier, the problems associated with congenital impairment of hearing are more complicated and more serious than those that follow an acquired impairment. The child or adult who becomes hard-of-hearing knew about sound, knows that a person talking influences another by the noises he produces, knows that different kinds of sound produce different effects, and also he has learned to talk while listening to the acoustic effects of his own speech and vocal activities. The deaf child has had no such incidental introduction to the world of sound.

### The Nature of the Problem

Figure 13-1 reminds us that a child with 50-dB hearing threshold level will hear either no speech at all or else only occasional loud bits, or perhaps some continuous speech from a mother that holds him close. Yet a 50-dB level is not uncommonly severe. It is more usual, following such diseases as maternal rubella or from hereditary deafness, that babies will show much higher thresholds. Children who are subsequently seen in nursery school or kindergartens for deaf children typically show thresholds as high as 70 dB in the low frequencies and 100 dB or more at 1000 Hz and above.

When we point out that the speech of a speaker a yard or so away will not be heard at all by these children, it is not only to comment on the difficulty they will have in understanding the speech of others. It is rather to emphasize that they are deprived of all sources of acoustic stimulation out of which the awareness of sound, the awareness of the possibilities of a communication, the raw stuff of language, and the learning of speech are built. Left unattended, without a hearing aid and without appropriate schooling, these children will become as if totally deaf, and their education, begun at a later time, will be difficult and will likely fall short of their maximum potential (see also Chapter 4).

Even the most optimistic teachers do not pretend that severe hearing losses can be overcome, that excellent training and the proper hearing aid will help the children to hear normally; but even the most pessimistic will recognize that carefully planned first steps plus the use of amplification will prepare such children for an optimum educational opportunity to realize their individual capabilities.

### Auditory Training Programs

The programs outlined above ememphasize *instruction* in a sound pedagogical framework of meaningful experience. Auditory training for babies and infants emerges from careful arrangement of circumstances rather than from teaching as such.

The infant with impaired hearing, moderate or severe, must be exposed to sound —patterned or changing sound. It should be made absolutely clear to parents that simply installing a hearing aid and thus "bathing the child in sound" is not a sufficient start in an auditory training program. After all, unless the sound environment is carefully planned and monitored, the hearing aid may function badly, may "squeal" or have high internal noise; and the child, while being bathed in sound, will not learn much of anything. Many writers on this subject in recent years have called attention to the analogy with vision, in which certain parts of the visual system may not develop properly unless the eyes are stimulated with patterned light. It is important to add that similar stimulation with homogeneous, unpatterned light did not prevent these failures of development. As important as the hearing aid itself is the construction of sequences of sounds, different from each other and interspersed with appropriate intervals of silence. Crude orienting responses to the sounds should be rewarded.

A second step involves sound discrimination and the association of different sounds with different objects. People talk to each other and to the child. The mother especially must talk, talk, talk—at close range—even though there may not be at first much overt reaction to the speech. The child's own beginnings in sound production must be rewarded at first, but then reinforcement should be withheld for the most appropriate or speechlike sounds.

Once again, we do not intend to write

a manual. Others have done that; and, unfortunately, in detail all such proposals are not entirely in agreement. The agreed general lines, however, as suggested in Chapter 16, include surrounding the child with meaningful, variegated, homelike sounds, including the sounds of speech, and providing sufficient amplification for these sounds to be audible. Family and teachers will strive to make the sounds, to encourage and reward responses to them, and to reinforce production of sound and speech. Both at home and in the nursery school, exchanges of sound that will lead to communication must be fostered and carefully built. Correction, whether of interpretation or of speech, must be accomplished carefully so as not to discourage the attempt. As one teacher puts it, "Better to say something incorrectly than to say nothing."

## USE OF HEARING AIDS

Although hearing aids have already been discussed in some detail in Chapters 10 and 11, there are some principles of use that need to be stated in the context of auditory training. After all, when the hearing loss is of such magnitude that inaudible speech sounds may be made audible only through amplification, then a hearing aid is *de facto* the vehicle of the auditory training.

Rehabilitative auditory training of an adult or older child who has sustained a moderate-to-severe hearing loss usually involves amplification through an individual, personal hearing aid. In former days a new patient was sometimes introduced to amplified sound through a larger desk unit with better reproduction than is possible even now in the wearable aids. The new hearing-aid user should be introduced to listening in favorable environments, with carpeted floors, draped walls and windows, and little extraneous noise. His first steps in listening should be taken with clear speech from only a few talkers. Only after the experience of successful listening should difficult sound discrimination, noisy backgrounds, multiple talkers, and everyday real situations be permitted. Personal hearing aids are still, even after many years of development, not high-fidelity systems.

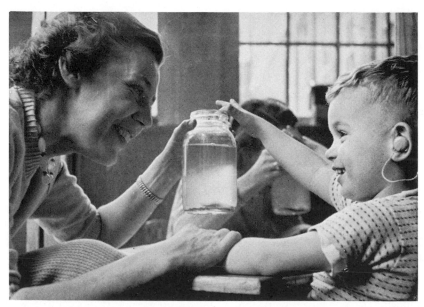

Fig. 13-2. Auditory and visual experiences are associated. (*Johns Hopkins University*)

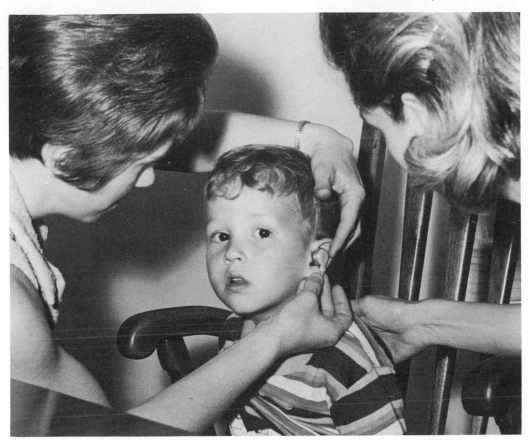

Fig. 13-3. A parent is instructed in seating the earmold. (*Central Institute for the Deaf, photo by Harold Ferman*)

The acoustic information is transmitted with changes due to frequency or amplitude distortion, to ringing, and to internal noise.

Early stages of auditory training should be conducted with relatively low-gain settings and high-input levels. The input should not be a shouted voice for the high levels, but rather a natural voice at close range.

### Early Education of the Deaf Child

Although high-fidelity group systems are widely used in schools for the deaf, the infant must learn in so many different rooms and environments that we probably have to give him a personal hearing aid. The personal aid does not usually have so high a gain or output level as the group systems, but at least it can be carried wherever the infant happens to go. Lower gain is not the only problem, however. An additional difficulty is that the microphone is located on the hearing aid, near the listener, and far from usual sources of sound. If mother is 2 or 3 yards away, her voice level at the hearing aid is only about 65 dB, too close to what is usually the background noise level. Her sounds will be better attended to and perhaps imitated if she stays as close to the child as possible. When he is in her arms, for example, her voice level is 85 or 90 dB, even for quiet speaking levels.

## Distance Is a Crucial Variable

This point will explain why there are more than a few experts who hesitate to put hearing aids on young babies whose exposure to sound will be uncontrolled. They do not want unfavorable listening conditions with too much background noise to be the first experiences with sound. Instead, they use amplification only under controlled circumstances, in special nursery schools or classrooms, where the sounds are carefully controlled and even programmed, as in a course sequence. Although this point of view is not held generally among all teachers, the basic principle is being implemented by better acoustic design in homes and schools and by better instruments to produce the sounds that are to be learned.

A great difference exists between the application of amplification to the training of infants and the use of hearing aids by hard-of-hearing adults. Except in rare cases, the aim for the latter is to permit a fair amount of discrimination of speech sounds. For the deaf child, such discrimination represents an unrealistically high goal. Instead, as pointed out in Chapter 16, one hopes that amplified sound will yield for the deaf child information about voice intonation, syllabic and verbal segmentation, other aspects of rhythmic structure, and some discrimination of speech sounds, based principally on the low-frequency sounds that are audible. The two goals should not be confused by the teacher, lest the tasks for her deaf students become frustratingly difficult, if not impossible.

As the young child enters a nursery school or regular school for the deaf, his spontaneous learning can gradually be changed to the more structured learning and teaching of a school curriculum. He may continue to use his personal hearing aid or he may be introduced to stronger better-quality sound through a group hearing aid. One advantage of most group systems is that the teacher can hold the microphone quite close to her lips so that, even without speaking loudly, she can present a voice level to the system that is much higher than the background noise. The classroom in which each child has his own personal hearing aid and nothing more is a most difficult learning situation because the desired source (teacher) is so much farther from the microphone than other less desired sources, such as other children, pencils on desks, feet on the floor, and so on.

## Signal Processing Systems

We know that certain parts of the acoustic spectrum are important for the various aspects of speech intelligibility. It is hardly surprising that many teachers and physicians consider useless the residual hearing of congenitally deaf children that is confined to the low frequencies. And it is true that if a child responds only to frequencies below 500 Hz, we can hope only to teach him to use such residual hearing for certain patterns of rhythmic structure, of intonation, and perhaps also of stress. In recent years, however, investigators in several countries have developed some ingenious systems for transforming the information that lies in the higher frequencies so that it becomes available in a special form in the low-frequency part of the spectrum. The principle is very plausible, but the details of its application are complicated, and much depends on just how much residual hearing each child may have. With some children considerable improvement in certain discriminations have been achieved, using devices specially designed to aid these particular discriminations, but tests of over-all speech discrimination and speech production have not yet shown a significantly better performance, even by selected groups of deaf children, than is accomplished by a similar teaching routine using an ordinary high-quality amplifying system.

## COOPERATION OR COMPETITION AMONG THE SENSES

When listening or speaking conditions are poor, people do not normally rely on hearing alone for understanding the speech of their fellows. In very noisy factories, workers with perfectly normal hearing use speechreading to help them communicate with each other. In even noisier surroundings, like the deck of an aircraft carrier, deck personnel use artificial hand signals to communicate with each other. An unfamiliar language heard on radio or by telephone is often more difficult to understand than it is in face-to-face speech. Even in the lecture hall, the student of a second language will get along much better if he sits near the front so that he can watch the face of the speaker. The hard-of-hearing or deaf people, about whom this book is written, are always listening under less than optimum conditions, and they, too, must rely on visual information to support the auditory information. The previous chapter has treated the learning of speechreading. Here we are concerned with the interaction between speechreading and auditory training.

The problem can be put very simply by example. Suppose that we want our student in auditory training to be able to distinguish the words *beet* and *boot*. The principal difference between these two words lies in the vowel, and the difference between those two vowels is given almost entirely by the presence of a second formant between 2000 and 3000 Hz for the vowel /i/ and the absence of such a high-frequency formant in the spectrum of the vowel /u/. Let us suppose further that the student's hearing aid has adequate amplification in the frequency region between 2000 and 3000 Hz and that he can therefore hear this part of the spectrum. Because of his high-frequency loss, he may never have heard that high-frequency formant before he was given a hearing aid. Now we must call his attention to its presence and train him in the distinction between these two vowels that will be based upon that high-frequency sound. But if the two words are *beet* and *boot*, even a normal listener can distinguish them perfectly well without any sound at all because the shape of the lips is so different for the two vowels. Should auditory training be carried out under "real life" circumstances in which the subject both hears and sees, or should we hide the face of the talker during auditory training? And, conversely, if the teacher wants to make clear the visible difference between those two vowels, should the subject be permitted to listen to them at the same time that he is learning to distinguish them visually? Teachers of auditory training have worked out various combinations and compromises, the details of which can be found in the readings listed at the end of this chapter.

This problem takes on an enormous significance, however, when we consider auditory training in the early education of the deaf baby. The association between the visible drum and its bang, or the seen bell and its dong, or the picture of the dog and its bark must be reinforced if the sound is to become a meaningful part of the experience of a young child. When speech sounds enter the picture, however, should we in any way limit the vision of the infant so that his attention will be focused entirely on the sounds of speech? Ramifications of this basic question become a professional dispute between those teachers who advocate the multisensory approach and those who advocate the unisensory approach. The former camp insists that the child must learn to take advantage of whatever cues are available to him, whereas the latter camp insists that the acoustic aspects of the environment should be presented almost to the exclusion of nonacoustic aspects because they presume that the visual and tactile senses have already developed normally, and their program aims to develop the auditory channel. If a severely hard-of-hearing baby is allowed to rely on visual and tactile information, he may never bother to attend to, and to learn, those auditory cues which are extremely difficult for him in the first place.

Unfortunately, there is no clear evidence that leads us to a choice between these camps. What does appear to be emerging from descriptions of the development of deaf children is that the multisensory approach will permit a child to enter more quickly into a communicating exchange with other people, and in this approach the auditory cues can be *emphasized* without any artificial attempt to exclude the nonauditory ones. On the other hand, it is likely that at more advanced stages in the education of the deaf or hard-of-hearing child, when analytic instruction is begun, specifically auditory training can be conducted in rather controlled or contrived circumstances.

With respect to speech production, it does appear that the auditory channel is the most suitable for monitoring and self-correction. In fact, if a deaf child is permitted to rely entirely on visual and tactile cues for speech recognition, he will begin to produce speech that looks right in the mirror or that feels right in the throat and mouth or to the fingertips, but which does not sound right. In fact some maintain that the peculiar characteristic of deaf children's voices does not appear until they begin their education in a school for the deaf in which an emphasis on visual and tactile cues forces the development of this unnatural voice. Here again, though the claim is plausible, the evidence is not at all clear.

## SUGGESTED READINGS AND REFERENCES

**American Annals of the Deaf,** 113 (March 1968).
> This issue is devoted to the proceedings of a conference on speech-analyzing aids for the deaf held at Gallaudet College, Washington, D.C., June 14–17, 1967. A substantial portion of the issue is concerned with the use of residual hearing by hearing-impaired children. Prepared papers and discussions are included.

**Guberina, P.** "Verbotonal Method and its Application to the Rehabilitation of the Deaf," *Report of the Proceedings of the International Congress on Education of the Deaf and the Forty-First Meeting of the Convention of American Instructors of the Deaf, U.S. Document No. 106,* U.S. Government Printing Office, Washington, D.C.: 279–293 (1964).

**Hirsh, I. J.** "Auditions in Relation to the Perception of Speech," in *Brain Function III: Speech Language and Communication,* E. C. Carterette (ed.). Los Angeles: UCLA Press, 93–115 (1966).

————. "Communication for the Deaf," *Report of the Proceedings of the International Congress on Education of the Deaf and the Forty-First Meeting of the Convention of American Instructors of the Deaf, U.S. Document No. 106,* U.S. Government Printing Office, Washington D.C.: 164–183 (1964).

————. "Perception of Speech," in *Sensorineural Hearing Processes and Disorders,* A. B. Graham (ed.). Boston: Little, Brown and Company, 129–137 (1967).

Johansson, B. "The Use of the Transposer for the Management of the Deaf Child," *J. Int. Audiology,* 5:362–371 (1966).

Ling, D., and W. S. Druz. "Transposition of High Frequency Sounds by Partial Vocoding of the Speech Spectrum: Its Use by Deaf Children," *J. Auditory Res.,* 7:133–144 (1967).

Oyer, H. J. *Auditory Communication for the Hard of Hearing.* Englewood Cliffs, N.J.: Prentice-Hall, Inc., 1961.

Perdoncini, G. "Our Auditory Training for Young Children," in *Proceedings of International Conference on Oral Education of the Deaf.* Washington, D.C.: Alexander Graham Bell Association for the Deaf, 577–580 (1967).

Silverman, S. R., "Clinical and Educational Procedures for the Hard-of-Hearing," in *Handbook of Speech Pathology,* L. E. Travis (ed.). New York: Appleton-Century-Crofts, 426–435, 1957.

Wedenberg, E., "Auditory Training of Deaf and Hard of Hearing Children," *Acta Otolaryng.* (Stockholm), Supplement 94, 1–129 (1951).

Whetnall, E., and D. B. Fry. *The Deaf Child.* London: William Heinemann, Ltd., 1964.

# CHAPTER 14

# DEVELOPMENT
# AND CONSERVATION
# OF SPEECH

## RAYMOND CARHART, Ph.D.

Speech is normally controlled by the ear. Nowhere is this more clearly shown than in the way a baby learns to talk. At first the baby can only cry. Some weeks after his birth he begins cooing, gurgling, and laughing. He then seems to enjoy lying in his crib and entertaining himself by listening to his queer noises. Without realizing it, he is building connections between his ear and his voice. As he listens to his own randomly produced sounds, he is beginning to learn muscular control of his speech mechanism. Before long he passes into the "parrot" stage, in which he amuses himself by repeating noises over and over. He keeps himself happy by saying trains of syllables like "ba ba ba ba" or "da da da da." He is now on the brink of learning his first words, for his parents respond to some of the syllable trains in his babbling. For example, when he says "da da da da," his mother may get his doll. She may also say "doll" as she hands it to him. This is an important moment. His babbling has controlled another person. He has also heard that person say a syllable which is very close to the sounds

he is making. On another occasion, his mother may say, "Do you want your doll?" as she hands him the toy. The child is likely to parrot her and say "da da da. . . ." His mother's pleased smile again rewards him. A few more experiences like this, and he will have learned to babble "da" whenever he wants his doll. He is now well on the road toward learning speech. All he needs is time: time for added experiences, time to learn new words through hearing them, and time to master vocal control by hearing his own speech.

The control which the ear exerts over speech is revealed differently by the adult. As was pointed out in Chapter 13, habits of hearing become so fixed that an older person has trouble mastering the pronunciations of a new language. His ear fails to distinguish new patterns from the ones to which he is accustomed. Erroneous impressions thus serve as the person's guide in speaking the new language. He talks with a foreign accent. For example, many Latin Americans have no need in their native Spanish to distinguish *b* and *v* except at the beginning of words. They consequently do not always use *b* and *v* correctly when they speak English.

## EFFECT OF HEARING LOSS ON SPEECH

Because it is natural for the ear to be the channel through which we learn to talk, a serious impairment in hearing will hinder a child's normal development of speech. Furthermore, because the ear serves as a guide to accurate control of the speech mechanism, degeneration of speech often follows hearing losses that occur later in life.

The most obvious example of the role played by hearing in acquisition of spoken language is furnished by the child who is born totally deaf. Unless special training is undertaken, of the kind described in Chapter 16, such a child never learns to talk. He grows up mute. His deafness closes for him the door through which he would normally acquire both knowledge of speech and control of the speech organs.

The child who hears low frequencies well but is insensitive to middle- and high-pitched tones faces a different problem. It is likely to be years before this child's deficiency is discovered. Because he can hear low frequencies, he reacts to many of the sounds in his world. People, seeing his response, reason that his hearing is normal. They fail to realize how distorted and imperfect are his impressions of sound. Confusion is this child's lot. He misses the acoustic elements which give speech its distinctive character. One outcome of this confusion is slow and uncertain development of his use of language. Moreover, the child incorporates in his own speech only the imperfect distinctions which he perceives in the speech of others. The result is a mushy and slurred pattern of talking which may border on the unintelligible.

Any substantial loss of hearing which exists at birth or occurs soon thereafter will hinder both language development and the establishment of adequate speech habits. Two factors are responsible. First, the hearing loss reduces sharply the number of listening experiences that the child has and thus slows up the process of learning to talk. Second, losses of certain types make it impossible for the child to distinguish some of the elements in speech. No child will learn to pronounce distinctions he does not hear, unless, of course, he has special guidance.

Speech defects may arise as the result of hearing losses that begin after childhood. If the ear can no longer serve as a monitor when one talks, slow degeneration of speech results. The sharpness and precision of enunciation disintegrate. The melodies of speech become monotonous. Intonations lose their life. The quality of the voice becomes rigid. Finally, control over the loudness of the voice suffers.

### The Nature of Speech

We can understand better the problems in speech which grow out of auditory impairment if we survey briefly the three essential aspects of speech.

*Phonetic elements.* Syllables, words, and connected phrases are formed by various combinations of simple sounds, which are known as *phonetic elements* or phonemes. The phonetic elements are the shortest units in human speech that can be recognized as having stable identity. In a general way, if we make allowances for the peculiarities of English spelling, the phonetic elements correspond to the letters of written language. However, the comparison is at best a rough one, since there are only 26 letters in the alphabet, but about 40 phonetic elements are used.

Phonetic elements are divided into three major classes: vowels, diphthongs, and consonants.

*Vowels* are relatively sustained and strong sounds. They are produced by initiating a tone in the voice box (larynx) and passing this tone through the mouth cavity, which is formed into a relatively open channel. Differences between vowels are achieved by shaping the mouth channel distinctively for each vowel. The tongue and the lips play a particularly important part in this shaping. Each vowel is actually a distinctive pattern of pure tones produced by the resonances of the various chambers of the mouth and nose. It is by means of this distinctive pattern that the listener identifies the vowel. Typical vowels (and their phonetic symbols) are those found in the following words: *seat* /i/, *sit* /ɪ/, *set* /ɛ/, *sat* /æ/, *saw* /ɔ/, *soot* /ʊ/, and *suit* /u/.

*Diphthongs* are blends of two vowels. They are produced by shifting the mouth channel from one vowel position to another while the sound continues. Acoustically, the tone initiated by the voice box is "resonated" as for a vowel, but in this instance the distinctive feature is the glide from the initial pattern of resonance to the final one. Typical diphthongs are those appearing in the following words: *boy* /ɔɪ/, *bay* /eɪ/, *bough* /aʊ/, and *buy* /aɪ/.

*Consonants* are of various types. All, however, have as a common feature the fact that the mouth channel is either closed completely or is formed into a more restricted passage than is employed to produce vowels and diphthongs. Furthermore, each consonant is characterized by a particular shaping and use of the speech organs. The tongue, lips, and soft palate are the primary structures whose positions determine this shaping. Consonants fall their manner of production and their acoustic character. We shall review each class separately.

*Semivowels* and *glides* are quite similar to vowels and diphthongs. The primary distinction is that the mouth channel is more constricted in producing semivowels and glides. Consequently, the resonances of these sounds are distinctive but less intense. Words exemplifying these conso-

nants are *rue* /r/, *lieu* /l/, *you* /j/ and *woo* /w/.

The *nasal consonants* are produced by completely blocking the mouth channel and allowing the tone from the voice box to escape through the nose. The sound patterns of the nasal consonants contain rather diffuse but definite resonances. These consonants are illustrated in the words *hum* /m/, *hun* /n/, and *hung* /ŋ/.

Most of the remaining consonants occur in pairs. One member of each pair is *voiced,* that is, it includes both the tone from the voice box and a second sound produced in the mouth. The other member of the pair is *voiceless,* that is, it consists only of the sound produced in the mouth. Typical pairs are *buy* /b/ and *pie* /p/, *vase* /v/ and *face* /f/, *zoo* /z/, and *sue* /s/.

Two major methods exist for initiating sounds in the mouth. One is to block completely the breath stream and then release it in a sudden gust which causes a pulse of noise. Consonants produced in this way are called *plosives.* The voiced plosives occur in *by* /b/, *die* /d/, and *guy* /g/. Their voiceless counterparts occur in *pea* /p/, *tea* /t/, and *key* /k/. By contrast, the fricative continuants are formed when the escaping breath stream produces a noise as it flows through an extremely constricted portion of the mouth channel. Acoustically, these consonants exhibit highly irregular sound patterns distributed over a wide pitch range. The voiced *fricatives* are exemplified in *vow* /v/, *zoo* /z/, *azure* /ʒ/, and *thou* /ð/. The voiceless fricatives are illustrated in *fin* /f/, *sin* /s/ *thin* /θ/, and *him* /h/. The acoustic features of phonetic elements are described in Chapter 13.

Finally, a few blends of consonants have been incorporated as phonetic elements in English. These blends combine elements of their parent sounds, yet they have independent identity. Typical illustrations are found in *what* /hw/, *check* /tʃ/, and *just* /dʒ/.

*Articulatory defects.* Speech deficiencies characterized by imperfect production of phonetic elements and transitions between them are called *articulatory defects.* Obviously, they may arise from many causes: physical deformity of the speech organs, disease, faulty habits, lazy enunciation, hearing loss, mental deficiency, and so on. Obviously, too, articulatory defects differ widely in severity and in type of error. Our present concern is limited to inadequacies arising because a hearing loss either prohibited the initial mastery of phonetic elements or removed the auditory control needed to maintain precise enunciation. In either event, since a prominent feature of the speech defect will be imperfect production of phonetic elements, an effective program of speech training must have as a major goal the elimination of articulatory errors.

*Nonphonetic elements.* Human speech possesses four aspects which are relatively unstandardized but which nevertheless contribute to the naturalness and acceptability of oral communication. These four aspects are *melody, quality, time,* and *force.* Each is a feature which, when properly used, helps to clarify meaning and add vitality.

The *melody* of speech is its "tune," or intonation pattern. Spoken language cannot escape having a melody. However, certain intonation patterns are conventionalized, and we expect them. An illustration is the rising inflection with which we designate a question. An unusual melody distracts the listener from the thought that is being expressed and thus may be considered a defect. For example, lack of variety, such as a monotonously pitched voice, imparts a lifelessness which reduces the effectiveness of speech.

*Quality* is the "flavor" of speech which distinguishes one voice from another. Quality is a very subtle feature which depends both upon physical conditions and upon habits of using the voice. Our interest in quality springs from the fact that an auditory impairment may lead to unfortunate habits, as, for example, in the strained and strident voice so often found in deaf children.

The *time* element of speech is the recurrence of patterns of duration of syllables that we may refer to as its "rhythm." We have learned to expect and to accept certain rhythms as "natural." Deviations from acceptable rhythms create the impression of artificiality, and, if extreme, may hinder understanding.

The element of *force* involves the emphasis given different syllables and words. Variations in force are achieved primarily by modifying loudness. Some patterns of emphasis are acceptable, whereas others are not.

In connected speech, the nonphonetic elements are completely blended and interwoven. We have already pointed out that proper blending helps clarify meaning and adds interest to spoken language. It follows that *a severe auditory impairment that makes it impossible for a person to hear the nonphonetic elements in his own speech may cause unnatural use of these elements and, hence, disturb the effectiveness of his oral communication.* The child with severe impairment will fail to learn proper control of melody, quality, time, and force. In the adult these same elements tend to degenerate slowly after he loses the power to hear them.

### Loudness of the Voice

The speaker ordinarily adjusts the loudness of his voice to the situation in which he is talking. In fact, the adjustment is so natural that few people even realize it takes place. The speaker has unconsciously learned to raise his voice when background noise is strong or when the listener is at a little distance. We find that our voices are tired after conversing while riding on the bus. Our efforts to talk over the din of traffic lead us unconsciously to shout, and a half hour of shouting tires the voice. By contrast, we unconsciously soften our voices in quiet surroundings. In other words, *we tend to maintain a favorable margin between the loudness of our speech and the background noise.* We thus achieve intelligibility without talking so that our listeners find our speech unpleasantly loud.

A person learns the proper balance between the loudness of his speech and his acoustic surroundings in the same way that he learns other features of acceptable speech, by the experience of hearing himself talk. Through his experience the ineffective levels of loudness are given up in favor of levels that result in successful communication.

A hearing loss disturbs the ability to adjust the level of one's voice to the needs of the moment. Two factors enter the picture. For one thing, the person with impaired hearing will miss much of the background noise. Thus, he has an imperfect gauge of the requirements of the moment. In the second place, the speaker with a hearing loss may receive a false impression of the loudness of his own voice. When the loss is of the sensory-neural type, his own voice sounds faint. Such a person has a tendency to talk loudly, regardless of the surrounding circumstances. In doing so his voice reaches a level where it seems of normal loudness to him. The reverse effect occurs when the loss is of the conductive type. Here the speaker's voice is transmitted effectively to his own ear by bone conduction. His voice seems to him so much stronger than other sounds that he often softens it until the balance between his voice and the background noise is more to his satisfaction. Such a person tends to talk more faintly than he should, and, as a consequence, he is hard to understand.

## SPEECH TRAINING FOR DEAF CHILDREN

As we have already pointed out, the child who suffers an early and complete hearing loss will remain a mute unless special methods of education are used with him (see Chapter 16). The difficulty and laboriousness of the educational task are tremendous. It is necessary to teach the child to put his speech mechanism to use. One must also build his vocabulary and the other basic skills of language. Ordinarily, when the training program begins, the child will have no adequate concept of either speech or language.

We discussed earlier the manner in which the child with normal hearing learns speech and language. The deaf child must be guided through a similar series of stages. However, two differences exist. First, successive stages cannot be attained as early in his life. Second, since the auditory channel for learning is restricted for the deaf child, other means must be used to stimulate the development of his language skills. The substitute means are less effective than hearing in accomplishing the goal, and the process is therefore extremely laborious.

There are three major channels which may be substituted for the ear: vision, the sense of touch, and the internal senses of movement and position. The reader will realize immediately that any superior program of training will interweave stimulation through these three channels and, of course, the auditory channel, as emphasized in Chapter 13. For convenience, however, the discussion that follows considers each separately.

### Visual Cues

*Visual cues* offer the deaf child his main approach to the experience of communication. He not only learns to interpret gestures; he also sees the facial activity

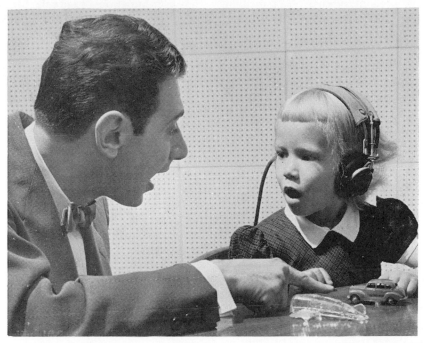

Fig. 14-1. The auditory and visual approaches are combined to teach speech. (*Central Institute for the Deaf*)

that is the visible aspect of speech. By proper guidance, he can be taught to attend to these facial activities as meaningful signals of the wishes and intentions of others. He can thus be started on the road to speechreading and mastery of language. An invention of the Bell Telephone Laboratories called "Visible Speech" seemed for a time to offer rich possibilities for training the deaf to speak properly. In this method a pattern of light and dark bands is formed on a moving, phosphorescent screen in response to the sounds of the voice. The pattern moves steadily from right to left. The height of the bright bands above the base line is determined by the frequency of the fundamental voice sound and the formants that give it the particular vowel qualities. It is possible to learn to read this form of visible, running frequency-analysis of speech, but the method has yet to be proved to be universally applicable in teaching deaf children to talk.

A recent symposium (1967) at Gallaudet College deals with a number of other electronic possibilities for presenting visual cues to speech, and a system of hand signals for certain features of sounds called "cued speech" (see Chapter 16) is also being tried out. All of these possibilities are still in the experimental stage.

### Tactile Cues

Through the sense of *touch*, the deaf child learns that the visible movements of speech are accompanied by a modulated flow of the breath and by vibration. Although he cannot hear the sounds produced as the breath is modulated by the larynx, tongue, and lips, the deaf child can be made aware of many tactile cues which will help him understand the nature of the process. For example, the skilled teacher places the child's hand in front of her mouth as she articulates plosive consonants such as /p/ or /b/. The child is trained to feel the momentary gust of air escaping from the mouth as the plosive is released. Similarly, a hand placed on the cheek receives vibratory sensations when vowels are produced. The nasal consonants produce agitation that can be felt on the nose, and all voiced sounds give rise to vibration that can be felt at the Adam's apple (larynx). These various tactile cues are among those used, not only to make the child aware of major phases in speech production but also to teach him to control his own speech mechanism. By alternately feeling the effects produced as the teacher speaks and then attempting to achieve the same effects with his own speech organs, the child learns techniques of sound production and enunciation. Some techniques use sounding boards, including pianos, and diaphragms which are caused to vibrate by speech and music.

Attempts are being made to improve tactile reception by filtering speech electronically and transmitting significant frequencies to each of the fingertips by bone-conduction vibrators. The Picketts (1963) described such an instrument called a "tactual vocoder" (voice coder) constructed in the Speech Transmission Laboratory, Royal Institute of Technology, Stockholm, Sweden. The Picketts conclude "that the skin offers certain capacities for transmitting speech information which may be used to complement speech communication where only an impoverished speech signal is normally received."

Another recently reported instrument is "Tactus" developed by M. Kringlebotn (1968) of Trondheim, Norway, which transposes frequencies down to the range of maximum tactile sensitivity, 100 to 400 Hz. Results of experimental use of this instrument are helpful when combined with speechreading and as an aid in speech development and improvement. We do know that the capacity for frequency discrimination of the vibrotactile sense is very limited and is in the wrong frequency domain for the discrimination of speech. Many of the past attempts to present speech to the vibrotactile sense have substituted a series of vibrators placed on the fingers or hand to serve as spatial representations of different frequencies. Whether the investment in time and money in these refined and sophisticated tactile approaches is justified, compared with the conventional methods described here and in Chapter 16, is now being studied in a number of laboratories and schools.

### Kinesthetic Cues

In the final analysis, the deaf child must control his speech primarily through the sensations he receives from effects occurring within his own body. These internal sensations are called *kinesthetic* cues. They are of various types, such as feelings of jaw movement, tongue movement, position of the lip, position of the soft palate, nasal vibrations, and laryngeal vibration. During the initial stages of training, the teacher may even manipulate the child's organs of speech so that they execute patterns of movement that the child must learn. The purpose is to get the child to feel the kinesthetic cues that characterize each movement. Furthermore, as the child is required to control his own speech through vision and touch, kinesthetic sensations will also occur. With the passing of time he learns to rely upon these kinesthetic sensations to tell him what he is doing. Thus, whereas the person with normal hearing judges the adequacy of his speech by the way it *sounds,* the deaf child must base the same judgment on the way it *feels.*

From what has been said, it is clear that teaching a deaf child to talk is an exacting task. The teacher must know both the principles of speech and the limitations of deaf children. The teacher must be adept at using visual, tactile, and kinesthetic cues to make the child try to speak. For these reasons, development of speech in deaf children can be best accomplished by teachers specializing in education of the deaf and the hard-of-hearing.

Parents and friends have three major responsibilities in encouraging the development of speech in a deaf child. The first responsibility is to seek out a competent teacher and place the child under her guidance. The second responsibility is to speak naturally, but with the addition of clarifying gestures, in the presence of the child. The parents thus keep before the child the fact that human communication is accompanied by activity of the structures in the face and neck. The third responsibility, once the child has begun to talk, is to respond positively to every effort he makes to speak. Even though the effort is imperfect, it is vital (if the speech can be understood at all) that parents and friends react appropriately. When they do so, the child soon learns to rely upon his speech efforts as a means of controlling other people and of adapting to his social environment. Thus, and only thus, will speech be made a functional tool in the child's everyday life.

## SPEECH TRAINING FOR HARD-OF-HEARING CHILDREN

When a child possesses a reasonable amount of residual hearing, his requirements for speech training are ordinarily different from what they would be if he were deaf. For one thing, the fact that he has some usable hearing means that he will probably acquire patterns of speech spontaneously. However, these patterns will be faulty and imperfect. Thus, one of his needs is *reeducation* designed to eliminate his faults. Furthermore, since he will have some understanding of language and its use, he needs encouragement toward fuller language development rather than the building of language skill from its very beginning.

*It is important for two reasons that speech training start as early in the child's life as possible.* In the first place, the period in life most favorable to the development of speech habits is thus utilized constructively. Moreover, early training will minimize the work required to counteract the faulty habits of speech, since these habits will be less firmly fixed than if training is delayed.

### Special Methods

Speech training for the hard-of-hearing child requires special methods that utilize both the child's residual hearing and his other sensory channels. Visual cues are particularly important. As in the case of the deaf child, these cues add awareness of speech activities. Furthermore, many of the phonetic elements that are particularly difficult to hear involve movements of the jaw and lips that are relatively easy to see. Visual cues thus offer opportunity for stressing the phase of enunciatory skill that the child particularly needs to learn. Attempts are still being made to translate the acoustic information in speech into a form in which it may be perceived by the eye, but the results in teaching the deaf by such methods have not been very encouraging.

Both the sense of touch and kinesthetic cues are important in the total training process, but these need not be used so copiously as with the deaf child. However, they can profitably be employed to help the child master articulatory movements that are difficult for him and to give him nonauditory means for controlling this everyday speech.

Auditory cues must be used to the fullest extent possible in teaching the hard-of-hearing child to talk better. Advantage can thus be taken of a natural bond between the ear and the voice. The child is helped to learn habits for controlling his own speech through the auditory experience he receives from it.

Obviously, the way in which auditory

cues are best used in speech training is an individual matter. Each child has unique potentialities and special needs that depend upon the details of his hearing loss. However, the general rule that must be met is to *bring sound to the child in the form that is most usable by him.* Here the principles discussed in the chapter on auditory training apply. Speaking close to the child's ear is often a practical means of presenting useful auditory stimulation. Moreover, the semiportable hearing aid is an excellent tool in the hands of a skilled teacher. Such an instrument allows the speech of both the teacher and the child himself to be amplified. Drill material of all types (from isolated sounds to connected passages) may be used. Sometimes drills are presented through the instru-

ment by the teacher. The pupil then repeats the drills. At other times, the child speaks the drills without previous example. Throughout the whole process the child's attention is directed to the auditory features of the errors he makes and the successes he achieves. The ear is thus made a functional channel to mastery of speech.

When the child begins to wear his own hearing aid, he has an additional advantage. The instrument will bring to him with greater clarity the patterns of speech he is using in life situations. He can thus rely more heavily upon his ear to guide his speech performance. The child who is properly prepared for this stage is encouraged to make his successful efforts habitual.

The reader will observe that instruction

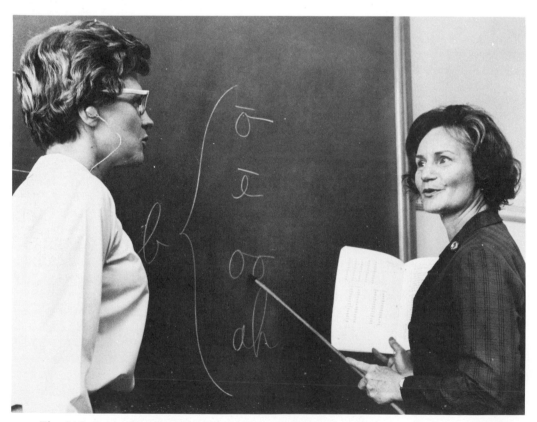

Fig. 14-2. Instruction in conservation of speech. (*Central Institute for the Deaf, photo by Harold Ferman*)

in speech and auditory training have much in common. Actually, it is profitable to combine the two. Furthermore, as with all phases of education for those with impaired hearing, the speech training that we have been discussing is most effective when carried on in a special school or by a qualified teacher of the acoustically handicapped.

### Help of Parents and Friends

Parents and friends can encourage speech development in the hard-of-hearing child. The first rule is to *see that the child gets plenty of auditory stimulation*, particularly by talking to him at close range or through a hearing aid. The second rule is to ensure that he realizes the communicative importance of speech. This result can be gained in part by using questions, comments, and explanations whenever possible during the everyday activities in which he participates. However, it also requires that the parents respond positively to any speech efforts the child himself makes in the initial stages of his training program, thus giving him the experience of controlling others through speech. In the later stages of the program, parents and teachers should *require as precise speech from the child as his accomplishment warrants*. At this stage, response to his speech efforts could be withheld whenever these efforts are inadequate. Here the guidance of the teacher is necessary in order to ensure that the parents require a fair level of performance; otherwise the child's progress may be frustrated by a feeling of failure when he is trying his hardest and doing his best.

## CONSERVATION OF ADEQUATE SPEECH

As we have already pointed out, the occurrence of a substantial loss of hearing may cause deterioration in speech. Such a situation exists when the auditory impairment does not occur until after normal patterns of speech have been firmly established. Thus, it is a situation that affects only older children and adults. Furthermore the deterioration in speech is neither instantaneous nor complete.

### Speech Insurance

The facts just mentioned call for a special type of training based on the concept of *speech insurance*. Stated differently, the person we are discussing enters the ranks of the hard-of-hearing with normal habits of speech. The main educational task is to teach him to *retain* these habits in order to conserve the skill he already has. *If training can be started soon enough after the hearing loss occurs, no deterioration in speech need result*. The technique is to give the person substitute channels for controlling his speech efforts, since his ear no longer serves as a fully effective monitor when he talks.

Only under two circumstances is it necessary to combine speech reeducation with the program of speech insurance. Sometimes the hearing loss has existed long enough so that deterioration in speech is evident, and sometimes the person has a speech defect that is independent of the hearing loss. In either event, faulty habits must be broken down. They must be replaced by adequate habits, and at the same time the substitute channels of control must be learned.

When the hearing loss is complete (or nearly so), speech insurance must depend mainly on learning effective use of kinesthetic cues. To this end, the person with extreme loss must first become acquainted with the nature of the speech process. He must understand the activity that he wishes to control. He must learn to preserve the phonetic elements of speech by becoming fully aware of the kinesthetic peculiarities of each element. Second, he must develop awareness of the bodily sensations associated with proper control of melody, quality, rhythm, and emphasis. In the third place, he must maintain physical alertness, facial expressiveness, and spontaneous gestures. Naturalness in speaking depends in part upon abandoning oneself to the act of communication. Finally, the person must learn to maintain effective control of the loudness of his voice.

## Problems of Partial Hearing Loss

Successful mastery of control of loudness is particularly difficult. However, two measures allow a reasonable solution to the difficulty. The person must first master the ability to talk at each of four or five general levels of loudness. He must learn to shift at will from one level to another. These levels, which are under kinesthetic control, must range from soft speech to very loud speech. Second, the person must study and classify typical sound environments. With the help of his instructor, he can learn what level of background noise he is most likely to encounter in each type of situation. He can then meet the requirements of loudness with reasonable success by speaking at the level (of the five he has learned) that is ordinarily demanded by the situation at hand. Furthermore, an alert talker will notice when his listeners are having difficulty responding to his speech and will raise his voice to the next level. He thus avoids relying rigidly on a set of rules in situations in which it happens that the rules do not apply.

When the hearing loss is partial, both the need for speech insurance and the techniques necessary to achieve it depend upon the degree and pattern of the hearing loss. The primary requisite is to retain, insofar as possible, control of speech by the ear. *Here a good hearing aid can be of great help,* since it may raise to a usable level many elements of the wearer's own speech that are inaudible to him without the instrument.

The task of speech conservation then divides itself into two phases. To the de-gree that components of speech remain inaudible even while the hearing aid is being worn, the person must be taught kinesthetic control of speech. Second, if some components that are made audible by the instrument are reproduced somewhat "unnaturally," he will require auditory training in interpreting his own speech. For example, when wearing a hearing aid, the person must learn to make allowances for changes in the way phonetic elements sound through his instrument. Otherwise, he may modify his articulation to satisfy his own unschooled ear and thus achieve an enunciation that is less effective for his listeners. Another example involves the loudness of speech. A peculiar situation often exists because the wearer's own voice seems extremely loud to him through the hearing aid. The balance between his own voice and the background noise is entirely different without the aid from what it is when he is using the instrument. This difference will work to his disadvantage unless he is taught to accept a balance that he does not particularly like but that is most acceptable to the listener.

## Progressive Hearing Loss

Special considerations enter the picture when the hearing loss has been diagnosed as one which is progressive. The auditory impairment may not at the moment be sufficient to endanger the patterns of speech. However, the future outlook may demand that a program of speech conservation be begun immediately. A full system of kinesthetic control over speech should be built while the patterns of speech are still good and while it is still easy for the person to understand instructions from the teacher. The person can thus be prepared to apply kinesthetic control when his hearing drops to the point where this control becomes necessary.

Training in the conservation of speech is best obtained from teachers who have been specifically prepared for their type of work. Such teachers are to be found in schools offering special work for hard-of-hearing children. They are also to be found in hearing clinics, aural rehabilitation centers, and similar organizations. Children needing guidance in speech conservation can often get help through schools, and both adults and children have access to speech and hearing clinics.

Family and friends can help the person who is fighting the threat of speech deterioration. As with other problems, the first step is to find a qualified teacher and enlist her participation. The second step is to cooperate fully with the teacher. The cooperation can be extensive, since the person in training can profit from much drill at home. The student needs the help of either a relative or a friend. Following specific instructions from the teacher, this assistant, who must have both normal hearing and normal speech, serves as a monitor who corrects errors made by the student as he works on his drills. And finally, members of the student's immediate social circle can build favorable morale by taking a positive and sympathetic attitude toward his misfortune and toward his efforts.

## SUGGESTED READINGS AND REFERENCES

**American Annals of the Deaf.** 113 (March, 1968).
>   This issue is devoted to the proceedings of a conference on speech-analyzing aids for the deaf held at Gallaudet College, Washington, D.C., June 14–17, 1967. A substantial portion of the issue is concerned with the use of instruments to transmit information about speech to the hearing-impaired aimed at the development and improvement of their speech. Prepared papers and discussions are included.

**Denes, P. B., and E. N. Pinson.** *The Speech Chain; the Physics and Biology of Spoken Language.* Baltimore: The Williams & Wilkins Company, 1963.
>   A popular but accurate treatment of our knowledge of communication by speech by workers at the Bell Telephone Laboratories.

**Fairbanks, G.** *Voice and Articulation Drillbook.* New York: Harper & Brothers, 1960.

**Gray, G. W., and C. M. Wise.** *The Bases of Speech.* 3d ed. New York. Harper & Brothers, 1959.

**Kringlebotn, M.** "Experiments with Some Visual and Vibrotactile Aids for the Deaf," *Amer. Ann. Deaf,* 113:311–317 (1968).

**Pickett, J. M., and R. H. Pickett.** Communication of Speech Sounds by a Tactual Vocoder," *J. Speech Hearing Res.* 6:207–222 (1963).

**Travis, L. E. (ed.).** *Handbook of Speech Pathology.* New York: Appleton-Century-Crofts, Inc., 1957.

**Zemlin, W. R.** *Speech and Hearing Science; Anatomy and Physiology.* Champaign, Ill.: Stipes Publishing Company, 1964.
>   A good treatment of the fundamentals of the subjects of the title.

# PART FIVE
# EDUCATION AND PSYCHOLOGY

# CHAPTER 15

## FROM ARISTOTLE
## TO BELL
## —AND BEYOND

### S. R. SILVERMAN, Ph.D.

The evolution of the present social point of view toward deafness has been marked by a growing recognition of its problems and by an increasing collective effort to do something practical toward their solution. We need go no further than the pages of this book for a forceful illustration of the variety of talents that are now cooperating in the attack. The removal of professional barriers, which now permits the physician, the researcher, the educator, the sociologist, the psychologist, the physicist, the psychiatrist, the industrial engineer, the audiologist, parents, and laymen to work together with mutual understanding, is one of the most promising developments of recent years. It forecasts a progressively broader and more intelligent base of social awareness of the entire question.

The development of an increasingly enlightened social attitude toward deafness, however, is no exception to the general rule that man's struggle toward enlightenment is slow, faltering, and, in many instances, haphazard. This development might be traced in the history of the educa-

tion of the deaf, but only fragmentary bits of information are available prior to the sixteenth century. Some of the bits are indirect and inferred, and it is difficult to trace any complete structure of systematic thought.

In the pre-Christian era, however, Aristotle and, later, Pliny the Elder observed that there was some relationship between congenital deafness and dumbness, but neither one elaborated on the relationship. It is still questionable whether Aristotle assumed a common organic basis for deafness and dumbness, but he placed strong emphasis on sound (speech) as the primary vehicle for conveying thought and therefore as the chief medium for education. Aristotle presumably believed, therefore, that since the deaf could neither give utterance to speech nor comprehend it from others, they were relatively incapable of instruction; and, furthermore, that the deaf were less capable of instruction than the blind. At any rate, Aristotle made no clear statement that dumbness is a consequence of deafness (of the congenital type) and that speech is an acquired skill whose patterns are learned through the ear. Of course, hearing is the normal channel through which speech is most readily perceived and consequently imitated. Note the stress on the *normal* channel, for we have also learned that it is possible for the deaf to acquire speech through touch, sight, and the sense of movement. Many deaf people receive information through the use of manual alphabets and the language of signs.

The idea that deafness and muteness depend on a common organic abnormality and that the deaf were poor educational prospects persisted through medieval times. It is probable that the derogatory use of "dumbness" in our modern slang, suggesting an inferior intellect, has its roots in the supposed mental incapacity of the deaf. And it was inevitable that the notion of the limited mental capacity of the deaf should exercise a powerful influence on their legal and civil status. Roman law classified the deaf and dumb with the mentally incompetent, and the Justinian Code (sixth century A.D.) excluded the deaf and dumb from the rights (entering into contracts, and so on) and obligations (witnessing in a court of law) of citizenship. In justice to Justinian's Code, it must be said that a sharp differentiation was made between deaf-mutes and those whose deafness was acquired and who had learned spoken and written language. Although the Code did not prohibit marriage for the deaf, its influence later caused medieval law to deny to the congenitally deaf and dumb the highly cherished right of primogeniture.

Although information concerning the attitude of religious institutions toward deafness during this early period is comparatively meager, fragments of evidence from church literature indicate that the church shared the prevailing notions of the times. Mosaic Law, through its Code of Holiness in the sixth century B.C., exhorted the faithful not to curse the deaf since their deafness was presumably willed by the Lord. In the second century B.C. the rabbis of the Talmud classified the deaf with fools and children. Although the rabbis were perfectly correct in calling attention to individual differences, their pronouncements reflect an inadequate understanding of deafness. It is strange that Jeremiah, usually recognized as the most forward-looking social philosopher among the prophets, made no mention of the deaf.

Similarly, the Christian Church looked with disdain on the intellectual capabilities of the deaf, although it did permit marriage by a ceremony conducted in the language of signs. We perceive a glimmer of enlightenment, however, in Bede's references (about the seventh century A.D.) to the feat of Bishop John of York in teaching a deaf-and-dumb youth to speak intelligibly. This accomplishment, however, is chronicled in the nature of a miracle, and the educational method is left to our imaginations. Nevertheless, the mere recording of the incident is a first, admittedly feeble, attempt (conscious or otherwise) to dispel the fog of misunderstanding in which deafness was enshrouded.

It was not until the middle of the sixteenth century that the mists began to lift. At that time an intellectually versatile Italian physician, Girolamo Cardano of Padua, in referring to the work of Rudolphus Agricola of Gröningen, proposed a set of principles that promised a more hopeful educational, and hence social, outlook for the deaf. He stated, in essence, that the deaf could be taught to comprehend written symbols or combinations of symbols by associating them with the object or picture of the object they were intended to represent. To this day, the association of meaningful language with experience is the keystone of techniques for teaching the deaf. The significance of Cardano's contribution lies not so much in his statement of basic principles of teaching as in his implicit rejection of the notion that the deaf cannot be educated and consequently are doomed to social inadequacy. It would not be too extravagant to attribute to Cardano the concept of an educational Magna Carta for the deaf.

Cardano's pronouncements initiated a series of serious, although sporadic, attempts to implement his principles. It is reasonable to credit these heartening developments in part also to the liberation of humanistic forces by the Renaissance and to the subsequent popularization of education in the vernacular induced by the Reformation. As early as 1555 we find oral education of deaf children of the nobility carried on by a Spanish monk, Pedro Ponce de Leon, in a convent of Valladolid. It was in Spain, too, that the first book exclusively on the deaf, by Juan Pablo Bonet, appeared in 1620. Bonet's pupils were taught articulation and language, supplemented by a manual alphabet and the language of signs. Other works in many tongues dealing with the education and intellectual and spiritual status of the deaf appeared soon after. John Bulwer, John Wallis, William Holder, and George Dalgarno carried on the work in the British Isles; Jan Baptiste Van Helmont and John Conrad Amman, in Holland; St. Francis de Sales, in Switzerland; Ernaud and Pereire, in France; and Otto Lasius and Arnoldi (among a host of others), in Germany.

In contrast to Aristotle's views comparing the intellectual capabilities of the deaf and blind, the beginning of enlightenment is best typified by a quotation from Dalgarno's *Didascalocophus,* published at Oxford in 1680:

Taking it for granted, That Deaf people are equal, in the faculties of apprehension, and memory, not only to the Blind; but even to those that have all their senses: and having formerly shewn; that these faculties can as easily receive, and retain, the Images of things by the conveiance of Figures, thro the Eye, as of Sounds thro the ear: It will follow, That the Deaf man is, not only, as capable, but also as soon capable of Instruction in Letters, as the blind man. And if we compare them, as to their intrinsick powers, has the advantage of him too; insomuch as he has a more distinct and perfect perception, of external Objects, then the other. . . . I conceive, there might be successful addresses made to a Dumb child, even in his cradle. . . .

Note the emphasis on equality with others, the suggestion that the deaf could be taught even in early childhood, and an implicit plea for what we now call early detection.

Two individuals, however, tower above all others in their contributions to advancing the cause of the deaf in the latter part of the eighteenth century—Abbé Charles Michel de l'Épée in France and Samuel Heinicke in Germany. De l'Épée found a fruitful outlet for his religious emotions, as many clergymen have since his time, in promoting the well-being of the deaf through education. It is to his everlasting credit that he founded the first public school for the deaf in 1775 in Paris. Heinicke, his contemporary in Germany, founded the first public school for the deaf in Germany; and it was the first recognized by any government.

De l'Épée and Heinicke disagreed about the merits of signs and "oralism" as methods of instruction, De l'Épée favoring signs and Heinicke writing prolifically on the advantages of speech and of speechreading. So widespread was the influence of these two men that the pattern of their controversy was reproduced subsequently in many countries, the United States included. Our purpose here, however, is not to evaluate the merits of their contentions but to stress their extremely important contributions to the liberalization of the social point of view toward deafness. By the end of the eighteenth century it had been convincingly demonstrated that the deaf were capable of instruction, and it was also clearly recognized that it was the moral and legal obligation of society to see that instruction was provided, even though the development of free public schools was slow. Such recognition was indeed a landmark of social progress.

The moral and intellectual advancement of the social attitude toward deafness in Europe naturally exerted its influence in the United States. Although there had been scattered instances of instruction of the deaf, of attempts to found permanent schools, and of mention of the deaf in the literature, it was not until 1817 that the first permanent public school for the deaf in the United States was founded, at Hartford, Connecticut. The establishment of this school was given its chief impetus by a young divinity student, Thomas Hopkins Gallaudet, who was sent abroad by a group of citizens to observe European methods in the education of the deaf. On visiting England he was disappointed in the help he received from the Braidwoods, who were said to be obtaining good results using the oral approach to deaf children. It appears that the Braidwoods, British educators of the deaf, were secretive about their methods.

Gallaudet therefore crossed the Channel to France and enlisted the services of Laurent Clerc, a French teacher of the deaf trained in the manual approach of De l'Épée, whom he succeeded in bringing to Hartford. Incidentally, Clerc, who was introduced to Gallaudet by Abbé Roch-Ambroise Sicard, De l'Épée's successor, was deaf himself and hence was the first deaf teacher of the deaf in the United States. The school at Hartford, called the American Asylum for the Education and Instruction of the Deaf and Dumb (now known as the American School for the Deaf), had to depend upon private funds for support, but in a relatively short time public assistance was made available. It was the forerunner of the great system of state-supported schools for the deaf which we have in the United States today. Later in the nineteenth century and early in the

twentieth century outstanding private and denominational schools were also established and were notable for their encouragement of oral methods of instruction.

Thanks to the indefatigable efforts of such trailblazers as Thomas Hopkins Gallaudet, for whom the federally sponsored college for the deaf in Washington, D.C., is named; Edward Miner Gallaudet, who carried on his father's work; Sarah Fuller, who promoted the day school for the deaf; Alexander Graham Bell and his father, Melville, who among other accomplishments elevated speech to the status of a science; Caroline Yale, who implemented many of the Bells' principles; and Max A. Goldstein, founder of the Central Institute for the Deaf, who drove home the needs of the deaf to the medical profession and who developed methods for training residual hearing, the great vision of universality of educational opportunity for the deaf has been transformed into reality. The ever-expanding opportunities for the deaf in publicly supported residential and day schools and in parochial and private institutions attest the wisdom of these great workers in the cause of the deaf. It is because of their foresight and energy that no deaf child need be denied an opportunity for education.

The happy combination of talents brought to bear on the problem of increasing the opportunities for the deaf is best epitomized in the person of Alexander Graham Bell. He established the Volta Bureau to disseminate information on deafness, and he opened new vistas in the teaching of speech to the deaf; and, of course, his invention of the telephone laid a firm foundation for the electrical transmission of sound. The writers of this book, consciously or otherwise, take inspiration and stimulation from his sympathetic understanding, his spirit of incisive inquiry, and his inventive genius. It was fitting that 1947 (the date of the first edition of this book), the hundredth anniversary of the birth of Alexander Graham Bell, should witness the emergence of the art and science of audiology, which in broad terms seeks the answer to the question, "How can we do a better job for the deaf and the hard of hearing?" There is no doubt that Bell is still with us as we seek more and better answers to this basic question.

As the schools for the deaf became more widespread and adequate, it was inevitable that the social point of view toward deafness should become proportionately more enlightened. The alumni of these schools were beginning to demonstrate how seriously the deaf had previously been underestimated. They have taken the initiative in promoting broad and intensive studies now underway dealing with the psychiatric and vocational needs of the deaf. The schools themselves are tending to become purely educational institutions, subject to boards of education and not to administrators of almshouses or to penal authorities.

Society now understands that the deaf not only can be educated but can also, with proper guidance and assistance, become economically and socially productive men and women. Agencies for vocational rehabilitation and guidance, emphasizing special training for adults in cooperation with schools and industry, have been established to facilitate the economic and social adjustment not only of the deaf but of the hard-of-hearing as well. And paralleling the enlarging educational and economic opportunities for the deaf, the unnecessary legal restrictions upon them have gradually been removed.

The progressive development of the education of the deaf generally reflected the popularization and liberalization of general education, particularly with respect to the spread of opportunity for education, the improvement of teacher training, and the application of better teaching techniques. The process has also worked in reverse. Educators of the hearing have consciously or otherwise borrowed from teachers of the deaf—especially the principle of "learning by doing." It is heartening to note also that recognized universities are increasingly introducing curricula dealing with educational, psychological, sociological, and physiological problems of deafness.

Perhaps the most tangible and significant expression of national concern for the hearing-impaired is the recent enactment of federal legislation aimed at improving and expanding the preparation of professional personnel, stimulating research, and fostering extended services. The major portion of the federal effort is concentrated in the Department of Health, Education, and Welfare, which administers these programs through the Social and Rehabilitation Services Administration, the National Institute of Neurological Diseases and Stroke, and the Office of Education.

A number of specific enactments and projects are worthy of mention to illustrate the growing commitment of the federal government to hearing-impaired children and adults. In October 1965 acting on a recommendation contained in a report to the Department of Health, Education, and Welfare entitled *Education of the Deaf,* Congress established the National Advisory Committee on the Education of the Deaf. NACED was charged:

1. To stimulate the development of a system for periodic gathering of informato make it possible to assess progress and identify problems in the education of the deaf
2. To identify emerging needs and suggest innovations that promise to improve the educational prospects of deaf individuals
3. To suggest promising areas of inquiry to guide the federal government's research effort in the education of the deaf
4. To advise the Secretary on desirable emphasis and priorities among programs

The Committee is now functioning and has

accomplished one of its first tasks, a National Conference on the Education of the Deaf in April 1967.

The nation is concerned with the increasing number of young people who enter the labor market without any marketable skills or with skills that, at best, are marginal. The technological revolution that goes on unabated and at a rapidly increasing pace is drastically reducing the employment opportunities for those with marginal or obsolescent skills. Realism compels us to recognize that in any economy persons with severely disordered communication find their economic opportunities limited. Aware that burgeoning technology compounds our problem and underlines our responsibility, Congress enacted legislation establishing a National Technical Institute for the Deaf to provide for a residential postsecondary technical education facility which would prepare young deaf adults for successful employment. In December 1966 the Secretary of H.E.W. entered into an agreement with the Rochester Institute of Technology, Rochester, New York, to establish and operate the Institute on its campus, thus making available to deaf students a broad modern range of educational opportunities with hearing students in the technical fields. Of course, the federal government continues to sponsor the century-old Gallaudet College which provides a liberal arts curriculum.

To focus attention on the needs of all handicapped children, Congress in November 1966 amended the monumental Elementary and Secondary Education Act of 1965 to establish a Bureau of Education for the Handicapped within the Office of Education to encourage and support professional training, research, improved demonstrations of services, and the dissemination of information. A measure of the impressive impact of federal support is the increase of badly needed trained teachers of hearing-impaired children. From 1950 to 1960 existing training centers graduated approximately 125 students annually. At the present time more than 500 graduates enter the profession. Similar relative increases in professional workers in audiology and speech pathology have resulted from training programs in the Social and Rehabilitation Services Administration and the United States Public Health Service.

The National Institute of Neurological Diseases and Stroke is engaged in an extensive collaborative perinatal project that may involve as many as 60,000 pregnancies. A central purpose is to study prenatal and perinatal factors which cause communicative disorders. Subsequent studies and evaluations are made of the children after birth and at various stages of development. Emphasis is thus being placed on the causes of deafness during pregnancy and early childhood and on the development of effective methods for early diagnosis and treatment.

Another encouraging development is the establishment of temporal bone banks in various laboratories to correlate histopathology of cases of deafness with prescribed information obtained during the life of the subject. Perhaps, the large number of cases of deafness labeled "cause unknown" will be reduced because of these investigations.

Increased organized activities on the national and international scene by academic, professional, philanthropic, and lay groups is further evidence of the growing interest in the hearing-impaired. This is revealed in the "Annual Directory of Services" of the *American Annals of the Deaf.*

Although man has traveled a long, tortuous road from the pre-Christian era in evolving an enlightened understanding of the social problems of deafness, a large portion of society still looks upon the deaf and the hard-of-hearing as queer, dependent, and sometimes ridiculous. We are all familiar with the cheap humor of which they are often the target. Since their handicap is not as visible as that of the blind and the crippled, the deaf often find themselves in embarrassing and humiliating situations because others do not understand their special problems.

The answer of the deaf to such mis-understanding is to continue their social and economic achievements as self-respect-ing and productive individuals. Our social action for the deaf, therefore, should not aim for special privileges for them but should constantly strive to provide oppor-tunity without discrimination for the deaf to help themselves.

This will happen if we realize that our attainments fall short of what is possible. We can close this gap by improving the quality of professional training, reducing the shortage of workers in the field, elimi-nating a persistent parochialism that is a residue from the days when the education of the deaf was in the hands of a dedicated but professionally inbred few, communicat-ing information to the public objectively, increasing and applying scientific knowl-edge, and by ennobling the legacy of com-mitment that characterized the early few.

## SUGGESTED READINGS AND REFERENCES

**Altshuler, K. Z. (ed.).** *Education of the Deaf: The Challenge and the Charge.* Washing-ton: U.S. Government Printing Office, Superintendent of Documents, 1967.
A report of a National Conference on Education of the Deaf arranged by the National Advisory Committee on the Education of the Deaf at the request of the Secretary of the Department of Health, Education, and Welfare of the United States in April 1967. The conference brought together educators, audiologists, physicians, legislators, psychologists, social workers, leaders of the deaf community, deaf students, and others to discuss the needs of deaf persons. The conference was organized around the special needs of particular age groups, 0 to 5, 6 to 16, 17 to 22, and 22 plus. Recommendations for action to meet these needs are contained in the report.

**Bender, R. E.** *The Conquest of Deafness.* Cleveland: Press of Western Reserve Univer-sity, 1960.
A recent historical treatment.

**Békésy, G. Von and W. A. Rosenblith.** "The Early History of Hearing-Observations and Theories," *J. Acoust. Soc. Amer.,* 20:727–748 (1948).
Author's summary: "The debris of broken systems and exploded dogmas form a great mound, a Mount Testaccio of the shards and remnants of old vessels which once held human beliefs. If you take the trouble to climb to the top of it, you will widen your horizon, and in these days of specialized knowledge your horizon is not likely to be any too wide." Oliver Wendell Holmes, 1882.

**Best, H.** *Deafness and the Deaf in the United States.* New York: The Macmillan Com-pany, 1943.

**Boatner, M. T.** *Voice of the Deaf: A Biography of Edward Miner Gallaudet.* Washington, D.C.: Public Affairs Press, 1959.
A sympathetic treatment of the life of the man associated with the founding and nurturing of Gallaudet College. Chapter 13 is particularly interesting because it discusses Gallaudet's relations with Alexander Graham Bell.

**Doctor, P. V. (ed.).** *Report of the Proceedings of the International Congress on the Education of the Deaf and of the Forty-First Meeting of the Convention of American Instructors of the Deaf, U.S. Document, No. 106.* Washington, D.C.: U.S. Government Printing Office, 1964.
A volume of 1269 pages reporting the presentations at an International Congress on the education of the deaf attended by more than 2000 persons from about 50 countries. The papers proceed sequentially from description and assessment of children through their educational experiences to their economic, psychological, and social accommodation to the world about them. The progression is from otologic, audiologic, psychologic, and educational assessment, through expressive and receptive communication (including speech, speechreading, hearing, and manual methods) to learning that involves language, reading, concept formation, and the content of the curriculum including vocational preparation. The final portion deals with organization and administration.

**Fellendorf, G. (ed.).** *Proceedings of International Conference on Oral Education of the Deaf.* Washington, D.C.: The Alexander Graham Bell Association for the Deaf, 1967.
Report in two volumes (2211 pages) of a conference observing the centennial of oral education of the deaf in the United States. It includes papers by world experts on identification of deafness, organization and administration of services, speech, auditory training, preparation of professional personnel, instruction in language, curriculum development, and educational trends.

**Farrar, A.** *Arnold's Education of the Deaf.* 2d ed. Derby: Francis Carter, 1923.
An account by a British author focused on the evolution of the education of the deaf from its European beginnings prior to the twentieth century.

**Garnett, C. B., Jr.** *The Exchange of Letters Between Samuel Heinicke and Abbé Charles Michel De L'Épee.* New York: The Vantage Press, 1968.
Authors summary: A monograph on the oralist and manualist methods of instructing the deaf in the eighteenth century, including the reproduction in English of the salient portions of each letter.

**Goldstein, M. A.** *Problems of the Deaf.* St. Louis: The Laryngoscope Press, 1933.
Essentially a collection of essays on topics pertinent to deafness, including an excellent historical chapter.

**Graham, A. B. (ed.).** *Sensorineural Hearing Processes and Disorders.* Boston: Little, Brown & Company, 1967.
Report of an international symposium (March 1965) that represents an interesting synthesis of information and opinions by recognized authorities on

processes of sensory-neural hearing mechanisms, psychoacoustic response to auditory stimuli, localization of auditory disorders, clinical diagnostic procedures, and pathology and manifestations of specific disease entities. In a historical sense, too, it is an important document for audiology.

**Hodgson, K. W.** *The Deaf and Their Problems*. New York: Philosophical Library, 1954. A historical study in special education by a British author including the growth of teaching systems and social attitudes toward deafness.

# CHAPTER 16

## DEAF CHILDREN

### S. R. SILVERMAN, Ph.D.
### H. S. LANE, Ph.D.

## DEFINITIONS

The approximately 39,000 deaf children of school age in the United States present a problem somewhat different from that of the more numerous hard-of-hearing children to be discussed in Chapter 17. Most deaf children either are born deaf or lose their hearing before patterns of language and speech have been established. By "deaf" children we here mean those who do not have sufficient residual hearing to enable them to understand speech successfully, even with a hearing aid, without special instruction. And even those children who lose their hearing after patterns of language and speech have been firmly established suffer more deterioration of speech than do hard-of-hearing children. On the other hand, a congenitally deaf child is not dumb. His mechanism for speech is normal, but he has simply never been taught to speak.

In their formative years children learn speech and language, both reception and expression, primarily through the ear. Sec-

tional pronunciations and accents learned as children are likely to be retained throughout life. The New Englander who uses the broad *a* in "park," as distinguished from the Midwesterner who rolls the *r* in the same word, is merely imitating what he has heard as a youth in his section of the country. In the same sense our use and understanding of language naturally depend at first upon hearing. The 2-year-old severely deaf child has no useful verbal language, whereas the hearing child of the same age has begun to develop a meaningful spoken and hearing vocabulary. Hence, means of communication with the deaf child must be developed through systematic and, in many instances, laborious procedures.

The detection and diagnosis of deafness and other abnormalities of communication have been discussed in Chapters 8 and 17, but it is important to keep clearly in mind the kind of child we are talking about when we refer to the "deaf child."

A great deal of unnecessary confusion among the laity and well-intentioned professional workers alike has surrounded the precise classification of hard-of-hearing and deaf children and unfortunately has frequently obfuscated discussions of their problems. The confusion seems to grow out of the differences in frameworks of reference to which classification and nomenclature are related. For example, some workers classify the child who develops speech and language prior to onset of deafness as "hard of hearing" even though he may not be able to hear pure tones or speech at any intensity. This child, it is argued, unlike the congenitally profoundly deaf child who has not acquired speech naturally, behaves as a hard-of-hearing child in that his speech is relatively natural or "normal" and, therefore, he should be classified as "hard of hearing." It is obvious that a not-too-precise educational standard has guided the labeling if not the definition of the child. If, however, we consider the same child from a purely physiological standpoint, it is grossly misleading to term him "hard of hearing" when for all practical purposes he hears nothing at all.

The situation is complicated further by the use of terms that suggest not only physiological communication and educational factors but also gradations of hearing loss and time of onset. To this category belong such terms as *deaf and dumb, mute, deaf-mute, semideaf, semimute, deafened, partially deaf,* and others. These terms are of little value from the physiological, communicative, or educational points of view, and it would be well to eliminate them from general usage (see also Chapter 4).

For purposes of our chapter we need to define the deaf child in terms of his educational and psychological potential. For some, the significant dimension would be the child's ability to talk. In England, for example, under the School Health Regulations, children have been described as (1) deaf, and (2) partially deaf. The former are those who have no "naturally" acquired speech when they are admitted to school;

the latter are those who have begun to talk naturally (however imperfectly) before being admitted to school. According to this scheme children with defective hearing are classified in three grades:

> *Grade I:* Children who are found to have defects of hearing (which in most cases are amenable to medical treatment) but who do not need hearing aids or special educational treatment.
>
> *Grade II:* Children who have some naturally acquired ability to talk but need special educational treatment, on either a part-time or a full-time basis. Many of these children need hearing aids.
>
> *Grade III:* Deaf children who are without naturally acquired speech when admitted to school. Many of these children are not totally deaf and can be helped by hearing aids in learning to talk and to speak distinctly.

For others, the important dimension is the hearing loss expressed by the child's ability to respond to various environmental sounds, speech, and pure tones. Itard, in the early nineteenth century, classified children according to their responses—to bells, drums, and flutes; Urbantschitsch some years later used a harmonica with a six-octave range ($E^{-1}$ to $e^4$) and an intensity regulator for the same purpose. Both of these workers also used speech stimuli, and Urbantschitsch's classification is fairly representative of the categories that emerge from these approaches: (1) total deafness, (2) tone-hearing, (3) vowel-hearing, (4) word-hearing, and (5) sentence-hearing. Others have translated this dimension to hearing for pure tones on the decibel scale by such schemes as are described in Chapters 4, 9, and 17.

Of course, the time of onset of deafness affects the psychological and educational developmental patterns and should be borne in mind in labeling and classifying a child. In 1937 the Committee on Nomenclature of the Conference of Executives of American Schools for the Deaf recognized the importance of ability to speak, ability to hear (as shown by their use of the word "functional"), and time of onset in proposing the following classification and definitions:

1. *The Deaf.* Those in whom the sense of hearing is nonfunctional for the ordinary purposes of life. This general group is made up of two distinct classes based entirely on the time of the loss of hearing: (*a*) *The congenitally deaf:* those who are born deaf. (*b*) *The adventitiously deaf:* those who were born with normal hearing but in whom the sense of hearing becomes nonfunctional later through illness or accident.
2. *The Hard-of-Hearing.* Those in whom the sense of hearing, although defective, is functional with or without a hearing aid.

Some object vigorously to the restricting influence of the definitions and classifications of impaired hearing contained in these proposals of the Conference of Executives and as suggested in Chapter 17. They maintain that the continuing increase of fundamental clinical and therapeutic audiological knowledge precludes any "static categorization." For example, study of the thresholds of tolerance for speech and for pure tones has suggested that there is a useful portion of the auditory area even beyond the range of classical audiometry. Some individuals who have heretofore been termed "totally deaf" as a result of audiometric tests may be reached by auditory stimulation using proper amplification. And it may prove to be more fruitful to classify the person with a physical disability on some psychological scale of behavior that expresses how he lives with his disability.

We are aware that delimiting definitions are hazardous, and we recognize that each child's capabilities must be assessed individually by the best methods avilable to us so that we are not restricted by the tyranny of classification. Nevertheless, we need some orientation as to the kind of child we are writing about in order that we may discuss him in general terms. This chapter will therefore be concerned with the child who, when we first encounter him, has not developed the expressive and receptive skills of communication before the onset of his deafness. He cannot talk, and he cannot understand the speech of others as does a child of the same age with normal hearing. We shall also include the child who has acquired some of these skills of communication before the onset of his deafness, but whose incompetence in language still calls for special educational techniques. For convenience, we shall refer to both of them as deaf children.

## MAGNITUDE OF THE PROBLEM

If we examine the results of mass testing surveys among schoolchildren, we find a range from 2 to 21 percent reported as having defective hearing. This great variability in reports of hearing impairment is undoubtedly due to differences in definitions of hearing impairment; in techniques, apparatus, and conditions of testing; and in the socioeconomic status and climate of the communities in which the surveys were carried out.

Our best estimate, supported by an extensive detailed study of Pittsburgh schoolchildren, is that 5 percent of school-age children have hearing levels, in one ear at least, outside the range of normal (see Chapter 9) and that one to two of every ten in this group require special educational attention. (These figures do not include children in special schools for the deaf.) The others are likely to respond to medical care, or their hearing loss is not apt to

TABLE 1

IMPAIRED HEARING IN THE PITTSBURGH STUDY POPULATION

Class of Handicap

| | A | B | C | D | E and F |
|---|---|---|---|---|---|
| Ages 5 to 10 years, inclusive | Not more than 25 dB* | 26–40 dB | 41–55 dB | 56–70 dB | More than 70 dB |
| Number 4064 | 3996 | 36 | 19 | 9 | 2 |
| Percent 100 | 98.3 | 0.9 | 0.5 | 0.2 | 0.05 |

←————— 0.3% —————→

←————————— 1.7% —————————→

* Impairment refers to the average hearing-threshold level for 500, 1000, and 2000 Hz. The original ASA-1951 categories have been translated to equivalent ISO categories (see Chapter 9).

reach the handicapping stage. The projections of Educational Statistics of the Office of Education, U.S. Department of Health, Education, and Welfare indicate a school-age population of 51,000,000 for 1968–1969, which will include 2,550,000 children with hearing levels outside the range of normal and 255,000 requiring special education services. Table 1 shows the Pittsburgh findings according to class of handicap developed in Chapter 9. Of course, account should be taken of children below school age. Our judgment is that the statistics would be about the same for them. We shall discuss in the following chapter how most of these hard-of-hearing children are handled.

Of interest is the number of all persons per 1000 population with binaural hearing loss. Figure 16-1 shows that there is a striking increase in the incidence of hearing impairments in the older age groups. Of course, the nature of the impairment may vary with age.

As we have described them, how many deaf children are there in the United States? This is difficult to state precisely because the enrollment in our schools for the deaf is likely to include children who are hard of hearing and is not likely to include all the children of preschool age and deaf children who are in schools for the hearing or in other kinds of schools. Our guiding figure is the reported enrollment of 38,391 children in all schools for the deaf in 1967–1968, a formidable even if not quite accurate figure.

## THE GOALS OF EDUCATION OF THE DEAF

How we go about educating deaf children is obviously related to the goals we have set for them, and these goals are in turn determined by what we consider to be the over-all potential of the deaf—educational, psychological, and social. Or, some of the sharp differences of opinion concerning the most desirable arrangements and methods for the education of deaf children really have their roots in fundamental differences of opinion on the long-range outlook for them. This outlook may be determined, among other considerations, by our own value system, by our experience with post-school accommodation and adjustment of deaf persons, by our own education and indoctrination, by our professional training, by our relation to deaf persons, or by some combination of these.

The overwhelming amount of literature on the subject (a bibliography would probably exceed 2000 titles), ranging from school papers and convention resolutions to lengthy sections of books, reveals an in-

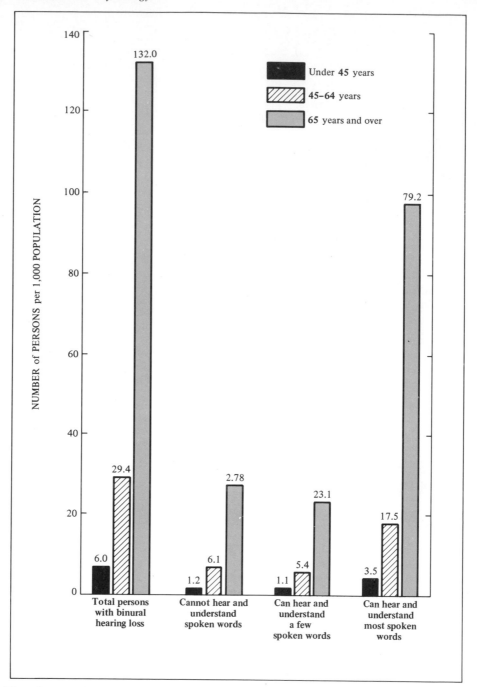

Fig. 16-1. Number of persons with binaural hearing loss per 1000 population, by age and speech comprehension group.

tense polemicism that rests mainly on a nonexperimental empirical foundation. Of course, there are many shades of opinion, but stated views and observed practices suggest what we may term three "schools of thought." We are aware that we may be indulging in caricature and that "it all depends on the individual child," but we believe that a sorting out of views is desirable if we are to understand the rationale for particular views of the education of deaf children.

One group appears to stress the limitations, especially the social limitations, of deafness. It is concerned about the exclusion of the deaf from certain types of desirable employment, the effect on the deaf of insurance practices and legislation, the implication of what amounts to minority status in certain educational and social contexts, the impact of isolation from other deaf people, the difficult if not impossible task for some of learning speech and speechreading, and the misunderstandings of the general public concerning the abilities and aspirations of the deaf. This group would suit the method of communication to the child, and its view is best summarized by the following statement:

> The aim of the education of the deaf child should be to make him a well-integrated, happy deaf individual, and not a pale imitation of a hearing person. Let us aim to produce happy, well-adjusted deaf *individuals,* each different from the other, each with his own personality. If a child cannot learn to read lips well or cannot speak well, it is far better to develop other modes of expression and communication, writing and gesturing, than to make him feel ashamed and frustrated because he cannot acquire the very difficult art of speech and lipreading. Our aim must be a well-balanced, happy *deaf* person and not an imitation of a hearing one.

The educational program should be geared to the production of contented members of a subculture secure in its sanctions, its modes of communication, and its opportunities for social expression.

A second group emphasizes the great possibilities of the deaf, as yet untapped, particularly for education and for participation in a world of hearing people. It stresses the importance of early education and the great possibilities of auditory training, and it is apt to emphasize the objective of "normalization." In essence, there is "one world" in which the deaf person must function, and that is a world of hearing and speaking people. There is no separate world for the deaf. The adherents of this view reject the validity of the subculture concept for deaf people and strive toward their complete assimilation in the world of the hearing.

A third school of thought points to the record of economic, academic, and social achievement of deaf persons *among the deaf and the hearing* as a strong, tangible justification for the belief that forward-looking, proper, and early fundamental training enables the deaf child to make the fullest use of his capabilities. Yet it is apparent, at least in our present state of knowledge, that there are situations in which the deaf will always be marginal, and our approach to them should be influenced accordingly. Realism urges us to spare parents and the child himself the psychological distress of failure to achieve the "normalcy" that was set up as an attainable goal.

Succinctly put, the first group says there are two distinct worlds, the deaf and the hearing. They communicate very little and only when necessary, and the deaf may not be too concerned with devaluation of their group. The second says there is only the world of the hearing, and deaf people must adjust to it through integration. For the third group the two worlds overlap. Some deaf people penetrate the majority culture more than others, perhaps because of their education, their native ability, their skill in oral communication, emotional makeup, their families, or for other reasons. These factors require more study in order that the knowledge we gain may enable us to set goals more rationally.

The prevalent attitudes influence not only the means of communication in the classroom and the content and nature of the curriculum, but they have a direct bearing on the organizational and administrative education arrangements, day or residential, integrated or segregated, that we make for deaf children and on the important and essential practice of guiding and counseling parents.

A reasonable guiding principle in our present state of knowledge is to reject the notion that deaf persons are an undifferentiated, monolithic mass and to avoid the stereotyping to which it gives rise. Deaf persons differ among themselves as do the hearing, and therefore there should be a reasonable and carefully thought-out range of educational options available to them. After all, this is the essence of our entire culture, and we achieve its aspirations to the extent that we increase the opportunities for people to be themselves.

At any rate, until more facts are available to fill the gaps now occupied by opinion, a rational attitude points to the recognition that deafness imposes certain unavoidable limitations that must be accepted. At the same time, proper education in its broadest sense strives to relate the deaf person to the world about him in a psychologically satisfying way.

## THE EDUCATION OF THE DEAF

We now turn to consideration of what we judge to be a "proper education." It is both convenient and logical to organize our discussion around the following topics:

1. The communication controversy
2. Organization of the education of the the deaf
3. The rise of the preschool movement
4. Psychological and educational assessment of the deaf child
   a. Intelligence
   b. Educational achievement
   c. Personality
   d. Language development and concepts

5. The skills of communication
   a. Speech
   b. Auditory training
   c. Speechreading
   d. Language
6. Curriculum development in schools for the deaf
7. Problems of parents

### The Communication Controversy

Because there is universal agreement among educators of the deaf that every deaf child should be given an opportunity to communicate by speech, our attention shall be directed solely to this approach, which is called *oralism.* Some educators also advocate supplementing, or, if indicated, supplanting oral instruction with other forms of communication. One of these other forms is the *manual alphabet,* which is a method of forming the letters from A to Z by certain fixed positions of the fingers of one hand. This is a form of "writing" in the air. A more structured form of the combined approach is known as the Rochester method after the school in which it was developed. Its aim is to supplement speechreading, and it is generally introduced after an oral groundwork has been laid.

The *language of signs* is another form of communication. This is a system of conventional gestures of the hands and arms that by and large are suggestive of the shape, form, or thought which they represent. A dictionary of signs based on a system of recording them with respect to location, configuration, and movement has been compiled. It is generally agreed that sign language is bound to the concrete and is rather limited with respect to abstraction, humor, and subtleties such as figures of speech which enrich expression. The *combined method,* which attempts to provide speech communication, the manual alphabet, and the language of signs, depends upon the aptitude of the child and the context of the communication. For example, the language of signs and the manual alphabet are frequently employed in public assemblies. The combined method is usually employed in public residential schools.

As we have seen in Chapter 15, the "oral-manual" controversy has deep historical roots. In our own country the influence of De l'Épée through Laurent Clerc and Thomas Hopkins Gallaudet established the tradition of manualism early in the nineteenth century, and it was not until well after the middle of that century that oralism began to take hold. At the present time 85 percent of children enrolled in schools for the deaf are reported to be instructed by the oral method of comunication, at least in their early years. The remainder are taught manually or by some combination of manual and oral methods. Although all organizations of educators of the deaf are on record officially as advocating an opportunity for all deaf children to learn to speak and to speechread, there is significant (and often heated) difference of opinion on what properly constitutes a fair opportunity. The criteria for transferring a child from an oral to a manual class, presumably because he shows no aptitude for oralism, are frequently vague and nebulous. Some educators make the transfer during the child's first year in school; others may wait until the child has been in school for three or four years; and still others provide oral instruction throughout but permit association in the dormitory with manually taught children. The latter plan obviously makes the oral instruction less effective because the speaking child must adjust himself to the child who cannot talk, and valuable practice in oral communication is lost.

Those who advocate some manualism generally contend that too often the results of exclusively oral teaching are unsatisfactory and that the deaf child cannot make himself understood to an untrained listener. Furthermore, it is argued that many children do not have the aptitude to benefit from oral instruction and that the time spent in this type of instruction could more profitably be used in concentrating on the child's "mental" development rather than on his means of communication. Also, some advocates of manualism believe that the deaf prefer to associate with other deaf and therefore have little or no need for oral communication.

The fundamental assumption of the oralists (advocates of oral instruction for the deaf), on the other hand, is that training in speech and in speechreading gives an easier adjustment to a world in which speech is the chief medium of communication. It does not confine the deaf man or woman to association with those who know the manual alphabet or to those who are willing to resort to pad and pencil. An employer is more inclined to favor a deaf man to whom he can give oral instructions over a man of equal ability with whom he must communicate by gestures or in writing. It is not always possible, especially in smaller communities, for the deaf to find employment or social companionship among other deaf people. Oralists feel that, in the main, orally trained children have done well and are likely to do better as more teachers are adequately trained in the methods of oral instruction.

*Recent trends.* Recent (1968) reports from the Soviet Union's Moscow Institute of Defectology suggest that oral skills may be facilitated by the introduction at the preschool level (unlike the Rochester method which introduces fingerspelling somewhat later) of "dactyl speech" or fingerspelling, which is free of phonetic ambiguity. Preliminary investigations appear to indicate that familiar words could be converted into oral language, speechreading, and speech even before the end of the first year of kindergarten. The aim is definitely oral and results in the gradual elimination of the need for fingerspelling except for special difficulties. Signs are excluded. It should be borne in mind that the Russian language is very phonetic. It is not known to what extent control groups were employed in these investigations, such as groups that had used early and extensive auditory stimulation.

There appears to be a significant movement to introduce the language of signs as a major mode of communication with young deaf children on the grounds that the capacity for thinking must be developed early and should not be confused with the capacity for using language. It is argued that we deter the development of thinking in deaf persons by emphasizing at the outset verbal means of communication, be they speech, the manual alphabet, or a combination of the two. In his book on the subject Furth indicates that by present methods we foster an "experiential deficiency which would be avoidable if nonverbal methods of instruction and communication were encouraged both at home in the earliest years and in formal school education." The assumption that this is the only alternative to certain conventional unproductive methods is open to question. For example, we must weigh carefully the accomplishment of parent guidance and the early intensive use of residual hearing, and also the impressive academic, vocational, and communicative attainments of many deaf persons.

The idea has been advanced that oral language be taught as a second language preceded by the language of signs and that the latter be used to bring out the advantages of oral language. The sign language, it is suggested, ought to be enriched so that it is less rigidly concrete and situation-bound.

The "oral-manual" controversy is not yet settled. It is encouraging, however, that numerous investigations are under way to study not only the linguistic, conceptual, and intellectual effects of modes of communication for deaf persons but also their influence on features of personality as emotional maturity and self identity.

## Organization of the Education of the Deaf

Perhaps the most significant fact about the education of the deaf in the United States is that it is universally available to all deaf children of school age. Of course, the quality of education may vary, but it is important that no child need be denied an opportunity for it. Where are these opportunities available?

Of 38,391 children enrolled in schools for the deaf in the academic year 1967–1968, 18,926 attended public residential schools for the deaf. These schools, open to qualified children without charge, are supported either directly or indirectly by state tax funds. Most of the public residential schools are supported by legislative appropriation and hence come under the control of state authorities. The educational services of the remaining schools are purchased by the states on a per diem or per capita basis and are controlled by their own boards. Examples of the first group are the Indiana and Illinois schools for the deaf; in the second group we find such schools as the Lexington (New York) and the Clarke (Massachusetts) schools for the deaf.

Other tax-supported institutions for the deaf are public day schools and classes. A school is usually large enough to be a separate entity; for example, Horace Mann School, Roxbury, Massachusetts. Day classes are usually groups within a larger school unit and there may be as few as one in a school or as many as ten; for example, in La Crosse, Wisconsin. In 1967–1968, 2300 children were being educated in public day schools, and 13,070 were in public day classes. The remaining children were being educated in denominational or private schools, such as Lutheran School (Detroit) and Central Institute for the Deaf (St. Louis). Such schools may be either day or residential. There were 409 children in schools and classes for the multiply-handicapped. The number of children in each class ranges generally from five to ten. Some deaf children have been absorbed into classes for the hearing. Deaf individuals attend high schools and colleges for the hearing. Most public residential schools provide education at the secondary level, and higher education exclusively for the deaf is available at Gallaudet College, Washington, D.C. Technical postsecondary education is provided at the National Technical Institute for the Deaf, which is an integral part of a larger technical institute for the hearing, the Rochester Institute of Technology, Rochester, New York.

Until we have more evidence to support the point of view of either the day or the residential school, we must study each child's situation thoroughly to determine what educational placement is likely to be most fruitful for him. This points up the crucial need for early identification, diagnosis, and careful assessment. In addition to information about a child's hearing, among the significant points to be considered are the etiology of the deafness, the child's age at its onset, his physical development, his behavioral development, his social maturity, his home environment, and the insight of his parents.

## The Rise of the Preschool Movement

The encouraging progress in the assessment of hearing of young children has stressed the value of preschool programs for deaf children. The period from birth to the age of 5 is particularly critical for the learning and over-all development of children, whether hearing or deaf. The importance of early auditory experience is now recognized, and hearing aids are being recommended with greater confidence than previously. It is worthy of mention that the extent to which auditory stimulation is combined with specific modes of visual communication such as speechreading, gesture, and fingerspelling varies and is the subject of much critical discussion.

Indirect evidence from neurophysiology, mentioned in Chapters 3 and 4, suggest that there is a critical early period of life when the nervous system is still plastic, and sensory experience exerts an important influence on its development. Psycholinguists, too, point to a critical period for the acquisition of language, particularly its syntactic features. Since the young deaf child is denied many of the normal experiences that lead to better socialization, it is all the more essential that he be given help and opportunity for his best development as early in life as possible. This means not just a sensible program for developing the skills of communication which so greatly contribute to socialization, but also a regimen that removes wherever possible the barrier which tends to isolate the deaf child from the world about him, from the world of his home, his parents, his sisters and brothers, and from other children. Formal and informal intercommunications (by whatever means) tend to lessen the child's feeling of apartness and hence to make him feel wanted and significant.

The child is thus motivated to communicate, and it is the task of the parent and the teacher to show him the usefulness of speech as a tool of communication. "The situations," according to the prominent British educators of the deaf, Professor and Mrs. Ewing, "do not happen enough by themselves; they must be anticipated and contrived frequently and deliberately" by all who are in close contact with the child.

Although it is not generally mandatory for tax-supported schools to provide preschool classes for deaf children, the need is beginning to be recognized. In the academic year 1967–1968, of 18,926 children enrolled in public residential schools for the deaf in the United States, 1028 were under the age of 6; of 15,370 children

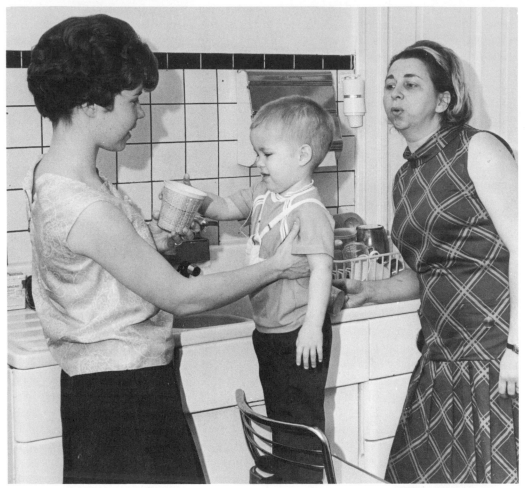

Fig. 16-2. Instructing a parent to take advantage of everyday opportunities to encourage communication. (*Central Institute for the Deaf, photo by Harold Ferman*)

in public day schools and classes, 2453 were of preschool age; and of the 3686 children in denominational and private schools, 1646 were under the age of 6. The proportions reflect the initiative of private groups in promoting programs for preschool deaf children.

It is appropriate, in discussing the young deaf child, to mention the increasing amount of information and guidance available for parents of deaf children. Although here and there an effort may be misguided, the proliferation of parent institutes and clinics, and of correspondence courses, reading lists, and literary output is one

of the most constructive and forward-looking developments in the education of the deaf. One parent put it succinctly:

. . . the tough thing about deafness is likely to be social isolation, social adjustment. There is no one in the world, and there never can be anyone, as important in determining any child's social adjustment as that child's own parents and his family at home. For that reason parents are important.

For the parents of very young deaf children there are now correspondence courses which offer guidance, practical suggestions, and information concerning the home care of the child before the nursery school years. Probably the first such correspondence course was established by the Wright Oral School in New York City; but the best known at the present time is operated by the John Tracy Clinic in Los Angeles. Intelligent and cooperative parents have found these courses most helpful in giving them specific step-by-step procedures in beginning steps and a good psychological approach to the deaf child. Other procedures include the development of visual discrimination by matching colors and pictures and the comparison of objects varying in size and shape, practice in discriminating odors and tastes, exercise in the imitation of bodily movements, and the use of materials that will aid the child in better muscular coordination. Training of this type is continued in the nursery school on a more extensive and advanced scale. Such a correspondence course is particularly useful for those who are too remote to obtain information and advice in person from one of the well-established schools for the deaf.

Children instructed by the parents who have followed a correspondence course of this type are better prepared to benefit immediately from a nursery school.

In general there appear to be no universally accepted specific aims or procedures in guiding parents of very young children. The emphases vary. For some, the primary aim is to create realistic "acceptance" of the child's condition, and counseling is weighted toward psychotherapy. For others, the emphasis is on conveying information in order to create an understanding of sensory deprivation and its effect on the total development of the child in general and of his communication deficit in particular. Wherever possible there is a growing trend toward carrying on parent "training" in homes and homelike settings, sometimes called demonstration homes, where, by demonstration and practice, parents learn to contrive and take advantage of natural situations in the home to sharpen perceptions and foster communication.

Of great interest to educators of deaf

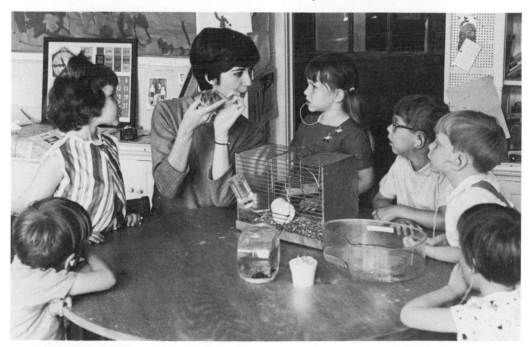

Fig. 16-3. Learning from experience in a preschool class. (*Central Institute for the Deaf, photo by Harold Ferman*)

children is the knowledge likely to be gained from the programs of early education such as Head Start directed at "culturally disadvantaged" children. Here too, vigorous schools of thought appear to be taking shape. On the one hand, there are those who would emphasize "cognitive" approaches that stimulate intellectual functioning. In its extreme form it has been labeled the "pressure-cooker" view, which aims to compensate for the lack of opportunity for perceptual development. Others would stress the child's social and emotional growth without too much "structured" teaching.

Most of these commendable efforts in orientation and guidance have been directed at parents of children of preschool age. This is natural, since the initial shock of the discovery of deafness must be intelligently cushioned, and crucial and immediate decisions must be made about the child's future. Even though we are discussing here children of preschool age, it should be realized that the placement of a child in a satisfactory educational situation in no way decreases the need for the guidance of parents. This was forcefully driven home to us in a survey made of the parents of present and former pupils at Central Institute for the Deaf. Parents of teen-agers and young adults wanted an opportunity to share information and experiences about such problems as choices of occupation, marriage with the deaf or hearing, the genetics of deafness, and the choice of companions for the deaf. In short, social adjustment is just as much a problem for the deaf youth as it is for the preschool child, and it is essential that parent institutes and clinics concerned with their problems be fostered also.

Such evidence as exists for the value of particular procedures and programs of parent counseling is meager and is generally anecdotal or based on studies (frequently retroactive) of children's records. It will be helpful, for the programs we undertake, to evaluate all of the following: *genetic counseling* for deaf married couples and parents of deaf children; the use of the *high risk register*; the *adaptations* necessary because of differences in the intelligence, motivation, and education of parents; the *emotional needs* of parents; the *special training* necessary for those who counsel parents; and the implications of the concept of *critical periods* in development.

## Psychological and Educational Assessment of the Deaf Child

*Intelligence.* What is intelligence? How we define it determines whether we feel confident in our ability to measure the intelligence of the deaf child. If it is the ability to carry on abstract thinking and to use abstract symbols in the solution of problems as defined by Terman, we are testing an area requiring verbal behavior. In fact, Terman considered the size of vocabulary to be the best single indicator of intelligence. Selection of mental tests that satisfy this definition would lead to the conclusions that deaf children are either mentally retarded *or* that their ability cannot be measured. However, if intelligence is defined as the aggregate or global capacity of the individual to act purposefully, to think rationally, and to deal effectively with his environment (Wechsler), then nonverbal tests can yield an estimate of mental ability.

The need for measures of mental ability of the deaf child preceded the development of intelligence scales. In 1889 at the New York School for the Deaf, Greenberger used colored picture books and blocks as a part of the procedure of admission of children to the school. Observation of facial expression and behavior with "test materials" enabled him to weed out the mentally defective child.

Pintner and Paterson (1915) attempted to apply the Binet-Simon scale to a population of deaf children and concluded that difficulties in the use of the scale occurred due to the lack of comprehension, the lack of environmental experience, and "the peculiar psychology" of the deaf child.

Pintner and his associates were pioneers in the psychological testing of the deaf. They attempted to use and modify existing tests developed for hearing children and finally constructed a performance test, a Non-Language Scale for group testing, and an Educational Scale for the deaf. The results of a national survey led to the conclusion that deaf children were mentally retarded (2 to 3 years) and educationally retarded (4 to 5 years or 3½ grades). These conclusions were accepted by most educators prior to 1930.

With the realization that a child with a hearing impairment must learn to understand language and to communicate, came the recognition that a test of mental ability must measure what the child is capable of learning. This required the selection of tests that were nonverbal in administration and response. Pantomime instructions were standardized, and gestures were substituted for such verbal instructions as: "Watch me carefully and do as I do" or "Put the blocks in the box quickly."

Test batteries, such as the Drever-Collins Scale, the Randall's Island Performance Series, the Ontario School Ability Examination, the Grace Arthur Point Scale, and the Hiskey or Nebraska test of hearing aptitude, were adapted or constructed for use with the deaf. These tests were administered to hearing populations, and their validity was determined by comparison with verbal tests. When the performance tests were administered to the deaf, results indicated a normal distribution of intelligence test scores.

The psychometrist using these tests needs to be skilled in getting rapport quickly, in stressing the importance of speed in some tests that are timed, in observing carefully the attention of the child, and in recording accurately significant behavior as well as test scores. Many performance test batteries use the same test items, and the test-retest reliability of some of these items is questionable. Therefore, the psychometrist must be alert to the child's familiarity with a test

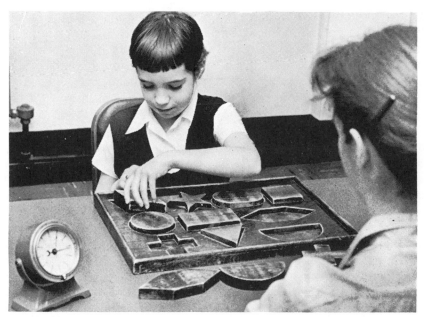

Fig. 16-4. A form board is used to test mental ability. (*Central Institute for the Deaf.*)

and be prepared to substitute other test batteries. It is especially important in clinical evaluation to avoid duplication of tests, as many parents take deaf children to clinics throughout the United States to get additional opinions and diagnoses.

Recently emphasis has been placed on qualitative differences in the mental ability of the deaf compared with the hearing instead of quantitative measures. There is a tendency to view intelligence on a continuum of concrete–abstract. According to Myklebust, when one type of sensation is missing, it alters the integration and function of others. Experience for the child is constituted differently, and the world of perception, conception, imagination, and thought has a new configuration. Oléron thinks that conventional tests have not served our purposes and that we need fresh approaches to study difficulties in perceptual analysis and organization, abstract thinking, and concept formation. The Snijders-Ooman Non-Verbal Scale (SONS) is used in Europe and is designed to include nonverbal items requiring conceptual thinking with a minimum of items requiring speed of performance.

Several investigators report the low predictive value of IQ's on performance tests for future academic achievement as evidence that the performance test is inadequate as a measure of the kind of intelligence needed to succeed academically. Otherwise, said educators have failed to produce academic achievement commensurate with intelligence.

The Hiskey-Nebraska Test of Learning Aptitude has been revised (1966) extending the chronological age limits from 3 to 18. Tests have been added but still scored as a learning quotient (IQ), indicating the use to predict learning skills observed in classrooms for the deaf. Birch and Birch used the Leiter International Performance Scale and the Goodenough Draw-a-Man, together with other test batteries, to predict which children will present serious teaching problems in speechreading, oral speech, and reading. On these tests the children test significantly lower than on the other test batteries.

The performance portion of the Wechsler Intelligence Scales has become one of the widely used tests to measure the intelligence of the deaf. Those used most frequently are Wechsler-Bellevue (W-B), the Wechsler Intelligence Scale for Children (WISC), and the Wechsler Adult Intelligence Scale (WAIS). All of these scales are constructed to have a verbal and a performance section with scores expressed in a verbal quotient, a performance quotient, and a full-scale quotient. It is assumed that in a normal population the mean of differences between the verbal and performance quotients is zero, with a normal distribution of differences. Therefore, psychometrists testing the deaf give only the performance portion and report a score on a test that is meaningful to educators and psychologists. The verbal portion may be significant as an index of readiness of the deaf child to be integrated into classes for the hearing. When the deaf child achieves a verbal quotient within normal limits, he should be able to cope with the language of the school curriculum for the hearing.

Early identification of deafness and parent-infant programs have created a need for tests from infancy to 3 years of age. Developmental scales such as the Gesell norms and the Vineland Social Maturity Scale serve as guides to which the teacher can supplement her observations of behavior. The Smith Non-Verbal Performance Scale constructed by Dr. Althena Smith at the Tracy Clinic is a behavior scale to be used to estimate levels of development with items (graded in difficulty) which present a broad clinical picture in children from 2 to 4 years of age.

Testing the multiply-handicapped deaf presents additional problems. There are no reliable measures for children with poor motor coordination. Tests of speed are not fair, and tests requiring precision of coordination are frustrating. The psychometrist can estimate ability, and this must be confirmed by a trial period of teaching.

The deaf child with learning difficulties will frequently show a wide range of abilities in the test items. Tests involving memory span are apt to be lower than other tests in the battery. The distribution and pattern of test scores in a battery of tests becomes significant in class placement in order to meet the individual differences of deaf children.

*Educational achievement.* Educational progress can be measured by scores on achievement tests, which should be administered at regular intervals, preferably annually, from the time the child reaches the equivalent of second grade until he is prepared to leave the school for the deaf. These tests measure ability in reading, arithmetic, social studies, science, language, spelling, and study skills. There is no need for special tests for the deaf to measure educational attainment in terms of grade and age equivalents. The value of these tests is to compare the educational level of the deaf child with national norms for the hearing. However, Wrightstone, Aranov, and Moskowitz (1963) have developed reading-test norms for the deaf using the revision of the Metropolitan Achievement Test, Elementary Reading Test 2. These norms enable educators to compare groups of deaf children.

There has been great concern about the gap between mental ability and educational level of deaf children from the time of the Educational Survey of Pintner to the present date. Hall and Fusfeld reported the educational test level of students entering Gallaudet to be a mean grade equivalent ranging from 9.2 in 1929 to 10.0 in 1932.

The average grade equivalents on the Stanford Achievement Test of deaf children over 16 years of age leaving school programs were tabulated by Boatner (1964) and can be summarized as follows:

|  | Total $N$ | Academic Diplomas | Vocational Certificates |
|---|---|---|---|
| Residential schools | 1145 | 8.2 | 5.3 |
| Day, private, denominational schools | 132 | 7.3 | 5.0 |

These statistics, however, fail to include deaf children leaving special schools before the age of 16.

The Babbidge report, citing the median-grade average of 920 students who left residential schools in the 1963–1964 school year revealed that at no age was a median seventh-grade achievement attained. Some congenitally deaf children achieve eighth grade, as measured by a battery of standardized tests, and qualify for admission to schools for the hearing at ninth grade. However, they are likely to have spent from 10 to 12 years in a special education program to accomplish this. It is important to emphasize that mean or median scores on a test battery do not give a meaningful measure of the child's achievement. Deaf children do not score equally well on all tests. Poorest scores are found in reading tests (paragraph meaning and word meaning) and in arithmetic reasoning or problem solving. Best scores are recorded in arithmetic computations and spelling.

The deaf child does not learn at the same rate as the hearing child. With the need to master new vocabulary and language, it takes about two or more years to achieve second-grade level and an additional one and a half to two years to complete third grade. This plateau in learning is discouraging but is not the fault of the child or teacher. It can be attributed to the time necessary to build a foundation for future progress.

The gap between mental ability and academic achievement can be reduced, but it is seldom eliminated. Recommendations to improve the educational level include:

1. Early identification followed by early parent-infant education and a preschool program
2. Maximum use of residual hearing
3. Improved reading with the desire to read for recreation
4. Improved reasoning ability through more opportunities to be placed in problem-solving situations
5. Higher aspirations of teachers and student teachers for better academic achievement of the deaf
6. Intelligent use of instructional media like visual aids
7. Continuous close cooperation of home and school

*Personality.* Results from the administration of personality tests are meager and contradictory and are complicated by language difficulties (see Chapter 20). Information concerning the personality of deaf children has been obtained from three types of tests: (1) behavior rating scales and questionnaires with the parent, houseparent, or teacher as informant, for example, the Vineland Social Maturity Scale or the Haggerty-Olson-Wickman Behavior Rating Scale; (2) questionnaires answered by deaf children, for example, the Rogers Test of Personality Adjustment, revised for the deaf by Brunschwig, or the California Test of Personality; (3) projective techniques such as the Rorschach Ink Blot Test, the Draw-a-Person Test, or the Make-a-Picture-Story Test (MAPS).

All of the questionnaires contain items that are not valid for use with the deaf because they require communication skills and normal hearing. When these items are eliminated, ratings indicate that the deaf have more emotional problems and less maturity. When a child fills in the questionnaire, the problems of reading comprehension, interpretation of qualifying vocabulary, such as "usually," "sometimes," and imagination influence his responses. In a study of the California Test of Personality as a tool for measurement, Vegly and Elliott (1968) found that items that were not understood presented semantic rather than syntactic problems. It was hypothesized that even after revision of items and test norms, deaf children would continue to show poorer adjustment.

Using the Rorschach Test, Levine found confirmatory evidence of mental "underdevelopment" and that personality development is closely linked to language development. Myklebust reported emotional immaturity with more emotional stress, conflict, and frustration for deaf children enrolled in day classes and more isolation for those in residential schools. On the Draw-a-Person Test used in his study, the deaf child showed perceptual distortions regarding himself and projected these to others. Hess has developed a nonverbal modification of the MAPS test for children 8, 9, and 10 years old. In a preliminary report the deaf differed from the adjusted and emotionally disturbed by showing faster and more impulsive reactions to new situations but with indication of adequate involvement. There was evidence of more expansive fantasy life, superficial personal attachment, and depressive emotional tone.

Personality tests are valuable tools in counseling the deaf because they may reveal problems that the school counselor did not suspect existed. They are essential in the vocational counseling program, and tests used for deaf adolescents and adults are described in Chapter 20 along with elaboration of other problems in assessing the abilities of deaf persons. At present there does not seem to be a personality of "the deaf" but rather individual differences that are significant both in teaching and in guidance of deaf children.

*Language development and concepts.* We know that language is fundamental for hearing-impaired children. A satisfactory description of language is essential for an improved understanding of how language is learned and, consequently, of how it should be taught is a satisfactory description of language. Investigators and teachers have not been satisfied by vague and frequently misleading assertions about deaf children being "2 to 5 years retarded" or about their having typical "deaf language." They have used such measures as sentence length and complexity, the frequency of occurrence of certain parts of speech and certain orders of words, the extent of vocabulary, so-called "type-token ratios" (the relation between the number of *different* words and *total* words in a sample of language), and subordination and abstractions. They have used the methods of structural linguistics to analyze the functional and lexical features of the spoken and written language of deaf children. This is one of many possible leads to better descriptions of language and to improved techniques of teaching vocabulary, syntactical patterns, and the semantic rules that relate words or sentences to things or events, not to mention the subtle and little-understood interweaving of the learning of language and the forming of concepts.

Psycholinguists are suggesting descriptive methods that enlighten us on how a child comprehends and manipulates language, particularly syntax. It has been suggested that children have a general capacity to acquire syntax, and this may be thought of as an inborn set of predispositions to develop a complex grammar from small amounts of information. The implications of this view for language instruction for deaf children are being explored.

How and if at all language competence is related to concept formation in deaf children is still an open question. The situation is complicated by generalizing about rather select groups of deaf children, taught by one "method" or another and educated in different environments, day or residential, manual or oral, or combinations of these. In general, the tasks presented to deaf children in studies of their ability to "conceptualize" have been weighted heavily in the direction of categorization. The studies show that deaf children can categorize "concrete" material as well as hearing children can but do less well in categorizing verbally. The tasks have been quite simple, and higher mental processes seem not to have been investigated. Throughout there is an assumption that verbal performance is equated with linguistic competence, but it may be reasonable to suggest that a sign or gesture, although not verbal, may have linguistic attributes.

In any event, a helpful way for parents and teachers to think of language development, suggested by Simmons, is shown in Figure 16-5.

## The Skills of Communication

It is obvious that the skills of *speaking,* of *understanding* speech (speechreading and "hearing"), and of *language* are interrelated in their development. For convenience, however, and without slighting the interrelations, we shall consider separately the following topics (treated generally in Chapters 12, 13, and 14): speech, auditory training, speechreading, and language.

*Speech.* Studies of the speech of deaf children have, by and large, dealt with differences between the speech of the deaf and of subjects with normal hearing. By a technique of kymographic recording, Dr. C. V. Hudgins, at Clarke School for the Deaf, found the following abnormalities in the speech of the deaf: slow and labored speech, usually accompanied by high chest

SOME STEPS of LANGUAGE DEVELOPMENT

SKILLS
Reading, writing,
spelling and composing

MATURE LANGUAGE
Involved syntax and reflection
vocabulary of 5000 +

CONNECTED LANGUAGE
Simple structure –   requests and
questions

LARGER EXPRESSIVE UNITS
Prepositional phrase
Participal phrase

LIMITED EXPRESSIVE LANGUAGE
Naming –  Adjectives
Few verbs

IMITATIONS
Actions including mouthing
Sounds including speech

FREE COMPREHENSION
Concepts
Connected language

SITUATIONAL COMPREHENSION
Concrete items
Visible actions

AWARENESS
Concepts
Vocabulary

EXPOSURE

Fig. 16-5. Some steps of language development. (A. A. Simmons, unpublished)

pressure with the expenditure of excessive amounts of breath; prolonged vowels with consequent distortion; abnormalities of rhythm; excessive nasality of both vowels and consonants; and imperfect joining of consonants, with the consequent addition of superfluous syllables between abutting pairs.

We gain a substantial insight into the speech of the deaf from the investigation of Dr. Hudgins and F. C. Numbers, who departed from the usual approach of comparing the speech of the deaf and of the hearing and studied the relation between errors of articulation and rhythm and the intelligibility of the speech of deaf schoolchildren. Ten sentences spoken by deaf children were recorded and then were analyzed by a group of auditors. They found two general types of error: errors of articulation involving both consonants and vowels and errors of rhythm.

Consonant errors were classified into seven general types, as follows: failure to distinguish between voiced and unvoiced consonants, consonant substitutions, excessive nasality, malarticulation of compound consonants, malarticulation of abutting consonants, omission of arresting consonants, and omission of releasing consonants.

The vowel errors were vowel substitutions, malarticulation of diphthongs, diphthongization of vowels, neutralization of vowels, and nasalization of vowels.

In general, our experimental and empirical evidence indicates that the deaf child who lacks an adequate auditory monitor is likely to develop, at least under present methods of instruction, a breathy, nasalized vocal quality, abnormal temporal and intonational patterns, and some surprisingly consistent errors of articulation. These observations do not imply that deaf children cannot be taught to speak intelligibly. Many do. They do, however, show where there is the greatest opportunity to improve our methods of teaching speech to deaf children.

FUNDAMENTAL ATTITUDE. As we have indicated previously, all educators of the deaf endorse the proposition that all deaf children shall have an opportunity to learn to speak. But the implementation of this notion in everyday practice reveals fundamental differences in attitudes.

For some educators, speech is a subject to be taught like a foreign language to those who can "benefit" from it. Practice and atmosphere are not aimed at vitalizing speech for the child. Rather, speech is viewed as an eminently desirable but not essential skill. For others (including ourselves), a corollary to the proposition of universality of opportunity to learn speech is inescapable: speech is a basic means of communication, and hence is a vital mechanism of adjustment to the communicating world about us. Therefore, we set the stage for speech *everywhere*—in the home, on the playground, in the schoolroom—from the moment we learn that a child is deaf, so that speech eventually becomes meaningful, significant, and purposeful for him at all times. We believe that parents, counselors, teachers, and all others who are responsible for the child's development should share this attitude. Only constant practice and actual use of speech will develop fully the deaf child's latent ability to communicate by speech. The absence of a "living speech environment" may account for some of the so-called "oral failures" in schools for the deaf.

THE MULTISENSORY APPROACH. Obviously the teacher must use all available sensory channels for teaching speech to a deaf child: the visual, the auditory, the tactile, and the kinesthetic.

When we consider the use to which we put *the visual system* in teaching speech, we tend to think primarily of speechreading. The child learns to watch with purpose the movements of the lips and the expressions of the faces of those about him and to imitate, however imperfectly, these movements in attempts to express himself. This really is the initial technique with deaf infants. Other well-known uses of vision include systems of orthography, color codes that differentiate the manner of production of phonetic elements, fingerspelling, models and diagrams that show position and movement of the mechanisms of speech, and acoustic translators of various sorts that display speech patterns visually and can carry information to the eye about time, frequency, and intensity. Now under consideration in some schools is the recently advocated system of "cued speech" which aims to improve the acquisition of speech and its production. It is a system of communication in which phoneme, syllable, or word is identified from lip movements with the aid of 12 cues supplied by the hands.

We know that the literature, even of the nineteenth century (Urbantschitsch, 1897), mentions the desirability of using *the auditory system* to aid in teaching speech to the deaf. Today we are better able to exploit this possibility because of the development of modern, wearable, and also group, hearing aids designed to deliver speech to the auditory area that the child still possesses. For the kind of child whom we are here discussing the auditory area is greatly restricted, but, as we have seen in Chapter 13, even a limited perception of stress patterns can help a child to achieve better rhythmic and voice quality and to better understand speech.

*The tactile or vibratory sense* is most commonly used by placing the child's fingertips or hands in contact with his own or the teacher's face or head during speech or during phonation. We have mentioned that some techniques use sounding boards, including pianos, and diaphragms which are caused to vibrate by speech and music. Surprisingly good differential sensitivity of the thoracic region of severely deaf children has been demonstrated. It has been suggested that translation of speech to the sense of touch by the principle of frequency analysis used in the visible-speech machine is possible. The argument is that the visible-speech instrument has shown how much and what kind of information must be transmitted to identify the words that are spoken. But rather than vision, the sense of touch is to be used. It is too early to assess the results of this approach, but it is unlikely, on general principles, that it will be any more successful than visible speech itself (see Chapter 14).

*The kinesthetic sense* is used in "getting the feel" of certain articulatory and vocal movements and in tongue and lip exercises. Some teachers employ rhythmic grossmuscle movements to reinforce kinesthetically the utterance of connected speech and of suitable nonsense syllables.

Many techniques to teach speech to the deaf are in common use. One reason for their variety is the wide difference of opinion concerning the relative emphasis that should be placed on each sensory pathway. Some believe that speech is better learned if attention is concentrated on one sense at a time and the others are deliberately excluded. The opposite view favors mutual reinforcement of the senses and a coordinated sensory input. In support of the latter view, it has been shown that a small fragment of hearing may be trained to supplement vision usefully in a visual-auditory presentation. In other words, the eye and the ear together perceive speech better than either one alone. Hence, it is argued, the bisensory approach is likely to produce better speech. The counterargument is that,

at least in the early stages, speechreading should be excluded from auditory training because the speechreading is likely to divert the child from full use of his hearing. Shutting the eyes of the child while he is learning to differentiate vibrations has also been suggested.

In developing techniques, it is desirable for the teacher to analyze the speech skill she is trying to cultivate and to select the combination of sensory channels best suited to stimulate the child. For example, the perception of the phonetic element $p$ is best accomplished through vision reinforced by feeling, and vowel differentiation is greatly aided by a combination of auditory, visual, and tactile stimulation. We believe that the sum of reinforced multisensory stimulation is greater than any of its parts. It is, in fact, "the nearest approach to the normal that can be made by the deaf child."

SYSTEMS OF ORTHOGRAPHY. Students of speech are aware of the irrationality of our symbols for discrete units of speech. The letters of our alphabet bear no consistent relation to the sounds they represent. Furthermore, most of our symbols represent more than one sound, and most of our sounds are represented by more than one symbol. This situation has led teachers of the deaf to devise systems of orthography that carry more information about speech units than do the unrelated letters of the alphabet.

The Bells created their system of *visible speech* in 1894. In this system consonants are represented by four fundamental curves that relate to the "articulators," that is, to the back of the tongue, the top of the tongue, the point of the tongue, and the lips. The insertion of a short "voice" line in the bow of the curve changes a voiceless consonant to a voiced consonant. For example, ɑ (which is $k$) becomes ɑ (which is $g$). There is also a system for modifying the fundamental symbols to represent the vowels. This system is described in the

Bells' book, entitled *The Mechanism of Speech.*

*The Northampton charts,* originated at Clarke School for the Deaf and popular with many teachers of the deaf, are arranged to give more phonetic significance to letters of the English alphabet. The charts do this by arranging the symbols in columns and rows according to the method of production of the sounds (see **Figure 16-6a and b**). Thus the consonants *p, b,* and *m* are in the same row because the lips are initially shut in the production of all three. They are in different columns because *p* is voiceless, *b* is voiced, and *m* is nasal. This arrangement shows the differences and similarities among sounds that are described by Dr. Carhart in Chapter 14. The multiplicity of letters and combinations of letters that represent the same sound are handled by arranging secondary spellings under the primary symbol, which is the one that occurs most frequently in the English usage. Thus *a-e* is the primary symbol for the diphthong in "cake." Here the dash represents any consonant. A secondary spelling under *a-e* is *ay,* as in "say."

The diacritical system used in our dictionaries assumes familiarity with the pronunciation of common key words. Where one letter may represent more than one sound, a differentiating symbol is used; thus *e* as in "be" is ē, and *e* as in "bed" is ĕ.

Phoneticians and linguists generally use the *International Phonetic Alphabet,* which has a single standard symbol for each sound and adds new symbols to the Roman alphabet to provide the necessary extra symbols.

Dr. A. Zaliouk, late Director of the Institute for the Deaf (in Haifa, Israel), devised a *visual-tactile system of phonetic symbolization* for teaching speech to the deaf. This uses two categories of symbols, static and dynamic. The static symbols represent the hard palate, the tongue, the teeth, and the lips, all of which participate in various "articulatory positions." The dynamic symbols indicate movement.

A recent addition to the pool of orthographic systems that may have value for deaf children is the *International Teaching Alphabet (i.t.a.),* of Sir James Pitman, as shown in Figure 16-7. It eliminates ambiguity by having only one symbol for each spoken sound and is arranged alphabetically. It is claimed that it "leads in" easily to reading and writing.

There have been other attempts, too numerous to mention, that have sought through shorthand or other means to convey phonetic information by a logical and consistent system of symbols. An ideal system of orthography would convey information on how to articulate, use the ordinary alphabet, be within the grasp of children, and be free of ambiguities. Obviously these criteria are in conflict, and some compromises must be made. For example, if we were looking primarily for symbols to convey information on how to articulate, we would probably choose the system of Bell or of Zaliouk. The Northampton charts, with their secondary spellings, represent the letters and combinations of letters used most frequently in the English langauge, and hence should show how to pronounce the written word. On the other hand, because there are so many secondary spellings and exceptions, the learned combinations may be confusing out of the context of the chart. The diacritical markings of the dictionary are obviously useful, but everyday printed English does not carry these marks. One of the drawbacks of the international phonetic alphabet is that some of its symbols are not letters of the alphabet. Some teachers prefer to start children with the Northampton charts and then to teach the diacritical marks when children reach the appropriate academic level. These comments on the various systems are by no means exhaustive, but they may be useful as a guide in choosing a system of phonetic symbolization.

UNITS OF SPEECH. The various approaches to teaching articulation to the deaf may

## CONSONANT SOUNDS

h—

wh    w—

p    b    m

t    d    n    l    r—

k    g¹    ng
ck
c

f    v
ph

th¹    th²

s¹    z
c(e)    s²
c(i)
c(y)

sh    zh    y—

ch    j
tch    g²—
       —ge
       dge

x = ks    qu = kwh

## VOWEL SOUNDS

oo¹    oo²    o—e    aw    —o—
(r) u–e    oa    au
(r) ew    —o²    o(r)
          ow

ee    —i—    a—e    —e—    —a—
–e    —y    ai    ea²
ea¹         ay
e–e

a(r)    —u—    ur
        —a    er
               ir

a—e    i—e    o—e    ou    oi    u—e
ai    igh    oa    ow¹    oy    ew
ay    —y    —o²
            ow

Fig. 16-6A. The Northampton Consonant Chart. In the consonant chart the left-hand column is occupied by the English breath consonants; the second column, by the voiced forms of the same sounds; the third, by the nasal sounds. The horizontal arrangement classifies these sounds according to formation. A dash following a letter indicates that the sound is initial in a word or syllable.

Fig. 16-6B. The Northampton Vowel Chart. In the vowel chart the upper line contains the back round vowels (those modified chiefly by the back of the tongue and the rounded aperture of the lips). The second line contains the front vowels (those modified chiefly by the front of the tongue). Remaining vowels are in the third line. The lowest line contains all the diphthongal sounds. Although ā and ō appear in the rows to which their radical (long component) parts belong, they are repeated here because their compound nature makes them diphthongs also.

An attempt is also made in these charts to teach the simple rules of pronunciation. For illustration, *a-e* (representing *a*) when contrasted with -*a*- (representing *ă*), is easily made intelligible by the introduction of the same consonants in both sets of blanks: r*a*te, r*a*t; h*a*te, h*a*t, and so on. Children will not find diacritical marks over the words in their books or in other material, but if they are familiar with the principles of pronunciation represented here, they will know that final *e* modifies the sound of the vowel preceding it, making *a*, *ā*; *e*, *ē*; *i*, *ī*; *o*, *ō*. The secondary spellings under each sound generally indicate frequently occurring variations for those sounds. Numbers above the sounds differentiate pronunciations for similar spellings. In this way words are made to pronounce themselves to the eye of the child. Eventually, the children learn the diacritical marks of the dictionary. (*Adapted from Caroline A. Yale, Formation and Development of English Elementary Sounds, Northampton, Mass., 1925, Gazette Printing Company.*)

CAN i.t.a. HELP THE DEAF CHILD, HIS PARENTS AND HIS TEACHER?

Sir James Pitman, K.B.E.  London

---

ｚhis iƨ printed in ｚhe iniſhial tee（hiŋ alfabet, ｚhe purpoƨ ov whi（h iƨ not, aƨ miet bee suppœƨd, tω reform our spelliŋ, but tω imprωv ｚhe lerniŋ ov reediŋ. it iƨ intended ｚhat when ｚhe beginner iƨ flωent in ｚhis meedium hee ſhωd bee confiend tω reediŋ in ｚhe tradiſhoňal alfabet

if yω hav red aƨ far aƨ ｚhis, ｚhe nue meedium will hav prωvd tω yω several points, ｚhe mœst important ov whi（h iƨ ｚhat yω, at eny ræt, hav eeƨily mæd ｚhe （hænj from ｚhe ordinary rœman alfabet wiｚh convenſhonal spelliŋs tω ｚhe iniſhial tee（hiŋ alfabet wiｚh systematic spelliŋ.

---

Here is the alphabet arranged systematically:-

| a<br>apple | ɑ<br>father | æ<br>angel | aʋ<br>author | b<br>bed | c<br>cat | ｃh<br>chair |
|---|---|---|---|---|---|---|
| d<br>doll | ɛɛ<br>eel | e<br>egg | f<br>finger | g<br>girl | h<br>hat | ie<br>tie |
| i<br>ink | j<br>jam | k<br>kitten | l<br>lion | m<br>man | n<br>nest | ŋ<br>king |
| œ<br>toe | o<br>on | ω<br>book | ꟺ<br>food | ou<br>out | oi<br>oil | p<br>pig |
| r<br>red | ɾ<br>bird | s<br>soap | ʃh<br>ship | ʒ<br>treasure | t<br>tree | ｔh<br>three |
| ｔh<br>mother | ue<br>due | u<br>up | v<br>van | w<br>window | wh<br>wheel | y<br>yellow |
| z<br>zoo | ƨ<br>is | | | | | |

Fig. 16-7. The I. T. A. by Sir James Pitman, K.B.E. From *The Volta Review,* December 1960. Used by permission of The Alexander Graham Bell Association for the Deaf, Inc., and Sir James Pitman.

(Duplicates C and k : z and ƨ : and wh for hw )

properly be placed on a continuum ranging from an elemental, analytical method to a patterned or "natural" approach. The former would emphasize the development of individual elements out of speech contexts, and the latter would begin with words and phrases "as it is natural for hearing children to do." The elementalists argue that in the absence of an appropriate auditory monitor, the kinesthesia of each phonetic element must be fixed before precise articulation can be achieved, lest fluency be attained only at the expense of good articulation. The "naturalists" contend that we must take advantage of the spontaneous articulation, temporal patterns, and voice qualities of young children. These generally are not isolated elements, and the naturalists believe that precision *can* be achieved within the framework of natural, spontaneous vocal output without sacrificing fluency.

Most present-day practice lies between these two extremes. It regards the syllable as the basic unit. The syllable is probably the simplest possible utterance in speech. Individual sounds cannot be uttered without somehow making a syllable. As Stetson, a great phonetician, expressed it:

When teachers and demonstrators give what they think are "separate sounds" they are actually uttering syllables; the vowels and on occasion the liquids and nasals constitute separate syllables, as in "oh, a, rr . . . , ll" . . . , long drawn out fricatives, ss . . . etc., become vowel substitutes, and other consonants are given with a brief vowel, as in "buh, puh." . . .

Of course, individual sounds may be corrected but they should not be considered learned until they are articulated properly in the kinds of syllables in which they are likely to occur. Furthermore, speech rhythm, which contributes to intelligibility, is primarily a matter of grouping, accentuating, and phrasing syllables. The babbled syllable and the building of connected rhythmic speech from syllabic units are used in many methods for the development of speech.

In studies of the development of sounds in young children with normal hearing it has been shown that by the tenth month practically all of the different sounds have appeared. Yet it is curious that even though a child may have produced *l* and *r* during his infantile babbling, he frequently cannot, at the age of 2 or 3, produce these sounds correctly in English words. Apparently he finds it difficult to use the phonetic elements of his babbling as the phonemes of his language. This relearning comes about by biologic maturation, perceptive development, both auditory and kinesthetic, and, in the case of the deaf child, by the use of whatever sensory channels are available.

EVALUATION OF SPEECH. Frequent critical evaluation of the *intelligibility* of the speech of deaf children is important, both as a guide to modifying existing methods of teaching and, particularly, as an objective assessment of the oral method. Evaluations can be made periodically during the school career of a deaf child, during which he is exposed to formal training in speech by one method or another. Other long-range procedures could be designed to discover how intelligible the speech of deaf pupils continues to be after they have graduated from schools for the deaf.

A child's improvement in speech intelligibility may be evaluated by periodic tests, but the available tests are not as objective or as valid as our corresponding tests of many other skills or of a child's mastery of subject matter. In one popular procedure a child reads a selection, and auditors indicate the extent to which the selection has been understood. Or carefully selected word samples are read and scored by the auditors. In a sense, the tests determine the extent to which the deviant talker imposes a loss of discrimination for speech on a normal listener. Although this may yield a limited but fairly reasonable appraisal of the mechanics of the child's speech, it does not simulate the pattern of usual oral intercourse which takes place without benefit of a printed or written visual aid. What is being evaluated is a form of *oral reading* and not speech in broad social terms. The translation of the child's *own* thoughts into intelligible speech is an ability neglected by this type of evaluation.

The use of memorized material without visual aid is subject to similar criticism, since the thoughts expressed usually are not the child's own; or, if they are, they have been memorized. This furnishes the child an advantage which he does not have in a normal social situation. The interview, in which the child is stimulated to talk freely, may yield a fairly accurate appraisal of speech if it is conducted skillfully. Very often in an interview, however, the child may correctly anticipate the questions; furthermore, the technique fails to appraise the child's ability to initiate speech. The use of speech recordings for periodic evaluation has considerable value. However, the limitations of printed or memorized selections and of the question-and-answer type of sample should be kept in mind. Of course, it would help to capture for study the casual conversation of children. We should be cautious about the inferences we make that relate tests of talker intelligibility to social usefulness of speech. The two are not always linearly related. Attitudes of talker and listener having to do with confidence, encouragement, frustration, motivation—all these play their role in the use a deaf person makes of his speech.

The outcomes of speech teaching which are most important in the long run are those that reveal the extent to which the benefits of the child's training in speech persist after he has left school. Unfortunately, we have no satisfactory evidence in this area, and the information that comes to us is frequently biased and invariably anecdotal. Good follow-up studies are a task which zealous oralists might profitably undertake.

Our discussion of teaching speech to the deaf suggests the following guides to practice:

1. An environment must be created or maintained for the child in which speech is experienced as a vitally significant and successful means of communication. Oralism is as much an atmosphere and an attitude as it is a "method" of teaching.
2. Spontaneity of speech should be encouraged, but formal instruction is necessary at the appropriate stage in a child's development. Good speech in deaf children does not come of itself.
3. The proper combination of the visual, auditory, tactile, and kinesthetic pathways should be exploited early, rationally, and vigorously.
4. The syllable is a suitable unit for the development of articulation and of desirable temporal patterns in speech. Through its use, adequate coordination of parts of the speech mechanism is more likely to be achieved.
5. A functional system of visual phonetic aids is essential.
6. Judicious correction of poor articulation, including individual phonetic elements, and of undesirable rhythm and voice quality is necessary. The acceptance of poor speech encourages its use. The teacher is the only accurate monitor of the child's speech, and she must let him know how he can improve it.
7. Periodic and long-range evaluations of the social effectiveness of the speech of the deaf, even though it be informal, is useful for both diagnosis and educational planning.

Future investigations of the speech of deaf children should be greatly stimulated by the availability of improved tools and methods for the investigation of speech as an acoustic event. Techniques are at hand for analyzing and synthesizing speech, for displaying it visibly and tactually and for repackaging it by selective filtering, frequency transposition, temporal expansion and compression (Chapter 11). Our understanding of the physiological mechanisms of speech is being enriched by the techniques of high-speed photography of the larynx during phonation and of x-ray views of the articulators in action. Helpful, too, is our study of speech that is deviant because of structural pathologies, such as cleft palate, vocal nodules, absent or partially removed larynx, or deficient innervation of speech musculature as in cerebral palsy.

*Auditory training.* The great advance

in electroacoustic instrumentation of the past three decades, both for testing hearing and for amplifying sound, has generated a sustained and substantial interest in auditory training. We must remind ourselves that in this chapter we are concerned with children who have a severely restricted auditory area. The auditory area that remains to them, if any, lies at high sound pressure levels near the threshold of pain (see Chapter 2). These levels can be reached for communication only by means of powerful, well-designed hearing aids. Both group hearing aids and individual hearing aids have been described in Chapters 10 and 11. There we have pointed out the necessity for proper limitation of acoustic output and the advantages and limitations of compression amplification in "packaging" speech for effective delivery to the child's restricted auditory area. Our understanding of the reception of speech has been aided greatly by the contributions of information theory and by our knowledge of pertinent acoustic properties of speech. Information theory concerns itself with the predictability of elements in communication or, in other words, guessing what comes next based on probabilities of occurrence of a phoneme, a word or a phrase according to the particular structure of a language. What is important for the hearing-impaired is that we now know how much can be "guessed" in the absence of much of a message. The cueing that may be possible with a small amount of residual hearing, properly amplified, may be greater than heretofore supposed.

The presence of low-frequency hearing in many children has stimulated various schemes of signal-processing that re-form the speech signal to improve its perceptibility. In general speech-compression systems of one sort or another are being tried that reduce the bandwidth much as is done in transmission by radio and telephone. For many children, listening over such systems requires that a new language be learned.

Several objectives of auditory training are within the reach of deaf children.

IMPROVEMENT IN SPEECH PERCEPTION. Deaf children are not likely to achieve much auditory discrimination for speech, certainly not enough to understand ordinary language through hearing alone. However, they can be taught to appreciate temporal patterns of speech and also to improve their control of the intensity and, in some instances, the pitch of their voices. Refined appreciation of phrasing and stress patterns may be expected to improve the child's ability to attain the "rhythmic grouping" which can contribute greatly to the intelligibility of his own speech. Auditory training improves speech perception, particularly when it is combined with speechreading. Failure of improvement in communication by speech after a regimen of auditory training may often be due to the fact that the training was not begun early enough. It should begin in the first year of life.

IMPROVEMENT IN LANGUAGE SKILLS. Although there is no definitive experimental evidence that auditory training improves language skills, it seems likely that the information carried by stressing and phrasing, not easily discerned by speechreading, adds to the meaning and significance of connected language. Vocabulary, particularly words with auditory associations, may be enriched. For example, if a child reads, "The baby cried," the word "cried," which has auditory connotations, has limited meaning for him even though he is able to draw a line between it and the word "baby" in his workbook and he has seen a picture of a baby crying. On the other hand, a recording of the cry of a baby played over an amplifying system, even though not perceived precisely, should enrich the meaning of the word "cry."

IMPROVEMENT IN PSYCHOLOGICAL COUPLING TO THE HEARING WORLD. Again, convincing experimental evidence is lacking. Nevertheless, consider the deaf child at a ball game. A thrilling play is made on the diamond that evokes a spontaneous outburst of yelling from the crowd. The child sees the hands clap and wave, the spectators rise from their seats, the mouths open, but he has not caught the full emotional impact of the moment because its basic richness lies in the yelling of the crowd and the accompanying noises. This is an auditory experience. If the child could perceive just the presence of these noises, however distorted, through a hearing aid, he would share more richly in the group experience. Not to be overlooked are the esthetic appreciations which may result from auditory exposure to the rhythm of music. Many deaf children who have been trained to appreciate rhythmic cadences seem to enjoy dancing and eurythmics.

Although it is likely that the future will reveal additional and greater values of auditory training, our statements of objectives within reach suggest that we must be cautious of the extravagant claims sometimes made for the use of hearing aids by deaf children, particularly the claim that if they are equipped from infancy with a hearing aid, they do not need special education.

Despite the unsolved problems that are still with us, there is no longer any question about the usefulness of the auditory system in the education of the deaf children. Dr. Hirsh, in Chapter 13, has delineated the fundamentals of auditory training for children. Out of our experience grow the following guides for practice in auditory training:

1. Most deaf children have a small but useful portion of the auditory area that lies above the range of usual audiometry. Consequently, many children who have been termed "totally deaf" as a result of audiometric tests actually can hear properly amplified sound. Audiograms may not tell the whole story of a child's ability to appreciate speech by his hearing. Formal auditory training is essential, however, to teach the deaf child to make use of this remnant of hearing. The hearing aid alone is not enough.

2. Auditory training appears to be more

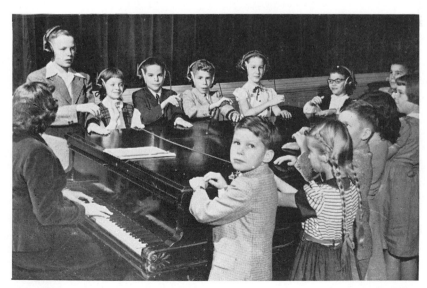

Fig. 16-8. Reinforcing auditory and visual stimulation with rhythmical tactile impressions from the piano. This procedure helps the fluency of speech. (*Central Institute for the Deaf.*)

effective, through mutual reinforcement, when hearing is combined with vision and/or touch. There are times when hearing alone is used to teach a child to concentrate on specified information-bearing cues.

3. The techniques of auditory training should be geared to a child's auditory capabilities. This requires frequent assessment of his hearing.

4. Auditory training, even without a hearing aid, should be begun as soon as it is determined that a child is deaf.

5. Formal instruction can make hearing aids more acceptable to children by giving them experiences that are meaningful. Such instruction should teach children to discriminate, even though grossly, various environmental sounds, and, within the limits of their hearing, teach them to understand speech by hearing.

6. Informally and wherever practicable, the child should have the benefit of amplified sound, either by a group hearing aid or a wearable one, in all of his classroom work, at home, and also at play.

7. Children should be taught as early as possible the use, the management, and the care of their own hearing aids.

*Speechreading.* As we have said repeatedly, children with normal hearing learn oral language primarily by hearing, which is reinforced by other sensory experience. The sounds are later associated with the visual symbols, that is, the movements of the talker's face, that partly represent language. This is speechreading. The deaf child is denied the possibility of learning this by association with auditory language, and is forced to learn his visual speechreading language directly. The extent to which he is able to do this may depend upon a number of factors, some of which are exceedingly complex and difficult to analyze. One group of factors concerns the speaker. These include his distance and position and direction from the speechreader and how well his face is illuminated. They include the character of his speech, his precision of articulation, how fast he talks, the mobility of his face, and the familiarity of the speechreader with the particular speaker. Then there are factors concerning the language material, such as the vocabulary and the language structure. Finally, there is the speechreader himself, his vision, his intelligence, his general information, and his ability to synthesize from contextual clues, to recognize discrete units of speech, to associate his own "feel" for speech with the speech he sees on the face, and the fundamental structure of his personality, which may determine his attitude toward speechreading.

Speechreading is further complicated by the ambiguities that result from hidden movements, such as $h$ and $k$, from homophonous words (words that look alike on the lips, such as "smell" and "spell"), and from the difficulty of appreciating patterns of stress, intonation, and phrasing.

Numerous attempts have been made to assess the role of these factors in speechreading to diagnose difficulties, to evaluate progress and methods of instruction, and to predict performance.

Among the possible factors that may be related to skill in speechreading and which have been investigated are intelligence, reading ability, perceptual ability, motivation, and rhythmic skills. These studies have led to no generalizations in which we have confidence. One of the major problems in studying these relations is the adequacy of tests of speechreading. The test constructers are faced with formidable variables that are unique to the population to be tested. Among these are the degree and kind of hearing loss, the time of onset of impaired hearing, the language ability of the subjects, the standardization of the test material itself, and particularly of the manner of its presentation. There is also the difficulty of establishing norms for a heterogeneous population. Furthermore, the validation of the tests appears to rely solely on ratings by teachers. This introduces new problems.

Instruction in speechreading for deaf children is usually not a thing apart. In the beginning, even before the child enters school, he is encouraged to watch the face of the talker. The deaf child is not as aware as the hearing child that he can get information, in its broadest sense, by watching the movements of the face. When formal instruction is begun, the child is taught to associate movements of the lips, jaws, and tongue with objects, feelings, and actions. The objective here is not merely the enlargement of speechreading vocabulary but cultivation of the idea that watching the face of the talker is useful. Finally, speechreading pervades every act of speech perception by the child and becomes an increasingly useful tool of communication as it is practiced in purposeful situations.

The inadequacy of our formal tools for assessment of the ability to speechread need not deter us from suggesting the following guides to practice in developing this valuable skill in deaf children:

1. An atmosphere of oral communication must be created and maintained. Speechreading must be shown to serve a purpose.
2. Even if the child is not expected to understand every word of a spoken message, he should be talked to, and he should be encouraged to take advantage of situational clues.
3. Speechreading should be reinforced by other sensory clues whenever practicable.

*Language.* In our discussion of the skills of communication to this point we have, in a sense, considered the development of the skills of talking and "listening,"

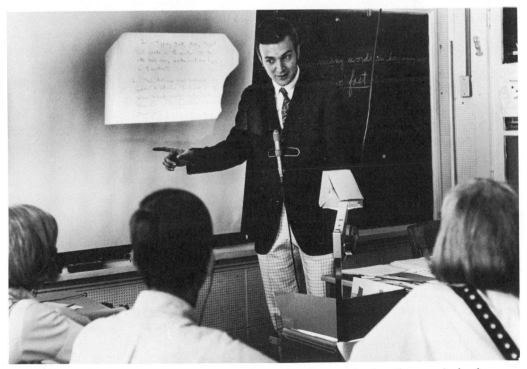

Fig. 16-9. A language class of deaf children using the combined auditory and visual approach. (*Central Institute for the Deaf, photo by Harold Ferman*)

namely, speech, auditory training, and speechreading. We now turn to the message itself, the stuff of oral communication. This is language. The "ear-to-voice link" is essential for talking and listening. It is the basis of a child's attachment of meaning, in speaking, in writing, in listening, and in reading, to words and combinations of words. The absence of hearing is catastrophic for the "natural" but complex development of association of language with experience.

It is the task of the teacher, nevertheless, to develop language in deaf children, although they do not have full use of the sensory channel that is considered essential for the growth of language. In the performance of this task she needs to be aware of the unique problems created by the total absence of hearing or by the severe distortions of auditory verbal experience. Among the major problems for the child are vocabulary, multiple meanings of words, the verbalization of abstractions, and the complexity of the structure of language.

VOCABULARY. It is difficult to determine when a child really "knows" a word. Does he have it in his spoken, his written, his reading, or his listening vocabulary? The different kinds of vocabulary account for differences in the estimates of the functional vocabulary of children. At any rate, it is interesting that one representative study shows that hearing children "know" 272 words at the age of 2, 1540 at 4, and 2562 at 6. Compare this with zero words that the deaf child is likely to know when he enters school, even at the age of 3 or, more frequently, at 6.

MULTIPLE MEANINGS. Single words in our language may have many meanings that are eventually clarified for hearing children, chiefly by the repeated auditory experience that is denied the deaf child. An average of almost four meanings per recurring word was found by count in twelve commonly used arithmetic textbooks. For example, the word "over" could mean "above" (the number over 5 is the quotient); "across" (over the Arctic Ocean); "again" (do your work over); "at an end" (the show is over); "more than" (over half the children); "besides" (left over); "during" (over a period of two years); "present" (turn the meeting over to); "on the other side" (turn the card "over"); "by means of" (over the radio).

VERBALIZATION OF ABSTRACTIONS. Of course, hearing children and, for that matter, adults may experience difficulty in attaching words to abstract concepts, but the deaf child is in particular need of formal and informal but nonetheless deliberate instruction in the meaning of such relatively simple abstractions as *hope* and *want*.

COMPLEXITY OF STRUCTURE. Smith has shown that by the age of 5 the spoken sentence of the average child has reached five words in length. For the superior child it is about ten words long. This increase in length is inevitably accompanied by the use of complex syntactical relations that clarify and enrich meaning. These involve such grammatical concepts as pronouns, connectives, tense, person, and word order, as well as relations among clauses and among phrases of various sorts. If the hearing child reaches these levels of complexity at the age of 5, we are again struck by the extent of the language gap between the deaf and the hearing. It was found by the Heiders at Clarke School, after their thorough comparison of sentence structure in the written compositions of deaf and hearing children, that the "whole picture indicates a simpler style (for the deaf) involving relatively rigid unrelated language units which follow each other with little overlapping structure or meaning."

In general, the deaf appear to be comparatively deficient in the flexible manipulation of our language in order to make the best use of it as a tool of communication. This may be due to their educational retardation; it may be due to the methods of teaching language, or, in addition to these, to the idea suggested by the Heiders that "the difference between the deaf and the hearing cannot be fully expressed in quantitative terms as the degree of retardation" and "that they represent differences not merely of skill in the use of language forms but in the whole thought structure."

METHODS OF INSTRUCTION IN LANGUAGE. Methods of instruction of the deaf in language can be divided conveniently into two major approaches: the natural method, sometimes known as the synthetic, informal, or mother method; and the grammatical method, sometimes referred to as the logical, systematic, formal, analytical, or artifical method.

Historically, the grammatical method preceded the natural method. It was based on the notion that after memorization of classifications of words and their conjugations and declensions, they could be used as building blocks for connected language. This approach evolved into a multiplicity of "systems" that were created primarily to provide a systematic set of visible symbols to guide deaf children in the use of language. We shall briefly describe three of the more popular ones.

*The Barry Five Slate System.* The assumption underlying this system, developed by Katherine E. Barry (1899) at the Colorado School for the Deaf, is that ability to analyze the relations among parts of sentences is necessary to the "clear thinking" essential to an understanding of language. Five slates or columns are visible on the walls of the schoolroom. The subject of a sentence goes on the first slate, the verb on the second, the object of the verb on the third, the preposition on the fourth, and the object of the preposition on the fifth. Children then learn the rationale of the verbalization of their actions according to the visual aid afforded by the slates. This system, many believe, tends to stultify idiomatic expression and actually may result in ungrammatical, stilted language.

*Wing's Symbols.* This system, devised in 1883 by George Wing of the Minnesota School for the Deaf, is based on a set of symbols, mostly numbers and letters, representing the functions of different parts of speech in a sentence. These symbols are placed over the word, phrase, or clause in order to demonstrate the form, function, and position of the parts of a sentence, rather than just to illustrate parts of speech. For example, *1* stands for the noun, *2* for a possessive, and *0* for the object. Advocates of the system believe that it is of great value as a corrective tool throughout the child's career and that it encourages correct grammatical usage.

*The Fitzgerald Key.* This system, first published in 1926, was developed by Edith Fitzgerald (1937), a congenitally deaf person, when she was head teacher at the Virginia School. Miss Fitzgerald advocated developing "natural" language but thought that this could be aided by developing the child's power of reasoning, judgment, and discrimination about language. This is accomplished by a set of key words and symbols related to language that was developed as it was needed by the children. There are six symbols, one each for verbs, infinitives, present participles, connectives, pronouns, and adjectives. For example, the symbol for a verb is =. Among the advantages of the method are its comprehensiveness, its flexibility, and the possibilities for self-correction.

The basic feature of the grammatical systems is the emphasis on getting the child to *analyze* functional relations among discrete units of language and, by repetition and visual aids, to impart to him an understanding of language principles or linguistic "rules," including the way in which the arrangement of words affects the meaning of a sentence. Methods that combine an analysis of the structure of language, a Key system, and expanding "kernel" sentences or patterns are also in use.

One of the early advocates of *the natural method* was D. Greenberger, who headed what is now the Lexington School for the Deaf in New York City. He believed that language was best learned by supplying it to children in the situations in which they had need for it. Practice was geared to actual and natural situations. A leading advocate of this approach is Dr. Mildred Groht, who suggests that prior to the time a language principle is to be introduced formally it should be used in natural situations through speechreading and writing. It is then drilled on in various ways that are interesting and purposeful for the child. In essence, the teacher creates situations which provide many and varied contacts with the principles of language. The method is claimed to be more consistent with the laws of learning of langauge by hearing children than is a formal, analytical method.

Until we gain more insight into how the deaf child conceptualizes, the teacher of language will need to use all the knowledge and ingenuity at her command to combine the best features of a grammatical method with the obvious excellent possibilities of the natural method. She will use such commonly accepted techniques as general conversation, composition, news items, trips, action work, topical essays, experience stories, letters, and descriptions of places, events, and persons. The child's progress in acquiring language will be governed only by the extent to which the teacher uses her own ingenuity, flexibility, and knowledge of how children grow and develop. Perhaps she may find some help in the following guides to practice:

1. Language teaching should be related to significant and meaningful experiences of children.

2. Language should constantly be made to serve a purpose for the child.

3. All sensory channels should be used to teach language.

4. Teachers need to be alert to the ideas that are developing in children so that they may provide the children with language with which to express them.

5. Children need many varied contacts with the same language in order to make it theirs.

6. Many children need formal, systematic aids to the acquisition of language. Many shun language when they feel insecure in its use.

7. Schools and homes should create an atmosphere in which language is used and books are read regularly.

### Curriculum Development in Schools for the Deaf

In general, the curricula of schools for the deaf resemble those in schools for the hearing, with appropriate adaptations for difficulties of verbal communication. However, the growing national concern for improving education of all children at all levels has expressed itself primarily in focusing attention, energy, and abundant resources on curricular revision and reform. Stimulated by these efforts, educators of the deaf are seeking ways to improve the performance of their schools. Efforts in curriculum development have centered around considerations of goals, processes, and materials, and their dissemination, implementation, and evaluation.

*Goals.* An obvious first question in goal setting is: Who sets them? Shall it be school administrators, teachers, parents, deaf adults, mature students, psychologists, social scientists, humanists, employers, psychiatrists, specialists in particular disciplines, funding agencies, or some combination of these? We appear to be a long way from examining on a rational basis the contributions that these and other elements have to make to our formulation of goals.

For example, what can students of mental health tell us about the wisdom of such long-range goals as complete integration of the deaf person in the world of the hearing, on the one hand, or production of contented members of a subgroup, on the other? Certainly the grand design of the educational experience we arrange for our children would be crucially influenced, if not fundamentally determined, by what we think about this issue.

Another question pertinent to goal setting is: How shall they be stated? Shall they be outlines of "content" like "how a plant grows"; shall they be skills like reading, writing, and so on, or behavioral objectives like identifying, describing, distinguishing, naming, stating, and applying a rule? Shall they go beyond the cognitive and apply to total human functioning?

What schemes are possible to bring these categories into some reasonable relationship?

Attainability is still another important aspect of goal setting. What is ideal and what are the realistic constraints imposed upon us by the limitations of deafness, by physical facilities, by financial needs, by geography, by the distressing unavailability of enough able and motivated teachers, and by the changing technological and social scene?

*Processes and materials.* Given a set of goals for a learner it is now the task of the technologists, be they "media specialists," discipline experts, educational psychologists, or just plain teachers in combination or individually, to develop processes and materials to attain the goals. Here we must be careful that the materials

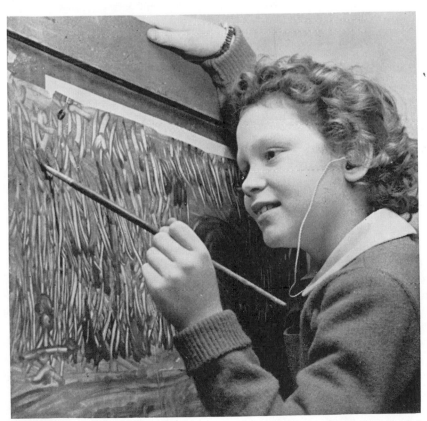

Fig. 16-10. Art is an excellent medium of expression for deaf children. (*Central Institute for the Deaf.*)

do not determine the goals and processes. All too frequently a kind of Parkinsonian principle operates. Goals are developed to use the materials available to attain them, often to the exclusion of more desirable goals.

The impressive array of processes and the increasing abundance of materials underline the growing importance of the educational technologists. The range and kinds of learning and teaching processes that are now or are soon likely to be available to us are indeed imposing. They include tutoring, small group discussions, lectures, laboratory demonstrations, individual programmed instruction, textbooks, slides, tapes, films, instructional television, and computer-aided instruction. The contemplation of these possibilities for curriculum improvement is as intriguing as the questions posed by them are formidable.

To assist in the dissemination and implementation of improved materials the Office of Education of the Department of Health, Education, and Welfare is supporting the development of regional centers for instructional materials for special education. In addition courses dealing with curricula in teacher education programs are being updated and elaborated. Yet there are subtle questions related to dissemination and implementation. For example, one of the appealing attributes of outstanding teachers of deaf children has been their spontaneity, their ability to sense an opportunity for learning by a child, and their skill in exploiting the siutation. In disseminating and stressing prepared materials are we likely to create a dependence on them that will stultify spontaneity and imagination? The textbook is a classic example of prepared materials (antedating modern technology). There are few among us who do not have grim recollections of teachers who "taught from the book." Nevertheless, we need not face a forced choice. Our deliberations on curriculum improvement point toward the preparation of professional "disseminators"

whose performance reflects an understanding of the learning problems of deaf children and how, for better or worse, they are taught.

*Evaluation.* In his summary of the 1967 National Conference on the Education of the Deaf the chairman said:

A nagging concern was the problem of evaluation, whether it be of curriculum, of a method of communication, teaching or guidance, or of a system of organization and administration. Common sense requires that the effectiveness of any procedure, or change therein, be tested by the most objective investigations we can devise, so that substantive grounds are established for eliminating, amending or modifying our arrangements and practices. In education this is devilishly difficult to accomplish. Many of the outcomes we seek resist satisfactory measurement, and some results must await the passage of years before an attempt at evaluation is even appropriate. Nevertheless, the conference time and time again pointed to evaluation as a crucial issue demanding more concentrated attention.

We may ask what needs to be evaluated? Dyer, in speaking of all schools, suggests a sobering thought:

The extraordinary fact is, however, that in spite of mountains of data that have been piled up from teachers' reports, tests, questionnaires and demographic records of all kinds, we still have only very hazy and superficial notions of what the effects of school experience really are.

Of course, we have academic achievement tests which, incidentally, may have an undue influence on our goals and which frequently are not too pertinent at certain levels to our particular problems in the education of deaf children. But little is done to evaluate the effective and social outcomes of school experience. A teacher may be doing an excellent job of teaching reading as measured by a reading test, but has she also taught some children to despise reading? Do we tend to evaluate only that for which we have tests, and do we accommodate assumptions to requirements of technique rather than to reality? Who shall do the evaluating? Should it be members of the closed system we call "the school"—the teachers, the administrators, the school psychologists, all of whom conventionally evaluate their own product? How about parent evaluations? Or extramural individuals or groups? Or employers of deaf persons? Or deaf persons themselves?

Ours is a time of "rising expectations" nurtured by "great advances in technology" with its inevitable idolatry of evangelistic technologists and its comforting faith in equating change with improvement, newness with validity, gimmickry with innovation, and public relations with evaluation. Nevertheless, we must continue to probe for strategies for curriculum improvement, with the recognition that it is a complex and demanding task.

The need for special provisions for children with handicapping conditions in addition to deafness is being recognized. In the academic year 1967–1968 there were, as we have said, 409 children in classes for the multiply-handicapped in day and private schools. Data on the number of these children in other schools is not available. Among the more frequently occurring complicating conditions are special learning disability, mental retardation, gross motor incoordination, and abnormalities of vision.

### Problems of Parents

In concluding our chapter on deaf children it is fitting to return to the problems of parents.

When parents become aware that their child is deaf, their initial reaction is one of profound grief. It is not pleasant to hear that one's child is deaf and that it is hopeless to expect a restoration of his hearing. Unfortunately, some parents refuse far too long to face the fact squarely. They begin a pilgrimage from one doctor to another, always hoping for a miracle and still not heeding advice about the necessity for special education. Instead, they may squander funds and waste valuable nursery-school years grasping for any and every "cure" they read about, from airplane rides to surgery.

Other parents surround the deaf child with an overwhelming, protective "love" as soon as deafness is recognized. They want to do everything for the child to compensate for his deprivation; they dress him, feed him, and amuse him, and shield him from contacts with other children. He is thereby deprived of opportunities for normal development, and his education is delayed.

Sooner or later all parents realize, as many do at the very first, that special education is necessary; but here they are naturally bewildered. "My child is deaf, but what do I do next?" Otologists, educators, and audiologists can help the parent make the educational arrangements best suited to the child's needs. Children differ, schools differ, communities differ. No single answer is correct for all deaf children in all places. We have outlined some of the principles of education for the deaf child, but the actual choice of a particular school is often a difficult problem.

Finally, however, a school for the deaf child is selected, and now comes the "long pull" for the parents, the extended period of learning how to work most effectively with the school throughout their child's educational career. Parents are more apt to enter willingly on this third and important stage of their evolving attitude if they realize that their earlier grief and bewilderment have been recognized, sympathetically understood, and met with kind, clear, but not too insistent, counsel. Here a heavy responsibility lies upon the school: first, to recognize the nature of the strong emotions that surround the relationship of the parents with their deaf child; second, to develop home cooperation by sending constructive and informative reports and by encouraging the parents to make frequent visits to the classroom.

Parents must seize upon every opportunity at home for the child to employ and practice the speech and the speechreading that he has learned at school. They can assist materially in the developing and correcting of the child's speech, in enriching his vocabulary, and in translating his experience into meaningful language. If the child is at a residential school, contacts with home should be maintained by letters and photographs. News from home is very essential to the deaf child's happiness. Reports from the teachers and at least an annual visit keep the parents informed concerning the child's progress.

As the deaf child reaches adolescence, his basic needs are the same as those of other children. He must soon be ready to earn money, to make decisions, to associate with the opposite sex, and to compete with the hearing. The schools and the home must prepare the deaf child for this broader environment.

Teachers, parents, and school executives must again cooperate in the selection of a school for further education or for vocational training after the boy or girl is graduated from the school for the deaf. Once more, many variables affect the decision: the age of the child, his intelligence, his ability to communicate, his academic record, his interests and skills, the schools available to him, and the vocational opportunities in his community. Parents should also make a sincere effort to help the deaf child make friends in his home community.

When the parents are able to observe the fruits of their long labors, they experience the comforting satisfaction that their efforts, augmenting those of the school, have played a tremendously significant role in the happy adjustment of their child. And on the part of the school, no Pollyanna philosophy but an attitude of realistic understanding of the parents' problem has facilitated the arduously long process of adjustment. Parents should not overlook their debt to the teachers, whose wisdom, patience, and understanding have made possible the deaf child's development and growth.

## SUGGESTED READINGS AND REFERENCES

**American Annals of the Deaf.** Published at Gallaudet College, Washington, D.C.
> The January issue each year is a statistical compilation of the hearing-impaired. It also contains a directory of personnel and services.

**Babbidge, H. D.** *Education of the Deaf: A Report to the Secretary of Health, Education, and Welfare by his Advisory Committee on the Education of the Deaf.* Washington, D.C.: U.S. Department of Health, Education, and Welfare, 1965.
> An assessment of the status and needs of the education of the deaf from preschool through adult levels. Recommendations for involvement of the federal government are included.

**Barry, K. E.** *The Five Slate System: A System of Objective Language Teaching.* Philadelphia: Sherman, 1899.

**Cornet, R. O.** "Cued Speech," in *Report of Proceedings of the Forty-Third Meeting of the Convention of American Instructors of the Deaf.* Washington, D.C.: U.S. Government Printing Office, 112–113, 1968.
A statement of a method of hand cues to assist in the reception and development of speech by the deaf.

**Boatner, E. B., E. R. Stuckless, and D. F. Moores.** *Occupational Status of the Young Adult Deaf of New England and Demand for a Regional Technical-Vocational Training Center.* West Hartford, Conn.: American School for the Deaf, 1964.
An investigation of the achievement of young deaf adults and an analysis of their needs.

**Craig, W. N., and H. W. Barkuloo (eds.).** *Psychologists to Deaf Children: A Developing Perspective.* Pittsburgh, Pa.: University of Pittsburgh, 1968.
Report of a meeting of psychologists who have to do with deaf children. Contains contributions on functions of school psychologists, predictive and evaluative measures, psychiatric and counseling services, and research findings and tasks.

**Davis, H. (ed.).** *The Young Deaf Child: Identification and Management. Proceedings of a Conference, Toronto, Canada. Acta Otolaryng. (Stockholm), Supplement* 206 (1964).
Report of a conference of American, Canadian, and European specialists dealing with the High Risk Register, prevention of deafness in very young children, identification, definitive tests of hearing of young children, differential diagnosis, medical and nonmedical management, parent training, biology of sensory deprivation, use of amplification, development of language, and improvements in electroacoustic instrumentation.

**Eagles, E. L., S. M. Wishik, L. G. Doerfler, W. Melnick, and H. S. Levine.** *Hearing Sensitivity and Related Factors in Children.* St. Louis: Laryngoscope (1963).
A detailed audiologic and otologic study of about 5000 Pittsburgh school children.

**Eagles, E. L., W. G. Hardy, and F. I. Catlin.** *Human Communication: The Public Health Aspects of Hearing, Language, and Speech Disorders.* Washington, D.C.: Public Health Service Publication No. 1754, U.S. Government Printing Office, 1968.
A concise (28 pages) document from the National Institute of Neurological Diseases and Blindness dealing with definitions, prevalence, effects, prevention, and management of children with communicative disorders. There are also sections on services and goals for adults and essentials for community health programs.

**Ewing, A. W. G. (ed.).** *Educational Guidance and the Deaf Child.* Washington, D.C.: The Volta Bureau, 1957.
A summary of investigations at Manchester University in England relating to the education of deaf children from infancy through school age.

**Ewing, I. R., and A. W. G. Ewing.** *Speech and the Deaf Child.* Washington, D.C.: The Volta Bureau, 1954.

In addition to the subject matter of the title, this book cites the School Health Regulations of England as they pertain to the definition and classification of hearing-impaired children.

**Fitzgerald, E.** *Straight Language for the Deaf.* Washington, D.C.: Gallaudet College Bookstore, 1949.

**Furth, H. G.** *Thinking Without Language: Psychological Implications of Deafness.* New York: The Free Press, 1966.

**Galloway, J. H.,** "The Rochester Method," in *Report of the Proceedings of the International Congress on the Education of the Deaf and of the Forty-First Meeting of the Convention of American Instructors of the Deaf.* Washington, D.C.: U.S. Government Printing Office, Document No. 106, 440–444, 1964.

An exposition of the Rochester Method by a former superintendent of the Rochester School for the Deaf.

**Groht, M.** *Natural Language for Deaf Children.* Washington, D.C.: The Volta Bureau, 1958.

Exposition of the "natural method" of teaching language to deaf children by a prominent teacher.

**Haycock, G. S.** *The Teaching of Speech.* Washington, D.C.: The Volta Bureau, 1942.

A systematic set of procedures for teaching speech to the deaf. Contains helpful suggestions for correcting faulty speech.

**Heider, F. K., and G. M. Heider.** "A Comparison of Sentence Structure of Deaf and Hearing Children," in *Psychological Monographs,* No. 232. Studies in the Psychology of the Deaf. Columbus: American Psychological Association, 42–103, 1940.

An investigation that analyzes the differences in structural features of language between deaf and hearing children.

**House, A. S. (ed.).** *Communicating by Language: The Speech Process.* Proceedings of a conference, Princeton, New Jersey, 1964. Bethesda, Maryland: U.S. Department of Health, Education, and Welfare, National Institute of Child Health and Development.

Report of a conference of investigators and clinicians dealing with the perception of speech, speech behavior, and the structure of the linguistic code, development and deficits in language skills, production of speech, disorders of speech production and perception, neural mechanisms and models, man-machine communication, and machine analogies of human communication.

**Hudgins, C. V., and F. C. Numbers.** "An Investigation of Intelligibility of Speech of the Deaf," *Genet. Psychol. Monogr.,* 25: 289–392 (1942).

An analysis of errors of articulation and temporal patterns in the speech of deaf children.

**Illinois Commission on Children.** *A Comprehensive Plan for Hearing-impaired Children in Illinois.* Report of a committee. Springfield, Illinois: Illinois Commission on Children, 1968.
A forward-looking plan for the statewide organization and administration of the management of hearing-impaired children.

**Kohl, H. R.** *Language and Education of the Deaf.* New York: The Center for Urban Education, 1966.
A critique of the education and achievement of profoundly deaf individuals in contemporary American society emphasizing the "relative failure" of oral teaching and advocating the teaching of sign language, with oral language taught as a second language.

**Kopp, H. (ed.).** "Curriculum: Cognition and Content," *Volta Review,* 70:September (1968).
The entire issue of September 1968 of the Volta Review is devoted to curriculum in schools for the deaf. Included are a formulation of issues, contributions on instruction in natural and social sciences, mathematics, language, art, health education, and pertinent features of learning theory. Educational media are also discussed.

**Lack, A.** *The Teaching of Language to Deaf Children.* London: Oxford University Press, 1955.
Systematic step-by-step procedures for teaching language to deaf children. Contains many specific suggestions for correlating spoken and written language.

**Lowell, E. (ed.).** *Curriculum Planning for the Deaf.* Sacramento: California State Department of Education, 1967.
Proceedings of a state conference. Contains an extensive bibliography.

**McGinnis, M.** *Aphasic Children: Identification and Education by the Association Method.* Washington, D.C.: Alexander Graham Bell Association for the Deaf, 1963.
A practical approach to instruction of hearing- and language-handicapped children who have difficulty in learning.

**Morkovin, B. V.** "Language in the General Development of the Preschool Deaf Child: A Review of Research in the Soviet Union," *ASHA* Monogr., 10:195–199 (1968).

**Myklebust, H. R.** *The Psychology of Deafness.* New York: 2d ed., Grune and Stratton, Inc., 1964.
Studies of psychological abilities of deaf children.

**Myklebust, H. R.** *Development and Disorders of Written Language.* New York: Grune & Stratton, Inc., 1965.

**Pitman, J.** "Can i.t.a. Help the Deaf Child, his Parents and his Teacher?" in *Proceedings of International Conference on Oral Education of the Deaf.* Washington, D.C.: Alexander Graham Bell Association for the Deaf, 514–542, 1967.

**Quigley, S. P. (ed.).** *Research on Behavioral Aspects of Deafness.* Proceedings of a conference, New Orleans, La. Washington, D.C.: Department of Health, Education, and Welfare, Vocational Rehabilitation Administration, 1965.
Report of a conference of investigators and educators dealing with research in language acquisition, personal adjustment, social and vocational adjustment, and learning problems.

————, **W. C. Jenné, and S. B. Phillips.** *Deaf Students in Colleges and Universities.* Washington, D.C.: Alexander Graham Bell Association for the Deaf, 1968.
A study of the factors related to success of deaf students in colleges and universities, the problems encountered by them, and suggestions for improving their opportunities and performance.

**Silverman, S. R.** "Education of Deaf Children," in Chapter 10, *Handbook of Speech Pathology,* L. E. Travis (ed.). Revision in press, New York: Appleton-Century-Crofts, Inc., 1969.
A comprehensive exposition of the education of the deaf in the United States. Contains an extensive bibliography.

**Smith, F., and Miller, G. A. (eds.).** *The Genesis of Language: A Psycholinguistic Approach.* Cambridge, Mass.: The M.I.T. Press, 1967.
Proceedings of a conference on language development in children. The aim of the conference was to "direct attention to the stages in the acquisition of grammar and phonology by children and to whatever biological and clinical evidence we have concerning the child's innate capacity for this acquisition."

**Smith, M. E.** "An Investigation of the Development of the Sentence and the Extent of Vocabulary of Young Children," *University of Iowa Studies in Child Welfare,* III, No. 5 (1936).

**Stepp, R. E.** (project director). "Symposium on Research and Utilization of Educational Media for Teaching the Hearing Impaired," *Amer. Ann. Deaf,* 110:508–620 (1965).
Report of a national conference at the University of Nebraska dealing with the use of media in the instruction of deaf children.

**Stokoe, W. C., D. C. Casterline, and C. G. Croneberg.** *A Dictionary of American Sign Language on Linguistic Principles.* Washington, D.C.: Gallaudet College Press, 1965.

**Streng, A.** "On Improving the Teaching of Language," *Am. Ann. Deaf,* 103:553–563 (1958).
Suggestions for teachers in improving the teaching of language to the deaf based on principles from the psychology of learning and from linguistics.

**Tervoort, B., and A. J. A. Verberk.** *Analysis of Communicative Structure Patterns in Deaf Children.* Report of Project RD-467-64-65 and Z.W.O. Onderzoek Nr. 585-15. Washington, D.C.: Vocational Rehabilitation Administration, Department of Health, Education, and Welfare, 1967.

An investigation of linguistic features of communication of deaf children based on filmed observations. Esoteric (the children's own system) and exoteric (the system being taught) systems of communication are compared.

**Urbantschitsch, V.** *Des Exercises dans la Surdi-mutité et dans la Surdité Acquise,* Translated by Egger, L. Paris: A. Maloine, 1897.
One of the first expositions of the possibilities and methods of auditory training.

**Vegely, A., and Elliott, L. L.** "Applicability of a Standardized Personality Test to a Hearing Impaired Population," *Amer. Ann. Deaf,* 113:858–868 (1968).

**Whetnall, E., and D. B. Fry.** *The Deaf Child.* London: William Heinemann, Ltd., 1964.
An exposition of the development of communication in deaf children emphasizing an early auditory approach.

**Wing, G.** (original author). *An Exposition of Wing's Symbols in their Relation to the Teaching of Language.* Faribault, Minnesota: Minnesota School for the Deaf, 1938.

**Yale, C. A.** *Formation and Development of Elementary English Sounds.* Northampton, Mass.: Gazette Printing Co., 1925.
A description and principles of the Northampton charts.

**Zaliouk, A.** "A Visual-Tactile System of Phonetical Symbolization," *J. Speech Hearing Dis.,* 19:190–207 (1954).

The reader is referred to Chapter 20 for suggested readings and references pertaining to the psychological and educational assessment of the deaf.

# CHAPTER 17

# HARD-OF-HEARING
# CHILDREN

S. R. SILVERMAN, Ph.D.
AND
H. DAVIS, M.D.

## THE NATURE OF THE PROBLEM

This chapter deals with children whose hearing impairments are mild enough for them to learn without great difficulty to communicate by speech and hearing. The distinction between these hard-of-hearing children and those whom we have called the deaf is not always entirely clear. The reason is that individual children may differ greatly in the use that they are able to make of the remainder of their hearing. It is not simply a matter of hearing level for speech but also of such different factors as the age of onset, the severity and the exact type of hearing loss, the intelligence of the child, the amount of training that the child has had, the age at which the training was begun, and particularly the auditory and language environment of the child. As we have learned from experience with "culturally disadvantaged" children who hear, an impoverished language environment retards development of skills of communication, a condition that is difficult to remedy

when the optimum time for acquisition has been passed. It is a matter also of the attitude of parents and their degree of understanding of the significance of the hearing impairment.

Even within the broad group of the hard-of-hearing there is a wide range of the ability to make use of hearing for communication by speech. As we have seen in Chapter 9, the relatively mild hearing losses with hearing levels for speech of less than 40 dB cause only a little handicap, except perhaps for faint speech or for hearing at a distance. At the other extreme, with hearing levels for speech of 70 dB or thereabouts, and particularly if the hearing loss is congenital or of early onset, the child may require painstaking instruction to learn to hear adequately, even with a hearing aid, and to understand and use language. Furthermore, the impairment of hearing is often not merely a loss of sensitivity that may be overcome by amplification, but it may involve also a loss of ability to discriminate between certain sounds. Such a failure of discrimination is common when there is a great loss of sensitivity for the high frequencies.

Just as there are gradations in the usefulness of hearing, so there are gradations in the quality and intelligibility of the speech of hard-of-hearing children. Many hard-of-hearing children speak so well that the lay observer notices no abnormality, whereas the severely impaired may be almost unintelligible to those who are not accustomed to this type of speech.

Many investigators have sought to define the relations of these various factors of hearing impairment: intelligence, personality, emotional stability, social behavior, and the like. Our best generalization from their studies is that it is impossible to draw a *single* composite picture of the hard-of-hearing child. There is too much variation, in both the severity of the hearing impairment and the many other pertinent factors. The personality structure of a child with hearing impairment is determined by many factors other than his difficulty in hearing.

In this chapter we shall discuss identification of hearing-impaired children, and we shall describe the hard-of-hearing child particularly in terms of his ability to understand speech, his ability to progress in school, and the extent to which these abilities are affected by his hearing loss. In making generalizations about the significance of various degrees of hearing impairment we shall assume that the hearing loss occurred before the child acquired speech and learned to use language. Obviously, if speech and language are acquired before the hearing loss occurs, the handicap imposed by the loss is much less severe. Hence the age of onset of the hearing impairment is an important factor.

Hearing-impaired children may be usefully divided into five classes, depending on their hearing levels for speech. These levels may be estimated quite accurately, as pointed out in Chapter 9, by averaging the hearing levels for pure tones at 500, 1000, and 2000 Hz. All levels are ISO.

Class 1: Hearing level for speech 40 dB or better. These children may have difficulty in hearing faint or distant speech but are likely to "get along" in school and to have normal speech.

Class 2: Hearing level for speech between 41 and 55 dB. These children usually understand conversational speech at a distance of 3 to 5 feet without great difficulty. They may have some defects in the articulation of their own speech, and they may have difficulty in hearing adequately in school if the talker's voice is faint or if his face is not visible to them.

Class 3: Hearing level for speech between 56 and 70 dB. These children understand conversational speech only if it is loud, and they have considerable difficulty in group and classroom discussions. Their language and, especially, their vocabularies may be limited, and abnormalities of articulation and voice production are obvious.

Class 4: Hearing level for speech between 71 and 90 dB. These children may hear the sound of a loud voice about 1 foot from the ear, and they may identify some environmental noises and may distinguish vowels, but, even with hearing aids, they have difficulty with consonants. The quality of their voices is not entirely normal, and they must be taught both speech and language. Many, but not all, children in this class should be considered "deaf" for educational purposes until or unless the combination of an adequate hearing aid and sufficient auditory training makes them only "hard of hearing."

Class 5: Hearing level for speech 91 dB or worse. These children are deaf, even though they may hear some very loud sounds. They never can rely on the auditory channel as a primary avenue of communication. Their speech and their language must both be developed through careful and extensive training.

The hearing levels that mark the divisions of these classes are substantially the same as those given in Chapter 9. It will be noted that a hearing level of 90 rather than 100 dB is here chosen as the level dividing the fifth from the fourth class. This choice agrees well with a more recent definition of "100 percent hearing impairment" for medicolegal purposes and is discussed in Chapter 9. The scale given by the Committee on Hearing also subdivides what is here the first class into "normal" and "near normal." For the purposes of the present chapter, however, we have grouped all of these children together because they are all likely to "get along" in school and to have normal speech.

## IDENTIFICATION OF THE YOUNG HEARING-IMPAIRED CHILD

The following section is taken verbatim with one minor addition from the proceedings of a conference "The Young Deaf Child: Identification and Management," held in Toronto, Canada, on October 8–9, 1964. The purpose of the conference was "to bring together a small hand-picked group of 'experts' to exchange information on and to evaluate methods for coping with impairment, whether it be by surgery, hearing aids, special education or the exploitation of other sensory channels." The medical conditions and terms listed below are described in Chapter 4.

### Auditory Screening of the Neonate

The first opportunity to detect severe auditory impairment in young children is during the neonatal period, within the first few days after birth. Positive evidence of hearing may often be obtained by simple tests based on a startle or arousal response elicited by sudden rather loud sounds. *Methods for routine screening of the newborn infant for auditory impairment have been developed, but before widespread programs are initiated the following points must be considered:*

1. The incidence of deafness or severe impairment of hearing in the newborn is very low. The percentage of children who fail to pass the screening test in the three most extensive studies ranges from 0.1 to 2.0 percent. Careful consideration must be given to the value and economy of a screening program whose yield is so low.

2. The validity and the reliability of screening tests of infant hearing are both difficult to establish. Much further research is required. The number of "false positives" and the number of cases missed, which are both rather high, must be considered; the former will cause unfounded anxiety, and the latter will give a false sense of security and thus delay later recognition of an auditory impairment. The chance of successful identification of auditory impairment and accurate assessment of its severity becomes progressively greater as the infant grows older.

3. The newborn infant is a very labile organism. He normally sleeps 20 to 22 hours of each 24-hour period, and on a routine basis it may be difficult to catch him in an optimal state for testing. The best state is asleep, but he may be difficult to arouse sufficiently from deep sleep. He is hyperactive and tense when hungry or cold.

4. Certain conditions which can affect the auditory system, such as anoxic brain damage and particularly hyperbilirubinemia, may not show their effects the first day or two. Hyperbilirubinemia in particular may not cause symptoms before the fourth or fifth day or even later.

5. After they leave the nursery for the new-born, only a small percentage of infants in most communities can be brought together for screening purposes. The maternity hospital thus offers a unique opportunity for screening. Against this must be weighed: (*a*) the economy of a neonatal screening program; (*b*) the question of whether effective remedial measures, special training, or management are available; (*c*) whether a delay in initiating the remedial measures or the special training and management is of critical importance, and, if so, (*d*) how long a delay is critical.

Opinions differ on the matter of how long a delay is allowable in the case of partial auditory impairment. There is no clear evidence that a delay of 6 months is critical from the point of view of development of language. Most participants in the conference agree that a year is probably critical, and many feel that the sooner auditory experience and training can be provided the better.

6. The possibility of injury to hearing as the result of misplaced and unnecessary use of amplified sound or of other loud and continued noise cannot be overlooked. Certainly the use of amplified sound for infants during the early weeks of life must be instituted with due caution. Indications of pain or discomfort are important guides, and an infant 6 months old can register them more clearly than a neonate.

### A Positive Program

It is not necessary to wait for the methods of routine auditory screening at birth to be perfected and validated or for its economic feasibility to be demonstrated. An effective program for the early identification of children likely to have problems in communication can and should be instituted immediately. Such a program might be developed in two steps.

1. *A high-risk register* should be instituted, containing the names of babies in whom, for one reason or another, the risk of an auditory handicap is substantially higher than it is in the general population. The indications for placing a baby in a high-risk register are given in detail below.

Babies at risk should be followed closely from the point of view of development of normal auditory behavior, and if deviations are suspected, definitive testing should be carried out. The children at risk should be seen fairly frequently during the first 2 years, say at 0, 3, 6, 9, 12, 18, and 24 months.

2. *All children attending well-baby clinics* or coming to pediatricians' offices might be screened during the latter part of their first year by a simple but well-planned test or else by a questionnaire pertaining to auditory behavior, such as the communicative evaluation chart developed by Anderson *et al.* Children who do not yield satisfactory responses on two test occasions or concerning whom doubt is raised by the questionnaire would then be referred for more definitive testing.

The success of such a program will depend on the education of physicians, public health personnel and, above all, parents with respect to normal expectations for the development of hearing and language and the possibility of auditory impairment. Among physicians it is particularly important to alert both obstetricians and pediatricians.

It would be ideal if impairment were detected and confirmed by 6 months of age, but a more practical time to try to identify the deaf child and institute appropriate special care and training is during the second half of the first year. This is a compromise between reliable detection of impairment and the earliest possible start on special auditory training.

## HIGH-RISK REGISTER FOR THE BETTER IDENTIFICATION OF CHILDREN WITH COMMUNICATION PROBLEMS

I. Antenatal
   a) Positive family history of deafness
   b) Familial biochemical abnormality associated with deafness
   c) Blood incompatibility (Rh factor)
   d) Virus infection during early pregnancy
   e) Bleeding, especially during the first trimester
   f) Drugs, notably any of the mycin group or quinine

II. Complications of Labor
   a) Premature delivery
   b) Fetal distress due to maternal shock, and so on
   c) Prolonged or precipitate labor
   d) Difficult delivery—traction on neck or birth injury

III. Neonatal Difficulty
   a) Apnea or cyanosis
   b) Cerebral birth injury
   c) Jaundice—hyperbilirubinemia (15 mg per cc and above)
   d) Multiple anomalies—from whatever cause
   e) Possible iatrogenic trauma, as noise of an incubator, drugs (notably streptomycin and kanamycin), and so on

IV. Factors in Early Childhood
   a) Infections, such as meningitis and measles
   b) Chronic respiratory infection and/or allergy
   c) Injuries
   d) Hypothyroidism
   e) Abnormality of external ear
   f) Appearance of Waardenburg's syndrome

V. Possible Social Factors
   a) Maternal mental retardation
   b) Sociocultural deprivation— poor child care, and so on

   c) Emotional problems

Items I, II, and III are the particular concern of the obstetrician; items III, IV, and V, of the pediatrician.

## THE SIGNIFICANCE OF THE PROBLEM

The problem of the hard-of-hearing child is one of serious social significance.[1] Specifically, the community should feel a concern for the unfortunate financial and social effects of the retardation in school of children whose handicap has been neglected or not recognized. Obviously, the repetition of grades is costly, and, in the long run, it is only a grossly superficial remedy which leaves the root of the problem quite untouched.

To those public school authorities and taxpayers who view with alarm the financial outlay necessary for a really constructive program for the hard-of-hearing child we may point out that the saving resulting from avoidance of repetition of grades offsets a large part of the cost of the program. In addition, we must reckon the cost of truancy and various forms of antisocial behavior which characterize the child who becomes bored with the schoolwork in which it is so difficult for him to participate.

But the financial aspects of the problem must in no way obscure the solemn moral obligation of every American community to provide for each child the opportunity to develop according to his maximum potentialities. This is the fundamental principle of our system of democratic education, and the community that shirks responsibility for an adequate program for the physically handicapped child stands guilty of its violation.

In the smaller community of the schoolroom itself the teacher is often not aware that the learning or behavior difficulty of a

[1] Chapter 16 contains statistics about the magnitude of the problem.

hard-of-hearing child is due to his impaired hearing and not to lack of mental ability or to some fault in her methods of teaching. For example, Goetzinger and his co-workers, in studying children with as good a hearing level as 30 to 45 dB, found that the hearing-impaired children had poorer auditory discrimination and more errors of articulation than children with normal hearing. Furthermore, the incidence of comments from teachers stressing poor work habits, poor attitudes, and emotional variability was much higher for the children with even mild hearing loss. Failure to understand the basic cause of the child's difficulties frequently leads to fruitless remedial measures that are time-consuming for both the child and his classmates. And when by good fortune the teacher recognizes the child's hearing impairment, her lack of special training and information and the requirements of other children in the room make quite impossible any adequate solution of the child's particular problem.

In the narrower confines of the family circle, too, the hard-of-hearing child presents a problem that requires wholesome and sympathetic understanding. Apparent inattention to the spoken word is often interpreted as sheer naughtiness. The misdirected punishment often results in tensions within the family which would be avoided if the parents were only aware of their child's handicap. Furthermore, repetition of grades in school delays the day when the child can become a self-supporting individual. In many families the prolonged dependence is a serious problem.

The desirability of identifying hearing losses early by various methods of screening audiometry and individual hearing tests, as well as the possibility of conserving hearing by proper diagnosis and by treatment of the medical conditions that are so disclosed, has been discussed in Chapters 4 and 7. In detecting hearing losses in children, informal procedures and simple intelligent observation can be of great value. Both teachers and parents should be informed of the clues in a child's behavior that suggest the possibility of a hearing loss. The symptoms include inattention, frequent requests for repetition of spoken words, cupping the hand to the ear, cocking the head, difficulty in copying dictation, indifference to music, abnormalities of speech, reluctance to participate in activities that require oral communication (such as dramatics), failure to follow oral directions, daydreaming, and poor scholarship. Not to be overlooked are truancy, lying, stealing, extreme introversion, and other forms of atypical behavior that frequently serve as compensations for the child who feels socially inadequate and wishes to attract attention to himself. Of course, such behavior may also depend on a host of other conditions. We merely note that the possibility of hearing impairment as a cause should not be overlooked by teachers or laymen. Medical indications, such as earache, bad tonsils, frequent colds, and so on, have already been discussed in Chapter 4.

## EDUCATIONAL NEEDS AND PROCEDURES

The educational needs of the hard-of-hearing child are different from those of the deaf child discussed in the preceding chapter. The hard-of-hearing child can learn to talk, to understand speech, and to learn language by more nearly natural means and by relying primarily on his sense of hearing. Furthermore, if his difficulties are recognized and if he is given proper assistance, his needs may well be met in a special class for the hard-of-hearing within the public school system, or even in the regular classroom itself. The assignment to a particular class will depend upon both his hearing level and the availability of special help. The aim should be to educate him with children with normal hearing whenever this is practicable.

The particular needs of hard-of-hearing children may be summarized as follows, according to their classification by hearing level for speech:

Class 1: Better than 40 dB. These children should be given the benefit of favorable seating in regular classrooms and may be assisted by special instruction in speechreading.

Class 2: 41 to 55 dB. These children should wear hearing aids and be given training in their use. They should be taught speechreading and also be given the benefit of speech correction and conservation of speech. They should also have the advantage of favorable seating in classrooms.

Class 3: 56 to 70 dB. Hearing aids and auditory training, special training in speech, and special language work are all essential. With such assistance and with favorable seating, some children can continue in regular classes. Others may derive more benefit from special classes.

Class 4: 71 to 90 dB. These children should be taught by means of educational procedures for the deaf child which were described in the preceding chapter, with special emphasis on speech, on auditory training, and on language. After a period of such instruction it is possible that these children may enter classes in regular schools.

Class 5: Worse than 91 dB. These are deaf children who require the special educational procedures described in the preceding chapter. Some of these children, however, eventually enter high schools for the hearing.

In Chapter 12, 13, and 14 Dr. Pauls, Dr Hirsh, and Dr. Carhart acquainted us with principles and techniques of speechreading, auditory training, speech correction, and conservation of speech that are suitable for hard-of-hearing children. Special help in these aids to communication may be available through a special class, an itinerant teacher, or a community speech-and-hearing center.

## GUIDANCE

Certainly we must not overlook the need for psychological, educational, and vocational guidance which should avert or eliminate the atypical forms of behavior that frequently characterize the hard-of-hearing child. He must be made to understand that speechreading lessons and his hearing aid are as necessary as geography, arithmetic, or any other school activity. In fact, they may be more so. He should be particularly encouraged to join in extracurricular and community activities, such as scouting, athletics, Hi-Y, 4-H, church functions, and other wholesome pastimes of youth. Success in any of these activities should do much to avert extreme introversion and preoccupation with the impairment of hearing.

Of course, extreme cases should be referred for psychiatric study. Vocational plans for the child should take into account the existence of hearing impairment. Obviously, we would not suggest preparation for any calling which demands a high degree of accuracy in oral communication. We are too well aware of the psychological distress which inevitably accompanies a trying occupational situation. Bookkeeping, for example, would be preferable to stenography. On the other hand, vocational guidance should stress the child's assets and not his liabilities. There are many occupations at all levels in which hearing impairment is not a barrier to success.

Throughout our discussion we have implied—and it is well now to stress—that, although the welfare of the hard-of-hearing child should be entrusted to specially trained personnel, all remedial measures should be carried out within the framework of the regular school and health system. It is psychologically and educationally desirable that the child should not be prevented from associating with children who hear normally. True, he must be segregated for speechreading lessons and auditory training, but these activities should be considered part of his school program. In fact, we suggest that academic credit be given for participation in such classes, since, for the hard-of-hearing child, they involve the development of communication skills as important as composition or public speaking. They should be so recognized and integrated with the curriculum. When the child is convinced that he is a person with a particular need that has been recognized, he has hurdled the chief obstacle to his eventual adjustment.

In summary, the management of hard-of-hearing children requires:

1. Public information about hearing impairment
2. Case finding through appropriate screening and identifying programs in hospitals, clinics for babies, and in schools
3. Complete medical diagnosis of hearing difficulties
4. Appropriate medical and surgical treatment
5. Thorough assessment of hearing after all indicated medical and surgical procedures have been completed, with particular attention to educational needs
6. Special educational measures that include auditory training, speechreading, speech correction and conservation of speech, vocational planning, and psychological guidance

## SUGGESTED READINGS AND REFERENCES

**Darley, F. (ed.).** *Identification Audiometry,* Monograph Supplement No. 9. Journal of Speech and Hearing Disorders, 1961.
Report of a conference dealing with definition, objectives, and program responsibility for identification audiometry from preschool through adult age.

**Davis, H. In Davis, H. (ed.).** *The Young Deaf Child: Identification and Managament, Proceedings of a Conference, Toronto, Canada.* Acta Otolaryng. (Stockholm), Supplement 206:13–15 (1964).
An exposition of possibilities and present-day limitations of auditory screening of the neonate and recommendations for a positive program. The recommendations for a high-risk register by Dr. Janet Hardy are discussed.

**Goetzinger, C. P., C. Harrison, and C. J. Baer.** "Small Perceptive Hearing Loss: Its Effect on School Age Children," *Volta Rev.,* 66:124–132 (1964).

**Mulholland, A. M., and G. W. Fellendorf.** *National Research Conference on Day Programs for Hearing Impaired Children.* Washington, D.C.: Alexander Graham Bell Association for the Deaf, 1968.

Report of a conference dealing with the day program movement and recommendations for organization, administration, and research.

**Silverman, S. R.** "Education for the Hard of Hearing," in Chapter 11, *Handbook of Speech Pathology,* L. E. Travis (ed.). Revision in press. New York: Appleton-Century-Crofts, Inc., 1969.

**Thomason, B. (ed.).** *Community Planning for the Rehabilitation of Persons with Communication Disorders.* Washington, D.C.: National Association of Hearing and Speech Agencies, 1967.
A guide for administrators, lay persons, and professionals.

# CHAPTER 18

# THE PSYCHOLOGY OF
# THE HARD-OF-HEARING AND
# THE DEAFENED ADULT

### D. A. RAMSDELL, Ph.D.

Anyone who has closely observed an adult soon after he has lost his hearing has noted that he becomes discouraged and struggles with feelings of depression. Sometimes he even becomes suspicious of friends and family. In order to understand the psychology of the deaf, it is necessary to understand why this personality change occurs and why it does not occur with equal severity in children who are born deaf or in those who become blind.

That loss of hearing does tend to result in this peculiar and serious personality change has long been known, but the reason for the change is not obvious. The depression is usually more serious than we should expect from the loss of easy two-way communication, particularly if we recall that the adult has already learned to talk, to read, and to write before the onset of deafness. Nor is the depression prevented by prompt instruction in speech-reading, although this assistance to communication is both desirable and helpful.

A study of the reactions of soldiers who lost their hearing in World War II has shown that the loss of communication is not the deaf man's only or most serious loss. Deafness produces a psychological impairment more basic and more severe than the difficulty in communication. The characteristic depression is caused by this more subtle impairment. Recognition and understanding of the cause are necessary if the depression is to be overcome and not attributed, as is so often the case, to a character weakness in the deafened. Fortunately, an understanding of the psychological factors involved is, in itself, a powerful means of overcoming the depression.

This chapter is written in the hope that it will help those adults who have suffered permanent impairment of hearing to understand the psychological problems involved and thereby overcome their depressive reactions, and that it will provide the families of the deafened with a clearer insight into the difficulties that deafness entails so that they, too, can help.

Before the person with normal hearing can attempt to understand the problem of deafness, he must make a conscious effort to imagine what it is like to become suddenly and totally deaf, cut off in a world of silence from the familiar sounds of everyday living. Most of us take normal hearing completely for granted because we hear without conscious effort. We do not even have to open an "earlid" in order to listen, nor do we have an "earlid" to close if we wish to experience for a moment what deafness is like.

One way to gain some idea of the deaf person's experience is to imagine what it would be like to start home in a silent world after your day's work. The outside door makes no noise as you close it after you and step out on the sidewalk. A heavy rain is falling silently. Five o'clock traffic is jamming the street; people are crowding past you, but you hear no sound. Newsboys in front of the building are arguing angrily over something, but you can only see the exaggerated movement of their lips as they shout at each other. Cars suddenly swerve to the curb and stop. Everyone turns to look behind you, startled by a sound that you have not heard. An ambulance rushes silently past. Everything moves with the unreality of pantomime. When you reach home, you see your family's smiles of greeting, you see their lips move, but the rich experience of hearing the tone and rhythm of their familiar voices is lost. They, too, are like actors on a silent stage. If you can imagine such a silent world, you know something of how the deaf man feels, in close visual contact with his family and his surroundings but forced to substitute sight for hearing.

The loss of any sense organ imposes limitations, but the nature and severity of those limitations depend upon the particular sense organ affected. The most obvious limitation of the deaf man is that he cannot hear the spoken word. He may partially compensate, to be sure, by learning speechreading and, if he has sufficient residual hearing, by using a hearing aid. But if he depends on speechreading, he is def-initely limited to clearly visible conversation directed to him. The deaf man's participation in the feelings and observations of others is restricted to those who deliberately address him. Without the full range of normal hearing, he misses the little asides that add immeasurably to the savor and zest of general conversation. He also misses the snatches of talk normally overheard as we ride the subway or bus or walk on a crowded street. Until these casual contacts are lost, it is impossible to realize how enormously they contribute to the feeling of group participation. The social handicap to communication with those around him therefore remains for the deaf man, even though it may seem to be partially overcome by speechreading or by the use of a hearing aid.

Because a blind man must also substitute one sense for another, blindness and deafness are popularly classed together. What we fail to realize is that the psychological effects of deafness are fundamentally different from those of blindness. The similarity between the two impairments is superficial, and the tendency to evaluate the effects of deafness in the terms used for blindness has retarded an understanding of the psychology of the deafened.

## THE THREE PSYCHOLOGICAL LEVELS OF HEARING

To understand the psychological changes which accompany the loss of hearing, it is necessary first to comprehend how normal hearing operates. In order to make the explanation as simple as possible, we shall discuss normal hearing as though it occurred on three levels:

1. On the social level, as we all realize, hearing is used to comprehend language. Words are symbols for objects around us and for activities. The word "tree" symbolizes the tree growing in the yard; the word "gallop" symbolizes the rapid gait

of a horse. Since language is symbolic in its nature, we shall call this level of auditory function the *symbolic* level.

2. Sound also serves as a direct sign or signal of events to which we make constant adjustments in daily living. At this level it is not the word "bee" (which is a symbol for the actual bee itself), but the sound of its angry buzz that makes us jump. We stop our car, not because someone says "policeman" (the symbol for the officer), but because we hear the shrill sound of his whistle. This level of auditory function we shall call the *signal*, or *warning*, level.

3. Finally, and most basically, sound serves neither as symbol nor as warning but simply as *the auditory background* of all daily living. At this level we react to such sounds as the tick of a clock, the distant roar of traffic, vague echoes of people moving in other rooms in the house, without being aware that we do hear them. These incidental noises maintain our feeling of being part of a living world and contribute to our own sense of being alive. We are not conscious of the important role which these background sounds play in our comfortable merging of ourselves with the life around us, because we are not aware that we hear them. Nor is the deaf man aware that he has lost these sounds; he only knows that *he feels as if the world were dead*. The real importance of this third level of hearing is the creation of a *background of feeling*, which the psychologist calls an "affective tone."

It was the constant reiteration, by hard-of-hearing patients at Deshon Army Hospital, of the statement that the world seemed dead which led to the investigation of this third level of hearing and of the psychological effect of its loss upon the deaf. This third level has not generally been recognized, although it is psychologically the most fundamental of the auditory functions. It relates us to the world at a very primitive level, somewhere below the level of clear consciousness and perception. The loss of this feeling of relationship with the world is the major cause of the well-recognized feeling of "deadness" and also of the depression that permeates the suddenly deafened and, to a less degree, those in whom deafness develops gradually. This level of hearing we shall designate as the *primitive* level.

The concept of levels of hearing has been chosen as the organizing principle of this chapter because this approach allows us to isolate and discuss the diverse but related auditory processes, together with their special implications for the deaf. "Hearing" is, of course, a combination of all these processes. At any given moment all are going on simultaneously. We hear on all the three levels at once. We hear the symbols of language, the signal of the ringing of the telephone, and we react to the background of sounds which we do not consciously discriminate and of which we are not aware. These diverse processes, however, vary independently, sometimes with a predominance of one, sometimes of another, but there is usually an interweaving contribution from each in the total pattern of hearing.

We shall begin our analysis of the psychological problems of the deaf at the most basic, least objective, and least structured level (the *primitive* level) and then explain the other two levels in the order of their objectivity—second, the *warning* level, and third, the *symbolic* level. Although such an approach may seem to be working backward, the reverse is true. Impairment or loss at the primitive "affective" level is most fundamentally and intimately connected with the emotional difficulties of the deaf.

### Hearing at the Primitive Level

At the primitive level of hearing, we react to the changing background sounds of the world around us *without being aware that we hear them.* This primitive function of hearing relates us to a world that is constantly in change, but it relates us to it in such a way that we are not conscious of the relationship, nor of the feeling it establishes of being part of our environment.

When we are at a concert listening to someone sing, we are not aware of the constantly changing pattern of sounds from the audience around us, the little noises of body movement, of breathing, of creaking seats, because our attention is on the singer. We are, however, reacting to these background sounds without realizing it. This constant reaction establishes in us states of feeling that are the foundation for our conscious experiences, a foundation which gives us the conviction that the world in which we live is also alive and moving. This process is a difficult one to describe, yet one so fundamental to an understanding of the primitive level of hearing that it must be labored in order to be made clear.

While we are focusing our attention on the singer at the concert, we do not consciously hear the background sounds from the audience or from the city outside. At any given moment, however, one of these background sounds may vary and attract our attention. The woman beside us may change the rhythm of her breathing by coughing. A horn on a car outside may become stuck and blow until we are aware of it. But the moment we become aware of such a background sound, it is no longer on the primitive level. As soon as we identify a sound, give it "thing" character, we are hearing on one of the other levels.

*The most distinctive feature of these background sounds is that they are constantly changing* because the world around us is in a state of constant activity. In the natural world there is constant motion: the wind blows; rain falls; animals move. In man's mechanical world, the same constant

motion occurs. The pattern of environmental sound from this continued activity changes with each moment and with the different times of day.

In the human body there is also constant change and activity. Even in our deepest sleep we breathe, we digest our food, our hearts beat, and the brain continues its activity. We have then two patterns of change always in motion, the pattern of environmental change in the world around us and the pattern of change in the human body. By far the most efficient and indispensable mechanism for "coupling" the constant activity of the human organism to nature's activity is the primitive function of hearing.

We as living organisms are not and can never be completely independent of our environment. We live in our environment in different degrees of security, and since the security is never complete, we must maintain a readiness to react, to withdraw, or to approach as need arises. The primitive function of hearing maintains this readiness to react by keeping us constantly informed of events about us which do not make enough noise to challenge our attention. *The feeling state established by the primitive function of hearing is therefore characterized by this readiness to react as well as by the comfortable sense of being part of a living, active world.*

We must remember that this "coupling" of the individual with the world is not a conscious process. It is even less conscious than beating time to martial music without realizing that our feet are moving. That this "coupling" does exist, that it establishes an unconscious feeling of aliveness in us, is demonstrated by the overwhelming feeling of deadness in the deafened. It is possible to maintain some degree of coupling with the environment through other senses than hearing, but none of the others is so effective—as the characteristic depression of the deaf indicates.

## The Depression of the Deaf

Observation of hundreds of patients has convinced this author that the answer to their persistent question, "Why do I feel so depressed, so caught in a dead world?" is to be found in the destruction of the sound-coupling which connects the individual at an unconscious level with the aliveness and activity of the world. Undoubtedly the loss of conversation makes the deaf man feel isolated from those around him, but the basic emotional upset is caused by the loss of hearing at the primitive level.

The depressive reaction is much the same whether the impairment in hearing has been sudden or gradual. Soldier patients who had suddenly become deaf were, however, so bewildered by their unexpected depression that they attempted to describe it. All of them were conscious of an undefined feeling of loss. Many of them felt vaguely sad and insecure. One of them stated that it was almost impossible to believe in the passage of time since he couldn't hear a clock tick. Several fell asleep every time they turned off the hearing aids that brought them some sound from the world around them. Even those who faced the practical difficulties of deafness in a realistic manner still suffered from the same undefined but permeating depression.

One reason for the overwhelming nature of the depression is that, until it is pointed out to him, *the deafened person is not aware of the loss he has suffered* at the primitive level of hearing or of its effect upon his feeling state. He is unaware of the loss because he is unaware that there is such a thing as this primitive level of hearing in the first place. Frequently, he attributes his depression to a lack of character, and often he feels that if he were man enough, he could shake it off. Bewilderment and self-accusation heighten the burden he has to bear.

*An extremely important step toward relieving the characteristic depression is taken when the deaf person realizes the reason for his emotional state.* The realization itself makes his depression more objective and thereby makes it possible for him to cope with it without bewilderment or self-blame. As long as he is blind to its cause, he suffers from the same vague feelings of discomfort that characterize the early stages of a disease before the symptoms have yet developed clearly. Diagnosis does not instantly remove a disease, but it makes the proper treatment possible. Similarly, knowing the cause of depression does not remove it, but fortunately *the mere understanding of the reason for a feeling state does much psychologically to relieve its intensity.*

The nature of the impairment of deafness at the primitive level and its consequent loss of coupling involve the deaf in a double threat. We have just described the aspect of experience in which its chief characteristic was that of feeling. But hearing at this low level also operates as a signal. It not only gives a quality of life to the present; it also serves as an indicator of what is to come. Even these undifferentiated feelings contain some reference to the future and serve to orient us unconsciously to meet it. They maintain in us a readiness to react to our environment. Without this orientation we suffer from a vague sense of insecurity which may be described in the words of a patient who said, "When I went deaf I lost my way of acting."

If the impairment of hearing is severe, the loss of the primitive hearing sense and its effect upon "feeling tone" are permanent and absolute unless a hearing aid can bring *some* sound from the outer world. When compensation for the loss in the primitive function is the objective, it is not essential that the hearing aid transmit sounds in their true character or speech which is intelligible, since the basic function operates with undifferentiated sounds. From a psychological point of view the use of a hearing aid is advisable even when it only serves to couple the individual to a world of sound patterns.

A type of compensation for severe loss in the primitive function has been developed independently and unconsciously by many recently deafened individuals. They substitute continuous muscular movement for the missing sensation of movement in the world. This continuous muscular activity is an overcompensation for the loss of those involuntary shifts in muscular tension which are the normal response to sounds heard at the primitive level. It is a good idea to make this muscular activity purposeful by keeping busy at something. Practical suggestions made later in the chapter will help the deaf person to substitute a satisfying activity for purposeless movement, such as pacing the floor.

### Sounds as Signs and Warnings

So far, major emphasis has been placed on the hearing of background sounds. Obviously, however, hearing at a higher level plays an even more important part in biological adjustment and survival. At this level, sound serves as a sign or signal and conveys factual knowledge about objects and activities within the range of hearing: there is a fan operating; someone is washing dishes; someone is coming up the stairs. Many of our adjustments are initiated by sounds of low intensity, that is, sounds that arise at a distance. The horn of the approaching automobile warns us far enough in advance to avoid an accident. The eye can see distant objects, but hearing has the advantage of being able to warn us of approaching events that are not directly in our line of vision. Because sound waves can bend around corners and travel through darkness, the ear can warn us of many things that we cannot see. A lack of hearing leaves us uninformed of events outside the visual field. At a given moment, we can see only a *fraction* of what it is possible to observe, whereas we can receive *all* the possible sound signals simultaneously and without interruption, except, of course, as one sound may drown out another. A pedestrian cannot watch at the same time the automobile approaching him from the right and the truck approaching him from the left, but he can *hear* them simultaneously.

Hearing informs us of the events taking place around us, and it can also tell us something about the direction from which a sound comes. We can thus locate the event in which we are interested. Not only do we need advance notice that an automobile is approaching, but we need to know from what direction it is bearing down upon us. Localization of the source is most accurate in the horizontal plane when we distinguish right from left. Discrimination is less accurate between front and back and still less accurate between up and down. Both ears are needed to perceive the direction from which sound comes, but in locating the source of a sound we are helped greatly by many additional clues and associations. The nature of the noise often restricts the number of possible directions from which it may come. An airplane in flight, for example, is always above, but an automobile is on the ground. If you know in which direction the nearby river lies, you will never be confused as to whether the sound of a boat whistle is coming from in front of or behind you, although you might be completely uncertain about the direction of a pure musical tone of unknown source.

The only noticeable handicap imposed by deafness in one ear is in the localization of the sources of sounds. For hearing language and background noises, one ear is almost as good as two. The man with one-sided deafness does not, however, suffer a complete loss of localization, since, as we have just mentioned, the principal cues for distance and some of the cues for direction do not depend upon binaural hearing. The accuracy of localization depends largely upon the recognition of the type of noise and its possible source. This substitute procedure, however, is not always accurate or quick enough in an emergency. The man with one-sided deafness is still liable to the right-left confusion that rarely occurs in a person with two normal ears.

Compensation for loss of hearing is easier at this warning level where sound is a sign or a signal than it is at the primitive level. Loss at this utilitarian level does not cause so basic an emotional upset. It does result in a feeling of insecurity because we are not able to hear warning signals or are uncertain of their source. Practical readjustments can be learned to help the individual meet the everyday demands of his environment. When the capacity to locate moving objects by their sounds is reduced or inadequate, a trained visual awareness will compensate to a considerable degree. A careful study of the conditions to be expected in certain situations, such as crossing a busy street, will give a feeling of security which approaches that of the hearing person.

### Aesthetic Experience

In addition to its function as signal or warning for biological survival, hearing contributes at the second level to our aesthetic experience. We listen to music and the sounds of nature for the pleasure that we derive from the sounds themselves. All people do not possess an equal need for this type of aesthetic auditory experience, nor do they suffer equally from the loss of the aesthetic experience of sound.

Just as there are differences in the degree of need, so there are differences in the kind of experiences sought. Some of us need visual, others need auditory, and others (apparently) do not need any aesthetic experience at all. If the loss of hearing occurs in someone with a pronounced aesthetic need in the auditory field, the absence of musical experience is felt as an impoverishment, and the lack is interpreted unconsciously as a lack in one's self.

In individuals with a pronounced aesthetic auditory need, this lack sometimes assumes acute proportions. A musician of this author's acquaintance who had a severe impairment declared that she would gladly sacrifice a year of her life if she could only once hear a symphony again. Such acute need is unusual, however, and occurs most often in those who have reinforced their natural auditory need by an occupation in the field of music.

Probably those who satisfy an aesthetic auditory need through the varied and multitudinous sounds of nature outnumber those who have found the answer to their need in music. The sounds of nature are available to everyone, whereas music is not. The sound of the sea, the singing of birds, the patter of rain furnish many people aesthetic experiences as poignant as those received through music. The silence of the natural world deadens it for them and superimposes upon the self the same lack felt by music lovers.

A hearing aid for those with some residual hearing, or even the vibratory sense by which the totally deaf can appreciate the rhythm of music, may enable a person with an auditory aesthetic need to capture enough of the desired sounds and rhythms to stimulate his imagination to recreate familiar and beloved auditory images either from music or from the natural world and thus satisfy his need in part.

### Sounds as Symbols

Animals as well as men depend on sound for warning; they also recognize the meaning of particular sounds, such as the trickle of water, the snapping of twigs, or the call of a mate. Man, however, can use ordered sounds as symbols for things not immediately present and even for abstract ideas. The use of sound as language sets human society apart as unique and different from animal societies. By the use of spoken language, man's sphere of influencing and being influenced is enormously increased and made more complex.

Hearing in its symbolic, linguistic function enriches human life in *three* ways: (1) Language makes possible the communication of experiences through a medium that is flexible and manifold almost to the degree to which experience itself is complex. (2) Language clarifies and organizes our thoughts by supplying a grammatical, syntactical, and logical framework and thus makes possible man's higher-order knowledge. (3) In the growing child, language serves to formalize and to bind those social prohibitions and permissions which make up the moral code: the *voice* of conscience, not a forbidding *glance*, directs our moral behavior.

Loss of hearing does not impair each of these three functions to an equal degree. The degree of hearing loss and the time of its onset are important in determining the effect of the impairment upon the personality. The adult who suffers a sudden and severe hearing loss is plunged into a world where sensory deficits form his principal handicap. The organizing of thought and the formulation of moral permissions and prohibitions have already been established; once established, they continue even with total deafness. The framework for higher-order knowledge and the moral code are not affected.

### Congenital Deafness

So far we have considered only the problems of the adult who either suddenly or gradually loses his hearing. The psychological effects of deafness are somewhat different in the child who is born deaf or who becomes deaf before he has learned the structure of language. His failure to learn to talk spontaneously or to be able to communicate any but the simplest ideas without intensive and special training has

been considered in Chapter 16. Fortunately, the greater difficulties in relation to communication are partly offset by a less devastating effect of the absence of the primitive auditory function. The child who has never established auditory "coupling" with the ongoingness of the world is not depressed by the absence of this coupling as the adult is by the loss of it. Nor has the child developed through training and experience any urgent aesthetic needs of an auditory nature. And once communication has been established, whether by visual reading, speechreading, the manual alphabet, or the language of signs, the deaf child is able to formulate successfully in nonauditory terms the structure for his thoughts and for his moral code.

### PRACTICAL SUGGESTIONS

Hearing loss presents obvious problems at the language level even for an adult. Unless the hearing loss is very mild, situations involving spoken language as a means of communication are difficult and remain difficult. *The first step toward surmounting the difficulty is to admit it frankly and realistically.* Much of the tension of social situations is eased for the deafened as well as for others if the impairment is regarded as factually and objectively as the need for glasses. Society accepts glasses for impaired vision and will accept with equal readiness the wearing of a hearing aid and also the need for face-to-face conversation to facilitate speechreading by those whose impairment is too severe for a hearing aid.

A few simple suggestions will help those with hearing loss to master practical situations which must be met. The complexity of even such a simple transaction as buying a railroad ticket may be great. Here the experience of those who have most successfully surmounted such difficulties has taught them to study the situation, to anticipate the difficulties which may arise, and to attempt by so doing to avoid confusion. If you wish to buy a railroad ticket from Columbus to Cincinnati, for example, you should if possible consult a timetable in which the three alternate routes are listed before asking for your ticket. You will then be familiar with the names of railroad lines and train schedules so that you can more easily recognize the words used in answer to your questions. Such advance knowledge makes it possible for you to ask pertinent questions and reduces the chance of your getting on the wrong train. A hearing aid in this situation is valuable, not only as an amplifier but also, if visible, as a sign and reminder of impairment. It relieves the wearer from the need of frequently mentioning his handicap and signifies to strangers that his difficulty in the situation depends on a physical and not an intellectual defect.

When a conversation is primarily the exchange of experiences with friends, no bluff at all should be attempted. The handicap should be frankly admitted so that the strain of keeping up with the conversation may be eased. An effort should be made, however, to participate whenever possible, and an attitude of dependence should be avoided. Here, as in the simple transaction of buying a ticket, a careful analysis of social patterns will provide a useful repertoire of anticipations which will facilitate in advance the adjustment to the inevitable difficulties of a social situation.

Social situations are not infinitely variable. There are not more patterns to learn than exist, for example, on a checkerboard. A mastery of social amenities is helpful and can be acquired without inducing a feeling of submission or dependency. Viewed realistically, the anticipation of the demands of a situation can become a competitive game.

Many who are deaf believe it important to be able to hear in order to make new friends. If the deaf who hold this belief would distinguish between friendship and casual acquaintance, they would realize that although friendship is undeniably carried on through the senses, it does not follow that the loss or impairment of only one of them destroys, makes impossible, or even lessens the depth of such a relation. The deaf man is in no way handicapped in the exchange of warm and affectionate experiences if he has developed the requisite deep sensibilities.

There are many situations in which none of us need or use our hearing. In such instances, when communication is unnecessary, the practical if not the emotional problems of the hearing and of the hard-of-hearing or deafened person are almost the same. For instance, all of us must face the problem of occupying leisure hours. For the hearing and for the deaf alike, idle time passes slowly, but occupied time passes quickly. The only difference in the problem for the two is that the hard-of-hearing or deafened person is more apt to fill his leisure hours with self-pity than with the chitchat of casual companions by which others may attempt to cover up a poor capacity for solitude.

Recreation should find a central place in the life of those suffering from hearing loss. They should habitually fill their leisure hours with some creative activity or avocation. If they do, they will soon realize that each person has his own individual and unique pattern of life and that it is worthwhile to find some definite interests and objectives as an outlet for this individuality. Since activity in a chosen field invariably leads to a relationship with others who share the same interests, those with hearing loss should make a careful survey of their interests and capabilities and discover the mechanical, artistic, or creative sphere in which they can express themselves. Those with mechanical ability can profitably spend their spare time repairing radios, electrical appliances, or watches. They can learn to refinish and upholster furniture or to rebuild antiques. An interest in furniture might lead eventually to cabinetmaking. A frequent approach to the artistic field is through model making. Models of airplanes, ships, houses, or trains may be made for personal pleasure alone or, if the individual develops sufficient skill, for the commercial market. Those with an interest in botany, biology, or medicine can apply their knowledge making models for classroom study. In the creative sphere, painting, writing, and modeling or sculpturing offer natural outlets. The amount of talent possessed is not important. If the individual is interested in one of these forms of creative work, he should try it as a means of personal expression and for the pleasure it brings. By identifying himself with a group interested in the same avocation, he may in part compensate for being unable to feel himself an intimate part of as large a social group as he could before hearing loss narrowed his conversational circle.

The experience of one man who developed a successful business from spare-time activity illustrates the professional possibilities of many avocations. Having time on his hands, he began by helping his mother, who was secretary of a large club, address the notices that she had to send out to its members. Friends of hers learned of his assistance and gave him letters to address for organizations with which they were connected. Requests for his aid increased. Today he runs a mailing and letter service that employs two assistants.

Interest in the problems of deafness, and assisting those who are similarly afflicted, is a common and very effective and useful form of social activity for the hard of hearing, provided that it does not turn into a form of mutual self-pity. Even better, if it can be achieved, is participation in more general social interests that do not depend on the handicap and do not make life and thoughts revolve about and continually emphasize it. More effort and skill may be required, but the most successful adjustment is the one that overrides and submerges the handicap in normal activity centering outside one's self.

### Feelings of Suspicion

There is an additional reason why it is psychologically healthful for the deaf to make a decided effort to center their interests and activities outside themselves. There is in many persons with normal hearing a tendency to feel that conversation interrupted upon their entrance into a room must have been about them or that half-heard remarks were critical and unfriendly. *Deafness accentuates this tendency and may make an oversensitive person unduly suspicious of hostility in those around him.* A word of explanation and warning is needed about such so-called *paranoid* reactions. Since the term "paranoid" is often used, perhaps erroneously, to characterize this hypersensitivity of the deaf, a simple explanation of the term is needed.

Not all persons can accept criticism without being hurt. It is possible for a friend to criticize your suit without implying any criticism of you. We all have a tendency, however, to interpret any criticism of something that is "mine" as a criticism of "me." If the tendency is strong, the person is described as sensitive. It is easy to imagine a person so sensitive that he is suspicious and anticipates that others are being critical of him. When the suspicion, reflecting a basic insecurity, is developed to this point, we speak of "paranoid reactions."

The tendency toward paranoid reactions exists to some degree in nearly all of us, but it is generally kept under control. Since control is lessened when a person is depressed, sensitiveness and suspicion are more easily aroused. *Deafness seems to be a powerful stimulus to any latent paranoid trend in the personality,* possibly because of the invariable association between depression and deafness.

We frequently observe that deaf people often think that conversations which they cannot hear are about them. They may often go so far as to think that derogatory remarks are being directed toward them in tones too low for them to hear. This is a typical "paranoid trend." Deafness alone, however, or even the insecurity that deafness may bring, is not enough to produce a paranoid trend. The person who becomes suspicious has a life pattern of placing his own insecurity in center stage and is preoccupied with the fear that others may see the lack which he feels. *A person secure in his own emotional life will develop no paranoid trends even when deafened.* The frequency of such paranoid trends shows, however, how many persons feel insecure in their social relations. Deafness may not be the fundamental cause of the trends, but it waters the seeds and encourages them to grow.

The conquest of this morbid symptom reduces to the problem of attaining a mature point of view that is centered outside one's self. If one has developed a genuine interest in other people and in outside activities, statements not heard will be interpreted as objective statements of fact, not as remarks about one's self.

### The Objective Attitude

The explanation of the psychology of hearing given in this chapter and the effect of impairment at the different levels have been realistically presented. There is no disguising the fact that anyone who becomes deaf or hard of hearing experiences an almost catastrophic loss when he must adjust himself to a completely or partially silent world. Only after he has faced this fact honestly and objectively can he determine the extent to which compensation is possible. An objective attitude furnishes the only sound basis upon which to build a readjustment.

Psychologically speaking, no permanent adjustment is possible until the individual realizes that the cause of his depressive state lies in the loss of the primitive function and until he faces the practical difficulties imposed by the loss at the two higher levels. Since depression and the feeling of deadness are the most destructive psychological effects of hearing impairment, it is fortunate that *the major step in recovering from these emotional states lies in a clear understanding of their cause.*

The suggestions made to facilitate mastery of the practical difficulties are by no means exhaustive. Each individual will work out his own, in accordance with the demands of his particular environment and his own personality and abilities.

The man with severe hearing loss will save himself much pain if he will realize that, although the difficulties imposed by deafness are now receiving recognition, he must not expect the general public to understand the problems of adjustment that are involved. Although this indifference is cruel, it does require him to develop a usefully independent and objective attitude toward his handicap.

## SUGGESTED READINGS AND REFERENCES

**Canfield, N.** *Hearing: A Handbook for Laymen.* New York: Doubleday & Company, Inc., 1959.
    An otologist talks to hard-of-hearing laymen.

**Meyerson, L.** "Somatopsychological Significance of Impaired Hearing," Chapter 5, in *Adjustment to Physical Handicap and Illness: A Survey of the Social Psychology of Physique and Disability,* R. G. Barker (ed.). New York: Social Science Research Council, 1953.

PART SIX
# SOCIAL AND ECONOMIC PROBLEMS

CHAPTER **19**

# THE VETERANS ADMINISTRATION AUDIOLOGY PROGRAM

## BERNARD M. ANDERMAN, Ed.D.

## HISTORY

The Veterans Administration is one of the heirs of the legacy of the World War II military audiology program. During that war, military centers, furnishing what was then termed "aural rehabilitation services," were established at Deshon (Pennsylvania), Borden (Oklahoma), and Hoff Army General (California) hospitals, for the Army, and at the United States Naval Hospital in Philadelphia for the Navy. The military programs met the requirements of their times in most commendable fashion and treated an estimated 15,000 servicemen for hearing impairment. Today, approximately 75,000 veterans of World War II and other conflicts have service-connected hearing impairments or diseases of the ear. The Veterans Administration program was established to assist them through audiological examination, treatment, and guidance.

Under Veterans Administration policy, outpatient beneficiaries may receive hearing aids and training when the disability is service-connected and when there is a need for them. For hospitalized patients, there must be a medically established need in the case of a service-connected condition, as well as in certain categories of adjunct or auxiliary treatment when the hearing condition is not service-connected.

The overwhelming majority of veterans who are furnished hearing aids and training are those whose condition is service-connected, and they are treated on an outpatient basis. A service-connected impairment is one which was incurred or aggravated in line of duty in the active military, naval, or air service. For purposes of outpatient medical services, any impairment of a veteran of the Spanish-American War is considered to be service-connected.

Facilities providing adequate audiolgical services were rare in the years immediately following World War II. Most veterans eligible for hearing aids were referred directly to dealers after medical examination but without intervening audiological evaluation. However, with the growth of

449

audiology, increasing numbers of clinics, both governmental and private, were established throughout the country.

The first Veterans Administration Audiology Clinic was established in the New York City Regional Office in 1946. A large unit, it was designed to meet the needs of the huge veteran population in southern New England and metropolitan New York. Other clinics were subsequently established in a number of large population areas. Twenty-eight are presently in operation, each serving the needs of neighboring localities as well as the one in which it is located. A list of the regional clinics and their locations is given in the Appendix. To provide needed audiological assistance for eligible veterans who lived at a distance from these centers, contracts were established with qualified university, hospital, and community clinics. As a consequence, more and more of the hearing aid selection for veterans has been carried out in clinics.

## PRESENT STATUS

The Veterans Administration audiology program has many facets. It provides direct services to eligible veterans, including auditory assessment and rehabilitation, and it carries on research, training, and consultation of considerable scope.

### Rehabilitation

The philosophy underlying the Veterans Administration rehabilitation effort is one which was originally developed in World War II military practice. At its core is a unified, integrated program involving the extensive use of educational techniques and personal counseling as well as the selection of hearing aids.

No single standard or model rehabilitation program has been provided by the Veterans Administration for its audiology clinics. Individual approaches have been developed in varying patterns to suit local needs and conditions. Then, too, many

veterans are served by the network of clinics that provide services under contracts.

A basic activity both in the Veterans Administration's own and in its contract clinics is the evaluation of hearing aids for eligible veterans. Testing is done under controlled conditions to determine whether or not the veteran is likely to benefit by wearing a hearing aid. Acoustic features of the instrument (described in Chapter 10) and audiological assessment of the veteran are considered in relation to his less tangible social, economic, and psychological needs. When the issuance of a hearing aid is indicated, selection is made from among a representative group of instruments which have been placed in the clinic stock. An important feature of the selection procedure is that the veteran receives the actual hearing aid used in the trial process. This provides the veteran with an instrument that has been found to suit his particular needs, and one whose limitations for the veteran, where present, have been ascertained. Thus the necessary adjustments can be made during his training.

The New York City Audiology Clinic is a good example of the application of the principles underlying the Veterans Administration Program of Rehabilitation. The veteran is given a course of instruction that is planned to restore his efficiency in communication as completely as possible. He is taught speechreading and speech conservation and is given auditory training and speech correction. The veteran is helped to understand the nature and extent of his impairment and is informed about the general problems related to loss of hearing. Psychological and social work assistance are offered when needed.

At the New York City Audiology Clinic group teaching has proved to be the most effective. The size of the class is limited so that attention may be given to individual needs while the benefits of group instruction and interaction are realized. The teachers have always striven to employ dynamic and meaningful teaching materials, geared to the level of the adult veteran. There is a choice of either a 4-week program consisting of 20 half-days, or a shorter program of 3 days' duration. Thousands of veterans have participated in this form of training in the New York City Audiology Clinic, slightly more than one-half electing to attend the 4-week sessions. The success of this program has, in part, been related to careful and sympathetic counseling of the veteran. The counseling has been carried out not only in the audiology clinic but also in the office of the prosthetic specialist in the Veterans Administration. The latter is himself a physically disabled veteran who has a background of special training and who relates effectively to handicapped veterans requiring a hearing aid.

A somewhat modified rehabilitation program has been in effect in the audiology clinic in the Los Angeles Outpatient Clinic of the Veterans Administration. There the extended program consists of 10 half-days, and the limited program runs for 3 half-days. Again, the goal is to improve the skills of communication while helping the veteran to attain a realistic estimate of his handicap due to hearing loss and of his progress in overcoming it. Frequently, special problems create the need for a special program of individual instruction, but group work is more typical. A social worker and a psychologist participate actively in the program. In common with the experience of the New York City Audiology Clinic, the office in Los Angeles has found that many veterans who have completed the program return later for further training. In Los Angeles, where the program developed more recently than that in New York, many veterans have attended, most of them for the extended course.

Numerous elderly veterans, including those who served in the Spanish-American War, have been referred to Veterans Administration Audiology Clinics. Clinicians who have assisted these patients are astonished by the large percentage who have been benefited. Unexpectedly large numbers of older veterans have learned to use hearing aids successfully, and many have participated enthusiastically in training programs. This experience runs counter to the notion that there is little that can be done for the amelioration of hearing loss in elderly persons.

It is now recognized that the immediate costs for rehabilitation are ultimately more than recovered in economic gains to the individual and to society. For example, a veteran who was experiencing job problems in his home city enrolled in the training program in Los Angeles. Before leaving he applied for a position in Los Angeles with a company that was known to be favorably inclined to the hard-of-hearing. The veteran was offered and accepted a job; he has since won several awards for outstanding sales ability. There have been many similar reports of benefits following the furnishing of a hearing aid, rehabilitation training, and counseling.

The military and veterans' programs are considered to have had a suitable yet important influence on public acceptance of hearing aids. Before World War II, hearing aids were not often seen in public and were especially shunned by young adults with hearing loss. A shift in attitude occurred when thousands of men in military service were furnished hearing aids before discharge during the final period of the war, and when, following its termination, additional thousands qualified for receipt of hearing aids as eligible veterans. It is likely that the example set by these groups encouraged the more general use of hearing aids. Perhaps, too, the attitudes of employers and the general public were favorably affected by veterans with impaired hearing who sought to overcome their handicap. Today, in Veterans Administration Audiology Clinics, one rarely encounters any reluctance to be seen wearing a hearing aid, a reluctance which was often strong among young veterans immediately after World War II.

## Assessment of Social Efficiency

Veterans Administration Audiology Clinics play a significant role in examining hearing function in claims for disability compensation. Immediately following World War II, these examinations were conducted in the various outpatient medical clinics, utilizing the traditional spoken-voice, distance-fraction tests.

Aware of the weaknesses in measuring hearing loss by the spoken-voice method, the Veterans Administration revised its procedures for evaluating hearing impairment. In 1952 it turned to a rating schedule based on pure tone and speech audiometry. The veteran generally went to the outpatient clinic nearest his home, where the examination was carried out. Although this procedure was demonstrably superior to the one previously employed, it too showed several weaknesses: poor acoustic conditions in many of the clinics, insufficient experience and training of some technicians, and limitations of the available audiometric equipment.

In 1955 came a fuller recognition of the fact that accurate assessment of auditory function was not a simple matter. A system was developed that took advantage of the growth which had occurred in the field of audiology. Within the Veterans Administration and available on a contract basis throughout most of the country were clinics with highly trained personnel and excellent equipment. An effort was made to take advantage of such facilities wherever possible.

The Veterans Administration, using selected audiology clinics, then instituted a program of reexamining veterans who had been receiving compensation for a service-connected hearing impairment. These audiology clinics, either under contract or as part of the Veterans Administration, were required to possess hearing evaluation equipment meeting specified technical standards. Further, a uniform minimum level of training and experience was established for all participating clinicians.

For purposes of compensation, a minimum battery of tests was established for examinations related to evaluation of hearing impairment. This presently includes air- and bone-conduction audiometry, electrodermal audiometry at one or more frequencies, speech reception threshold, and speech intelligibility tests, for each ear. When these tests give results which are equivocal, additional tests must be performed. These include the Stenger and the Doerfler-Stewart tests and tests based on the principle of delayed speech. These tests are described in Chapters 7 and 8. Highly trained supervisory personnel continually monitor the test findings, the status of equipment, and the performance of staff audiologists. This testing program has since been extended to the evaluation of veterans who present new claims for loss of hearing.

The audiological reexamination program has been important in many ways. It has provided the Veterans Administration with a significant advance in procedures for determination of hearing impairment and, because of its insistence on minimum standards for personnel and equipment, the Veterans Administration has helped in the development of competent clinics in the few areas where they were not previously available.

## The Problem of Nonorganic Deafness

One of the most interesting aspects of the Veterans Administration audiology program is its concern with the problem of functional or psychogenic deafness.

(The Veterans Administration uses the broad term "nonorganic," which includes "functional" and psychogenic deafness.) Psychogenic deafness and the other forms of central dysacusis are described in Chapter 4. It is noted there that the incidence of psychogenic deafness in the general population seems to be very small. In all probability this is partly due to the failure to employ appropriate procedures routinely, since the detection of psychogenic deafness requires both an awareness of the problem and a willingness to use the necessary techniques, even though the tests may be more elaborate than those for threshold audiometry.

Nonorganic deafness has been observed quite frequently in Veterans Administration Audiology Clinics. Its difference from organic hearing loss is often a subtle one. For this reason, the decision to have examinations for rating purposes conducted in audiology clinics has proved wise because it has encouraged audiological evaluations of a most exacting nature. Were they to be done in a cursory manner, nonorganic deafness might not be recognized, and the possibilities of award of compensation and issue of a hearing aid might very well lead veterans to accept easily the idea that they have an organic impairment when actually they do not. This is especially likely when one reflects on the nature of nonorganic or "functional" hearing loss. Typically, it appears in conjunction with a mild organic impairment.

Electrodermal audiometry is particularly useful in the audiological test battery, principally because it may suggest that the impairment is not organic. Other tests which have been successfully employed for this purpose in addition to the minimum battery of pure-tone audiometry, speech audiometry, and electrodermal pure-tone audiometry, are Stenger, shifting-voice, electrodermal speech audiometry, Doerfler-Stewart, delayed sidetone, and Békésy audiometry—all tests described in Chapters 7 and 8. Psychological and psychiatric procedures have also proved helpful in evaluation.

Nonorganic deafness has long been a poorly understood and rarely discussed phenomenon outside the military and veterans' sphere. Partly because of the use of contract clinics for Veterans Administration examinations, there has developed a much more widespread knowledge and appreciation of the condition. The awareness of what it is and that it exists in the civilian population, including children, is increasing.

## Interdepartmental Relations

Veterans Administration Audiology Clinics have had the advantages of good physical plants as well as versatile and modern equipment. Quite naturally, therefore, they have worked closely with the Departments of Otolaryngology, Neurology, Psychology, Psychiatry, and related specialties. As the evaluation of auditory function has become more complex and revealing, the possible professional contribution of the clinical audiologist has grown. Such associations have been fostered in research and training also.

## Research

Audiological research in the Veterans Administration has a strong orientation to clinical needs. Research activities help create a stimulating professional environment, which in turn results in improved treatment of patients. Audiology clinics have shared in the general growth of research throughout the Veterans Administration's Department of Medicine and Surgery. Research projects typically develop secondarily to regular clinical duties. In some situations, however, the primary activity is research. The study of hearing aids, nonorganic deafness, and hearing problems related to aging are among the research interests.

### Training

Veterans Administration Audiology and Speech Pathology Clinics have encountered difficulties in securing the services of qualified personnel, largely because of the national shortage. To help alleviate this situation, a training program has been established in cooperation with several dozen universities offering graduate training in audiology, speech pathology, and speech and hearing science. At this time, well over 100 graduate students from affiliated universities are in receipt of stipends from the Veterans Administration. The amount of financial assistance and the level of the trainee's appointment are dependent upon his professional ability, prior graduate education, and previous experience. Supervised training, in a progressive medical environment, is furnished in a wide range of clinical assignments and research methodologies. Trainees are under no obligation to accept Veterans Administration staff positions upon completion of their program. Many excellent former trainees have decided to continue their careers in the Veterans Administration, but others have helped to meet the growing national health needs by taking positions in other environments.

### Hearing Aid Procurement

Since World War II, the Veterans Administration has been furnishing hearing aids to large numbers of eligible veterans. Its Department of Medicine and Surgery quite naturally is keenly interested in the quality of commercially available hearing aids and, as it does with other prosthetic and sensory-aid devices, it actively supports research and other programs aimed at fostering improvements.

As we have said, the Veterans Administration prefers to furnish the veteran with the actual instrument which is selected in the hearing-aid evaluation. A complicating factor in the whole procedure is the large number of manufacturers, each of whom is likely to have a variety of models which are subject to periodic change. The decision as to which instruments to stock in the audiology clinics is thus a difficult one. It would be undesirable for the stock to lag significantly behind current models, yet too-frequent addition of new but very different models could result in a continually increasing inventory of out-of-date hearing aids. Furthermore, not every change necessarily represents an improvement over the existing models.

For a number of years the Veterans Administration procured its hearing aids on the basis of negotiated contracts with the various manufacturers. Many companies were represented and, as a result, the variety of models in stock was so extensive that it created administrative problems in the clinics without compensating professional advantages.

In 1956 the hearing-aid procurement policy was changed. One goal was to reduce to a smaller and more manageable level the number of different models that the individual clinics were required to stock. In addition, and insofar as possible, it was hoped to achieve lowered costs while obtaining hearing aids of the highest quality.

A special consultant group was organized to assist in the management of this new program. The plan is to evaluate annually the performance characteristics of hearing aids submitted to the Veterans Administration for proposed inclusion in its clinic stock. Competitive bids are then invited from the manufacturers whose instruments score highest in the performance tests. Final procurement thus rests on a relation between performance scores and bid prices, or cost-per-point-of-quality.

The cooperation of the National Bureau of Standards has been enlisted for the actual measurement of the performance characteristics. The bureau tests the various models of hearing aids for a number of acoustic features and submits the results to the Veterans Administration. The Auditory Research Laboratory, Veterans Administration Hospital, Washington, D.C., then subjects the data to statistical and comparative analyses from which a final performance score is derived.

The Veterans Administration has retained the right to eliminate from consideration any instruments which it regards as clinically unacceptable. In addition, each manufacturer desiring to participate in the program must have been actively engaged in the business of manufacturing hearing aids for a period of not less than three years. Furthermore, because hearing aids must occasionally be procured through local commercial dealers rather than from the factory, each manufacturer must have established dealers or distributors in most of the major cities of the United States. The plan has never contemplated the development of formal specifications. Instead, emphasis is placed on actual comparative performance of the instruments, in the hope of stimulating research and benefiting from continuing design improvements in the hearing aid industry. To meet needs which may arise, the Veterans Administration has also reserved the right to procure hearing aids having special desirable characteristics apart from the basic program.

The manufacturers are, of course, free to decide which of their models to submit for evaluation. A maximum number of models per manufacturer has been established, however. The manufacturers are given a description of the tests which will be made. It is their responsibility to decide which tone settings, adjustments, and battery voltages they wish to specify for a particular model. They are advised to select those settings that will yield a frequency response curve that is close to a 5 dB per octave rise. Three randomly selected samples of each hearing aid model are then given the entire series of tests.

The tests for evaluation include measurements of maximum power output, frequency response, gain, battery drain, nonlinear distortion, and signal-to-noise ratio. (These various characteristics and the importance of each have been described in Chapters 10 and 11.) The models are then classified, on the basis of gain and maximum power output, into three categories: mild, moderate, and strong. The results from the other measurements of the three samples of each model are then averaged to yield a performance score for that model on each test item. The raw scores representing the various physical measures are then weighted according to a ranking that has been assigned to their relative importance. This ranking and the consequent weighting of the scores is based on the advice of the special consultants, and every effort is made to ensure that they also reflect the needs and the experience of the audiologists in the various Veterans Administration clinics.

The cost of each model to the Veterans Administration is divided by the quality-point score of that model. The cost-per-point-of-quality establishes a ranking for the various models in each of the three categories of mild, moderate, and strong. The clinical needs of the Veterans Administration are being successfully met by procuring a selected number of instruments for each of these three categories.

It should be clearly recognized that this description is intended to furnish a general outline of the Veterans Administration goals and policies in this field. It has not been a complete analysis of the program for procurement of hearing aids. Further, there is a continuing review of objectives and evaluation of results. Important changes and minor modifications have been introduced annually.

The Veterans Administration intends that its hearing-aid test program should assist in reducing the number of different models that must be stocked in its clinics. It further seeks to provide a means for competitive bidding while still assuring the acquisition of hearing aids which have high performance ratings. The physical features evaluated are those which the Veterans Administration considers to be important in a large procurement program. The cost factor is related to quantity purchasing. The hearing aids are ultimately selected on the basis of a series of factors which are most meaningful to the Veterans Administration, but these factors do not necessarily guide directly the choice of a hearing aid for each individual consumer.

### Prospects

The 28 regional clinics discussed earlier are fairly large in terms of size of staff, scope of program, and quantity and complexity of instrumentation. Together with a few contract clinics, this network provides nationwide coverage for hearing-impaired veterans who are eligible for the services. Attention is now being directed to the needs of hospitalized patients for whom it is not feasible to rely on the regional clinics. Efforts are being made to provide basic instrumentation in additional Veterans Administration hospitals where audiological evaluations are recognized as having diagnostic importance. As the age of hospitalized veterans rises, there has been an accompanying increase in the number of brain-damaged and laryngectomized patients. Speech pathologists are being added to the regional clinics and to other hospital programs to furnish urgently needed speech and language services to patients who have had strokes, laryngeal cancer, and other serious communicative difficulties. In striving for a communicative disorders program of the highest quality, the Veterans Administration hopes to benefit its patients as well as contribute to the field of audiology and speech pathology.

## SUGGESTED READINGS AND REFERENCES

**Bergman, M.** "The Audiology Clinic," *Acta Otolaryng.* (Stockholm) 1950, Supplement 89, 1–107.
   This is a description of the Audiology Clinic in the Veterans Administration Regional Office, New York.

**Ventry, I. M., and J. B. Chaiklin (eds.).** Multidiscipline Study of Functional Hearing Loss." *J. Auditory Res.,* 5:179–272 (1965).
   The interesting subject of nonorganic hearing loss is carefully explored in this report of a series of investigations at the Veterans Administration Hospital, San Francisco. An unusually exhaustive bibliography is given.

# CHAPTER 20

## VOCATIONAL GUIDANCE FOR THE DEAF

BOYCE R. WILLIAMS, LL.D.
McCAY VERNON, Ph.D.

Deaf people have generally maintained a good public image in the world of work as compared to other groups of disabled persons, and they have shown advantageously in competition with workers with normal hearing. In fact, the deaf population in a national survey by Lunde and Bigman (1959) reported a higher average of earned income than its hearing counterpart. This apparent success has not been due to good vocational guidance, but probably to the normal vigor, mobility, and intelligence of deaf people, and to their prevocational shop experience in residential schools for the deaf. Nevertheless, unemployment is frequent among the lower half of the population, and underemployment is common to almost all deaf people. The reasons for this situation are complex and may have their roots in the unavailability of appropriate services or in the poor quality of services that are available. Furthermore, the burgeoning technology, particularly as it is expressed in automation, has brought about major

changes in the world of work. The deaf population may be faced with a vocational crisis, the successful resolution of which will demand massive changes in our approach to the counseling, education, and training of deaf persons.

This chapter will first delineate assets, liabilities, communication problems, and work patterns of deaf and severely hard-of-hearing people. Then the various services available to them will be described. Counseling and psychodiagnosis, related problems, and pertinent recommendations will be discussed. The major focus is to relate the deaf client to the contemporary world of work and to emphasize the needs and directions for vocational guidance. A final section treats characteristics and problems of certain subgroups within what is broadly defined as the hearing-impaired population.

## COUNSELING DEAF PERSONS

Counseling deaf persons requires a consideration of their characteristics, the services available to them, testing procedures, the actual counseling process, and placement and follow-up.

### The Deaf Client

The counselor must know that persons who are deaf represent essentially the same broad spectrum of human assets and liabilities that characterize people in general. For example, the deaf person seeking counseling may range from a brilliant, highly motivated doctoral student needing financial assistance for graduate study to an illiterate, multiply-handicapped, indifferent youth from a rural area who has had no opportunity for any formal education or for even rudimentary socialization. He must know also that, although the deaf population has the same range of variability that exists in the normal-hearing, deafness can be so pervasive in its effects that for certain functions there are levels of achievement, potential abilities, and behaviors related to vocational counseling which are unique to deaf persons.

It is essential that counseling and vocational planning incorporate an awareness of the similarities and differences. This section will consider topics pertinent to vocational guidance and the effects of profound hearing loss. They include intelligence, education, communication, motor skills, work patterns, social patterns, and personality.

*Intelligence.* The intelligence of deaf persons has been extensively studied since the advent of IQ tests in the early 1900's, as described in Chapter 16. This research clearly supports the view that deaf people as a group have essentially the same level of intelligence as the general population. The public's occasional association of deafness with "dumbness" or stupidity is without basis in fact. Among other things, it rests upon the age-old fallacy of assuming the lack of speech to be related to inferior intellect and upon the equally invalid as-

sumption that the difficulties of many deaf people with written language reflect their intelligence instead of simply their lack of having had the opportunity to learn language through hearing, as we have seen in Chapter 16. Furthermore, the public is generally unaware of the extent to which profound deafness may complicate even simple human relations.

Another and perhaps more sophisticated fallacy is that the deaf person has a reduced capacity for abstract thought. At a very practical level, the deaf person's language limitations may make it difficult for the counselor to pose abstract questions to him and for him to express verbally his more abstract concepts to the counselor. However, Furth (see Chapter 16) and Vernon point to investigations that demonstrate a potential for abstract thought among deaf people equal to that of the hearing. For example, there are a number of deaf mathematicians. The tendency of the deaf client to be concrete in his counseling sessions is likely to be caused by inadequate education and language, and not by a lack of capacity for abstract cognitive thought.

It is important that professionals in vocational guidance and related fields recognize that deaf people have the same range and variability of intelligence as the general population and that they, in turn, communicate this to employers and educators. Certainly, this should influence the level of vocational aspiration of the deaf.

*Education.* The educational achievement of deaf persons stands in sharp contrast to the facts just established about their intelligence. Although some attain Phi Beta Kappa or the Ph.D. degree, the average deaf person is grossly undereducated. This is, in part, a failing of the educational system which has not developed the intellectual capacity of deaf students and, to some extent, is evidence of the tremendous impediment to academic and other learning resulting from deafness.

The most extensive current survey of the educational achievement of the deaf included 93 percent of deaf students 16 years or older in the United States (Boatner, 1965), (see Chapter 16). It found that only 5 percent achieved tenth-grade level or better (most of these being hard of hearing or postlingually deafened), 60 percent were at grade level 5.3 or below, and 30 percent were functionally illiterate.

Another study by Wrightstone, Aronow, and Moskowitz in 1962, based on 73 school programs for the deaf and representing 54 percent of all school-age deaf children 10 to 16 years of age, reports their reading scores on the Metropolitan Achievement Test: 88 percent of the 16-year-olds were below grade 4.9 in reading. Furthermore, the average gain in reading from age 10 to 16 was less than one year (grade 2.6 to grade 3.4). Fortunately, some of these students receive extensive prevocational training which may prepare them to enter skilled or semiskilled occupations for advanced vocational training. However, many do not.

It is evident that the average deaf person represents a unique client for vocational guidance. He may have the same intelligence and cognitive abilities as the hearing, yet he generally lacks the educational achievement normally required to realize his potential. Fitting this unique, uneven pattern of characteristics into an appropriate vocational situation is a major challenge. The counselor must guard against a natural tendency for the educational inadequacies of his deaf client to divert him from the client's strengths. The counselor must also keep in mind that the grade designation used in schools for the deaf may be more related to age and years in school than to achievement. A deaf "twelfth grader" may very well be 20 years old and be achieving at fourth-grade level.

*Communication.* Central to an understanding of deafness is knowledge of its impact on communication. Despite the crucial significance of this, many professionals in education, speech, audiology, medicine, and other allied specialties are likely to have little insight into the psychological, social, and vocational implications of the difficulties of communication for deaf persons. The professionals meet so few deaf people outside clinics or schools that they often have a naive "Pollyanna-like" perception of deafness, its problems, and solutions. If deaf people spent their entire lives in clinics and schools instead of facing the taxing challenge of economic and psychic survival, such deficiencies in professional insight would not be critical.

The communication controversy has been treated in Chapter 16, and the reader is encouraged to pursue this important issue further through suggested reading (Furth, 1966, 1–16; Di Carlo, 1964, 85–115; Williams, 1965; Vernon and Mindel, 1969).

Most young people today who are deaf were born that way or else acquired hearing loss early in life before they were old enough to have learned to talk and to use language. They are not likely to develop *normal* speech. As we have seen in Chapter 16 intelligible speech can be acquired, but in many cases the prelingually deafened client will not be able to talk intelligibly to the counselor or to potential employers. Although speech is an invaluable asset in all aspects of life and work and is an important criterion in assessing individual employability, the counselor simply must recognize that many bright, capable deaf persons cannot speak understandably. Unfortunately, as we have said, a few counselors and employers may wrongly equate the inability to speak with ignorance. The counselor must also be alert for the deaf person who has good basic speech that is deteriorating for want of remedial attention, as pointed out in Chapter 14.

Speechreading is a valuable skill for communication, but, as we have seen, it has limitations, and many deaf persons do not acquire it at all, or enough of it to be practically useful. We have seen in Chapter 12 that many sounds of English are not visible on the lips or may be confused with other sounds. The difficulties are compounded by such factors as poor lighting, protruding teeth, cigarettes in the mouth, moustaches, bad speech habits, small immobile mouths, and distracting head movements. Consequently, few deaf people, particularly those seeking counseling, are expert speechreaders. Fortunately, many routine jobs do not require extensive communication. When it is necessary in higher employment levels suitable for above-average deaf persons, they frequently find many ways to compensate. Nevertheless, ability in speechreading can be an important vocational asset. In Chapter 16 we have seen how early deafness affects the acquisition, the vocabulary, and the structure of language and frequently results in poor or inadequate communication even by writing.

In view of the frustrations of deaf persons with speech, speechreading, and writing, many of them turn to the language of signs and fingerspelling. Often deaf persons who lack any appreciable ability at oral or written communication can express fluently and receive understandably complex ideas in the language of signs. The client should have the right to choose the means of communication with which he is most comfortable. Although competence with the language of signs and fingerspelling is not a vocational asset except in unusual situations, it does give the counselor better knowledge of his client's potential and more assurance in guiding him to an appropriate job.

In years past, most deaf youths attended residential schools, at least during their high-school years. In these schools, those who could not communicate orally were given an opportunity to learn how to communicate manually. Today many deaf young people attend day classes or day-school programs with hearing students. This works out successfully for some. They develop intelligible speech, can read and write, and are able to use speechreading for many practical communication purposes. However, a large proportion of these students do not learn to speak intelligibly; they cannot read and write enough to convey more than rudimentary daily needs; and they do not speechread.

Vocational counselors are facing more and more of these cases, especially in larger cities. They are often confronted by clients who have no dependable means of communication despite 12 years of schooling. With these persons it is necessary to start almost from scratch and to give them intensive instruction in the language of signs in order that counseling may become possible. As it may take a year or more of intense exposure to become fluent in manual communication, these young people represent an unfortunate, frustrated group.

*Motor skills.* Motor functioning, especially as it relates to manual dexterity, is particularly important for deaf persons because approximately five-sixths of deaf workers are in manual work. Myklebust's (1960) investigations and those of others suggest that the deaf as a group are not inferior in manual dexterity. Furthermore, he thinks that in areas such as simultaneous movement, locomotor coordination, and motor speed, in which the deaf have scored lower than the hearing, the deficit may be correctible with training. Only in the sense of balance, dependent upon the vestibular mechanism, which in some deaf persons has been destroyed by the condition causing the deafness, do many deaf people have a motor disability which must be considered in vocational guidance.

The favorable performance of deaf persons in motor skills may be a mixed blessing. It has certainly provided entry to the manual work in which five-sixths are employed. The appeal of immediate income has also diverted substantial numbers of young people of those five-sixths from advanced training, and consequently deprived them of higher-level employment.

*Work patterns.* Historically, deaf people have had high rates of employment, mostly in unskilled and semiskilled areas. The foregoing discussion of their intelligence and motor ability suggests that this pattern is actually one of underemployment. The lack of better vocational guidance, of better education, and of better opportunities for advanced training, interacting with the problems inherent in deafness, have resulted in widespread underemployment and very few deaf people in the professions. Discrimination by employers is another factor that has tended to diminish opportunities, despite the fact that those employers who give deaf applicants a chance report satisfactory work records. Deaf workers as a group are highly stable in job tenure, except for some young deaf persons who may lack maturity when first entering the world of work.

*Social patterns.* Vocational guidance must constantly be sensitive to realities of social life for most deaf clients. The main reality is that the communication problem causes most deaf people to have the overwhelming majority of their social contacts and close friendships with other deaf people with whom they can communicate. This enables deaf people to develop the emotionally satisfying close personal ties and friendships that are rarely possible when communication is inaccurate and frustrating.

Vocational guidance workers must consider these factors very carefully. Usually urban areas, where social contacts with other deaf persons are possible and where job opportunities that are not too demanding in communication are most available, are the most favorable. Work, which is task-oriented, is a different matter. In work, the deaf person generally is employed with hearing people with whom he communicates primarily through writing. He also uses speech and speechreading when possible. Clichés about a "deaf" versus a "hearing" world represent a naive sort of thinking that has colored vocational guidance in the past by failing to recognize that the "work" world of the deaf is usually predominantly "hearing," whereas their "social" world is primarily "deaf."

*Personality.* Most deaf persons are able to relate to hearing people in a pleasant, satisfactory, though frequently limited, way. Among the undereducated people with whom deaf persons are likely to work, they are sometimes the butt of crude, insensitive jokes. They may be taken advantage of in situations in which bad shifts or unpleasant duties must be assigned. The more mature deaf person has experienced this often enough either to be able to cope with it and stand up for his rights, or to have learned to live with it philosophically. The younger employee may react impulsively with understandable anger. However, the anger may not be channeled constructively, and the counselor must take remedial steps.

Just as the deaf employee may have to tolerate considerable unpleasantness from some hearing workers, certain undesirable traits may be more common to the deaf workers. These again are due to his communication problem, which leads to a lack of a full understanding of what is going on around him. One consequence of this may be a rigidity or stubborness about accepting changes, which may have its roots in insecurity. He may fail to be aware of his unpleasant voice or the shuffling noises he creates.

Beyond anecdotal accounts, as we have seen in Chapter 16, investigations of the personality traits of those who are deaf have been meager and have in many cases frequently led to misinformed judgments. Many have used personality tests, such as the Minnesota Multiphasic Personality Inventory, which are grossly inappropriate

(Rosen, 1967). We have seen the inadequacy of most verbal tests of personality. In general, there seems to be no more "psychotic-type personality" pathology among the deaf than among the hearing. However, organic factors seem to assume a more dominant role, but little is really known about qualitative differences that may exist.

In summary, vocational guidance for deaf persons is a unique challenge. The tendency has been to use primarily the manual skills which are readily learned while ignoring the intellectual capacity and general potential which is far more difficult to exploit. The result has been a degrading, frustrating kind of underemployment. This problem is now being constructively attacked by the Social and Rehabilitation Service of the Department of Health, Education, and Welfare. This attack is another reflection of the national concern with deafness elaborated on in Chapter 15.

### Services for the Deaf

Vocational services for the deaf are available in educational institutions, in vocational rehabilitation agencies, state employment facilities, in public and private organizations, in higher education, and in mental health establishments.

*Ongoing vocational guidance for the deaf in educational institutions.* Important changes have occurred in the vocational guidance available to deaf youth in recent years. Until the late 1930s or early 1940s deaf students of secondary age were in residential schools where they received extensive prevocational or, in rare cases, vocational training. The guidance available to them was informal and revolved primarily around the few shops maintained

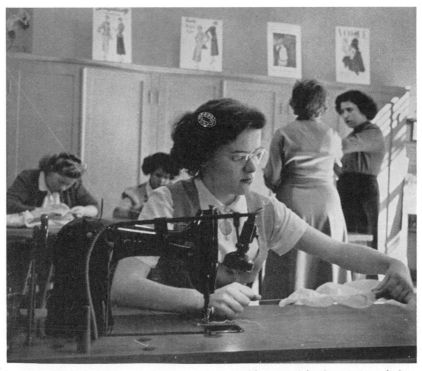

Fig. 20-1. Deaf girls learn to operate power machines used in the garment industry.

in the school (for example, wood, metal, leather, print) or around counseling directed toward preparation for Gallaudet College.

This approach had advantages and disadvantages. On the one hand, it gave many deaf youths an entry-level skill in a trade —usually printing, shoe repairing, or woodworking. However, it seriously restricted a deaf individual and his associates in the setting of appropriate occupational goals, because of the very limited range of experience in school and because of the lack of opportunities for postschool training. Thus, a kind of environmental constraint has operated to curb individual range and levels of choice. In the case of the college-bound, Gallaudet as a liberal arts college offered a substantial major only in teaching, which for a deaf professional person offered a very limited opportunity for advancement. In fact, the professional training at Gallaudet was so narrow that a large percentage of the graduates entered printing, resulting in gross underemployment.

In recent years day-school programs have increased for secondary-age deaf youths. For them vocational guidance is critical. As a rule, these programs emphasize academic courses, often far above the educational abilities of their deaf students except for the brighter ones. Token effort is made to handle this major problem by having a "resource teacher" who meets for a period a day with a group of the deaf students. Vocational types of courses may or may not be available, and serious and appropriate vocational guidance is not likely to be practiced. The dropout rate may be high, and opportunities for vocational success limited.

Residential schools, with the exception of a few, have failed to keep their vocational programs up to date. Consequently, most residential schools may offer one or two well-taught prevocational skills (one is usually printing) and fairly extensive industrial arts or exploratory types of programs. The presence of deaf vocational teachers in these schools, the classes in vocational guidance, and the closeness of many of the students to members of the deaf community in the world of work generally give residential students better vocational guidance than those in other schools.

The result of the changes in educational patterns is that many deaf youths are getting no vocational guidance or training. A few of those who attend residential schools are getting entry-level skills in a trade. Others are given a superficial familiarity with tools and shop practice and some vocational guidance. This seems to contribute to the rising number of unemployed and underemployed deaf youth.

The clients from residential schools may have weak educational backgrounds, but they do know how to communicate manually and have generally had some vocational guidance and training. Hence, their future may be brighter than those from day schools. However, there are bright students from day and residential schools who leave secondary schools with a bona fide high school education and a readiness for guidance and further education. In between are many deaf youths with *average* potential which is grossly underdeveloped, but which is sufficient to benefit from vocational guidance and training, leading to skilled or semiskilled work.

### Vocational Rehabilitation Services

Each of the 50 states, the District of Columbia, Guam, Puerto Rico, and the Virgin Islands has a vocational rehabilitation program that serves eligible deaf clients. In the years 1957 to 1966 a total of 19,119 deaf and 43,971 hard-of-hearing persons were vocationally rehabilitated by this service.

The determination of eligibility and the actual extension of services are functions

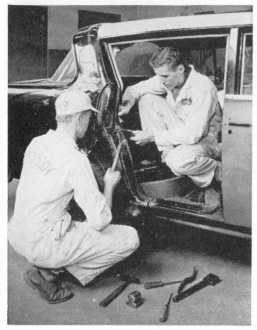

Fig. 20-2. Deaf boys learn to repair automobile bodies. (*New Jersey School for the Deaf.*)

rehabilitation services will render the individual able to engage in a remunerative occupation or in an occupation more in keeping with his total characteristics. Eligibility also is ordinarily limited to disabled persons of working age or nearly so.

Rehabilitation services are provided in accordance with a plan worked out by the client and his counselor, assisted by the vocational guidance team that is available. They may include in any appropriate combination:

1. Thorough physical, mental, and aural examinations
2. Extended evaluation, up to eighteen months for a severely handicapped deaf person, to determine employment potential
3. Communication development, including hearing aids, speechreading, speech correction and conservation, auditory training, reading, writing, the manual alphabet, and the language of signs
4. Individual counseling and guidance including attention to problems of personal adjustment as they influence employment
5. Training for jobs—in school, on the job, by correspondence, or by tutor.

of the state vocational rehabilitation agencies. Eligibility rests upon the presence of a physical or mental impairment, the existence of a substantial handicap to employment as a result of the impairment, and reasonable expectation that vocational

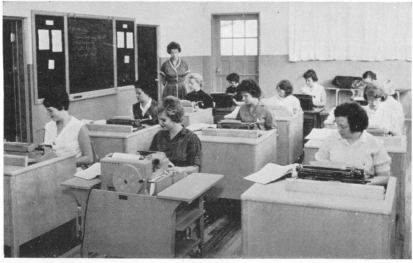

Fig. 20-3. Deaf girls learn to operate business machines. (*New Jersey School for the Deaf.*)

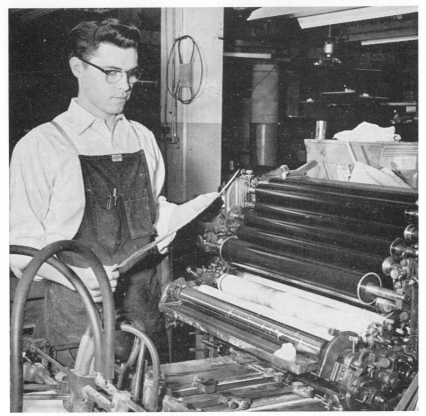

Fig. 20-4. A deaf printer checks proofs. (*Commercial Letter Service, Inc., St. Louis.*)

6. Maintenance and transportation during rehabilitation
7. Necessary tools, licenses, and equipment
8. Placement in the right job
9. Follow-up to make sure that the rehabilitated worker and the job are properly matched.

The 54 general state rehabilitation agencies have more than 7000 highly skilled counseling and placement workers in over 1600 offices throughout the country. More and more counselors as they gain experience are becoming knowledgeable about serving deaf clients with increasing effectiveness.

### State Employment Services

Almost 2000 local employment offices in all of the states and territories are important service centers for unemployed deaf persons. Their aims are:

1. Equal job opportunity and equal pay in competition with other job seekers
2. Jobs appropriate to individual physical and other qualifications
3. Satisfaction in the job
4. Jobs that are safe for the individual and his co-workers

Their services include:

1. Selective placement—matching the individual's qualifications to job requirements
2. Employment counseling, including determination of need for services to improve employability
3. Development of job opportunities for individuals for whom no suitable vacancies exist

4. Preparation of client and employer for the job interview so that the handicap is seen in proper perspective
5. Advice on job modifications needed to meet with client's capacities
6. Follow-up to ensure mutual job satisfaction

Staffs are skillful in selective placement procedures, have current knowledge of the job market, and are experts in employer-employee adjustments.

### Public and Private Facilities

Important new organizations for vocational guidance are found in various contexts of the vocational rehabilitation movement. Centers for serving the most severely handicapped deaf persons have been established in recent years in Alabama, Arizona, Arkansas, California, Florida, Georgia, Illinois, Indiana, Massachusetts, Michigan, Mississippi, Missouri, Ohio, Pennsylvania, and Washington. In most instances these are places which can carry out extended evaluation to determine employment potential and intensive training to improve communication and capacities for satisfactory interrelationships and ultimate independence. More such centers are being planned.

The deaf resident of a metropolitan area who is in need of, but unable, because of his communication problem, to avail himself effectively of public services that surround him is an old story to knowledgeable workers for the deaf. Coordinating and referral centers in New York City, Pittsburgh, Kansas City, and Seattle are developing new patterns of service for vocational guidance that are likely to be adopted by other urban areas.

### Higher Education

For many years higher education for a deaf person meant attendance at Gallaudet College, which offers majors in fields such as chemistry, mathematics, education, biology, literature, psychology, and so on. Admission is based on passing entrance examinations which are administered throughout the United States, Canada, and other countries.

In recognition of the educational lag which often results from deafness, Gallaudet College has established a Preparatory Department where students of college potential who are not ready for college work are given a year of intensive advance academic courses. Vocational guidance for deaf youth of college potential should include evaluation of the possibility of matriculation at Gallaudet. Unfortunately, many young people who are deaf but who do not attend residential schools or large day programs are never told of Gallaudet and lose this opportunity for higher education.

The limitations of a liberal arts curriculum and its inappropriateness for many deaf college students has led to the recent establishment of the National Technical Institute for the Deaf (N.T.I.D.), a part of the Rochester Institute of Technology. Here deaf students may earn diplomas, or associate of arts, and baccalaureate degrees in many technical fields, including engineering, graphic arts, and commercial photography. Some of the courses are taken only with other deaf students, but a large part of the program involves classes with the normally hearing. The first class at N.T.I.D. enrolled in 1968.

Some deaf students also attend regular colleges with hearing students. There are no special programs for them in these institutions (see Quigley, 1968). A college education under these circumstances is demanding academically, socially, and psychologically. Generally students who succeed in graduating from these colleges are exceptionally able, and have a good command of language. Often they communicate well orally but some may require outside support and help.

At San Fernando Valley State College

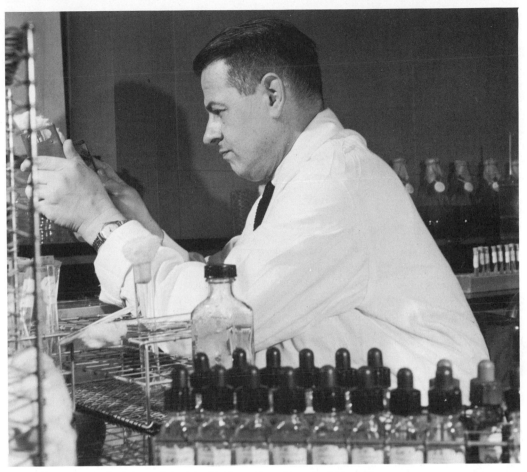

Fig. 20-5. A deaf bacteriologist. (*Indiana State Board of Health*)

and Riverside Junior College in California and at Northern Illinois University and a few other colleges and some technical schools, arrangements have been made to take in a number of deaf students and provide for them the needed tutoring, interpreting, note taking, and so on, that are usually necessary if a deaf person is to benefit adequately from attendance in an existing regular institution of higher learning. Of particular recent significance is the growth of opportunities for graduate work. San Fernando Valley State College, Gallaudet, and the University of Arizona have provided these opportunities, and the National Technical Institute for the Deaf is likely to do so. If the expanding opportuni-ties in higher education are to be utilized fully, vocational guidance must be instituted more effectively and earlier in the secondary schools.

### Mental Health

Until 1958 there was no professional treatment available for psychologically disturbed deaf persons. They were simply placed in state hospitals for the mentally ill or the mentally retarded. Here they were maintained custodially, isolated from other deaf people, often for the remainder of their lives. Neither hospital staff nor other patients could communicate with them. They had no way to express their feelings or to establish human relations.

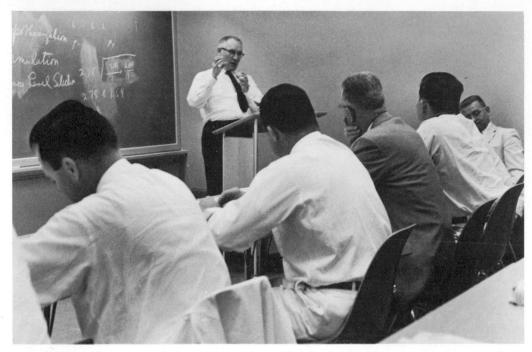

Fig. 20-6. A deaf scientist lectures to a class of hearing pupils. (*Used by permission of The Alexander Graham Bell Association for the Deaf, Inc. Volta Review, Dec. 1960*)

Finally, in the late 1950's Dr. Edna Levine interested the psychiatrist, Franz Kallmann, in the problem. Under their initial leadership, John D. Rainier and Kenneth Z. Altshuler have established an inpatient and outpatient service for the deaf in New York State. Their investigations are recorded in two books: *Family and Mental Health Problems in a Deaf Population* (1963) and *Comprehensive Mental Health Services for the Deaf* (1967), both of which demonstrate the value and need of providing a treatment milieu and psychotherapy for deaf people who are mentally ill.

Now similar facilities are being established at the Psychosomatic and Psychiatric Institute of Michael Reese Hospital in Chicago, the Langley-Porter Neuropsychiatric Institute in San Francisco, St. Elizabeth's Hospital in Washington, D.C., and at other facilities in New Hampshire and Texas. Social workers, psychiatrists, psychologists, and others are learning manual communi-

cation in order to be able to communicate with and to treat the deaf. More such services are needed.

## Psychological Evaluation

Psychological tests for deaf children have been discussed in Chapter 16. Here we shall concentrate on tests for deaf clients of vocational guidance. A psychological evaluation should consist of measures, in part or entirely, of the following kinds of information: (1) intelligence; (2) personality; (3) educational achievement; (4) communication skills; (5) aptitudes; and (6) interests. In many cases, all of these data may not be needed; or, if needed, can be obtained in part from school records or from sources other than the psychological examination.

Before discussing each of these areas of evaluation separately, it is helpful to establish certain basic general principles. Four basic concepts underlie effective psychological examinations of deaf clients.

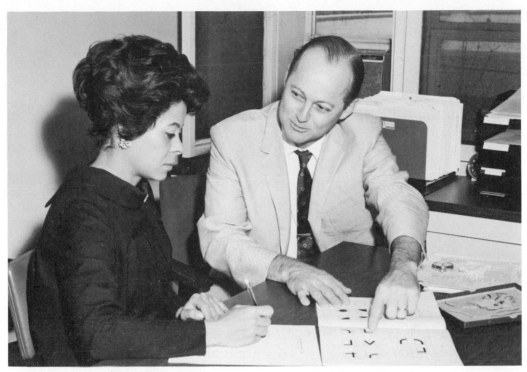

Fig. 20-7. Psychological testing of a deaf adult. (*Michael Reese Hospital*)

These principles also apply to the hard of hearing or those adventitiously deafened, but to lesser degrees. However, since it is the prelingually deafened client who is likely to be the greatest challenge, the primary focus of this section is on the evaluation of this type of client.

1. Psychological tests that involve the use of verbal language to measure intelligence, personality, and aptitude are not generally valid because they measure the deaf person's language limitations that are due to his deafness. Thus, they do not really measure how bright he is, what he can do, or his emotional stability. This is also emphasized in Chapter 16.

2. Tests given by persons not experienced with deaf or hard-of-hearing clients are subject to appreciably greater error than those administered by one familiar with individuals who are deaf.

3. Group testing of deaf and hard-of-hearing clients is a questionable procedure and should at best be done only for screening.

4. Often the congenitally hard-of-hearing client is, from a psychodiagnostic point of view, much more like a congenitally deaf client than his speech and his apparent response to sound would suggest. It is, therefore, crucial in a psychological evaluation that he be given tests appropriate for a person with a profound hearing loss, as well as tests for a person with normal hearing. When large differences appear between the sets of test responses, they often show that the client did better on the non-language tests appropriate for the deaf person. It is the latter findings which should be judged the more valid in such a circumstance.

*Intelligence testing.* An intelligence

TABLE 1
EVALUATION OF SOME OF THE INTELLIGENCE TESTS MOST COMMONLY USED
WITH DEAF AND HARD-OF-HEARING ADULTS

| Tests | Appropriate Age Range Covered By the Test | Evaluation of the Test |
|---|---|---|
| 1. Wechsler Performance Scale for Adults (1955) | 16 years to 70 years | The Wechsler Performance Scale is at present the best test for deaf adults. It yields a relatively valid IQ score and offers opportunities for qualitative interpretation of factors such as brain injury or emotional disturbance (Wechsler, 1955, pp. 80–81). It has good interest appeal, is relatively easy to administer, and is reasonable in cost. |
| 2. Progressive Matrices (Raven, 1948) | 9 years to adulthood | Raven's Progressive Matrices is good as a second test to substantiate another more comprehensive intelligence test. The advantage of the Matrices is that it is extremely easy to administer and score, taking relatively little of the examiner's time and is very inexpensive. It yields invalid test scores for impulsive deaf subjects who tend to respond randomly rather than with accuracy and care. For this reason, the examiner should observe the client carefully to assure that he is making a genuine effort. |
| 3. The Revised Beta (Levine, 1960, pp. 203, 206, 269) | Adults | The Revised Beta is a nonlanguage test involving mazes, spatial relations, matching, and similar performance type items. It provides an adequate measure of the intelligence of adults who are deaf. |

test, to be valid with a majority of deaf clients, must be a nonverbal performance type of instrument. Unfortunate consequences have resulted when verbal tests have been given to deaf people. There have been cases of above-average deaf persons being put in hospitals for the retarded and of deaf people being denied proper vocational guidance and training because inappropriate tests were employed. A verbal test of intelligence usually does not measure accurately the intelligence of a deaf person. It may measure the language handicap that results from his hearing loss. Performance tests, however, do measure a deaf person's intelligence. For example, it

is possible for a deaf person to score at the genius level on the performance scale of an IQ test and at the retarded level on the verbal scale of the same test. In Table 1 three intelligence tests for use with deaf clients are suggested and briefly reviewed.

*Personality.* Personality evaluation of deaf individuals is a far more complex task than intelligence testing. For this reason, test findings should be carefully interpreted in light of case histories and personal experiences with the client. In fact, it is often wise for counselors experienced with deafness to view with skepticism results reported by examiners who are unfamiliar with deafness when these findings differ from their own impressions of a deaf person.

Due to the communication problems inherent in severe hearing loss, personality tests are more difficult to use with deaf subjects than with the general population. Not only do these tests depend on extensive verbal interchange or reading skill, but they also presuppose a rapport and confidence on the part of the subject that is often difficult to achieve because the person examined does not fully understand what is being said or written. Paper-and-pencil personality measures are perhaps suitable for hearing-impaired persons with well-developed expressive and receptive language; however, such individuals are the exception, and even here the problems of test administration and interpretation render the results questionable. When projective measures such as the Rorschach or Thematic Apperception Tests are used, fluency in manual communication by the examiner is mandatory.

There is some question whether the norms for the personality structure of hearing people are appropriate for deaf and hard-of-hearing subjects. Conceivably, deafness alters the perceived environment sufficiently to produce an essentially different organization of personality, in which normality would then differ from what it is in the case of a person with adequate hearing. This is presently an unresolved problem, but it should be considered in any discussion of the personality of those with severe hearing loss.

The use of interpreters who express the psychologist's directions in fingerspelling and the language of signs is a questionable procedure. What is required is an interpreter who is fluent not only in manual communication but also in psychology and testing. Obviously, such an individual would be doing the examining himself and not interpreting for another. Therefore, results reported when an interpreter is involved are not likely to be valid.

It is important to note that the confusion and disassociation reflected in the writing of deaf clients with low-level verbal skills rarely indicate an equally disturbed thought process. It is usually largely the result of language deficiency. Psychologists unaware of this have been known to equate the written language of semiliterate deaf persons with that of the schizophrenic. This confusion has frequently led to unfortunate diagnoses.

Few personality tests have had wide successful application with deaf or hard-of-hearing adults because of the difficulties that we have pointed out. Five tests are suggested and reviewed briefly in Table 2.

*Educational achievement.* In many cases vocational guidance requires a measure of the level of educational achievement of a deaf client. The Metropolitan Achievement Test is an appropriate test for this purpose. It has norms for deaf and hearing subjects and is easy to administer, but the examiner must make certain that the client understands and successfully completes the same items for each subtest. Another critical point in using this or any achievement test is to choose a battery that is at a level appropriate to the person being tested. A failure to make *absolutely certain* that sample items are understood and that the level of the test battery is appropriate invalidates the entire procedure.

In interpreting results of achievement tests with deaf persons, it is important to keep in mind that only about 5 percent of graduates from day and residential schools for the deaf attain a tenth-grade educational level; 41 percent, seventh or eighth grade; 27 percent, fifth or sixth grade; and approximately 30 percent are in fourth grade or below. Most of those in the last category are termed functionally illiterate by present standards. These figures help a counselor understand some of the educational deficiencies resulting from deafness.

*Communication skills.* Because, as we continue to emphasize, communication

TABLE 2
PERSONALITY TESTS USED WITH DEAF AND HARD-OF-HEARING ADULTS

| Tests | Appropriate Age Range Covered By the Test | Evaluation of the Test |
|---|---|---|
| 1. Draw-A-Person (Machover, 1949) | 9 years to adulthood | A good screening device for detecting severe emotional problems. It is relatively nonverbal and is probably the most practical projective personality test for use with deaf subjects. Its interpretation is highly subjective, and in the hands of a poor psychologist it can result in rather extreme diagnostic statements about deaf clients. |
| 2. Thematic Apperception Test (TAT) or Children's Apperception Test (CAT) (Stein, 1955) | Can be used with subjects of school age through adulthood who can communicate well manually or who can communicate skillfully in written language. | This is a test of great potential, if the psychologist giving it and the deaf subject taking it can both communicate with fluency in manual communication. Otherwise, it is of very limited value unless the deaf subject has an exceptional command of language. The test could be given through an interpreter by an exceptionally perceptive psychologist, although it is more desirable if the psychologist can do his own communicating. |
| 3. Rorschach Ink Blot Test (Rorschach, 1942) | Can be given to deaf subjects if they are able to communicate fluently manually or communicate with exceptional skill orally. | In order for the Rorschach to be used, it is absolutely necessary that the psychologist giving it and the deaf subject taking it be fluent in manual communication. Even under these circumstances it is debatable whether it has great value unless the subject is of above-average intelligence. It would be possible with a very bright deaf subject, who had a remarkable proficiency in English, to give a Rorschach through writing, but this would be a dubious procedure. |
| 4. The House Tree Test (H-T-P) (Buck, 1949) | School age through adulthood | This is a procedure similar to the Draw-A-Person test. It requires little verbal communication and affords the competent clinician some valuable insight into basic personality dynamics of the subject. |
| 5. Bender-Gestalt (Bender, 1938) | Best for ages 12 years through adulthood | A useful projective test for personality and also for the detection of brain damage. Because of the rather high prevalence of brain damage among people who are deaf, it is often valuable to administer a Bender-Gestalt to clients who have severe learning problems or who give evidence of bizarre behavior. |

is the major handicap of deafness, it is important that an evaluation include an assessment of communication.

There are three aspects of communication that should be appraised in a deaf person. The first and by far the most important is the ability to *read and write*. It has been found that these modes of communication are most widely used in their job setting by persons who are deaf. The degree of skill of the deaf person will go a long way toward determining the type and level of occupational skills open to him.

*Speech* and *speechreading* are the other key aspects of communication to be evaluated. These skills have considerable potential value to a deaf person in the world of work. To be able to speak intelligibly is especially important and helpful. Speechreading is an asset, but even skilled speechreaders sometimes resort to the written word. At present, counselor judgment of speech and speechreading is likely to be the preferred method of evaluation. It is assumed that hearing will have been previously assessed as described in Chapter 7. Certainly a hearing aid and auditory training should be considered if there is any possibility that they can help.

*Aptitude and interest testing.* As there are hundreds of tests of aptitude and interest which are vital parts of client evaluation on the market, it is not feasible to list or discuss them individually. These are treated by Levine (1960) and Myklebust (1962). However, certain information about manual dexterity, mechanical aptitude, and spatial relations is particularly pertinent for deaf persons because they are important for the work that many deaf people do.

Interest tests are almost without exception highly verbal and, therefore, can generally not be used effectively with a deaf person. There are pictorial tests designed for use with clients who are deaf, but they are narrow in scope and offer limited data for a psychological evaluation.

*Case history.* The past is still the one best predictor of the future. Complete background information on a client is essential, especially for deaf persons for whom conventional tests may be of questionable validity. Among the factors to consider are the client's performance on past jobs, whether or not he had habitually demonstrated any particular problems or assets, what kinds of circumstances led to his success or failure, and what specific educational and vocational skills he mastered. In the case of young deaf clients from residential or large day schools, it is often possible to obtain complete and significant information from their schools. Integrated educational programs, where the deaf and hearing attend together, may also offer valuable information if they employ teachers or consultants who are qualified to work with deaf youth.

### The Counseling Process and Follow-Up

Counseling with a client who is deaf involves: first, a basic ability to counsel; second, an understanding of deafness; and third, a knowledge of available services.

Serious doubts have been raised about the value of abstract depth counseling and therapeutic approaches. With most deaf clients there appears to be no question that counseling should be concrete. The use of highly verbal techniques, such as classical psychoanalysis, have failed even in the hands of skilled therapists. Some nondirective techniques, modified to take account of deafness, have been used effectively with deaf persons.

Only the counselor who is extensively experienced in serving the deaf and who is a real master of manual communication may achieve good results through counseling interviews conducted in his office. Most often counseling best takes place in job evaluation centers or at the job interview. Thus, environmental manipulation, stimulation of employers and family, and supportive counseling are more important tools for most counselors serving the deaf in these times of shortage of experienced workers than abstract counseling procedures, which depend so heavily upon accurate and, at times, subtle communication.

Locating a job and then applying for it often represent major, if not insurmountable, obstacles to many otherwise capable deaf persons. The majority of deaf clients have these difficulties. We consider job placement to be an essential function of counseling the deaf. Successful job placement of a qualified deaf person may require that the counselor accompany him to the interview, serve as an interpreter, and provide for the interviewer, the supervisor, and co-workers brief, meaningful, and reassuring orientation to deafness. This should avoid any suggestion of paternalism or other behavior that may tarnish his image as an employee and co-worker.

The placement process is not complete for any deaf person without adequate follow-up on the job. The kind and extent of follow-up will vary according to the needs of the client. In many instances simple checks with client and employer are sufficient. Deaf persons who are severely handicapped by undertraining or marginal capability for adjustment will very likely need more intensive follow-up that includes several months of periodic visits with supportive counseling on the job.

In the case of the counselor who cannot finger-spell or use the language of signs, an interpreter should be available to assist those clients needing this service. Interpreters can be readily located by writing to National Registry of Interpreters for the Deaf, 2025 Eye Street, N. W., Washington, D. C. 20037, or by contacting the local club for the deaf.

It must be recognized that although the use of the language of signs can greatly facilitate communication, it is limited by the basic linguistic competence of the deaf client and the manual skills of the counselor or interpreter. Simply making a lot of signs does not ensure communication, nor does it overcome the basic vocabulary problem of a semiliterate deaf client.

Deaf clients often need guidance regarding the feasibility of their job wishes, especially when levels of aspiration are not in keeping with abilities. Sometimes work evaluation programs are the best way to convey what is realistic. At other times, lengthy and repeated counseling interviews may be necessary before it is possible to counsel in terms of more suitable goals.

Often help in manners and appearance is necessary. For example, a deaf person may make offensive noises and not know it. He may smoke at the wrong time. His personal hygiene may be offensive. Likewise, knowing how to dress for an interview or how to fill out the forms is important. A guidance counselor must assume responsibility for his client's ability to do these things right. These seemingly minor factors can mean the difference between success and failure in obtaining and keeping employment.

### Special Groups

Included in the group that seeks help from the counselor for the deaf will be the multiply-disabled, the hard-of-hearing, and those who acquired deafness later in life.

*Multiply-disabled.* The problem of the deaf individual with other disabilities is an increasing one. From 15 to 35 percent of deaf youths 16 years of age or younger are excluded from admission to, or are dropped from, educational programs because of cerebral palsy, mental retardation, agnosias, mental illness, visual defects, orthopedic and other disabilities.

Vocational guidance in the conventional sense does not apply to most multiply-disabled deaf persons. They require special facilities and programs for early education and training coordinated with existing programs of vocational rehabilitation. Among these facilities are terminal workshops

(Chouinard & Garrett, 1965, p. 7) and transitional workshops (Thompson, 1960) that are oriented to psychological and vocational adjustment. For some multiply-disabled deaf persons these facilities must provide structured living and working environments on a 24-hour-a-day basis.

In contrast to comprehensive services of these types, the common practice today is to exclude or drop these youths from existing educational programs for the deaf. Then, at the age of 16 or so, with sharply limited education, with the disability of deafness and one or more other disabilities, they are referred to a rehabilitation counselor. Because of the almost total lack of appropriate resources, the counselor may find these deaf people "nonfeasible" or place them in a sheltered workshop or some other similar program not geared to the problems of the deaf. The end result is that these deaf persons often live at home, dependent on their parents until the latter are no longer able or willing to sustain them, or they must subsist on welfare. Some may be improperly committed to hospitals for the mentally ill or mentally retarded for want of proper diagnosis and services. Others may run afoul of the law and be imprisoned.

Until programs are developed for these people, vocational guidance in the conventional sense is much like therapy for a person with leukemia. Diagnoses can be made, and some alleviation of medical symptomatology is often possible, but at present the outlook is not encouraging. This need not be the case, as was demonstrated recently by the Michigan Association for Better Hearing in Lansing when 36 of 39 multiply-handicapped deaf men were prepared for and placed in employment.

*Hard of hearing.* The person who can understand enough speech to follow reasonably well the general trend of thought in a one-to-one situation is hard of hearing. Although the more refined audiologic criteria described in Chapter 9 may apply, this is a functional definition of a hard-of-hearing person for psychological and guidance purposes.

Two paradoxes soon become evident to the counselor working in guidance with congenitally hard-of-hearing persons. One is that as a group they often have much more in common with the deaf than one would have thought prior to having actual experience with them. This is particularly true in terms of educational achievement, language skills, general knowledge, and certain behavioral patterns. Second, the hard-of-hearing seem to reflect more psychological disturbance than the deaf. They frequently share the problem of marginal people in any group, that of identification. The person born hard of hearing may not be able to find full acceptance among the normal-hearing or the deaf. Whereas association with the hearing ideally offers a wider range of friends and interests, it may be at the price of frequent rejection or a subservient role. Association with the deaf is sometimes perceived as psychologically threatening in the sense that deafness is a magnification of their own real or perceived deficiencies. Furthermore the small number of deaf people restricts the opportunities for identification with them.

The problems of vocational guidance with the hard-of-hearing that are different from those encountered with the normal-hearing or the deaf are most often manifestations of the identity conflict. Effective guidance and counseling is, therefore, often a long-term process aimed at fundamental changes in the self image. Rarely is such service provided hard-of-hearing persons. Consequently, it is common to see them go through life overcompensating for their hearing loss or magnifying its significance, both of which lead to vocational and personal dissatisfaction.

*Acquired deafness.* As we have seen in Chapter 18, deafness is often a severe psychological trauma to the person who loses his hearing after he has completed school, started a career, and married. In contrast to the person deafened in his school years, who generally enters a special educational program, meets other deaf persons, and plans a career and marriage with a knowledge of his handicap, the individual who is deafened later has often already made job and marriage choices that may be incompatible with deafness.

The loneliness and the insecurity in social situations are common reactions to this stress. Neurotic defenses often appear. These may include controlling social situations by doing all the talking and thereby avoiding having to listen, denial of hearing loss, withdrawal from social contact, or an extreme dependent or paranoid pattern which exploits the handicap.

Although some differences in reaction are noted when the hearing loss is sudden as contrasted with when it is chronic, the basic problem of vocational guidance is the same. The appropriateness of the vocational placement of the client must be considered in terms of the new factor of his deafness. In certain lines of work, this poses no major problem, but often complete retraining or additional education is required along with basic adjustments in marriage and social life. Vocational guidance has a primary responsibility to help the client very directly in terms of vocational or educational aspects of his adjustment, but because these general social and personal problems are so often related, it is often necessary to provide extensive counseling on the total over-all reaction to the stress of the hearing loss.

## THE DEAF AND TRENDS IN THE WORLD OF WORK

Vocational counseling requires a clear understanding of current employment trends and their implications for the deaf client. John A. Sessions (1966), labor authority of the AFL-CIO, has predicted that unless this understanding develops and the necessary changes in education and training are brought about, approximately 70 percent of deaf persons will be unemployed within the next ten years, and most of the remaining 30 percent will be frozen in various unskilled and menial jobs. What are the major trends in our contemporary society and in its near-term future that would have this effect on the deaf person in the labor force? What kind of counseling and training can counteract the effect of these changes?

1. *The shift is to many more white-collar jobs and to relatively fewer manual, semiskilled, and unskilled kinds of work, and to relatively fewer blue-collar positions.* Only 17 percent of the deaf are in white-collar work as contrasted with 46.8 percent of the general population. Furthermore, opportunities in manufacturing, in which over half of the employed deaf work, are decreasing. Not only has the over-all number of jobs in manufacturing not kept pace with the general economy, but the proportion of white-collar workers in manufacturing has increased from 16 percent in 1947 to 25 percent in 1966, with strong evidence for an even greater shift to this direction in the future. As indicated earlier, deaf people are employed in the manual occupations related to production, not in the white-collar positions which include accountants, engineers, scientists, teachers, nurses, and secretaries. Very few deaf people have worked in these occupations in the past.

2. *Seventy percent of Americans now live in the cities and suburbs as compared to the recent past when the proportion was about half.* This urbanization of population may impose certain hardships upon the deaf, but from a counseling point of view it offers one major advantage. With deaf people concentrated in a community, it is easier to

provide them with professional vocational counselors who are specifically qualified to deal with their problems. In the past deaf clients were so widely scattered that the provision of specialists was not practicable because too much of their time would have been spent in travel.

3. *Advancing technology is changing the world of work. Of the 22,000 jobs listed in 1965 in the Dictionary of Occupational Titles, over 6000 were new since 1959 and over 8000 that had existed then are extinct.* This means that flexibility and the capacity to be retrained are primary requirements for vocational survival. Because of their communication and educational problems, deaf people often have great difficulty in conventional retraining programs and may, therefore, be relatively inflexible vocationally. Furthermore, it is no longer reasonable to prepare a deaf person for a job when he is young and then to expect him to be able to rely for the rest of his life on these same skills for employment. Counselors must recognize the need for special programs to retrain older deaf workers, many with families and financial responsibilities.

4. *Employment in the service sector will experience the fastest growth.* For example, the number of jobs in state and local government will increase 48 percent. Miscellaneous service industries, such as educational, health and medical care, recreation, hotels, repair services, and so on, will require many new workers, and this trend will continue. One of every two new jobs created in the past decade has been in the service industries.

The outlook of the deaf client is not too encouraging. Civil service examinations usually require language skill far above the level of a majority of the deaf population. In the miscellaneous service industries from 55 to 88 percent of the positions are white-collar jobs. This is the very area in which deaf people are currently least well represented and (presumably) least well prepared by aptitude and training. It is interesting that in the service industries 10 percent of the people have managerial positions from which the deaf are almost totally excluded.

5. *Educational requirements for employment are rapidly increasing.* The average worker today has spent 33 percent more years in school than his predecessor, and this trend is increasing. The number of jobs open to the functionally illiterate, which includes at least 30 percent of deaf school-leavers, is rapidly shrinking and in their place are jobs requiring at least a high school education. Even the jobs the illiterate can do well may not be open to them because when industry hires it wants flexibility in a worker and, therefore, often demands at least a high school education.

These five major trends in the world of work create for the deaf a vocational crisis, but the problem is not insoluble. As we have said, deaf people have the same intelligence as the normal-hearing, their work habits are good, and employers who hire them like them. We need to provide suitable educational options that accommodate to problems of communication. Then we must build on this, counseling and guidance services that enable the deaf person to achieve all that he is capable of achieving.

## SUGGESTED READINGS AND REFERENCES

Boatner, E. B., E. R. Stuckless, and D. F. Moores. *Occupational Status of the Young Deaf Adult of New England and Demand for a Regional Technical-Vocational Training Center.* West Hartford, Conn.: American School for the Deaf, 1964.

Chouinard, E. L., and J. F. Garrett (eds.). *Workshops for the Disabled: A Vocational Rehabilitation Resource.* U.S. Office of Vocational Rehabilitation. Washington, D.C.: U.S. Government Printing Office, 1956.

Di Carlo, L. M. *The Deaf.* Englewood Cliffs, N. J.: Prentice-Hall, Inc., 1964.

Furth, H. G. *Thinking Without Language.* New York: The Free Press, 1966.

Lunde, A. S., and S. G. Bigman. *Occupational Conditions among the Deaf.* Washington, D.C.: Gallaudet College Press, 1959.

Levine, E. *The Psychology of Deafness.* New York: Columbia University Press, 1960.

Myklebust, H. R. *The Psychology of Deafness* (2d ed.). New York: Grune and Stratton, Inc. 1964.

————. "Guidance and Counseling for the Deaf," *Amer. Ann. Deaf,* 107:370–415 (1962).

Ott, J. T. (ed.). *Proceedings of a National Workshop on Improved Opportunities for the Deaf,* Knoxville, Tenn., 1964. Washington, D.C.: U.S. Department of Health, Education, and Welfare, Vocational Rehabilitation Administration, 1965.
Report of a workshop emphasizing the needs and opportunities for deaf people in the world of work.

Quigley, S. P., W. C. Jenné, and S. B. Phillips. *Deaf Students in Colleges and Universities.* Washington, D.C.: Alexander Graham Bell Association for the Deaf, 1968.

Rainier, J. D., K. Z. Altshuler, F. J. Kallmann, and W. E. Deming (eds.). *Family and Mental Health Problems in a Deaf Population.* New York: New York State Psychiatric Institute, 1963.

————, and K. Z. Altshuler. *Comprehensive Mental Health Services for the Deaf.* New York: Columbia University Press, 1967.

————, and ———— (eds.). *Psychiatry and the Deaf.* New York: New York State Psychiatric Institute, 1967.

> Report of a 1967 workshop of psychiatrists from all parts of the country who "came together to learn about, to discuss, and to exchange views gained from their psychiatric and psychological work with the deaf."

Rosen, A. "Limitations of Personality Inventories for Assessment of Deaf Children and Adults as Illustrated by Research with the Minnesota Multiphasic Inventory," *J. Rehab. Deaf,* 1:47–52 (1967).

Sessions, J. A. *Automation and the Deaf.* A paper presented to the Leadership Training Program in Deafness, San Fernando Valley State College, San Fernando, Calif., June 1966.

Thompson, N. Z. *Experimental Evaluative Instrument Based on Standards for Sheltered Workshops.* Washington, D.C.: National Institute on Workshop Standards 1960.

Vernon, M. "The Relationship of Language to the Thinking Process," *Arch. Gen. Psychiat.* (Chicago), 16:325–333 (1967a).

————. "A Guide for the Psychological Evaluation of Deaf and Severely Hard-of-Hearing Adults," *Deaf American,* 19:15–18 (1967b).

————, and D. W. Brown. "A Guide to Psychological Tests and Testing Procedures in the Evaluation of Deaf and Hard-of-Hearing Children," *J. Speech Hearing Dis.,* 29:414–423 (1964).

————, and E. D. Mindel. "Psychological and Psychiatric Aspects of Deafness," in D. Rose (ed.), *Audiological Assessment.* Englewood Cliffs, N.J.: Prentice-Hall, in press, 1969.

Wrightstone, J. W., M. S. Aronow, and S. Muskowitz. "Developing Reading Test Norms for Deaf Children," *Amer. Ann. Deaf,* 108:311–316 (1963).

# APPENDIX

In this appendix are presented several collections of words or sentences that are widely used as tests of hearing. Some of them are also useful for auditory training and as test material in the selection of hearing aids.

The principles of the tests that employ these words and sentences are explained in Chapter 7, and their use in the selection of hearing aids is discussed in Chapter 11. It is pointed out in Chapter 7, for example, that a "discrimination score" obtained with monosyllabic word lists has a totally different meaning from a "hearing level for speech" measured with the two-syllable word lists. The principles of the different types of test will not be discussed again, but a brief statement introduces each set of lists, telling something of their properties, how and where they were constructed, their general fields of usefulness, and whether they are available in recorded form.

Some of the shorter lists are given in full; others are represented only by samples, but by more generous samples than could properly be included in the text. It must be remembered, however, that word lists or sentences alone do not make a test of hearing. The loudness and clarity with which they are spoken and the acoustic conditions of the test are equally important. These lists are only the materials. As explained in Chapter 7, they must be correctly and intelligently used.

## 1. SPONDAIC WORDS (CID)

Auditory tests W-1 and W-2 were developed at Central Institute for the Deaf as modifications of Auditory Test No. 9 of the Psycho-Acoustic Laboratory of Harvard University. The test material is a list of 36 words, each composed of two syllables that are equally stressed (spondees). The words were chosen for familiarity and also for equal intelligibility when spoken at the same intensity as measured by the VU meter. Six different scramblings of the 36 words have been recorded.

Tests W-1 and W-2 are particularly suited to measuring the hearing threshold level for speech. In Test W-1 all of the spondaic words are recorded at the same intensity. The carrier phrase is recorded at a level 10 dB higher. A 1000-Hz calibration tone is also recorded at this level. In W-2 the intensity of the words descends systematically by 3 dB for each successive group of three words. With this form of test it is only necessary to count the number of words repeated correctly. Each word correct lowers the threshold level by 1 dB.

Phonographic recordings of these tests may be purchased from the Technisonic Studios, Inc., 1201 South Brentwood Blvd., Richmond Heights, Missouri 63117. These tests are described in an article entitled "C.I.D. Auditory Tests W-1 and W-2," by R. W. Benson, H. Davis, C. E. Harrison, I. J. Hirsh, E. G. Reynolds, and S. R. Silverman, in *Journal of the Acoustical Society of America*, 23:719 (1951), and, in more detail, "Development of Materials for Speech Audiometry," by I. J. Hirsh, H. Davis, S. R. Silverman, E. G. Reynolds, E. Eldert, and R. W. Benson in *Journal of Speech and Hearing Disorders*, 17:321–337 (1952). (These tests were

## SPONDAIC WORDS OF AUDITORY TESTS W-1 AND W-2

| | | | |
|---|---|---|---|
| 1. airplane | 10. eardrum | 19. iceberg | 28. railroad |
| 2. armchair | 11. farewell | 20. inkwell | 29. schoolboy |
| 3. baseball | 12. grandson | 21. mousetrap | 30. sidewalk |
| 4. birthday | 13. greyhound | 22. mushroom | 31. stairway |
| 5. cowboy | 14. hardware | 23. northwest | 32. sunset |
| 6. daybreak | 15. headlight | 24. oatmeal | 33. toothbrush |
| 7. doormat | 16. horseshoe | 25. padlock | 34. whitewash |
| 8. drawbridge | 17. hotdog | 26. pancake | 35. woodwork |
| 9. duckpond | 18. hothouse | 27. playground | 36. workshop |

developed under contracts with the Office of Naval Research and the Veterans Administration.)

Tape recordings of test W-1 (7.5 inches per sec. on a 7-inch reel) are available from the Los Angeles Foundation of Otology at 2130 West Third Street, Los Angeles, California 90057. This recording is known as the "LAFO speech test tape." In addition to 35 W-1 spondee words in two arrangements and the calibration tone, each tape carries four W-22 PB word lists, described below, and a sample of "connected discourse" (Declaration of Independence). The talker is not the same as the C.I.D. talker, but the form of the tests and the word lists are the same, except for the omission of "airplane" from the LAFO version.

## 2. PB (PHONETICALLY BALANCED) WORD LISTS

One of the 50-word phonetically balanced word lists prepared by the Psycho-Acoustic Laboratory is presented first in this sec-

tion. All 20 of the 50-word lists are given in the article by J. P. Egan entitled "Articulation Testing Methods" in *The Laryngoscope*, 58:955–991 (1948), and in U.S.A. Standard S3.2-1960, entitled "Method for Measurement of Monosyllabic Word Intelligibility." Each list consists of 50 common English monosyllables. For articulation testing, the words should be arranged in different random order for each presentation. The special merits of these lists and the uses to which they may be put are described in Chapter 7. The words range in difficulty from quite intelligible to rather difficult.

Several of these lists, slightly modified, including the example below, were recorded for experimental use at Central Institute for the Deaf. Rush Hughes was the talker. These recordings are unduly difficult, hovever, even for listeners with normal hearing, largely because of Hughes's particular manner of speaking; and the college-level vocabulary is not ideal for clinical use. Nevertheless the articulation

### PB-50—LIST 5

| | | | | |
|---|---|---|---|---|
| 1. add | 11. feed | 21. love | 31. rind | 41. thud |
| 2. bake | 12. flap | 22. mast | 32. rode | 42. trade |
| 3. bathe | 13. good | 23. nose | 33. roe | 43. true |
| 4. beck | 14. Greek | 24. odds | 34. scare | 44. tug |
| 5. black | 15. grudge | 25. owls | 35. shine | 45. vase |
| 6. bronze | 16. high | 26. pass | 36. shove | 46. watch |
| 7. cheat | 17. hill | 27. pipe | 37. shy | 47. wink |
| 8. choose | 18. inch | 28. puff | 38. sick | 48. wrath |
| 9. curse | 19. kid | 29. punt | 39. solve | 49. yawn |
| 10. drive | 20. lend | 30. rear | 40. thick | 50. zone |

### PB-50—LIST 1

| | | | | |
|---|---|---|---|---|
| 1. ace | 12. deaf | 21. it | 31. owl | 41. toe |
| 2. ache | 13. earn | 22. jam | 32. poor | 42. true |
| 3. an | (urn) | 23. knees | 33. ran | 43. twins |
| 4. as | 14. east | 24. law | 34. see (sea) | 44. yard |
| 5. bathe | 15. felt | 25. low | 35. she | 45. up |
| 6. bells | 16. give | 26. me | 36. skin | 46. us |
| 7. carve | 17. high | 27. mew | 37. stove | 47. wet |
| 8. chew | 18. him | 28. none | 38. them | 48. what |
| 9. could | 19. hunt | (nun) | 39. there | 49. wire |
| 10. dad | 20. isle | 29. not (knot) | (their) | 50. you |
| 11. day | (aisle) | 30. or (oar) | 40. thing | (ewe) |

### PB-50—LIST 2

| | | | | |
|---|---|---|---|---|
| 1. ail (ale) | 12. ease | 24. knee | 33. own | 44. too |
| 2. air (heir) | 13. eat | 25. live | 34. pew | (two, to) |
| 3. and | 14. else | (verb) | 35. rooms | 45. tree |
| 4. bin | 15. flat | 26. move | 36. send | 46. way |
| (been) | 16. gave | 27. new | 37. show | (weigh) |
| 5. by (buy) | 17. ham | (knew) | 38. smart | 47. well |
| 6. cap | 18. hit | 28. now | 39. star | 48. with |
| 7. cars | 19. hurt | 29. oak | 40. tare | 49. yore |
| 8. chest | 20. ice | 30. odd | (tear) | (your) |
| 9. die (dye) | 21. ill | 31. off | 41. that | 50. young |
| 10. does | 22. jaw | 32. one | 42. then | |
| 11. dumb | 23. key | (won) | 43. thin | |

### PB-50—LIST 3

| | | | | |
|---|---|---|---|---|
| 1. add (ad) | 11. done | 21. is | 31. out | 41. this |
| 2. aim | (dun) | 22. jar | 32. owes | 42. though |
| 3. are | 12. dull | 23. king | 33. pie | 43. three |
| 4. ate (eight) | 13. ears | 24. knit | 34. raw | 44. tie |
| 5. bill | 14. end | 25. lie (lye) | 35. say | 45. use |
| 6. book | 15. farm | 26. may | 36. shove | (yews) |
| 7. camp | 16. glove | 27. nest | 37. smooth | 46. we |
| 8. chair | 17. hand | 28. no | 38. start | 47. west |
| 9. cute | 18. have | (know) | 39. tan | 48. when |
| 10. do | 19. he | 29. oil | 40. ten | 49. wool |
| | 20. if | 30. on | | 50. year |

### PB-50—LIST 4

| | | | | |
|---|---|---|---|---|
| 1. aid | 11. clothes | 21. his | 31. ought | 40. they |
| 2. all (awl) | 12. cook | 22. in (inn) | (aught) | 41. through |
| 3. am | 13. darn | 23. jump | 32. our | 42. tin |
| 4. arm | 14. dolls | 24. leave | (hour) | 43. toy |
| 5. art | 15. dust | 25. men | 33. pale (pail) | 44. where |
| 6. at | 16. ear | 26. my | 34. save | 45. who |
| 7. bee (be) | 17. eyes | 27. near | 35. shoe | 46. why |
| 8. bread | (ayes) | 28. net | 36. so (sew) | 47. will |
| (bred) | 18. few | 29. nuts | 37 stiff | 48. wood |
| 9. can | 19. go | 30. of | 38. tea (tee) | (would) |
| 10. chin | 20. hang | | 39. than | 49. yes |
| | | | | 50. yet |

scores obtained in the clinic with these recordings were made the basis of the Social Adequacy of Hearing Index (see Chapter 7). In spite of this historic interest the use of these recordings is not recommended.

CID Auditory Test W-22 is a set of recordings of phonetically balanced word lists that represent a more restricted and simpler vocabulary than the original Psycho-Acoustic Laboratory lists. The talker is Ira Hirsh. These recordings are considerably more intelligible than the earlier experimental Rush Hughes version. Test W-22 is described in detail, including the criteria for phonetic balance, in the article entitled "Development of Materials for Speech Audiometry" cited in Chapter 7.

CID Auditory Test W-22 and the Rush Hughes version of the PB-50 test can be obtained from Technisonic Studios, 1201 South Brentwood Blvd., Richmond Heights, Missouri 63117.

The LAFO speech test tape, described in the previous section, contains these same word lists, spoken by a different talker. The address is Los Angeles Foundation for Otology, 2130 West Third Street, Los Angeles, California 90057.

## 3. FAMILIAR MONOSYLLABLES

For testing young children and for subjects with restricted vocabularies we need lists of very familiar words. Exact phonetic balance is not important in this situation. Four lists of familiar monosyllables, approximately balanced phonetically, were developed at Clarke School for the Deaf by the late C. V. Hudgins. They are known as the PBF lists. They have not been recorded.

## 4. PHONEMICALLY BALANCED (CNC) LISTS

There are three rather distinct objectives of speech audiometry and its word lists:

### LIST PBF 1

| | | | |
|---|---|---|---|
| 1. box | | 26. end | |
| 2. eyes | | 27. there | |
| 3. range | | 28. tone | |
| 4. soap | | 29. drive | |
| 5. pants | | 30. then | |
| 6. wheat | | 31. ford | |
| 7. rat | | 32. rag | |
| 8. prove | | 33. are | |
| 9. pan | | 34. guess | |
| 10. toe | | 35. pest | |
| 11. bad | | 36. bead | |
| 12. bar | | 37. such | |
| 13. frog | | 38. dish | |
| 14. this | | 39. heat | |
| 15. slip | | 40. hid | |
| 16. hurt | | 41. price | |
| 17. bite | | 42. pile | |
| 18. hose | | 43. net | |
| 19. rise | | 44. fork | |
| 20. farm | | 45. ride | |
| 21. smile | | 46. trade | |
| 22. crush | | 47. crash | |
| 23. rub | | 48. no | |
| 24. gift | | 49. not | |
| 25. is | | 50. plans | |

### LIST PBF 2

| | | | |
|---|---|---|---|
| 1. niece | | 26. bill | |
| 2. fuse | | 27. bounce | |
| 3. tan | | 28. mad | |
| 4. bought | | 29. shoe | |
| 5. trash | | 30. our | |
| 6. rap | | 31. loose | |
| 7. vest | | 32. start | |
| 8. rib | | 33. boot | |
| 9. tongue | | 34. pump | |
| 10. cloud | | 35. wish | |
| 11. awe | | 36. five | |
| 12. shake | | 37. flood | |
| 13. charge | | 38. course | |
| 14. throb | | 39. tip | |
| 15. howl | | 40. grease | |
| 16. glass | | 41. log | |
| 17. else | | 42. hop | |
| 18. bean | | 43. night | |
| 19. them | | 44. arm | |
| 20. ways | | 45. job | |
| 21. hit | | 46. that | |
| 22. quart | | 47. smash | |
| 23. set | | 48. bud | |
| 24. did | | 49. nut | |
| 25. need | | 50. tank | |

## LIST PBF 3

| | |
|---|---|
| 1. trip | 26. jam |
| 2. dig | 27. why |
| 3. check | 28. dog |
| 4. nest | 29. may |
| 5. town | 30. whirl |
| 6. fame | 31. size |
| 7. eight | 32. thick |
| 8. law | 33. clown |
| 9. take | 34. class |
| 10. far | 35. fog |
| 11. noise | 36. air |
| 12. dim | 37. guard |
| 13. tenth | 38. sled |
| 14. drop | 39. flash |
| 15. barge | 40. oak |
| 16. wedge | 41. neck |
| 17. vow | 42. path |
| 18. stood | 43. horse |
| 19. shout | 44. cake |
| 20. look | 45. praise |
| 21. leave | 46. past |
| 22. who | 47. sad |
| 23. fresh | 48. laugh |
| 24. please | 49. deck |
| 25. purse | 50. late |

## LIST PBF 4

| | |
|---|---|
| 1. judge | 26. tent |
| 2. slap | 27. earn |
| 3. bee | 28. gas |
| 4. move | 29. raise |
| 5. meat | 30. curse |
| 6. thin | 31. on |
| 7. race | 32. blonde |
| 8. howl | 33. rip |
| 9. hog | 34. fan |
| 10. sour | 35. food |
| 11. hook | 36. cod |
| 12. aim | 37. float |
| 13. skid | 38. frown |
| 14. bus | 39. pack |
| 15. creak | 40. hot |
| 16. bush | 41. beast |
| 17. pipe | 42. struck |
| 18. pinch | 43. bike |
| 19. oils | 44. badge |
| 20. test | 45. yes |
| 21. cart | 46. roe |
| 22. fed | 47. stitch |
| 23. mat | 48. touch |
| 24. stars | 49. mend |
| 25. tick | 50. new |

one is to assess the adequacy of the listener's hearing for social purposes; another is to analyze his auditory impairment for diagnostic purposes; and another is the analysis of normal speech from the linguistic point of view. Interest in this last objective has led to the study in detail of the phonetic and phonemic structure of English speech in general and of word lists that might be used as laboratory tools for the study of communication by speech. Several such lists have been prepared, and the new ways of using them are suitable for clinical use as well.

An analytical study by I. Lehiste and G. E. Peterson in the *Journal of the Acoustical Society of America*, 31:280–286 (1959), shows in detail the distribution of vowels, initial consonants, and final consonants in 10 of the original PB-50 lists and compares them with the corresponding distribution of the phonemes in

the entire "corpus" of reasonably familiar English monosyllables that have the form consonant (C)–nucleus or "vowel part" (N)–consonant (C). The authors prepared 10 new CNC lists of 50 words each that match quite well the phonemic composition of the larger group. These authors distinguish between "phonetic," related to acoustics and physiology, and "phonemic," related to linguistics and the hearing of speech. Later they (G. E. Peterson and I. Lehiste) published a revision of their lists in the *Journal of Speech and Hearing Disorders*, 27:62–70 (1962). These lists provided a foundation for the Northwestern University Auditory Tests Nos. 4 and 6.

The Northwestern University Auditory Test No. 6 is the most carefully prepared and thoroughly studied set of CNC word lists so far published. There are four lists of consonant-nucleus-consonant words which have the phonemic balance of the Peterson-Lehiste lists and which experimentally have high interlist equivalence and also test-retest reliability. The "articulation functions" (see Chapter 7) of a particular recording of these lists have been established for normal-hearing subjects and also for subjects with sensory-neural hearing loss. For normal-hearing listeners the function rises linearly from about 8 percent correct at 4 dB below the speech reception threshold (spondees 50 percent correct) to 75 percent correct at 8 dB above SRT. The slope of this part of the curve is 5.6 percent per decibel. The function then bends horizontally to a plateau of 99 percent correct, attained at 32 dB above SRT. The slope and the final plateau are both lower for subjects with sensory-neural impairment.

The four lists of Test No. 6 are given below. The words that also appeared in the original PB-50 lists are marked with asterisks. The description of the lists appeared in a technical report of the USAF School of Aerospace Medicine (T. W. Tillman and R. Carhart, SAM-TR-66-55 in June 1966). The authors feel that this test is not merely a list of words but a particular recording of them. This test was developed strictly for research purposes and there is no expectation that the recorded version will be made available commercially.

## CNC MONOSYLLABIC WORDS COMPRISING THE FOUR LISTS OF N.U. AUDITORY TEST NO. 6

| List I | | List II | | List III | | List IV | |
|---|---|---|---|---|---|---|---|
| bean* | met | bite | merge* | bar* | mouse | back* | mob |
| boat | mode* | book* | mill | base* | name | bath* | mood* |
| burn | moon | bought* | nice* | beg | note* | bone | near |
| chalk | nag* | calm | numb | cab* | pain | came | neat* |
| choice | page | chair | pad* | cause | pearl* | chain* | pass* |
| death* | pool | chief | pick* | chat* | phone | check* | peg* |
| dime* | puff* | dab* | pike | cheek | pole | dip* | perch* |
| door | rag* | dead* | rain | cool | rat* | dog* | red* |
| fall* | raid* | deep* | read* | date | ring | doll | ripe* |
| fat* | raise* | fail | room | ditch* | road* | fit* | rose* |
| gap | reach* | far* | rot* | dodge* | rush* | food | rough* |
| goose | sell* | gaze | said | five* | search | gas* | sail |
| hash* | shout* | gin* | shack* | germ | seize | get* | shirt |
| home | size* | goal | shawl | good* | shall | hall | should |
| hurl* | sub | hate* | soap* | gun* | sheep* | have* | sour* |
| jail | sure | haze | south* | half | soup | hole* | such* |
| jar | take | hush* | thought* | hire* | talk | join | tape |
| keen | third | juice | ton* | hit* | team | judge* | thumb* |
| king | tip* | keep | tool | jug* | tell* | kick* | time* |
| kite* | tough* | keg | turn* | late | thin* | kill* | tire* |
| knock | vine* | learn | voice | lid* | void* | lean | vote* |
| laud | week* | live | wag* | life* | walk* | lease | wash* |
| limb | which | loaf | white* | luck | when | long | wheat* |
| lot | whip | lore | witch | mess | wire* | lose | wife* |
| love* | yes* | match | young | mop* | youth* | make | yearn |

* Also in original PB-50 lists.

# 5. MULTIPLE-CHOICE WORD LISTS

A multiple-choice word-intelligibility test was developed by Professor John W. Black of Ohio State University in collaboration with the United States Naval School of Aviation Medicine. It has been used extensively in tests of talkers speaking under various conditions of interest to military aviation. The talker is given a list of words to read. The listeners mark prepared blanks on which each word read by the talker appears as one of four rather similar possible choices. Twenty-four of these lists are published in the *Journal of Speech and Hearing Disorders*, 22:213–235 (1957). The first of these lists is given here as a sample. The word in each group actually read by the talker is italicized.

| | | |
|---|---|---|
| groove | modern | *vice* |
| drew | moderate | fight |
| crew | modesty | mice |
| *grew* | *modest* | bite |
| say | forbade | *chink* |
| *stay* | *pervade* | kink |
| stayed | surveyed | check |
| spade | survey | chin |
| stung | drunk | *intent* |
| *stun* | *grunt* | intend |
| sun | brunt | content |
| stunned | runt | intense |
| quench | busy | wade |
| went | physics | waves |
| *whence* | *physic* | *wave* |
| when | visit | way |
| *pass* | clearly | *fine* |
| past | weary | find |
| cast | quarry | sign |
| task | *query* | kind |
| popular | nurse | *get* |
| *poplar* | first | gap |
| hopper | birth | guess |
| opera | *burst* | guest |
| *immense* | named | only |
| commence | *name* | woman |
| emit | main | pullman |
| cement | knave | *omen* |
| latter | *last* | swain |
| ladder | lash | *slain* |
| *lattice* | laugh | flame |
| rabbit | glass | plain |
| crash | gold | pail |
| crab | bowl | poor |
| *craft* | cold | *polo* |
| crack | *bold* | palace |

|     | A     | B     | C      | D     | E     | F     |
|-----|-------|-------|--------|-------|-------|-------|
| 1   | bat   | bad   | back   | bass  | ban   | bath  |
| 2   | bean  | beach | beat   | beam  | bead  | beak  |
| 3   | bun   | bus   | but    | buff  | buck  | bug   |
| 4   | came  | cape  | cane   | cake  | cave  | case  |
| 5   | cut   | cub   | cuff   | cup   | cud   | cuss  |
| 6   | dig   | dip   | did    | dim   | dill  | din   |
| 7   | duck  | dud   | dung   | dub   | dug   | dun   |
| 8   | fill  | fig   | fin    | fizz  | fib   | fit   |
| 9   | hear  | heath | heal   | heave | heat  | heap  |
| 10  | kick  | king  | kid    | kit   | kin   | kill  |
| 11  | late  | lake  | lay    | lace  | lane  | lame  |
| 12  | map   | mat   | math   | man   | mass  | mad   |
| 13  | page  | pane  | pace   | pay   | pale  | pave  |
| 14  | pass  | pat   | pack   | pad   | path  | pan   |
| 15  | peace | peas  | peak   | peal  | peat  | peach |
| 16  | pill  | pick  | pip    | pig   | pin   | pit   |
| 17  | pun   | puff  | pup    | puck  | pus   | pub   |
| 18  | rave  | rake  | race   | rate  | raze  | ray   |
| 19  | sake  | sale  | save   | sane  | safe  | same  |
| 20  | sad   | sass  | sag    | sack  | sap   | sat   |
| 21  | seep  | seen  | seethe | seed  | seem  | seek  |
| 22  | sing  | sit   | sin    | sip   | sick  | sill  |
| 23  | sud   | sum   | sub    | sun   | sup   | sung  |
| 24  | tab   | tan   | tam    | tang  | tack  | tap   |
| 25  | teach | tear  | tease  | teal  | team  | teak  |
|     |       |       |        |       |       |       |
| 26  | led   | shed  | red    | bed   | fed   | wed   |
| 27  | sold  | told  | hold   | fold  | gold  | cold  |
| 28  | dig   | wig   | big    | rig   | pig   | fig   |
| 29  | kick  | lick  | sick   | pick  | wick  | tick  |
| 30  | book  | took  | shook  | cook  | hook  | look  |
| 31  | hark  | dark  | mark   | lark  | park  | bark  |
| 32  | gale  | male  | tale   | bale  | sale  | pale  |
| 33  | peel  | reel  | feel   | heel  | keel  | eel   |
| 34  | will  | hill  | kill   | till  | fill  | bill  |
| 35  | foil  | coil  | boil   | oil   | toil  | soil  |
| 36  | fame  | same  | came   | name  | tame  | game  |
| 37  | ten   | pen   | den    | hen   | then  | men   |
| 38  | pin   | sin   | tin    | win   | din   | fin   |
| 39  | sun   | nun   | gun    | fun   | bun   | run   |
| 40  | rang  | fang  | gang   | bang  | sang  | hang  |
| 41  | tent  | bent  | went   | dent  | rent  | sent  |
| 42  | sip   | rip   | tip    | dip   | hip   | lip   |
| 43  | top   | hop   | pop    | cop   | mop   | shop  |
| 44  | meat  | feat  | heat   | seat  | beat  | neat  |
| 45  | kit   | bit   | fit    | sit   | wit   | hit   |
| 46  | hot   | got   | not    | pot   | lot   | tot   |
| 47  | nest  | vest  | west   | test  | best  | rest  |
| 48  | bust  | just  | rust   | must  | gust  | dust  |
| 49  | raw   | paw   | law    | jaw   | thaw  | saw   |
| 50  | way   | may   | say    | gay   | day   | pay   |

## 6a. THE RHYME TEST (Fairbanks)

A more precise test of *phonemic differentiation* known as the rhyme test was described by G. Fairbanks in the *Journal of the Acoustical Society of America*, 30: 596–599 (1958). The test was designed to emphasize auditory-phonemic factors and to minimize linguistic factors. It somewhat resembles a multiple-choice word test, but instead it is of the completion type; and it also is oriented more to the study of speech communication than to assessment of the listener or clinical diagnosis.

The stimulus words are drawn from a vocabulary of 250 common monosyllables which consists of 50 sets of 5 rhyming words each. One word from each set is read to the subject. On his response sheet are given the 50 stems, with a space in front of each where the subject enters one letter to complete the spelling of the word he believes he heard. The author imposed several constraints related to ambiguities of spelling and pronunciation. The test is simple but rather limited in scope.

## 6b. RHYME TEST (House, et al.)

A modification of the Fairbanks rhyme test is described by A. S. House, C. E. Williams, M. H. L. Hecker, and K. D. Kryter in the *Journal of the Acoustical Society of America*, 37:158–166 (1965). The title includes the phrase "Consonantal Differentiation with a Closed-Response Set." The test was designed to be used in group-articulation testing of voice-communication systems.

The materials consist of six equivalent word lists in which no strict account is taken of word familiarity, nor of relative frequency of occurrence of sounds in the language, nor of some of Fairbank's constraints related to spelling. The listener's task is a multiple choice, not a completion task. The answer sheet provides a closed set of six alternatives. This procedure virtually eliminates learning time and also word-frequency effects. The lists are not phonetically or phonemically balanced, but they have reasonable phonemic similarity and contain representatives from the major classes of speech sounds. The words are nearly all of the consonant-vowel-consonant type.

Across the six lists the vowel in the nucleus is the same. In some sets the *final* consonant is the same; in others the *initial* consonant is the same. On the response sheet each set of six words is arranged in two lines of three words each and is enclosed in a rectangular box. The subject draws a line through one to indicate his choice.

The properties of these lists under conditions of various signal-to-noise ratios are given in some detail in the original article. The word lists appear below.

## 7. QUESTION-ANSWER TYPE OF SENTENCE LISTS

The following sentences are the basis of Auditory Test No. 12, prepared by the Psycho-Acoustic Laboratory. The questions are relatively simple and can be answered by a single word. This feature makes them useful when a written test for use in group testing is desired. If only one subject is being tested, he may be allowed to repeat the entire sentence. This procedure allows him to concentrate more fully on his listening.

These sentences have been recorded phonographically in groups of four at successively lower intensities. In this form the test is useful for obtaining a *threshold* for speech. The threshold level determined by this test is normally about 4 dB above the threshold measured by the spondaic two-syllable words. This test, together with Test No. 9 (spondaic words), is described in detail in the article entitled "The Development of Recorded Auditory Tests for Measuring Hearing Loss for Speech," by C. V. Hudgins, J. E. Hawkins, J. E. Kar-

they are not satisfactory for clinical use. The scoring is a little less certain; and for many listeners, the difficulty may be in understanding or remembering rather than in correct hearing. A small sample from one list is given below.

1. What is meant by "A stitch in time saves nine"?
2. What is the first letter of your last name?
3. Why is there a spring in a window shade roller?
4. What is meant by the expression "during rush hours"?
5. How many judges make up the Supreme Court?
6. Why is it necessary to build foundations for houses?
7. Name the tool with which a burglar opens a window.
8. Of what benefit was the Red Cross to soldiers during the war?
9. What man is called the "Father of his country"?
10. What instrument do we use to drive nails into wood?

## 10. EVERYDAY SPEECH (CID)

A set of sentences has been prepared at Central Institute for the Deaf to represent "everyday American speech." The specifications for such a sample were laid down by a Working Group (chairman, Dr. Grant Fairbanks) of the Armed Forces-National Research Council Committee on Hearing and Bio-Acoustics. Some of the more important characteristics are as follows:

1. The vocabulary is appropriate to adults.
2. The words appear with high frequency in one or more of the well-known word counts of the English language.
3. Proper names and proper nouns are not used.
4. Common nonslang idioms and contractions are used freely.
5. Phonetic loading and "tongue-twisting" are avoided.
6. Redundancy is high.
7. The level of abstraction is low.
8. Grammatical structure varies freely.
9. Sentence length varies in the following proportion:

| | |
|---|---|
| Two to four fords | 1 |
| Five to nine words | 2 |
| Ten to twelve words | 1 |

10. Sentence forms are in the following proportion:

| | | | |
|---|---|---|---|
| Declarative | 6 | Imperative | 2 |
| Rising interrogative | 1 | Falling interrogative | 1 |

The sentences have been recorded but have not yet (1969) been released for general use until the properties of the speech sample have been thoroughly studied. Ten talkers were employed, five male and five female. None were trained speakers. Much effort was devoted to obtaining natural, spontaneous, everyday inflection, tempo, and emphasis, with a realistic range of individual variation.

No "test" has been developed from this material. It represents a sample of American speech of high face validity against which more specific tests of intelligibility or of "correct hearing" may be validated. In scoring the "correctness of hearing" of the new speech material, a system based on the correct repetition of 50 key words in each list of ten sentences has proved satisfactory.

The actual sentences, with the key words italicized, are as follows:

## LIST A

1. *Walking's my favorite exercise.*
2. *Here's a nice quiet place to rest.*
3. *Our janitor sweeps the floors every night.*
4. It *would* be *much easier if everyone* would *help.*
5. *Good morning.*
6. *Open* your *window before* you *go* to *bed!*
7. *Do* you *think* that *she should stay out so late?*
8. *How do* you *feel* about *changing* the *time when we begin work?*
9. *Here we go.*
10. *Move out* of the *way!*

## LIST B

1. The *water's too cold* for *swimming.*
2. *Why should I get* up *so early* in the *morning?*
3. *Here* are *your shoes.*
4. *It's raining.*
5. *Where are* you *going?*
6. *Come here when* I *call you!*
7. *Don't try* to *get out of it this time!*
8. *Should we let little children go* to the *movies* by *themselves?*
9. *There isn't enough paint* to *finish* the *room.*
10. *Do* you *want* an *egg* for *breakfast?*

## LIST C

1. *Everybody* should *brush* his *teeth* after *meals.*
2. *Everything's* all *right.*
3. *Don't use up all* the *paper* when you *write your letter.*
4. *That's right.*
5. *People ought* to *see* a *doctor once* a *year.*
6. *Those windows* are *so dirty I can't* see *anything outside.*
7. *Pass* the *bread* and *butter please!*
8. *Don't forget* to *pay* your *bill before* the *first* of the *month.*
9. *Don't let* the *dog out* of the *house!*
10. *There's* a *good ballgame* this *afternoon.*

## LIST D

1. *It's time* to *go.*
2. *If* you *don't want these old magazines, throw* them *out.*
3. *Do* you *want* to *wash up?*
4. *It's* a *real dark night so watch your driving.*
5. *I'll carry* the *package* for *you.*
6. Did *you forget* to *shut off* the *water?*
7. *Fishing* in a *mountain stream* is my *idea* of a *good time.*
8. *Fathers spend* more *time* with their *children than* they *used to.*
9. *Be careful not* to *break* your *glasses!*
10. *I'm sorry.*

## LIST E

1. *You can catch the bus across the street.*
2. *Call her on the phone and tell her the news.*
3. *I'll catch up with you later.*
4. *I'll think it over.*
5. *I don't want to go to the movies tonight.*
6. *If your tooth hurts that much you ought to see a dentist.*
7. *Put that cookie back in the box!*
8. *Stop fooling around!*
9. *Time's up.*
10. *How do you spell your name?*

## LIST F

1. *Music always cheers me up.*
2. My *brother's in town for a short while on business.*
3. *We live a few miles from the main road.*
4. *This suit needs to go to the cleaners.*
5. *They ate enough green apples to make them sick for a week.*
6. *Where have you been all this time?*
7. *Have you been working hard lately?*
8. There's *not enough room in the kitchen for a new table.*
9. *Where is he?*
10. *Look out!*

## LIST G

1. I'll *see you right after lunch.*
2. *See you later.*
3. *White shoes are awful to keep clean.*
4. *Stand there and don't move until I tell you!*
5. *There's a big piece of cake left over from dinner.*
6. *Wait for me at the corner in front of the drugstore.*
7. *It's no trouble at all.*
8. *Hurry up!*
9. The *morning paper didn't say anything about rain this afternoon or tonight.*
10. The *phone call's for you.*

## LIST H

1. *Believe me!*
2. *Let's get a cup of coffee.*
3. *Let's get out of here before it's too late.*
4. I *hate driving at night.*
5. *There was water in the cellar after that heavy* rain *yesterday.*
6. *She'll only be gone a few minutes.*
7. *How do you know?*
8. *Children like candy.*
9. *If we don't get rain soon, we'll have no grass.*
10. *They're not listed in the new phone book.*

## LIST I

1. *Where can I find* a *place* to *park?*
2. *I like those big red apples* we *always get* in the *fall.*
3. *You'll* get *fat eating candy.*
4. The *show's over.*
5. *Why don't* they *paint their walls* some *other color?*
6. *What's new?*
7. *What are* you *hiding under* your *coat?*
8. *How come I should always* be the *one* to go *first?*
9. *I'll* take *sugar* and *cream* in my *coffee.*
10. *Wait just* a *minute!*

## LIST J

1. *Breakfast* is *ready.*
2. *I don't know* what's *wrong with* the *car, but* it *won't start.*
3. *It sure takes* a *sharp knife* to *cut this meat.*
4. *I haven't read* a *newspaper since we bought* a *television* set.
5. *Weeds are spoiling* the *yard.*
6. *Call me* a *little later!*
7. *Do* you *have change* for a *five-dollar bill?*
8. *How are* you?
9. I'd *like some ice* cream *with my pie.*
10. I *don't think I'll have* any *dessert.*

# VETERANS ADMINISTRATION CLINICS

The following is a list of VA audiology and speech pathology clinics of a regional nature.

ARIZONA
   VA Hospital, Tucson
ARKANSAS
   VA Hospital, Little Rock
CALIFORNIA
   VA Outpatient Clinic, Los Angeles
   VA Hospital, San Francisco
COLORADO
   VA Hospital, Denver
DISTRICT OF COLUMBIA
   VA Hospital, Washington
FLORIDA
   VA Hospital, Coral Gables (Miami)
   VA Hospital, Bay Pines
GEORGIA
   VA Hospital, Atlanta
ILLINOIS
   VA Hospital, Chicago (Westside)
IOWA
   VA Hospital, Iowa City
KENTUCKY
   VA Hospital, Louisville
LOUISIANA
   VA Hospital, New Orleans
MASSACHUSETTS
   VA Outpatient Clinic, Boston

MICHIGAN
   VA Hospital, Ann Arbor
MINNESOTA
   VA Hospital, Minneapolis
MISSOURI
   VA Hospital, Kansas City
NEW JERSEY
   VA Hospital, East Orange
NEW YORK
   VA Hospital, New York
   VA Hospital, Syracuse
OHIO
   VA Hospital, Cleveland
OKLAHOMA
   VA Hospital, Oklahoma City
PENNSYLVANIA
   VA Outpatient Clinic, Philadelphia
   VA Hospital, Pittsburgh
PUERTO RICO
   VA Center, San Juan
TEXAS
   VA Hospital, Dallas
   VA Hospital, Houston
WASHINGTON
   VA Hospital, Seattle

# BRIEF GLOSSARY OF AUDITORY TERMS

Several terms or usages employed in this book, particularly in Chapters 4, 5, 6, 7, 8, 9, and 16, are relatively new but are believed to be clarifications of, or improvements over, certain older usages. The following definitions (arranged in logical rather than alphabetical order) form a self-consistent system and are in agreement with current U.S.A. Standard Acoustical Terminology (S1.1–1960) and, to the best of our ability, with relevant authoritative statements by the Committee on Conservation of Hearing of the American Academy of Ophthalmology and Otolaryngology and the American Medical Association. The index should be consulted for terms not included in this list.

**Hearing Impairment.** This is the most general term for malfunction of the auditory mechanism. It does not distinguish either the anatomical area primarily involved (central versus peripheral) or the functional nature of the impairment (sensitivity, frequency range, discrimination, sense of loudness or of pitch, recognition of meaning, and the like). In a medicolegal context "hearing impairment" implies a severity sufficient to "affect personal efficiency in the activities of daily living," specifically in respect to communication.

**Hearing Handicap.** This term is a companion to "hearing impairment." It expresses the *result* of the impairment in terms of "personal efficiency in the activities of daily living." The basis of compensation is the degree of handicap (percentage handicap), not the extent of anatomical or physiological impairment. Such impairments are often too limited to produce a handicap in daily living.

**Disability of Hearing.** This medicolegal term (sometimes misused for impairment or handicap) is avoided in this book because of its special connotation related to earning power. Impairment is only a contributing factor to disability.

> *Disability:* actual or presumed inability to remain employed at full wages.
>
> *Impairment:* a deviation or a change for the worse in structure or function, usually outside the range of normal.
>
> *Handicap:* the disadvantage imposed by an impairment sufficient to affect one's personal efficiency in the activities of daily living.

**Normal-hearing Persons.** A normal-hearing person is one whose ears, on otological inspection, show no indications of present or past otological disease or anatomical deviation that might interfere with acoustic transmission, who has no history of past otological disease or abnormality, who has no hearing complaints, and who understands and cooperates in the tests of hearing that may be applied. Unless otherwise specified, normal-hearing persons are assumed to be of either sex and between 15 and 65 years of age. Many psychoacoustic relations have been established for such individuals, including threshold of sensitivity as a function of frequency; discrimination of loudness, of pitch, of words, and the like; as well as the relation of subjective loudness to physical intensity, and so on. For all quantitative tests of hearing a group of normal-hearing individuals shows a range of performance. The performance of the group is usually expressed as the mean or the median accompanied by some measure of the dispersion (scatter), such as the standard deviation.

**Actuarial Hearing Thresholds.** The median threshold of sensitivity of normal-hearing persons varies as a function of many parameters of the stimulus, such as frequency, manner of listening (open acoustic field or under an earphone), the place and manner of measuring the sound-pressure level, and the psychoacoustic method employed in the test. These must all be specified. It also varies according to the age and sex of the individuals. "Actuarial hearing thresholds" are the average (median) expectations of hearing sensitivity for normal-hearing persons according to age and sex.

**Range of Normal Hearing.** The scatter of actual determinations of hearing sensitivity of normal-hearing persons with respect to the median expectation for age and sex determines the range of normal hearing. The limit is sometimes taken as two standard deviations, sometimes as the 95th percentile.

**Normal Threshold of Hearing.** *This term should be avoided because of its medical and medicolegal implications.* There is no single normal threshold of hearing; there are instead *various ranges of normal hearing* related to the various median actuarial hearing thresholds.

**Sound-pressure Level (SPL).** This is the ratio, expressed in decibels, of the effective (root-mean-square) sound pressure of a particular tone or noise to a standard reference pressure which is the same for all frequencies and bandwidths. The usual reference pressure for airborne sound is 0.0002 dyne per square cm. This is also written as $2 \times 10^{-4}$ microbar ($\mu$bar), or, in the meter-kilogram-second (MKS) system, as $2 \times 10^{-5}$ newton per square meter ($N/m^2$).

**Reference Zero Level for Pure-tone Audiometry.** A single sound-pressure level is needed for each frequency and for each combination of earphone and coupler, to serve as the reference or zero level for the decibel scale of intensity of standard audiometers. A particular set of levels has been recommended for this purpose by the International Organization for Standardization (ISO). This set is in widespread international use and is apparently replacing the older "American Standard" reference level (ASA–1951) in the United States. The ISO values are the weighted averages of 15 recent determinations in 5 countries of the median hearing thresholds of well-motivated normal-hearing young adults (18 to 30 years), using comparable psychoacoustic methods. The ISO reference levels for pure-tone audiometers do not, however, define or constitute a legal standard for normal hearing (see Chapter 9).

**Hearing-threshold Level (for Pure Tones).** This is the ratio, expressed in decibels, of the threshold of an ear at a specified frequency to a standard reference zero level for pure-tone audiometers. Practically it is the reading in decibels, on a standard audiometer, that corresponds to the listener's hearing threshold.

**Audiogram (Threshold Audiogram).** An audiogram is a graph that shows hearing-threshold level as a function of frequency.

**Speech Reception Threshold (SRT).** This term specifies the sound-pressure level, measured as described in Chapter 7, at which certain test words or sentences reach the threshold of intelligibility for a particular subject. The most commonly used material is a set of spondaic words, described in the Appendix, and the threshold of intelligibility is usually defined as 50 percent correct repetition of the words. Ambiguity is reduced if the value is given as sound-pressure level, that is, SPL.

**Reference Level for Speech Audiometers.** The average sound-pressure level of the speech reception threshold for several groups of young normal-hearing adults was determined experimentally, using a particular set of recorded spondaic words. This value, 22 dB SPL, was given in the American (USA) Standard for Speech Audiometers (1953) as the standard reference zero level. (This value will probably be adjusted to 20 dB in the next revision of the USA Standard for Audiometers.)

**Hearing-threshold Level for Speech.** This is the ratio, expressed in decibels, of any individual's threshold (50 percent correct) for the spondaic words to the reference zero level for standard speech audiometers.

For the calculation of *percentage handicap of hearing,* which in principle depends on the individual's speech reception threshold, it is customary to use the average hearing-threshold level for the three pure tones, 500, 1000, and 2000 Hz, instead of a direct determination of the hearing-threshold for speech (see Chapter 9).

**Hearing Loss.** This term has acquired three distinct meanings:

1. The symptom or condition of impaired hearing, particularly impairment of the sensitivity of hearing as tested by either pure tones or speech. For this meaning the terms "hearing loss" and "hypoacusis" are employed in this book.
2. The *hearing-threshold level* as defined above. This term should always be used instead of "hearing loss" when a numerical value in decibels is given. *The set of standard reference levels employed* (ISO, ASA–1951, or other) *must be specified.*
3. A change for the worse in an individual's threshold of hearing. This meaning carries the connotation of disease, injury, or deterioration, as in the common phrase "to suffer a hearing loss." To avoid these connotations the term *threshold shift* is often employed. It is helpful to specify whether the threshold shift is *temporary* or *persistent.* The consistent use of the distinctive terms "hypoacusis," "hearing level," and "threshold shift" is particularly helpful and desirable in medicolegal contexts.

**Deafness (Anacusis).** Deafness is the traditional term for a severe or complete loss of auditory sensitivity. For adults it should only be used if the hearing-threshold level for speech, estimated as recommended above, is 93 dB (ISO) or worse. This implies a hearing loss sufficient to make auditory communication difficult or impossible without amplification. For children the cutoff level is often set as low as 70 dB for educational purposes, as explained in Chapter 16.

**Dysacusis.** Any impairment of hearing that is not primarily a loss of auditory sensitivity is called dysacusis. The cause of dysacusis may be a malfunction or injury of either the central nervous system, the auditory nerve, or the sense organ. Dysacusis is not relieved, like hypoacusis, by simple amplification of speech, and therefore is not measured in decibels.

Among the many types of dysacusis are:

*Discrimination loss* for words, syllables, or phonemes

*Reduced intelligibility* for sentences

*Auditory Agnosia* or *Central Auditory Imperception*. This condition is explained in Chapter 4. It is also called "sensory aphasia," "receptive aphasia," "auditory aphasia," or "word deafness."

*Phonemic Regression*. This is the symptom, found in the elderly, of loss of the ability to comprehend all of the words in a sentence, or even single words, spoken at normal tempo, in spite of relatively good sensitivity for pure tones or slow speech.

*Recruitment*. The recruitment of loudness (Fowler) is an abnormally rapid increase in subjective loudness as a function of sound-pressure level.

*Binaural Diplacusis*. In this condition a single pure tone, presented alternately to the right and left ears, is judged to have a different pitch in each ear.

*Monaural Diplacusis*. In this condition a single pure tone, presented monaurally, is heard as a group of tones, a noise, or both.

**Aphasia.** Aphasia is loss or impairment of the capacity to use words as symbols of ideas. The predominant defect may affect the ability to speak (*motor aphasia* or *expressive aphasia*), or the failure may be a lack of comprehension of the spoken word (*sensory aphasia* or *receptive aphasia*), or both. Receptive aphasia may be visual (*alexia*) as well as auditory.

**Dysmathia.** Dysmathia means "difficulty in learning." It is contrasted with dysacusis which means "difficulty in hearing." Dysmathia may occur in children with or without dysacusis or hypoacusis.

**Dyslogomathia.** Dyslogomathia means specifically *difficulty in learning language*. It is recommended as a more accurate substitute for "congenital aphasia" or "childhood aphasia" (see Chapter 4).

**Combined Hearing Impairment.** This term implies the combination of hypoacusis (a peripheral reduction of sensitivity) with a central dysacusis. This term is not applied to a combination of conductive and sensory-neural hearing loss (mixed hearing loss).

**Air Conduction.** Air conduction is the process by which sound is conducted to the inner ear through the air in the outer ear canal as part of the pathway.

**Bone Conduction.** Bone conduction is the process by which sound is conducted to the inner ear through the cranial bones. No reference zero levels for bone conduction have been proposed for the forthcoming USA standard for audiometers, but considerable progress has been made toward an ISO recommendation based on a standard "artificial head-bone." In the meantime manufacturers of audiometers will presumably continue to calibrate bone-conduction audiometers in such a way as to minimize the "air-bone gap" for normal-hearing persons.

**Air-bone Gap.** The air-bone gap is the difference in decibels between the hearing-threshold levels for a particular frequency as determined by air conduction and by bone conduction.

**Conductive Hearing Loss.** A hearing impairment due to interference with the acoustic transmission of sound to the sense organ, usually in the outer or middle ear, is known as conductive hearing loss. The term "middle-ear hearing loss" is preferable to "conductive hearing loss" in most contexts because of the possibility of inefficient conduction of sound in the inner ear. In the past conductive hearing loss and middle-ear loss have been practically synonymous. In pure middle-ear conductive hearing loss the hearing-threshold levels measured by bone conduction are usually near normal, and the air-bone gaps are large, up to 60 dB.

**Sensory-neural Hearing Loss.** The term implies a hearing impairment due to abnormality of the sense organ, the auditory nerve, or both. Some or all hearing-threshold levels by bone conduction are abnormal. The air-bone gaps are small or absent, with pure inner-ear hearing loss.

**Mixed Hearing Loss.** A combination of conductive with sensory-neural hearing loss, or a combination of middle-ear with inner-ear hearing loss is known as mixed hearing loss. This term is restricted by custom to peripheral hearing losses.

# INDEX OF NAMES

# INDEX OF SUBJECTS

# INDEX OF ORGANIZATIONS